THE AMERICAN HERBAL PRODUCTS ASSOCIATION HERB SAFETY RATING SYSTEM

Herbs incl[...] [...]ding to the American H[...] [...]b safety rating system.

The AHPA supports standardization of the labeling of commercial herbal products as a means of achieving product safety. In 1997 the AHPA published the *Botanical Safety Handbook,* which is based on case reports; toxicologic, pharmacologic, and clinical studies; and information drawn from a number of books considered to be authoritative references on botanicals. This publication provides data on hundreds of herbs and plant-based products sold in the United States.

The AHPA has created a unique rating system, outlined in the *Botanical Safety Handbook,* that classifies herbal products according to their relative safety and potential toxicity based on the following four categories. The classification of an herb in any given category is dependent upon the reasonable use of the herb.

Class 1 Herbs which can be safely consumed when used appropriately.

Class 2 Herbs for which the following use restrictions apply, unless otherwise directed by an expert qualified in the use of the described substance:
2a For external use only.
2b Not to be used during pregnancy.
2c Not to be used while nursing.
2d Other specific use restrictions as noted.

Class 3 Herbs for which significant data exist to recommend the following labeling: "To be used only under the supervision of an expert qualified in the appropriate use of this substance." Labeling must include proper use information as follows: dosage, contraindications, potential adverse effects and drug interactions, and any other relevant information related to the safe use of the substance.

Class 4 Herbs for which insufficient data are available for classification.

Mosby's Handbook of Herbs&Natural Supplements

Second Edition

Linda Skidmore-Roth, RN, MSN, NP

Consultant
Littleton, Colorado

Formerly, Nursing Faculty
New Mexico State University
Las Cruces, New Mexico
El Paso Community College
El Paso, Texas

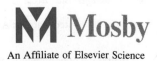

An Affiliate of Elsevier Science

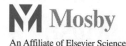

Mosby

An Affiliate of Elsevier Science

11830 Westline Industrial Drive
St. Louis, Missouri 63146

Mosby's Handbook of Herbs & Natural Supplements, Second Edition
ISBN 0-323-02535-8

NOTICE

Knowledge regarding the proper use of herbs and supplements is ever changing. Standard safety precautions must be followed, but as new research and clinical experience broaden our knowledge, changes in use may become necessary or appropriate. Readers are advised to check the most current product information provided by the manufacturer of each product to be administered to verify the recommended dose, the method and duration of administration, and contraindications. It is the responsibility of the licensed practitioner, relying on experience and knowledge of the patient, to determine dosages and the best treatment for each individual patient. Neither the publisher nor the editor assumes any liability for any injury and/or damage to persons or property arising from this publication.

Previous edition copyrighted 2001

International Standard Book Number 0-323-02535-8

Executive Editor, Nursing: Darlene Como
Senior Developmental Editor: Tamara A. Myers
Publishing Services Manager: Deborah L. Vogel
Design Manager: Bill Drone

Printed in the United States of America

Last digit is the print number: 9 8 7 6 5 4 3 2 1

CONSULTANTS

Joyce K. Anastasi, PhD, RN, FAAN, LAc
Associate Professor
Columbia University School of Nursing
New York, New York

Mary L. Conley, PhD
Owner
The Conley Farm
Natural Healing Practices
Burtonsville, Maryland

Linda Coulston, BSN, RN
Case Manager
Hospital of the University of Pennsylvania
Wissahickon Hospice
Philadelphia, Pennsylvania
Consultant
Bubbling Well for Integrative Health Care
Morton, Pennsylvania

Georgia M. Decker, MS, RN, CS-ANP, AOCN
Integrative Care, NP, PC
Albany, New York

Metanasa Drammgh
Health Educator
JOY Foundation
Denver, Colorado

Mary V. Fenton, RN, DrPH, FAAN
Professor
School of Nursing
University of Texas Medical Branch
Galveston, Texas

Karta Purkh Singh Khalsa, CN, AHG
Seattle, Washington
Linda U. Krebs, RN, PhD, OACN
Assistant Professor of Nursing
University of Colorado Health Sciences Center
Lakewood, Colorado

Sue H. Mustalish, RN, HNC
Nurse Herbalist
East Fallowfield, Pennsylvania

Jamie S. Myers, RN, MN, AOCN
Oncology Clinical Nurse Specialist
Research Medical Center
Kansas City, Missouri

Becky A. Ridenhour, PharmD
St. Louis College of Pharmacy
St. Louis, Missouri

PREFACE

It is estimated that almost half of all health care consumers in the United States take some form of herbal or natural product supplement alone or in combination with conventional medicines. Yet the therapeutic value of many of these products is unproven. Additionally, some products may interact with prescription medications, and some products may be harmful to patients with certain conditions. Of perhaps even greater concern is the fact that the majority of patients who use alternative medicines never mention their use to their health care providers.

Because of the prevalence of the use of herbal products, health care professionals need access to reliable, unbiased information about herbs and other alternative medicines. *Mosby's Handbook of Herbs and Natural Supplements,* second edition, does not advocate for or against the use of herbal products and other natural supplements. Rather, this book acknowledges the widespread use of these types of remedies with the goal of providing health care professionals with current, reliable, unbiased information with which to advise clients on the responsible and intelligent use of herbal products as a part of their overall health treatment and maintenance plan.

This book contains detailed monographs of almost 300 herbs and natural supplements, multiple appendixes filled with key information, a glossary, a botanical atlas, and a comprehensive index, all designed to be easy to use and to provide the depth of information today's health care professionals demand.

Herbal Monographs

Mosby's Handbook of Herbs and Natural Supplements provides the user with an essential reference that allows easy access to extensive information on nearly 300 herbal and natural supplements. A unique feature of this handbook is the consistent format, which allows for quick reference without sacrificing the depth of detail necessary for a thorough understanding of the material presented. The following information is provided whenever possible:

Common Name. Each herb or supplement is arranged alphabetically by the most common name in natural order. Hence, black hellebore is located within the B's and white cohosh within the W's.

Scientific Name. The scientific, or botanical, name immediately
follows the common name whenever applicable. The scientific
name provides positive identification for various species or
substances that might share a common name. Occasionally,
more than one species is listed when various herbs are chemically similar. Gentian, for example, has two scientific names:
Gentiana lutea and *Gentiana acaulis*.

Other Common Names. Most herbs and natural supplements
are known by a variety of additional names. The most common of these are listed here and in the index of the book
to aid the reader in locating and identifying a particular herb
or natural supplement.

Herb Class. The American Herbal Products Association
(AHPA) has assigned a safety rating to many of the herbs and
supplements in use today. These ratings are broken into four
main classes with several subclasses and usually identify
specific plant parts or forms of each herb. More information
on herbal safety and the AHPA system can be found in the
Herbal Safety appendix.

Origin. This section briefly states the origins of each herb or
supplement.

Uses. The uses section has been divided into two categories
whenever possible. *Reported Uses* are the uses for which the
remedy is known or has been used in the past. The *Investigational Uses* category provides information on current research and possible new uses for a variety of herbs and
supplements.

Product Availability and Dosages. The common *Available
Forms* and *Plant Parts Used* are listed in this section of the
monograph, followed by *Dosages and Routes*. Whenever possible, the dosages are divided by use; age group, including
specific pediatric and geriatric doses; and any limiting conditions, such as renal impairment or pregnancy. Because of
great variance in reported dosages, references are cited whenever possible.

Precautionary Information. Precautionary information includes *Contraindications, Side Effects/Adverse Reactions,*
and the *Interactions* box. The contraindications information
includes an explanation of situations in which a particular
herb or supplement should not be used. This information
may also include warnings for specific groups of people based
on lack of research in a particular area. Herb class information is repeated here for clarity. Side effects and adverse reactions are broken down by body system, with the most

common side effects listed first. Any life-threatening side effects are printed in bold type using small capital letters, making them easy to find. The interactions are conveniently broken into four categories—drug, food, herb, and lab test interactions—making it quick and easy to look for particular types of interactions.

Client Considerations. Client considerations are based loosely on the nursing process and are organized into *Assess, Administer,* and *Teach Client/Family* categories. Considerations are consistently organized under these headings to highlight information in a format convenient for client care.

Pharmacology. *Pharmacokinetics* for various herbs and natural supplements, including information on peak, half-life, binding, and excretion, are covered here. Immediately following the pharmacokinetic information is a table of *Chemical Components.* This table lists the potentially active chemical constituents for each herb and any possible actions those components might have.

Actions. In this section of the monograph, the actions of each herb and supplement are explained, together with any research or studies performed.

References. Each monograph has been individually referenced, with detailed references listed at the end of the monograph.

Icons. Throughout the monographs, certain icons are used to highlight key information. The Alert icon ◉ calls out key information regarding toxicity, dangerous interactions, and other significant reactions that may threaten a client's health. The Popular Herb icon ✎ is used to show that an herb has been designated by the Herbal Research Foundation as an herb in common use in the United States. The Pregnancy icon 🍼 identifies information of special interest to pregnant or lactating patients. The Pediatric icon 👣 highlights information for pediatric patients. Some medicinal herbs are quite rare and should not be harvested; these herbs are marked with an Endangered Herb icon 🌱. Finally, certain herbs are only safe to use topically, or should be ingested only in very rare circumstances; the words "Do Not Ingest" are noted at the tops of these herb monographs.

Appendixes

Herb Resources. This appendix contains a list of herbal resources located on the World Wide Web, including key organizations, not-for-profit research agencies, and additional educational resources. Next to each web site address is a brief description of the site and the types of information that can be found there.

CAM Programs in the United States and Canada. This appendix contains a select group of Complementary and Alternative Medicine programs, schools, and organizations throughout the United States and Canada.

Poison Control Centers. This list contains contact information for poison control centers for the continental United States, Hawaii, and Alaska.

Herb/Drug Interactions. This table is a single, handy resource for reviewing all known drug interactions for the herbs and supplements listed in this book.

Botanical Atlas. Eight beautiful botanical plates illustrate plant parts and types for ease of identification.

Pediatric Herbal Use. This extensive appendix covers current pediatric herbal use and research.

Herbal Safety. Both the American Herbal Products Association (AHPA) and the Food and Drug Administration (FDA) have published information on herbal safety. An explanation of each system and a list of the herbs in this book that also appear in the FDA Poisonous Plant Database appear in this appendix.

Glossary

The glossary explains the special vocabulary of herbal medicine. Terms such as *tincture, infusion, extract,* and *decoction* are defined clearly and succinctly.

Index

The comprehensive index allows the user to look up each herb by any of its common or scientific names, as well as by any of the conditions it may be used to treat. That is, the reader can use the index to find a comprehensive list of herbs used in the treatment of cancer, HIV, or other conditions.

INTRODUCTION

In today's health care climate, reduced insurance coverage, constraints on access to care, and increased costs of prescriptions and services are the norm. People are living longer than ever before, and chronic diseases such as arthritis, diabetes, cancer, Alzheimer's, and HIV/AIDS are on the rise. Conventional prescription drugs used to treat these conditions are often expensive, and because at least a portion of the cost may not be reimbursed by insurance carriers, consumers are paying more out of pocket for them. At the same time, people are becoming increasingly interested in preventive strategies and holistic approaches to health, such as eating a nutritionally sound diet, maintaining fitness, and reducing stress. Interest in "natural" treatments and products continues to grow.

For these reasons and many others, health care providers today are encountering increasing numbers of clients who are using one or more of the so-called "nontraditional" treatment methods that comprise complementary and alternative medicine, or CAM. These include not only herbal medicine but many other healing philosophies such as homeopathy, naturopathy, therapeutic massage, acupuncture, Ayurvedic medicine, and traditional Chinese medicine, to name but a few. Traditional medical systems are beginning to incorporate many of these services into their offerings and insurance carriers to provide coverage for some of them. More than ever, traditional care providers need to be well informed about the various CAM modalities that their clients may be using, in order to make intelligent care decisions themselves and to help their clients make informed choices as well.

Americans spent $3.24 billion on herbs in 1997 and were projected to spend $4.3 billion in 2000 (Johnston, 1997; Yakutchik, 1999). Two studies done in 1997 suggest that approximately 42% of adult Americans in the general population had used one or more CAM approaches as of that date (Eisenberg, 1998) and that approximately 34% had used herbal remedies (Johnston, 1997). Two more recent studies confirm rising rates of CAM use even for more narrowly defined subsets of the general patient population. A study focusing on health maintenance organization (HMO) patients found that 40% of the patients surveyed had used herbal remedies to treat or prevent a health condition (Bennett, 2000), while a study using a cross-section of patients in the rural South found that 44% had used one or more CAM approaches during the year preceding the study (Oldendick, 2000). Use of CAM, including herbs, appears to be even more widespread among other groups of patients. For example, a recent study found that 61% of elderly Hispanic and non-Hispanic white patients had used herbal remedies (Dole, 2000). Another study reported a similarly high percentage of CAM use for patients with HIV/AIDS, 68% (Piscitelli, 2000).

Of the CAM modalities, herbal medicine is probably the most popular, and the most ubiquitous. Even so, it has yet to be subjected to the same level of scientific scrutiny as traditional medical treatments, and as a result, it has not yet gained wide acceptance by mainstream medicine. Much confusion and misinformation surround herbal medicine. Because herb use is not widely accepted or understood by mainstream medical caregivers, clients often do not disclose their herb use to their health care provider. Many use prescription drugs concurrently with herbal remedies and face possible health risks as a result of adverse reactions. As stated in the *Preface,* the intention of this handbook is to educate health care providers with the "need-to-know" information about common herbs that their clients may be taking and to acquaint them with the known interactions and risks. A well-informed, nonjudgmental care provider is most likely to inspire the client's trust and gain not only a more accurate picture of the client's herb use but also an opportunity to provide valuable information about herb safety issues as outlined in this introduction.

Key Concerns for the Health Care Provider

It is beyond the scope of this book to undertake an exhaustive treatment of herbalism and the herb industry. The remaining sections of this introduction are intended to provide a concise summary of the background and facts needed to help the caregiver provide the best possible care for the client. These sections include a brief overview of the risks and benefits of herbal medicine; an introduction to the herb industry and the corollary issues of regulation, manufacturing quality control, and safety; and a brief discussion of client education. First, though, the caregiver should be aware of several important caveats, each of which is treated in more detail in the sections that follow.

Limitations of the Research

Scientific information available to caregivers today about herbs and their effects is increasing but is still scanty, mainly because the primary research itself is limited. In the United States, scientific study of herbs and their medicinal effects has begun in earnest only within the past two decades. The reasons for this are described below in more detail (see section entitled "The Herb Industry"). Much of the information that is available is anecdotal and largely unscientific, not having been subjected to the same rigorous controls and replicative studies as are mandated for prescription and over-the-counter drugs.

It is also crucial for the provider to understand the ongoing nature of herb research and the speed with which knowledge in this field is accruing. Because of the burgeoning interest in herbal remedies and their widespread use, more and more scientific study is being devoted to herbal medicines. Adverse effects that are unknown today may be revealed tomorrow. Thus it is not safe to assume that if this book lists no interactions for a particular herb, then no risk exists. A more likely scenario is that insufficient study has been done to determine potential adverse effects. Caution is necessary.

Manufacturing, Storage, and Quality Issues

In the United States, herb manufacturers are not held to the same stringent standards as are manufacturers of pharmaceuticals. Herb manufacturers are not required by law to demonstrate the safety, efficacy, or quality of their products. Herb manufacture remains unregulated and is likely to continue to be so in the current political and economic climate. Some manufacturers voluntarily adhere to so-called "good manufacturing practices" (GMPs) and make every effort to produce a quality product, while others do not. In addition, the content of active chemical constituents in an herbal product can vary widely from manufacturer to manufacturer. Chemical analysis of samples labeled as the same herbal product, but purchased from various suppliers or outlets, has revealed wide variations in quality and chemical content. The manner in which an herb is grown, harvested, processed, and stored also affects the strength and quality of the product, as do many other factors (see "Manufacturing and Quality Issues").

Lack of Standardization

Unlike prescription drugs, most herbs do not yet have standardized dosages, nor do manufacturers always produce preparations of consistent strengths. Even the crude herb itself may vary in chemical composition from one batch of the plant to another, or even from plant to plant. Disagreement among trained herbalists about dosages is common, and dosages often depend on the use to which the herb is being put, the part of the herb being used, its strength, the route of administration, and many other factors. Also, because the industry lacks regulation, some herbs may be manufactured with dosages standardized to their active chemical components, while others are not (see "Manufacturing and Quality Issues"). In practical terms, this means that a consumer taking a nonstandardized herbal product made by one manufacturer may receive a much higher or lower dose (or perhaps even none) of the active chemical than another consumer taking the same herb, made by a different manufacturer whose products are standardized. However, even if all herbal products were standardized to their active constituents, consensus on appropriate dosages for various age groups and various health conditions does not yet exist. Current research is insufficient to allow safe generalizations.

Potential Toxicity

Many herbs are potentially toxic if used incorrectly. For example, an herb may be safe and effective when used topically in the amount specified but may be highly toxic if taken internally. Some herbs contain potent liver toxins, systemic toxins, carcinogens, mutagens, or teratogens. Special caution is needed when treating pediatric, geriatric, and pregnant clients who are or may be using herbs. For example, it is not safe to assume that a child should receive a proportionally smaller dosage of an herb than an adult would use. The effects of herbs on children remain largely unknown, with a few herbs known to pose an outright risk. Commercial herbal preparations may also be contaminated by various toxic substances during the manufacturing process. Many of the toxic effects of herbs have yet to be determined, both because of insufficient research and because no law requires that adverse effects from herbal products be reported.

With these cautions in mind, the provider should also realize that many herbs may produce beneficial effects when used as directed. Research continues to confirm the efficacy of many popular herbs, echinacea and ginkgo being only two of many examples. Although many clients who use herbal products self-diagnose and self-administer, the safest course of action is to use herbal preparations only under the supervision of a trained herbalist, and to disclose the use of all herbal products to the health care provider.

An Overview of Phytomedicine

Phytomedicine, or the use of plants or plant parts for therapeutic purposes, is an ancient discipline that is practiced worldwide. In fact, a 1985 report by the World Health Organization estimated that herbal remedies constitute the primary form of health care for about 80% of the world's people (Farnsworth, 1985). Phytomedicine is a part of the broader scheme of pharmacognosy, or the study of chemical constituents taken from natural sources for their medicinal purposes.

Risks and Benefits of Phytomedicine

From the point of view of the trained herbalist, one of the benefits of herbs is that they are often used to help achieve homeostasis within the body, as well as to treat or cure certain conditions outright. The herbalist may administer one or more herbs to help bring the body back to its natural balance, seeking to correct the underlying condition. In contrast, traditional drugs may be used to treat symptoms without resolving the underlying health problem. Herbalists also cite their belief that herbs, when used properly, cause fewer and milder side effects than traditional drugs and pose less risk overall. From the consumer's standpoint, another advantage of the use of herbs compared with prescription drugs is their lower out-of-pocket cost. An additional factor is their easy availability. Consumers can purchase herbs without a prescription at a wide variety of retail outlets, as well as over the Internet. Access to herbs is virtually unlimited and unrestricted.

Some of these same benefits may also be viewed as risks, however. For example, purchasing herbs over the Internet allows the consumer to obtain herbs from foreign countries that may be unavailable in this country because of their high potential for toxic effects. Such products may be of questionable quality, and the consumer often ends up taking them without supervision. The easy availability of herbs may also be a detriment when one considers the long-term consequences, in the sense that consumers may delay seeking conventional diagnosis and treatment of a serious health condition by attempting to self-treat with herbs. Many consumers may also hesitate to report their herb use to the health care provider, possibly placing themselves at further risk of adverse reactions. The potential for abuse of herbs with narcotic properties is also high.

Adverse reactions are possible, either from the active chemical components of the herb itself, from adulterants or contaminants that may be introduced into the product during faulty manufacturing processes, or from interactions of herbs with prescription drugs. Additional risks are posed by the lack of regulation of the herb industry. Because herbs are unregulated, no law mandates the reporting of adverse reactions as is the case with prescription drugs. Databases of such information are available via the Internet, and many reputable manufacturers report adverse reactions voluntarily, but neither the consumer nor the care provider can assume that such databases are comprehensive. As mentioned previously, the lack of standardized dosage ranges and preparations poses still another risk, as does the inadequacy of scientific research on the effects of herbs in general.

The Herb Industry

Lack of regulation is probably the single biggest factor affecting the reliability of commercial herbal products in the United States. Because many of today's pharmaceuticals are already plant-derived, such as digitalis (from foxglove), one may wonder why the pharmaceutical industry is so tightly regulated while the herbal industry is not. The answer is based primarily in economics.

In the United States, clinical trials to demonstrate the safety, efficacy, and reliability of a drug are expensive and time consuming. Currently, the drug approval process takes anywhere from 8 years to as many as 18 years, with costs in the hundreds of millions of dollars. Because of the great expense, manufacturers typically want to patent their product in order to recover their investment and make a profit. However, naturally occurring products such as herbs cannot be patented. Hence, no economic incentive exists, and to date U.S. pharmaceutical manufacturers have pursued only limited research on whole plants or their crude extracts. Such has not been the case in Germany.

The Herb Industry in Germany

Many professionals consider the German Commission E monographs to be one of the definitive sources of information on herbs. Commission E is a German governmental body much like the Food and Drug Administration (FDA) in the United States. In 1978, the German Federal Health Agency established the Commission and charged it with the mission of investigating the safety and efficacy of herbal remedies commonly used in

Germany. As of this writing, the Commission has published monographs for more than 400 herbs.

Unlike U.S. law, German law allows herb manufacturers to market herbs with drug claims if the herb is proven to be safe and effective. A manufacturer's product is considered safe and effective if it meets the standards outlined in the Commission E monograph for that herb, or if the manufacturer can furnish additional evidence attesting to the safety and effectiveness of the herb. This evidence may come from the literature, from anecdotal information, or from clinical studies. The ability to make appropriate claims for herbal products has enabled many manufacturers to achieve commercial success and invest in further research that in turn helps to increase the credibility of herbal products in mainstream medicine. In Germany, some herbs are sold over the counter as in the United States, while others are available by prescription only. The over-the-counter or prescription status of an herb is based on its use and safety. Prescription herbs in Germany are reimbursable by insurance (Murray, 1999).

With an eye to future regulation of herb manufacture throughout Europe, an organization formed in 1989 known as the European Scientific Cooperative on Phytotherapy (ESCOP) has been working to achieve consistent regulation of all drugs, including herbal medications. Much like the German Commission E, ESCOP has been developing monographs describing the therapeutic uses of herbs, based on sound clinical and scientific evidence. Plans call for the monographs to be integrated eventually into the European Pharmacopeia. Leading scientific authorities from all over Europe are collaborating to carry out ongoing research efforts of ESCOP.

Regulation in the United States

In the United States, three major laws regulate the quality, safety, and efficacy of medicinal products. The Food and Drugs Act of 1906 spoke to the quality issue, the Federal Food, Drug, and Cosmetic Act of 1938 addressed safety, and a 1962 amendment to the 1938 Act mandated proof of therapeutic efficacy. This amendment permitted products that had been approved before 1962 to remain on the market as long as their manufacturers did not make claims of therapeutic efficacy directly on the product labels or containers. Some herb manufacturers began to try to get around this stipulation by placing books, pamphlets, advertisements, and other promotional information either on or near the shelves where the products were displayed.

To address this problem, the Dietary Supplement Health and Education Act (DSHEA) was signed into law in 1994. Currently, herbs and other supplements such as vitamins and minerals fall within its purview. This law defined herbs as dietary supplements, thus preventing them from being regulated as food additives (which must undergo an approval process) unless the manufacturer makes claims for therapeutic efficacy. For products approved for market after the law was enacted in 1994, the manufacturer is responsible for proving safety. For products approved before 1994, the FDA is responsible. Manufacturers are permitted to distribute information about the therapeutic efficacy of herbs, but with limitations. The information is not allowed to endorse any particular products, it may not be misleading, and it must be physically separated from the product. Product labels are permitted to make general health claims, but not therapeutic claims. They may contain detailed directions for use; list precautionary information such as warnings, side effects, contraindications, and safety data; and describe the properties of the product. Labels must clearly state that the product is a dietary supplement and must contain a disclaimer stating that the FDA has not evaluated any health claims. The disclaimer must also include the statement "This product is not intended to diagnose, treat, cure, or prevent any disease."

The U.S. Government and Herb Research

The DSHEA also established the Office of Dietary Supplements (ODS) within the National Institutes of Health (NIH). While not a regulatory agency, the ODS is responsible for coordinating research on dietary supplements and is also a clearinghouse for information on legal and regulatory issues relating to supplements. In 1998, Congress established another branch of the NIH, the National Center for Complementary and Alternative Medicine (NCCAM), to help ensure high-quality scientific research into CAM practices, including herbalism. The NCCAM conducts and supports basic and clinical research, as well as training in research methods, on CAM modalities, and it provides information about CAM to both health care providers and consumers. The missions of the NCCAM include the following:

"Evaluating the safety and efficacy of widely used natural products, such as herbal remedies and nutritional and food supplements. . ."

[and] "Supporting pharmacological studies to determine the potential interactive effects of CAM products with standard treatment medications. . ." (NCCAM, 2000).

It appears unlikely that herb manufacture in the United States will be subject to further regulation in the near future. Consumers place a high value on their freedom of choice, and many view regulation as an attempt by the government and the medical community to monopolize treatment options. Manufacturers are also unlikely to support further governmental control. Therefore the health care provider is advised to remain abreast of the regulatory status of herbal products and to advise the client who uses them to purchase only from reliable manufacturers or suppliers.

Manufacturing and Quality Issues

Many factors affect the ultimate quality, strength, shelf life, and use of an herbal product. Some influences occur before the crude herb ever reaches the manufacturer. Others occur in manufacturing during the various stages of production. All can significantly affect the quality of the final product that ends up on the consumer's shelf.

Preproduction Considerations

Where, when, and how an herb is grown do much to determine the strength of its chemical components. All of the following factors can influence the quality and potency of an herb:

- Habitat
- Ambient temperature
- Rainfall
- Hours of daylight at the latitude where the plant is grown
- Altitude
- Wind conditions
- Soil characteristics

Another factor that may affect the potency of an herb is whether the plant grows naturally in its native habitat or whether it is cultivated. Many herbalists believe that herbs grown in their natural habitat are far superior to cultivated herbs in terms of their constituents and chemical properties. However, the use of naturally occurring herbs involves risks as well, such as the possibility of identifying the species incorrectly and of obtaining herbs with varying degrees of potency. Cultivation offers its own benefits. Growing conditions can be controlled, ensuring greater consistency in the end product, and the harvester is assured of obtaining the correct herb (Murray, 1999).

The Production Process

Some herbs are used in their crude state, while others undergo various forms and degrees of refinement. Although manufacturing processes differ widely, the production process used to take the crude herb to extract form usually involves the following steps (Murray, 1999):

- **Collection/harvesting:** The harvesting of naturally occurring herbs is called "wild crafting." Cultivated herbs may be harvested either by hand or by machine, depending on the scale on which the herbs are grown. The time of harvest is critical because harvesting either too early or too late can yield a product that may be too weak or too strong for effective use. Because different parts of the plant may be put to entirely different medicinal uses, the harvester must also make sure to harvest the right part or parts of the herb for a particular use.

- **Garbling:** The usable portion of the plant is separated from the nonusable part or parts, and other materials such as dirt and insect parts are also separated and discarded.

- **Drying:** Herbs that are to be stored after harvesting must be dried in order to prevent breakdown of their active components and contamination by microorganisms. A mild heat is used to prevent destruction of the active constituents of the herb.

- **Grinding:** The herb is broken down mechanically into smaller pieces, ranging from coarse to fine depending on intended use. (Crude herbs may also undergo grinding before use.)

- **Extraction:** The extraction process involves using a solvent (in the United States, usually alcohol or water, or sometimes a lipophilic solvent or liquid carbon dioxide) to separate the desired chemical components from the plant parts. This process yields various solutions such as tinctures, fluid extracts, and solid extracts. Solid extracts may be either soft solids (in viscous form, containing some moisture) or dry solids, which may be ground into powder.

- **Concentration:** Solutions produced by extraction may undergo evaporative concentration to remove the solvent and produce a pure extract.

- **Drying of extracts:** Methods such as freeze-drying or atomizing may be used to dry extracts to solid form. Because their moisture has been removed, such products are less susceptible to contamination by microorganisms.

- **Addition of excipients:** Herbal manufacturers often compound herbal preparations such as capsules or tablets using the same inert ingredients (e.g., starch) that the pharmaceutical industry uses.

Because the manufacture of herbs is unregulated, the quality of an herbal preparation is not assured. The herb used in the manufacturing process may be contaminated by various toxins, including pesticides and heavy metals from the soil in which the plant is grown or contaminants from polluted air. Some herbs, especially rare or hard-to-obtain ones, may be adulterated by adding less expensive, lower-quality ingredients to them to "cut" the herb, much as is done with illegal drugs. Careless or unskilled processing may also degrade the quality of the herb via exposure to moisture, light, or excess heat. Voluntary adherence to quality control and good manufacturing processes can do much to solve these problems. The consumer who uses herbal preparations is well advised to research the reputation of the manufacturers or suppliers of all products used, and to follow carefully all instructions for storage and handling.

Standardization

For the health care provider's purposes, as well as the consumer's, it is important to distinguish between the terms *concentration* and *potency* as they are used in the herb industry because they do not mean the same thing. To understand the difference between the terms, it is necessary to understand how the strength of an herbal extract is expressed, and why.

If the active chemical components of an extract have been identified, the strength of the extract is usually expressed in terms of the content of these chemical components. If the active components are unknown, however, the strength of the extract is expressed simply in terms of concentration (Murray, 1999). The caveat here is that concentration simply reveals the physical *quantity* of herb used in proportion to the quantity of solvent. It does not reveal the potency of the extract. Consider, for example, a scenario in which one manufacturer produces a 1:5 extract using a high-quality herb, while another manufacturer uses the same species of herb, but of a lower quality, and also produces a 1:5 extract. The extract made from the high-quality herb will contain more of the active chemical components than will the one made from a low-quality herb—that is, it will have a much higher potency. Thus it is possible for the potency of two extracts of the same herb with the same concentration to vary greatly.

How, then, can the consumer be assured of receiving a consistent dose of a refined herbal product such as an extract? At this time, the safest practice is to purchase standardized products (also known as guaranteed potency products), which are manufactured to contain a specified content of the active chemical components of the herb. Standardization thus assures the consumer that each dose of the preparation contains a consistent amount of the active component or components.

It should be noted that a standardized extract contains not only the active chemical constituent to which the extract has been standardized, but also the other components of the herb. This can be important because research has shown that using the isolated active component alone often does not produce the same therapeutic effect as does using a preparation containing all of the components together. This so-called synergistic action of herbs is not yet fully understood (Murray, 1999). Even so, the use of standardized products currently provides the greatest assurance of receiving an accurate, reliable dose of the active constituents of an herb, and of safely achieving the desired therapeutic effect.

Working With the Client Who Uses Herbs

As stated earlier, the purpose of this handbook is not to advocate either for or against the use of herbs. Its primary intention is to help ensure that the caregiver is as well informed as possible, given that herb research itself is in its infancy and that findings are emerging faster than publications can keep up with them. It is recommended that the caregiver take the following approach with clients:

- Encourage the client to disclose his or her use of herbal treatments by maintaining a nonjudgmental stance about CAM modalities in general and herbalism in particular. Obtain as complete a history of herb use as possible, including all products taken, amounts, and brand names.
- Determine whether the client is using herbal treatments instead of, or as an adjunct to, conventional treatments. Also, determine whether the herb is being used prophylactically or to treat an existing health condition.
- Advise the client of the risks of delaying conventional diagnosis and treatment of potentially serious health conditions.
- Inform the client of the various benefits and risks of phytomedicine as outlined in this introduction, particularly

the potentially serious adverse reactions that can occur when herbs are used with other drugs the client may be taking.

- Instruct the client who uses herbs to remain alert for any unusual symptoms and to document and report these symptoms to the caregiver immediately.
- Advise the client that herb use may incur serious risks in pediatric, geriatric, and pregnant clients, as well as those with chronic liver disease or other health conditions that affect the ability of the body to process the chemical constituents of herbs. If the client still wishes to use herbs, recommend that he or she proceed only under the supervision of a trained herbalist.
- Explain the importance of considering quality control, manufacturer/supplier reliability, and product safety when purchasing an herbal product.
- In general, advise the client to keep all herbal products away from moisture, heat, and light unless otherwise instructed by the product label or a qualified herbalist. Such precautions will help prevent degradation of the product and contamination by microorganisms.

For client and caregiver alike, reliable sources of information about herbs, herb manufacture, and herb research include the National Center for Complementary and Alternative Medicine web site (http://nccam.nih.gov) and the Office of Dietary Supplements web site (http://dietarysupplements.info.nih.gov). The ODS maintains two useful databases, one covering federal government-supported research on dietary supplements, including herbal products, and the other a database of published international scientific literature on dietary supplements. The database covering federally supported research is known by its acronym CARDS, which stands for Computer Access to Research on Dietary Supplements. The international database is IBIDS, which stands for International Bibliographic Information on Dietary Supplements. Both may be accessed from the ODS web site, and both allow consumers, caregivers, educators, and researchers alike to locate credible scientific information on herbal supplements.

References

American Botanical Council: Herbal information web page/terminology, *American Botanical Council* web site, August 21, 2000.

American Herbal Products Association: AHPA association information web page, *American Herbal Products Association* web site, September 6, 2000.

Bennett J, Brown CM: Use of herbal remedies by patients in a health maintenance organization, *J Am Pharm Assoc* 40(3):353-358, 2000.

Dole EJ, Rhyne RL, Zeilmann CA, et al: The influence of ethnicity on use of herbal remedies in elderly Hispanics and non-Hispanic whites, *J Am Pharm Assoc* 40(3):359-365, 2000.

Eisenberg DM, Davis RB, Ettner SL, et al: Trends in alternative medicine use in the United States, 1990-1997, *JAMA* 280:1569-1575, 1998.

Farnsworth N et al: Medicinal plants in therapy, *Bull World Health Org* 63:965-981, 1985.

Johnston BA: One-third of nation's adults use herbal remedies: market estimated at $3.24 billion, *Herbalgram* 40:49, 1997.

Murray MT, Pizzorno Jr JE: Botanical medicine—a modern perspective. In Murray MT, Pizzorno Jr JE, editors: *Textbook of natural medicine, vol 1,* London, 1999, Churchill Livingstone, pp 267-279.

National Center for Complementary & Alternative Medicine: General information, *NCCAM* web site, August 21, 2000.

National Center for Complementary & Alternative Medicine: Major domains of complementary & alternative medicine, *NCCAM* web site, August 21, 2000.

Oldendick R, Coker AL, Wieland D, et al: Population-based survey of complementary and alternative medicine usage, patient satisfaction, and physician involvement, *South Med J* 93(4):375-381, 2000.

Piscitelli SC: Use of complementary medicines by patients with HIV: full sail into uncharted waters *Medscape HIV/AIDS* 6(3), 2000.

Yakutchik M: The science behind some popular herbs, *OnHealth* web site, September 14, 1999.

CONTENTS

Herbal Monographs

Appendixes

Acidophilus
(a-suh-dah'fuh-lus)

Scientific name: *Lactobacillus acidophilus,* alone or combined with *Lactobacillus bulgaricus*

Other common names: Acidophilus milk, Bacid, Lactinex, MoreDophilus, Probiata, Probiotics, Superdophilus, yogurt

Origin: Acidophilus is commercially prepared.

Uses

Reported Uses

Acidophilus is used to increase the normal flora in the gastrointestinal tract in uncomplicated diarrhea, antibiotic-induced diarrhea, *Clostridium difficile* diarrhea, to treat or prevent vaginal candida infections with or without antibiotics, and to treat bacterial and other candida and urinary tract infections. *Lactobacillus acidophilus* may decrease *Campylobacter pylori,* and some *Lactobacillus* spp. may decrease lipoprotein concentrations. Yogurt is used topically to treat thrush in the infant.

Investigational Uses

Preliminary research is exploring the use of *Lactobacillus* to stimulate nonspecific immunity (Miettinen, 1996) and to prevent recurrent superficial bladder cancer (Aso, 1995), proliferation of breast cancer (Biffi, 1997), colonic preneoplastic lesions (Rao, 1999) and inhibition of *Helicobacter pylori* (Lorca, 2001). New studies have shown a decrease in growth of *Gardnerella vaginalis* (Aroutcheva, 2001) and rotavirus positive and negative status in children with acute diarrhea (Lee, 2001).

Product Availability and Dosages

Available Forms

The following forms contain added cultures of 500 million to 10 billion organisms: capsules, dairy products (acidophilus milk, yogurt), granules, powder, tablets, vaginal suppositories, chewable tablets.

Dosages and Routes

Dosage information is for replenishment of normal bacterial flora and suppression of bacterial infection. No dosage information is available for other uses.

Adult

- PO: 1-10 billion organisms (or an amount of product containing the equivalent) divided tid-qid
- Vaginal suppository: insert one suppository in vaginal fornix qhs

Infant

- Topical: apply yogurt topically in mouth to treat oral thrush

Precautionary Information

Contraindications

Dairy products are not recommended for use by lactose-sensitive individuals. Acidophilus-containing products may be used during pregnancy and lactation and may be given to children. Do not give in the presence of high fever.

Side Effects/Adverse Reactions

This product is well tolerated by most individuals.
Gastrointestinal: Flatus

Interactions with Acidophilus

Drug

Antibiotics: Acidophilus should not be used concurrently with antibiotics.
Warfarin: Acidophilus may decrease warfarin action; use together cautiously.

Food	Lab Test
None known	None known

Herb

Garlic: Acidophilus may decrease the absorption of garlic. If taken concurrently, separate the dosages by 3 hours.

Client Considerations

Assess

Replenishment of Normal Bacterial Flora/Suppression of Bacterial Infection

- Assess for recent antibiotic use if candida infection is present vaginally or if thrush is identified. Provide a list of dairy

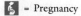 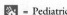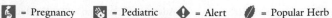

products that contain *Lactobacillus* (e.g., acidophilus milk, yogurt).
- Assess for lactose-intolerant clients. Discourage the use of supplemental dairy products and recommend the use of *Lactobacillus* in supplement form instead.

Hypercholesteremia
- Assess the client's lipid profile: cholesterol, total triglycerides, low-density lipoprotein (LDL), and high-density lipoprotein (HDL).
- Assess the client's diet for foods high in cholesterol, LDL, and HDL.
- Assess whether the client is taking medication to treat hypercholesteremia.
- Assess for the use of garlic (see Interactions).

Administer
- Instruct the client to take acidophilus PO as a supplement, or in milk or yogurt. Take on an empty stomach in AM or 1 hr before each meal.
- Refrigerate *Lactobacillus* in supplement form to prevent spoilage. Nonrefrigerated products often are not viable by the time they are purchased. Instruct the client to continue to refrigerate supplements.
- Administer *Lactobacillus* GG to individuals with candida infections who cannot tolerate other products.

Teach Client/Family
Replenishment of Normal Bacterial Flora/Suppression of Bacterial Infection
- Instruct the client to take all antibiotics as prescribed, even if candida infection occurs.
- Teach the client about the use of *Lactobacillus* in the diet for infection prevention and maintenance. Unless contraindicated, provide information about dairy products that naturally contain *Lactobacillus*.

Hypercholesteremia
- Inform the client that acidophilus may be added to the diet without altering the medication therapy, diet, or exercise regimen.

Pharmacology
Pharmacokinetics
Pharmacokinetics and pharmacodynamics are unknown.

Actions

Replenishment of Normal Bacterial Flora and Suppression of Bacterial Infection

Lactobacillus is part of the normal flora living in the gastrointestinal tract. It acts by competing for nutrients with other organisms such as *Candida,* thus preventing the other organism from reproducing and flourishing to infection. Most people obtain sufficient quantities of *Lactobacillus* by including dairy products such as milk and yogurt in their diet. *Lactobacillus* is also responsible for assisting in the digestion and absorption of several vitamins, including the fat-soluble vitamins and proteins. Research shows that *Lactobacillus* GG promotes local antigen-specific immune responses in the immunoglobulin A (IgA) class, protects the body from invasive pathogens, prevents cell membrane permeability defects, and controls the absorption of antigens (Majamaa, 1997). This supplement also inhibits the growth of vaginal microorganisms such as *Escherichia coli, Candida albicans,* and *Gardnerella vaginalis* (Hughes, 1990).

Treatment of *Clostridium difficile* Diarrhea

Research shows that *Lactobacillus* GG is a reliable alternative to antibiotic therapy for relapsing *C. difficile* diarrhea (Bennett, 1996). Of the 32 patients included in this study, all reported improved symptoms, and 84% were cured with a single treatment. Because *Lactobacillus* remains in the gastrointestinal tract longer than other bacteria, it is useful for treating a variety of gastrointestinal conditions.

Hypocholesteremic Action

It is believed that *Lactobacillus* decreases cholesterol by assimilating it. However, one study showed no improvement in cholesterol levels when subjects took *Lactobacillus* four times a day for 21 days (Lin, 1989). The fact that this study used a strain of *Lactobacillus* other than *L. acidophilus* could account for the differing results.

Other Possible Actions

A few other recent studies have investigated the potential role of *Lactobacillus* in preventing recurrent superficial bladder cancer (Aso, 1995), increasing the production of tumor necrosis factor-alpha (TNF-alpha), increasing interleukin-6 and interleukin-10, and inducing nonspecific immunity (Miettinen, 1996). The consumption of *Lactobacillus* has been shown to decrease enzymes in the colon that may play a role in causing cancer (Marteau, 1990). However, research has not yet confirmed this hypothesis. Also, use of *Lactobacillus* has been shown to decrease *H. pylori* in vitro by acid production and low pH (Lorca, 2001).

References

Aroutcheva AA et al: Antimicrobial protein produced by vaginal *Lactobacillus acidophilus* that inhibits *Gardnerella vaginalis, Infect Dis Obstet Gynecol* 9(1):33-39, 2001.

Aso Y et al: Preventive effect of a *Lactobacillus casei* preparation on the recurrence of superficial bladder cancer in a double-blind trial, *Eur Urol* 27:104-109, 1995.

Bennett R: Treatment of relapsing *Clostridium difficile* diarrhea with *Lactobacillus* GG, *Nutr Today* 31(suppl):35s-38s, 1996.

Biffi A et al: Antiproliferative effect of fermented milk on the growth of a human breast cancer cell line, *Nutr Cancer* 28:93-99, 1997.

Hughes VL et al: Microbiologic characteristics of *Lactobacillus* products used for colonization of the vagina, *Obstet Gynecol* 75(2):244, 1990.

Lee, MC et al: Oral bacterial therapy promotes recovery from acute diarrhea in children, *Acta Paediatr Taiwan* 42(5):301-305.

Lin SY et al: *Lactobacillus* effects on cholesterol: in vitro and in vivo results, *J Dairy Sci* 72(11):2885, 1989.

Lorca, GL et al: *Lactobacillus acidophilus* autolysins inhibit *Helicobacter pylori* in vitro, *Curr Microbiol* 42(1):39-44, 2001.

Majamaa H et al: Probiotics: a novel approach in the management of food allergy, *J Allergy Clin Immunol* 99(2):179-185, 1997.

Marteau P et al: Effect of chronic ingestion of fermented dairy product containing *Lactobacillus acidophilus* and *Bifidobacterium bifidum* on metabolic activities of colonic flora in humans, *Am J Clin Nutr* 52(4):685, 1990.

Miettinen M et al: Production of human tumor necrosis factor alpha, interleukin-6, and interleukin-10 is induced by lactic acid bacteria, *Infect Immun* 64:5403-5405, 1996.

Rao CV et al: Prevention of colonic preneoplastic lesions by the probiotic *Lactobacillus acidophilus* NCFMTM in F344 rats, *Int J Oncol* 14:939-944, 1999.

Aconite
(a'kuh-nite)

Scientific names: *Aconitum napellus* L., *Aconitum columbianum, Aconitum chinense, Aconitum carmichaeli*

Other common names: Blue rocket, bushi, friar's cap, helmet flower, monkshood, mousebane, soldier's cap, wolfsbane

Class 3

Origin: Aconite can be found in Asia, Europe, and North America.

Uses

Reported Uses

Aconite is used primarily in Europe and Asia. Because of its extreme toxicity, many trained practitioners in the United States do not use this product. The root is the plant part used in traditional medicine. In Asia, aconite has multiple uses and is usually mixed with other herbs. Circa 1500 B.C., aconite was used to make poisonous arrows. In homeopathic and Oriental medicine, aconite extract is used as a hypotensive and analgesic and to relieve cancer pain. It is also used to decrease fever and to treat arthritis, bruises, fractures, and rheumatism. Aconite is extremely heating and therefore is used to treat cold extremities and poor digestion.

Product Availability and Dosages

Available Forms

Dried root (prepared); homeopathic; liniment; tincture of dried root: 1:10, 1:20; tincture of fresh leaf: 1:2; a few Chinese forms of this herb are sold only to practitioners

Plant Parts Used: Leaves, roots, flowers

Dosages and Routes

Use of this herb is not generally recognized as safe, and it is not found over the counter. Maximum dosage is 25 mg tid *(Aconitum napellus)*.

Adult
- PO tincture of fresh leaf: 1-5 drops qid to relieve pain (Moore, 1995)
- Topical liniment: maximum 1.3%

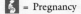 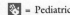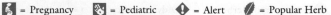

A

Precautionary Information

Contraindications

Aconite should never be used during pregnancy and lactation and it should not be given to children. Aconite can be absorbed through the skin if handled improperly. Because of its extreme toxicity, this herb should be administered only by a trained practitioner. Class 3 herb.

Side Effects/Adverse Reactions

The following result from moderate to high doses.
Cardiovascular: Hypotension, bradycardia, CARDIAC ARRHYTHMIAS, TACHYARRHYTHMIAS, DEATH
Central Nervous System: Weakness, tingling in extremities
Ear, Eye, Nose, and Throat: Blurred vision, THROAT CONSTRICTION, oral numbness
Gastrointestinal: Nausea, vomiting, anorexia, diarrhea
Metabolic: Metabolic acidosis, hypokalemia
Musculoskeletal: Weakness, paresthesia

Interactions with Aconite

Drug

Antiarrhythmics (beta-blockers): Increased toxicity and death may occur when aconite is used with these and other cardiac agents; do not use concurrently.
Antihypertensives: Increased toxicity and death may occur when aconite is used with these and other cardiac agents; do not use concurrently.
Cardiac glycosides (digoxin): Increased toxicity and death may occur when aconite is used with these and other cardiac agents; do not use concurrently.

Food	Herb	Lab Test
None known	None known	None known

Client Considerations

Assess

- Assess for client use. Many other natural products have the same uses as aconite, without the extreme toxicity.

 Endangered Herb   Adverse effects: BOLD = life-threatening

• Assess for the use of antiarrhythmics, antihypertensives, and cardiac glycosides. Toxicity and death may occur (see Interactions).

Administer

• Inform the client that aconite is not available over the counter. Only practitioners trained in the use of aconite may administer this herb.

Teach Client/Family

 • Warn the client never to use aconite during pregnancy and lactation and not to give it to children.
• Because of its extreme toxicity, warn the client never to use aconite except under the direction of a qualified herbalist.
• Warn the client not to touch the aconite plant; toxicity and death can occur.

Pharmacology

Pharmacokinetics

Pharmacokinetics and pharmacodynamics are unknown.

Primary Chemical Components of Aconite and Their Possible Actions		
Chemical Class	**Individual Component**	**Possible Action**
Alkaloid	Aconitine	Paralysis of nerve endings and central nervous system; antiinflammatory; analgesic
	Hypaconitine (Kimura, 1988)	Neuromuscular blocker
	Lappaconitine	Analgesic; irreversibly blocks heart sodium channels (Wright, 2001)
	Mesaconitine; Oxoaconitine; Picraconitine; Aconine; Napelline	

Continued

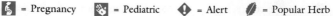

Primary Chemical Components of Aconite and Their Possible Actions—cont'd		A
Chemical Class	**Individual Component**	**Possible Action**
Acid	Malonic acid; Succinic acid; Itaconic acid; Aconitic acid	
Sugar		
Starch		
Fat		
Resin		

Actions

Except for toxicology studies, very little research is available on the pharmacologic actions of aconite. Most qualified practitioners use this product only after proper processing. It is commonly used in traditional Chinese medicine.

Cardiovascular Action

Cardiovascular action results from the ability of aconite to raise membrane permeability for sodium ions, thus prolonging cardiac repolarization. When minute quantities of the herb were given to rabbits intraperitoneally, severe nerve damage and damage to the myelin sheath occurred (Kim, 1991). This herb is considered cardiotoxic. A recent study (Wright, 2001) identifies the irreversible blocking of heart sodium channels by one component (lappaconitine) of the herb piconite.

Stimulation of Immunity

Aconitum carmichaeli increases the secretion of interleukin-1b, tumor necrosis factor-alpha (TNF-alpha), and interleukin-6 in human mononuclear cells (Chang, 1994). Neither the mechanism of immune stimulation nor the exact site of action has been identified.

Analgesic and Antiinflammatory Actions

In mouse studies, aconite alkaloids have been shown to be much more potent and effective than hydrocortisone and indomethacin for reducing inflammation. Lappaconitine, an alkaloid of aconite, has been identified as a central-acting, non-opioid analgesic that decreases the pain response during both the first and second pain phases (Ono, 1991). In Ayurvedic medicine, aconite root generally is considered safe. However, before use the herb is processed using an elaborate detoxification method to make it safe. The level of toxicity drops significantly during such controlled processing (Mahajani, 1990). Another way toxicity is reduced is by cooking the root with other herbs, foods, and salt. Toxicity still occasionally occurs, but its occurrence is rare.

References

Chang J et al: The stimulating effect of radix aconiti extract of cytokines secretion by human mononuclear cells, *Planta Med* 60:576-578, 1994.

Kim SH et al: Myelo-optic neuropathy caused by aconitine in rabbit model, *Jpn J Ophthalmol* 35:417, 1991.

Kimura M et al: Hypaconitine, the dominant constituent responsible for the neuromuscular blocking action of the Japanese-Sino medicine "buchi" (aconite root), *Jpn J Pharmacol* 48:290-293, 1988.

Mahajani SS et al: Some observations on the toxicity and anti-pyretic activity of crude and processed aconite roots, *Planta Med* 56:665, 1990.

Moore M: *Materia medica*, Bisbee, Ariz, 1995, Author.

Ono M et al: Pharmacological studies on lappaconitine: antinociception and inhibition of the spinal action of substance P and somatostatin, *Jpn J Pharmacol* 55:523-530, 1991.

Wright SN: Irreversible block of human heart (hH1) sodium channels by the plant alkaloid lappaconitine, *Mol Pharmacol* 59(2):183-192, 2001.

Agar
(ah'gur)

Scientific names: *Gelidium cartilagineum, Gracilaria confervoides,* and others

Other common names: Agar-agar, Chinese gelatin, colle du japon, E406, gelose, Japanese gelatin, Japanese isinglass, layor carang, vegetable gelatin   Class 2d

Origin: Agar is found in several species of red marine algae in oceans around the world.

Uses

Reported Uses

Agar is used as bulk laxative and as a treatment for neonatal hyperbilirubinemia (Vales, 1990). However, most naturopaths

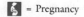 = Pregnancy   = Pediatric    = Alert   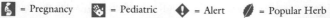 = Popular Herb

and herbalists would not use this product to treat neonatal hyperbilirubinemia. Agar is commonly found in foods and is safely and regularly used as a thickener in place of gelatin by those with gelatin sensitivity.

Product Availability and Dosages

Available Forms

Flakes, powder, strips

Plant Parts Used: Thallus

Dosages and Routes

Adult

Bulk Laxative

• PO: 4-16 g (1-2 tsp) powder mixed with fruit or 8 oz liquid, taken qd-bid; do not use dry

Precautionary Information

Contraindications

Until more research is available, agar should not be used during pregnancy and lactation and should not be given to children. Agar should not be used when coma or gastrointestinal obstruction are present. Avoid use in those with swallowing difficulties. Class 2d herb.

Side Effects/Adverse Reactions

Gastrointestinal: Bowel obstruction, esophageal obstruction
Respiratory: Choking, aspiration (if client is not alert or if insufficient liquids are given)
Systemic: Decreased absorption of vitamins and minerals

Interactions with Agar

Drug

Electrolyte solutions: Agar causes dehydration when used with electrolyte solutions; do not use concurrently.
Tannic acids: Agar causes dehydration when used with tannic acids; do not use concurrently.
Thyroid products: Because of the high iodine content of agar, avoid concurrent use with thyroid products.

Continued

 Endangered Herb   Adverse effects: **bold** = life-threatening

Interactions with Agar—cont'd		
Food	Herb	Lab Test
None known	None known	None known

Client Considerations

Assess

- Assess the client's bowel pattern and determine whether laxatives are used frequently; monitor for bowel obstruction.
- If the client is using agar for its anticholesterol action, assess the client's lipid levels: triglycerides, cholesterol, HDL, and LDL.
- Assess for the use of thyroid products; the iodine in some agar products may interfere with thyroid hormones (see Interactions).
- Assess for the use of electrolyte solutions and tannic acids (see Interactions).

Administer

- Instruct the client to take agar PO on an empty stomach to prevent improper absorption of vitamins.

Teach Client/Family

- Until more research is available, caution the client not to use agar during pregnancy and lactation and not to give it to children.
- Teach the client the signs and symptoms of bowel obstruction.
- Explain that vitamins and minerals may not be absorbed properly while taking agar.
- Instruct the client about lifestyle changes that prevent constipation: increased fluids, bulk in the diet, and exercise.

Pharmacology

Pharmacokinetics

Very little is known about the pharmacokinetics of agar, although this herb is known to increase the excretion of cholesterol, decrease the digestion of fat, and decrease the retention of nitrogen. Gastrointestinal absorption is poor.

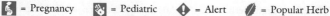

Primary Chemical Components of Agar and Their Possible Actions		
Chemical Class	**Individual Component**	**Possible Action**
Calcium salt **Sulfuric acid** **Polysaccharide**	Agarose	Increases bulk in the colon
Alginic acid	Agaropectin	Hypocholesteremic

Actions

Laxative Action

Agar swells in the intestine, thus stimulating peristalsis and increasing bulk content in the colon. It is not broken down and therefore passes through the gastrointestinal system almost unchanged.

Hypocholesteremic Action

For many centuries in Japan, seaweed was thought to decrease atherosclerosis. In 1960, Kameda's study showed a decrease in blood pressure using *Laminaria* spp., and the next year Kameda's results with rabbits showed a decrease in both blood pressure and cholesterol (Kameda, 1960, 1961). However, subsequent studies using rats were unable to duplicate these results. Several more recent studies have used various types of seaweed, including *Porphyra tenera*, which has been shown to decrease cholesterol levels significantly in rabbits. The anticholesterol action of agar takes place in the gut, where it interferes with the absorption of cholesterol (Fahrenbach, 1966).

References

Fahrenbach MJ et al: Hypocholesterolemic activity of mucilaginous polysaccharides in white leghorn cockrels, *Proc Soc Exp Biol Med* 123:321, 1966.

Kameda T et al: *Fukushima Igaku Zussi* 10:251, 1960.

Kameda T et al: *Fukushima Igaku Zussi* 10:251, 1961.

Vales TN et al: Pharmacologic approaches to the prevention and treatment of neonatal hyperbilirubinemia, *Clin Perinatol* 17:245-273, 1990.

Agrimony
(a'gruh-mow-nee)

Scientific names: *Agrimonia eupatoria, Agrimonia pilosa* var., *Agrimonia japonica*

Other common names: Church steeples, cocklebur, langya-cao, liverwort, longyacao, philanthropos, potter's piletabs, sticklewort, stickwort

Origin: Agrimony is grown in Asia, Europe, and the United States.

Uses

Reported Uses

Agrimony in the form of tea or gargle is used to treat sore throat. Agrimony may be used topically as an astringent, to help stop bleeding, and to treat cuts and abrasions. Little research exists on its use in humans. Some herbalists report that agrimony has antiasthmatic, sedative, antiinflammation, decongestant, and diuretic properties, although no scientific studies support these claims. Diuretic and uricosuric use have been reported (Giachetti, 1986). Most other uses are based solely on anecdotal reports. However, agrimony has been used for decades as a hemostatic to promote blood coagulation. It has been used to decrease vaginal bleeding, discharge, and for urinary tract infections. Ointments made from agrimony may shrink hemorrhoids and soothe sores, insect bites, and athlete's foot. It may be used for its antibacterial action to treat vaginal trichomoniasis.

Investigational Uses

Agrimonia pilosa is currently used in China to treat cancer (Sugi, 1997). A new study (Min, 2001) showed an inhibitory effect against HIV-1.

Product Availability and Dosages

Available Forms

Gargle, tablets, tea, ointment, capsules

Plant Parts Used: Flowers, leaves, stems

Dosages and Routes

Adult

Ophthalmic
- Topical eyewash: 30 g/500 ml licorice root, fennel seed, eyebright, and agrimony (dilution 1:1) (Mills, 2000)

Sore Throat
- PO gargle: 3 g in water

Other
- PO tablet: 3 g qd or equivalent (Blumenthal, 1998)
- PO tea: 3 tsp in 1 cup boiling water, up to 4×/day
- Topical: apply as poultice as needed

Precautionary Information

Contraindications

Until more research is available, agrimony should not be during pregnancy and lactation, and it should not be given to children. Agrimony should not be used by persons with hypersensitivity to this plant or to roses.

Side Effects/Adverse Reactions

Cardiovascular: Palpitations, flushing of the face
Integumentary: Photosensitivity, photodermatitis
Systemic: Hypersensitivity, rash, allergic reactions

Interactions with Agrimony

Drug
Anticoagulants (warfarin, heparin): Agrimony may decrease clotting times when used with anticoagulants; avoid concurrent use (PO) (theoretical).

Food	Herb	Lab Test
None known	None known	None known

Client Considerations

Assess

- Assess the client for hypersensitivity reactions such as rash or breathing difficulty. If such reactions are present, discontinue use of agrimony and administer antihistamines.
- Assess for the use of anticoagulants (see Interactions).

Administer

- Instruct the client to take agrimony PO in tea or tablet form.
- Instruct the client to dilute the herb in warm water for use as a gargle.
- Instruct the client to store eyewash frozen in sterile blocks, or use immediately.

Teach Client/Family

- Until more research is available, caution the client not to use agrimony during pregnancy and lactation and not to give it to children.

Pharmacology

Pharmacokinetics

Pharmacokinetics and pharmacodynamics are unknown.

Primary Chemical Components of Agrimony and Their Possible Actions		
Chemical Class	**Individual Component**	**Possible Action**
Tannin	Ellagitannins	Wound healing; astringent
	Trace gallotannins	Antiinflammatory
Agrimonin	A; B; C; Pimic acid Agrimonii	Nonhemostatic
	Agrimonic acid; Pedunculagin; Casuarictin; Potentillin (Okuda, 1984)	Antitumor
Furanocoumarin		Photosensitivity; anticoagulant
Polysaccharide		
Silic acid		
Urosolic acid		
Agrimonolide		
Flavonoid	Luteolin; apigenin	
Essential oil		
Vitamin	B_1; K; C	
Seeds Also Contain		
Acid	Oleic acid; Linoleic acid; Linolenic acid	

 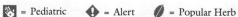

Actions

Most of the research on agrimony was done in the 1950s and 1960s. Very little research has been done in recent years.

Hemostatic Action

Some early studies reported that agrimony promotes blood coagulation. In one study, when *Agrimonia* was given to rabbits intravenously, platelets and calcium increased, and clotting time decreased (Yao, 1957). However, other early studies reported that *A. pilosa* does not promote coagulation but instead increases clotting time. Even at high doses (15 mg/kg), agrimony given intravenously to rabbits had this result (Qu, 1957). Frogs treated with agrimony experienced elevated blood pressure and respiration, as well as increased heart rate and cardiac contractility (Wu, 1941). Mice treated with agrimony experienced prolonged tail bleeding time and, as a result of antiplatelet action, acute pulmonary thromboembolism (Hsu, 1987). This conflicting research indicates that strict controls need to be in place in order to replicate these studies.

Antiinflammatory Action

The antiinflammatory action of agrimony has been demonstrated on rabbits. In one study, when the irritated conjunctivas of rabbits were treated with agrimony, a definite decrease in inflammation occurred. This effect may have resulted from high levels of the tannin phlobaphere, a potent astringent in the herb (Eda, 1972).

Antibacterial Action

A study of 40 women with vaginal trichomoniasis showed that a decoction of agrimony extract inhibited the growth of gram-positive bacteria (Wang, 1953). When a 200% concentrated extract was applied over the vaginal wall and a cotton ball treated with the herb was inserted into the vagina for 3 to 4 hours, 37 of the women were cured with one treatment. In another study using a decoction of *Agrimonia eupatoria,* agrimony inhibited the growth of *Mycobacterium tuberculosis* (Peter-Horvath, 1965) and even destroyed streptomycin– and para-aminosalicylic-acid–resistant strains. The only strains not affected were those resistant to isoniazid.

Other Actions

One study showed that *A. pilosa* inhibited carcinoma in laboratory animals, but not in human fibroblasts (Kampo Kenkyu,

1979). Another study demonstrated the antitumor activity of agrimonii, one of the tannins in agrimony, on test mice (Miyamoto, 1985, 1988). A single dose of 10-30 mg/kg resulted in almost complete resolution of the tumor. One recent study (Min, 2001) evaluated several Korean plants for anti-HIV-1 activity. *Agrimonia pilosa* showed anti-HIV-1 activity.

References

Blumenthal M, editor: *The complete German Commission E monographs: therapeutic guide to herbal medicines,* Austin, Tex, American Botanical Council; Boston, Integrative Medicine Communication, 1998.

Eda A: Chinese traditional and herbal drugs communications, *Fushun Fourth Hospital* 1:37, 1972.

Editorial Dept: *Kampo Kenkyu* (2):51, 1979.

Giachetti D et al: Diuretic and uricosuric activity of *Agrimonia eupatoria* L., *Boll Soc Ital Biol Sper* 62(6):705-711, 1986.

Hsu M et al: Effect of hsien-ho-t'sao *(Agrimonia pilosa)* on experimental thrombosis in mice, *Am J Chin Med* 15:43-51, 1987.

Mills S, Bone K: *Principles and practice of phytotherapy,* Edinburgh, 2000, Churchill Livingstone, p 134.

Min BS et al: Inhibitory effects of Korean plants on HIV-1 activities, *Phytother Res* 15(6):481-486, 2001.

Miyamoto K et al: Isolation of agrimoniin, an antitumor constituent, from the roots of *Agrimonia pilosa* Ledeb, *Chem Pharm Bull* 33:3977-3981, 1985.

Miyamoto K et al: Induction of cytotoxicity of peritoneal exudate cells by agrimoniin: a novel immunomodulatory tannin of *Agrimonia pilosa* Ledeb, *Cancer Immunol Immunother* 27:59-62, 1988.

Okuda T et al: Tannins of rosaceous medicinal plants I: structures of potentillin, agrimonic acids A and B, and agrimoniin, a dimeric ellagitannin, *Chem Pharm Bull* 32:2165-2173, 1984.

Peter-Horvath M: *Chem Abstracts* 62:3105g, 1965.

Qu DQ et al: *Abstracts of the 1956 Symposium of the Chinese Pharmacy Association (Shanghai Branch),* ed 1, Shanghai Branch, 1957, p 254.

Sugi M: Cancer therapy by Chinese crude drugs. In Kondo K: *Cancer therapy in China today,* Tokyo, 1997, Shizensha, p 95.

Wang Y et al: *Acta Botanica Yunnanica* 2:312, 1953.

Wu YR et al: *Zhendan Med J* 6:28, 1941.

Yao JC et al: *J Acad Military Med Chin PLA* (1):144, 1957.

Alfalfa
(al-fal'fuh)

Scientific name: *Medicago sativa* L.

Other common names: Buffalo herb, lucerne, purple medic, purple medick

Origin: Alfalfa grows throughout the world.

Uses

Reported Uses

Alfalfa is used to treat digestive disorders, including constipation, and arthritis, to increase blood clotting, as a diuretic, to relieve inflammation of the prostate, and to treat acute or chronic cystitis. Its seeds are made into a poultice and applied topically to treat boils and insect bites. Alfalfa is primarily used as a nutritive tonic and alkalizing herb. It may be used during pregnancy to increase nutrition or alleviate anemia. Alfalfa is used to boost normal vitality and strength, stimulate the appetite, and help in weight gain. It is an excellent source of beta-carotene.

Investigational Uses

Researchers are experimenting with the use of alfalfa to protect against carcinogens in the gastrointestinal tract, decrease cholesterol levels, prevent menopausal symptoms, and treat atherosclerosis. It may also be a good source of vitamin K.

Product Availability and Dosages

Available Forms

Capsules, flour, flowering tops, infusion, fluid extract (from leaves), poultice (from seeds), sprouts, tablets

Plant Parts Used: Flowers, germinating seeds, whole herb, leaves

Dosages and Routes

Adult

- PO fluid extract: 5 ml tid maximum; 1-2 ml tid-qid (Smith, 1999)
- PO powder: 5-300 grains (a food status)
- PO capsules: 3-6 caps qd

Precautionary Information

Contraindications

Because it acts as a uterine stimulant, alfalfa should not be used during pregnancy except under the direction of a qualified herbalist. It should not be used by persons who are hypersensitive to this herb or who have lupus erythematosus. The seeds of alfalfa should not be eaten, because they contain a toxic amino acid.

Side Effects/Adverse Reactions

Cardiovascular: Hypotension
Integumentary: Photosensitivity
Systemic: Systemic lupus erythematosus (SLE)-like syndrome (from sprouts), BLEEDING, BLOOD DYSCRASIAS

Interactions with Alfalfa

Drug

Anticoagulants (heparin, warfarin): Alfalfa may increase prothrombin time and prolong bleeding when taken with anticoagulants.
Antidiabetics (including insulin): Alfalfa may potentiate hypoglycemic action; use cautiously.
Estrogen: May increase action; avoid concurrent use.
Oral Contraceptives: May alter action; avoid concurrent use.

Food	Herb	Lab Test
None known	None known	None known

Client Considerations

Assess

- Assess for allergic reactions. If present, discontinue use of this herb and administer antihistamine or other appropriate therapy.
- Assess for SLE-like symptoms. If these symptoms occur, determine whether the client is using alfalfa sprouts, and if so, the amount and duration of use (Malinow, 1982; Roberts, 1983).
- Assess for use of anticoagulants, antidiabetics, estrogen, and oral contraceptives (see Interactions).

🜪 = Pregnancy   🜪 = Pediatric   ◆ = Alert   ∅ = Popular Herb

Administer
- Instruct the client to take alfalfa PO as powder, tablets, capsules, fluid extract, or flowering tops, or in food as flour or sprouts.

Teach Client/Family
- Because alfalfa acts as a uterine stimulant, caution the client not to use this herb during pregnancy unless under the direction of a qualified herbalist.
- Inform the client that a SLE-like syndrome has occurred in persons using alfalfa sprouts.
- Teach the client to report bleeding, hot flashes, lupuslike symptoms to health care provider.

Pharmacology

Pharmacokinetics

Pharmacokinetics and pharmacodynamics are unknown.

Primary Chemical Components of Alfalfa and Their Possible Actions		
Chemical Class	Individual Component	Possible Action
Caroteinoid	Lutein	Cancer prevention
Saponin	Aglycones	Antiatherosclerotic
	Medicagenic acid; Hederagenin	
Isoflavonoid	Formononetin Glycosides; Genistein; Daidzein	Estrogenic
Coumarin	Coumestrol	
	Lucernol; Sativol; Trifoliol	
Chlorophyll		
Minerals	Copper; Iron; Manganese; Zinc	Antidiabetic
Vitamins	A, C, D, E, K, B-Complex	
Carotene	Alpha; Beta	
Electrolytes	Calcium; Phosphorus; Potassium; Sodium; Magnesium	

Continued

Primary Chemical Components of Alfalfa and Their Possible Actions—cont'd		
Chemical Class	**Individual Component**	**Possible Action**
Seeds Also Contain		
L-canavaine		Increased immune response
Betaine	Stachydrine	Estrogenic
	Homostachydrine	
Trigonelline		
Fatty oil		

Actions

Antiatherosclerotic Action

Several research studies have focused on the ability of alfalfa to counteract the atherosclerotic effect of dietary cholesterol. In one study, monkeys that were fed high levels of cholesterol with alfalfa added showed a decrease in cholesterolemia and plasma phospholipids. The distribution of their plasma lipoproteins also normalized, as did the extent of aortic atherosclerosis (Malinow, 1978). In a subsequent study of monkeys fed semi-purified food and alfalfa saponins, the monkeys showed a decrease in cholesterol levels with no change in high-density lipoprotein (HDL) levels and an increase in fecal excretion of neutral steroids and bile (Malinow, 1981, 1983). Another study using rabbits showed similar results, with prevention of hyper-cholesteremia and atherosclerosis. Alfalfa saponins and seeds also produced similar results in rabbits (Malinow, 1980).

Estrogenic Action

In one study, chromatography was used to examine several types of alfalfa tablets for the presence of coumestrol, a phytoestrogen. This phytoestrogen was found in all of the alfalfa tablets studied (Elakovich, 1984).

References

Duke JA: *CRC handbook of medicinal herbs,* Boca Raton, Fla, 1985, CRC Press, pp 299-300.

Elakovich S et al: Analysis of coumestrol, a phytoestrogen, in alfalfa tablets sold for human consumption, *J Agric Food Chem* 32(1):173-175, 1984.

Malinow MR et al: Effect of alfalfa in shrinkage (regression) of atheroscle-

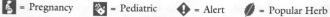

§ = Pregnancy   ※ = Pediatric   ◆ = Alert   ∅ = Popular Herb

rotic plaques during cholesterol feeding in monkeys, *Atherosclerosis* 30:27-43, 1978.

Malinow MR et al: Alfalfa saponins and alfalfa seeds, *Atherosclerosis* 37:433-438, 1980.

Malinow MR et al: Cholesterol and bile acid balance in *Macaca fascicularis, J Clin Invest* 67:156-162, 1981.

Malinow MR et al: Systemic lupus erythematosus-like syndrome in monkeys fed alfalfa sprouts: role of a nonprotein amino acid, *Science* 216(23):415-417, 1982.

Malinow MR et al: Experimental models of atherosclerosis regression, *Atherosclerosis* 48:105-118, 1983.

Roberts JL et al: Exacerbation of SLE associated with alfalfa ingestion, *N Engl J Med* 308(22):1361, 1983.

Smith E: *Therapeutic herb manual,* Williams, Ore, 1999, Author.

Allspice
(awl′spise)

Scientific names: *Pimento officinalis, Eugenia pimenta*

Other common names: Clove pepper, Jamaica pepper, pimenta, pimento

Class 1

Origin: Allspice is a tree that grows in Central America, Mexico, and the West Indies.

Uses

Reported Uses

Allspice is used to treat indigestion, flatulence, muscle pain, and dental pain. Contemporary use is limited, and allspice is rarely used therapeutically.

Investigational Uses

Researchers are experimenting with the use of allspice as an antimicrobial and as a treatment for diabetes and hypertension.

Product Availability and Dosages

Available Forms

Extract, pimento water

Plant Parts Used: Berries (dried, unripened, rind), powdered fruit

Dosages and Routes

Dosages vary.

🌀 Endangered Herb   Adverse effects: BOLD = life-threatening

Adult

Indigestion/Flatulence
- PO: 2 tsp powder mixed in 8 oz water bid-tid
- PO: 3 drops of essential oil on sugar

Pain
- Topical: mix oil or powder in water to make a paste, apply prn

Precautionary Information

Contraindications

Until more research is available, allspice should not be used therapeutically during pregnancy and lactation and it should not be given therapeutically to children. Allspice use is not recommended for use by persons with colitis, irritable bowel syndrome, Crohn's disease, diverticulitis, or cancer. Class 1 herb.

Side Effects/Adverse Reactions

Central Nervous System: Seizures (high doses)
Gastrointestinal: Nausea, vomiting, gastroenteritis, anorexia
Integumentary: Rash, hypersensitivity reactions (topical)

Interactions with Allspice

Drug

Minerals: Allspice may interfere with the absorption of minerals such as iron and zinc. Do not use concurrently with mineral supplements.

Food	Herb	Lab Test
None known	None known	None known

Client Considerations

Assess

- Assess the client's use of mineral supplements; allspice may interfere with their absorption (see Interactions).
- If allspice is being used to treat hypertension, assess the client's cardiac status: blood pressure, pulse, character, and edema. Also, assess for other medications the client may be taking to treat this condition.

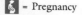 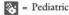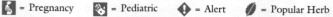

Administer

- Instruct the client to take powder PO or use as a topical treatment.

Teach Client/Family

- Until more research is available, caution the client not to use allspice therapeutically during pregnancy and lactation and not to give it therapeutically to children.
- Teach client to limit the time that allspice is used to prevent seizures.

Pharmacology

Pharmacokinetics

Very little is known about the pharmacokinetics in humans. Two metabolites, homovanillic acid and homomandelic acid, have been identified.

Primary Chemical Components of Allspice and Their Possible Actions		
Chemical Class	Individual Component	Possible Action
Volatile oil	Eugenol	Antifungal; antioxidant; central nervous system depressant; prostaglandic activity; digestive enzymes
	Methyleugenol; Caryophylene	Antioxidant; central nervous system depressant; prostaglandic activity; digestive enzymes
Vitamin	A; C; Thiamine; Riboflavin; Niacin	
Flavonoid	Quercetin	Antiinflammatory
Glycoside		
Sesquiterpene		
Mineral		
Tannin		Wound healing; antiinflammatory
Resin		
Sugar		
Gum		(Ayedoun, 1996)

Actions

Most of the primary research available has focused on several possible actions of *Pimenta dioica*.

Antibacterial and Antifungal Actions

One study showed that allspice is effective against yeasts and fungi (Hitokoto, 1980). Eugenol, one of the chemical components of allspice, may be responsible for this action.

Cardiovascular Action

One study showed that allspice acts as a hypotensive, presumably because of the ability of tannic acid to exert a depressant effect on smooth muscle and cardiac tissue. However, it is also possible that allspice extract produces a negative inotropic effect (Súarez, 1997). *P. dioica* has been shown to act as a central nervous system depressant, as well as a hypotensive. When aqueous extract of allspice was given to rats intravenously at doses of 30, 70, and 100 mg/kg, the larger fraction produced the greatest hypotensive effect, with no significant changes in heart rate or ECG (Súarez, 1997). However, further studies are needed to determine whether the substance in *P. dioica* that is responsible for the hypotensive effect is tannin or some other component.

References

Ayedoun AM et al: Aromatic plants from tropical West Africa, IV: chemical composition of leaf oil of *Pimenta racemosa* (Miller) *JW Moore* var. *racemosa* from Benin, *J Essent Oil Res* 8:207-209, 1996.

Hitokoto H et al: Inhibitory effects of spices on growth and toxin production of toxigenic fungi, *Appl Environ Microbiol* 39:18-22, 1980.

Súarez A et al: Cardiovascular effects of ethanolic and aqueous extracts of *Pimenta dioica* in Sprague-Dawley rats, *J Ethnopharmacol* 55:107-111, 1997.

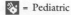 = Pregnancy   = Pediatric   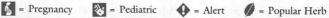 = Alert   = Popular Herb

Aloe
(a'low)

Scientific names: *Aloe vera* L., *Aloe perryi, Aloe barbadensis, Aloe ferox, Aloe spicata*

Other common names: Aloe barbadensis, aloe vera, Barbados, aloe, bitter aloes, burn plant, Cape aloe, Curacao aloe, elephant's gall, hsiang-dan, lily of the desert, lu-hui, socotrine aloe, Venezuela aloe, Zanzibar aloe   Class 1 (Leaf Gel)
Class 2b/2d (Dried Juice)
Class 2d (Topical)

Origin: Aloe is a succulent found throughout the world. It is native to Africa.

Uses
Reported Uses
Aloe is used topically to treat minor burns, sunburn, cuts, abrasions, bedsores, diabetic ulcers, acne, and stomatitis. It is used internally as a stimulant laxative; however, there is little scientific evidence for any internal use. Aloe may also be used to relieve radiation burns suffered by cancer patients and may help slow the development of wrinkles.

Investigational Uses
Researchers are experimenting with the use of the leaf gel (dried juice), taken internally, as a treatment for diabetes mellitus, HIV, cancer, ulcers, colitis, bleeding, asthma, and the common cold.

Product Availability and Dosages
Available Forms
Capsules: 75, 100, 200 mg extract or powder; cream; gel: 98%, 99.5%, 99.6%; jelly; juice: 99.6%, 99.7%; shampoo and conditioner

Plant Parts Used: Large, blade-like leaf, secretory cells below leaf epidermis, roots (rarely)

Dosage and Routes
Adult
All dosages listed are PO.
Active Bleeding Ulcer

- Juice: 1 L/day (Murray, 1998)

HIV/AIDS

- 800-1600 mg/day (acemannan) (Pizzorno, 1999)

Laxative

- Dried juice: 50-300 mg hs (Federal Register, 1985)

Renal Calculi

- Dried juice: take a dose just below that of the laxative dose (Murray, 1998)

Adult and Child

Skin Irritation/Wounds

- PO capsules: 100-200 mg hs
- PO extract: 50-100 mg hs
- Topical leaf gel: apply prn; do not use on deep wounds

Precautionary Information

Contraindications

Dried aloe juice should not be used internally during pregnancy and lactation; should not be given to children younger than 12 years of age; and should not be used by persons with kidney disease, cardiac disease, or bowel obstruction. Aloe should not be used topically by persons who are hypersensitive to this plant, garlic, onions, or tulips. It should not be used topically on deep wounds. Dried aloe juice is not for long-term use. Class 1 herb (leaf gel); class 2b/2d herb (dried juice); class 2d herb (topical).

Side Effects/Adverse Reactions

Gastrointestinal: Spasms, INTESTINAL MUCOSA DAMAGE (IRREVERSIBLE), HEMORRHAGIC DIARRHEA (internal use of dried juice)

Genitourinary: Red colored urine, NEPHROTOXICITY (internal use of dried juice)

Integumentary: Contact dermatitis, delayed healing of deep wounds (topical use)

Metabolic: Hypokalemia (frequent internal use)

Reproductive: UTERINE CONTRACTIONS CAUSING SPONTANEOUS ABORTION, PREMATURE LABOR (internal use of dried juice)

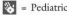

Interactions with Aloe

Drug
Antiarrhythmics, antidiabetics, cardiac glycosides, loop diuretics, potassium-wasting drugs, systemic steroids, thiazides: Aloe products taken internally may increase the effects of antiarrhythmics, cardiac glycosides, antidiabetics, loop diuretics, potassium-wasting drugs, systemic steroids, and thiazides.

Food
None known

Herb
Jimsonweed: The action of jimsonweed is increased in cases of chronic use or abuse of aloe.
Licorice: Licorice may cause hypokalemia when used with aloe taken internally; avoid concurrent use.

Lab Test
Serum potassium: Aloe may lower test values with long-term aloe use.

Client Considerations

Assess

General Use
- Assess whether the client is taking cardiac or renal medications (antidysrhythmics, cardiac glycosides, loop diuretics, antidiabetics, thiazide diuretics). Assess whether systemic steroids or potassium-wasting drugs are being used. Inform the client that aloe products taken internally may increase the effects of these drugs.
- Assess for the use of licorice and jimsonweed (see Interactions).
- Assess for internal use. Caution client that dried juice aloe products taken internally can be dangerous and should be used only under the supervision of a qualified herbalist.
- ◆ Assess for pregnancy and lactation. Under no circumstances should dried juice aloe products be taken during pregnancy and lactation.

🞅 Endangered Herb   Adverse effects: BOLD = life-threatening

Antidiabetic Use
- Assess all prescription antidiabetic agents used by the client.
- Assess fasting blood glucose, 2 hr pp (60-100 mg/dl normal fasting level; 70-130 mg/dl normal 2 hr level).
- Assess blood and urine glucose levels during herb use to determine adequate control.
- Assess for hypoglycemia and hyperglycemia.

Laxative Use of Dried Juice Products
- Assess for repeated laxative use of aloe or traditional products.
- Assess blood and urine electrolytes if herb is used often.
- Assess for cramping, gastrointestinal spasms, and hemorrhagic diarrhea.
- Assess for cause of constipation: identify whether fluids, bulk, or exercise is lacking from lifestyle.

Skin Disorders
- Assess area to be treated with topical aloe products. Identify characteristics of burns, rashes, inflammation, and color of area. Aloe products should not be used on deep wounds; healing can be delayed.
- Assess for route of use. Caution the client not to use by injection; persons have died using this route (Anon, 1998).

Administer
- Instruct the client to use aloe internally only under the direction of a qualified herbalist. Electrolyte imbalances may occur.
- Juice of the plant can be used topically by cutting off a leaf, warming, and squeezing gel onto affected area.
- Refrigerate 100% aloe vera gel after opening.

Teach Client/Family
- Caution the client not to use aloe internally during pregnancy and lactation and not to give it internally to children younger than 12 years of age.
- Caution the client not to use aloe topically if hypersensitive to this plant, garlic, onions, or tulips.
- Caution the client not to use aloe topically on deep wounds.
- Caution the client that dried aloe juice is not for long-term use.

Pharmacology
Pharmacokinetics
Pharmacokinetics and pharmacodynamics are unknown.

🔥 = Pregnancy   🔅 = Pediatric   ❶ = Alert   𝟙 = Popular Herb

Primary Chemical Components of *Aloe* Species and Their Possible Actions*

Chemical Class	Individual Component	Possible Action
Vitamin	A; B group; C; E	Antioxidant; immunostimulant
Enzyme	Carboxypeptidase	Antiinflammatory; analgesic
	Bradykinase	Blocks histamine
Mineral	Magnesium lactate	
	Sodium; Potassium; Calcium; Magnesium; Manganese; Copper; Zinc; Chromium; Iron	
Polysaccharide	Glucomannans	Immunomodulation
	Acemannan	Antiviral; anti-HIV
Anthraquinone	Barbaloin; Isobarbaloin; Anthrone-C glycosides	Purgative effect (large amount); aids absorption from the gastrointestinal tract (small amount)
Lignin		Penetrative ability
Saponin		Antiseptic
Salicylic acid		Antiinflammatory (internal use); keratolytic (topical use)
Amino acid		

Aloe spp. contain more than 75 different constituents.

Actions

Aloe products have been used for centuries for a variety of purposes.

Antiinflammatory and Wound Healing Actions

The topical actions of topical aloe products are well documented. Numerous studies have demonstrated their antiinflammatory, wound-healing properties (Udupa, 1994; Heggers, 1993; Bunyapraphatsara, 1996a, 1996b). Aloe products have been used to reduce inflammation by inactivation of bradykinin, to inhibit prostaglandin A2, to oxidize arachidonic acids, and to block thromboxane A. The wound-healing action of aloe may result from its causing increased blood flow in the affected area.

Other research demonstrates that aloe products have additional medicinal effects. One study (Hutter, 1996) indicates that *Aloe barbadensis,* when used topically on mice, produces effects equivalent to those of topical hydrocortisone. Tests have demonstrated the antiinflammatory activity of aloe vera gel extract when used to treat induced edema of the rat paw. The extract reduced edema and the number of neutrophils migrating into the rat's peritoneal cavity (Vazquez, 1996). In addition, aloe has been shown to be an effective treatment for aphthous stomatitis (Plemons, 1994).

Laxative Action

The laxative effects of aloe result from its ability to inhibit absorption without stimulating peristalsis (Ishii, 1990, 1994a, 1994b).

Antiviral Action

Aloe increases immunity by acting on cytokine. It stimulates phagocytosis in neutrophils, activates complement systems, stimulates B-lymphocytes to make a specific antibody, and also stimulates T-lymphocyte activity (Carrington Laboratories; Sheets, 1991). Montaner (1996) found that CD4 counts and P24 antigens are not affected by acemannan, one of the polysaccharide components of aloe, at 1600 mg/day.

Antidiabetic Action

Aloe gel acts as a thromboxane inhibitor (TXA2), promotes vasodilation, and maintains homeostasis within the vascular endothelium (Heggar, 1993). Studies have shown that aloe gel reduces blood glucose levels significantly within 2 weeks, but not to normal levels (Ajabnoor, 1990; Bunyapraphatsara, 1996a, 1996b; Yongchaiyudha, 1996).

Other Possible Actions

At this time research is minimal on the use of aloe to treat asthma and peptic ulcer. However, studies are underway, and action for these disorders is possible.

References

Ajabnoor MA: Effect of aloes on blood glucose levels in normal and alloxan diabetic mice, *J Ethnopharmacol* 28:215-220, 1990.

Anon: License revoked for aloe vera use, *Nat Med Law* 1:1-2, 1998.

Bunyapraphatsara N et al: Antidiabetic activity of *Aloe vera* L. juice, II:

---

clinical trial in diabetes mellitus in combination with glibenclamide, *Phytomedicine* 3:245-248, 1996a.

Bunyapraphatsara N et al: The efficacy of aloe vera cream in the treatment of first, second and third degree burns in mice, *Phytomedicine* 2:247-251, 1996b.

Carrington Laboratories: *Pharmacologic effects and mechanisms of action of acemann,* Irving, Tex, Author.

Federal Register: 50 FR2124 et seq, Jan 15, 1985.

Heggers JP: Beneficial effects of aloe in wound healing, *Phytother Res* 7:s48-s52, 1993.

Hutter JA et al: Antiinflammatory C-glucosyl chromone from *Aloe barbadensis, Am Chem Society* 59:541-543, 1996.

Ishii Y et al: Studies of aloe, III: mechanism of cathartic effect, *Chem Pharm Bull* 38:197-200, 1990.

Ishii Y et al: Studies of aloe, IV: mechanism of cathartic effect, *Biol Pharm Bull* 17:495-497, 1994a.

Ishii Y et al: Studies of aloe, V: mechanism of cathartic effect, *Biol Pharm Bull* 17:615-653, 1994b.

Montaner JSG et al: Double-blind placebo-controlled pilot trial of acemannan in advanced human immunodeficiency virus disease, *J Acquir Immune Defic Syndr Hum Retrovirol* 12:153-157, 1996.

Murray M, Pizzarno J: *Encyclopedia of natural medicine,* ed 2 (revised), Roseville, Calif, 1998, Prima.

Pizzorno J, Murray M: *Textbook of natural medicine,* London, 1999, Churchill Livingstone, p 587.

Plemons JM et al: Evaluation of acemannan in the treatment of recurrent aphthous stomatitis, *Wounds* 6:40-45, 1994.

Sheets MA et al: Studies of the effect of acemannan on retrovirus infections, *Mol Biother* 3:41-45, 1991.

Udupa SL: Anti-inflammatory and wound healing properties of aloe vera *Fitoteraphia* 65:141-145, 1994.

Vazquez B et al: Antiinflammatory activity extracts from aloe vera gel, *J Ethnopharmacol* 55:69-75, 1996.

Yongchaiyudha S et al: Antidiabetic activity of *Aloe vera* L. juice, I: clinical trial in new cases of diabetes mellitus, *Phytomedicine* 3:241-243, 1996.

American Hellebore
(uh-mehr'i-kuhn heh'luh-bowr)

Scientific name: *Veratrum viride*

Other common names: False hellebore, green hellebore, Indian poke, itchweed, swamp hellebore

Class 3 (Root)

Origin: American hellebore is a perennial found in the United States.

Uses

Reported Uses

American hellebore traditionally has been used to treat pneumonia, seizure disorders, and nerve pain.

Investigational Uses

Research is underway to determine the usefulness of American hellebore for the treatment of hypertensive crisis, myasthenia gravis, and pregnancy-induced hypertension.

Product Availability and Dosages

Available Forms

Fluid extract, powder, tincture

Plant Parts Used: Dried rhizome, roots

Dosages and Routes

Adult

All dosages listed are PO.

Hypertensive Disorders
- Fluid extract: 1-3 minims q2h until stabilized
- Powder: 2 grains
- Tincture: 20-30 minims

No other dosage information is available.

Precautionary Information

Contraindications

American hellebore should not be used during pregnancy except under the direct supervision of a competent herbalist. Until more research is available, this herb should not be used during lactation and it should not be given to children.

🍼 = Pregnancy   👶 = Pediatric   ❗ = Alert   🌿 = Popular Herb

Precautionary Information—cont'd

Contraindications—cont'd

American hellebore should not be used by persons with hypersensitivity to it or those with cardiovascular disorders such as hypotension, cardioversion, cardiac glycoside toxicity, or pheochromocytoma. Class 3 herb (root).

Side Effects/Adverse Reactions

Cardiovascular: Hypertension, hypotension, BRADYCARDIA, ARRHYTHMIAS

Central Nervous System: Dizziness, paresthesia, SEIZURES

Gastrointestinal: Nausea, vomiting, anorexia, abdominal cramps

Ear, Eye, Nose, and Throat: Salivating, dysgeusia

Integumentary: Hypersensitivity reactions

Respiratory: Shortness of breath, RESPIRATORY DEPRESSION

Toxicity: NAUSEA, VOMITING, DIARRHEA, ABDOMINAL PAIN, CHANGE IN VISION, BURNING THROAT, COMA, PARALYSIS, DYSPNEA

Interactions with American Hellebore

Drug	Food	Herb	Lab Test
None known	None known	None known	None known

Client Considerations

Assess

- Assess for hypersensitivity reactions. If present, discontinue use of this herb and administer antihistamine or other appropriate therapy.
- Determine the reason the client is using American hellebore and suggest safer, more conventional alternatives. Because the therapeutic and toxic levels of this herb are very close, this herb is rarely used.

Administer

- Instruct the client to store American hellebore products in a cool, dry place, away from heat and moisture.

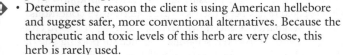

Teach Client/Family

- Caution the client not to use American hellebore during pregnancy except under the direct supervision of a competent herbalist. Until more research is available, caution the client not to use this herb during lactation and not to give it to children.
- Because its therapeutic and toxic levels are very close, advise the client to avoid using American hellebore altogether. Safer alternatives are available.

Pharmacology

Pharmacokinetics

Pharmacokinetics and pharmacodynamics are unknown.

Primary Chemical Components of American Hellebore and Their Possible Actions		
Chemical Class	**Individual Component**	**Possible Action**
Alkaloid	Veratridine	Topical analgesic; parasiticide
	Veracintine	Antineoplastic
	Pseudojervine; Rubijervine; Jervine; Neogermitrine; Cevadine; Protoveratrine; Protoveratridine	Steroidlike
Resin		

Actions

Cardiovascular Action

American hellebore produces many cardiovascular effects, including reduced blood pressure and increased blood flow to the vital organs. It has been used to treat hypertensive conditions such as pregnancy-induced hypertension and hypertensive crisis (Arena, 1986). However, scientific evidence supporting any of the anecdotal claims for American hellebore is lacking.

Because its toxic and therapeutic levels are so close, it is not a commonly used herb.

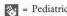

Other Actions

American hellebore historically has been used in Rome to make poisonous arrows.

References

Arena JM et al: *Poisoning toxicology: symptoms, treatments,* ed 5, Springfield, Ill, 1986, Charles C Thomas.

Angelica
(an-jeh'li-kuh)

Scientific names: *Angelica sinensis* (see Dong Quai); *Angelica acutiloba, Angelica archangelica, Angelica atropurpurea, Angelica dahurica, Angelica edulis, Angelica gigas, Angelica keiskei, Angelica koreana, Angelica polymorpha, Angelica pubescens, Angelica radix*

Other common names: American angelica, European angelica, garden angelica, Japanese angelica, wild angelica   Class 2b/2d

Origin: Angelica is a member of the parsley family grown in Iceland and several other northern areas.

Uses

Reported Uses

Angelica is used to improve circulation; to treat headaches, backaches, osteoporosis, asthma, allergies, and skin disorders; to increase gastric juices for digestion; and as a diuretic, an antispasmodic, and a cholagogue. It has also been used as a folk remedy to treat stomach cancer (Duke, 1985). In addition, it has been used as a mild antiseptic; as an expectorant; to ease rheumatic pains, stomach cramps, muscle spasms; and as a treatment for bronchitis.

Investigational Uses:

Angelica has been shown to possess sedative and antibacterial actions.

Product Availability and Dosages

Available Forms

Drops, fluid extract, tincture, whole herb, capsules, liniment

---

🍀 Endangered Herb   Adverse effects: BOLD = life-threatening

Plant Parts Used: Fruit, roots (used by most herbalists), seeds, whole herb, leaves

Dosages and Routes

Adult

Counterirritant

- Topical essential oil: dilute and apply 10-15 drops to inflamed areas (Blumenthal, 1998)

Other

- PO dried root: 1-2 g tid (Pizzorno, 1999)
- PO dried root infusion: 1-2 g tid (Pizzorno, 1999)
- PO fluid extract: 0.5-2 ml tid (1:1 dilution) (Pizzorno, 1999)
- PO tincture: 1-3 ml tid (1:5 dilution) (Moore, 1995)

Children

GI problems/to stimulate the appetite

- PO tincture 1.5 g of 1.5 g/ml
- PO fluid extract 1.5-3 g of 1:1 g/ml

Precautionary Information

Contraindications

Angelica should not be used during pregnancy; can induce miscarriage. Persons with diabetes (angelica can increase blood sugar.), peptic ulcers, or bleeding disorders should use this herb cautiously. Class 2b/2d herb.

Side Effects/Adverse Reactions

Cardiovascular: Hypotension

Gastrointestinal: Anorexia, flatulence, spasms of the gastrointestinal tract, dyspepsia

Integumentary: Photosensitivity, PHOTOTOXICITY, photodermatitis

Systemic: BLEEDING MAY OCCUR WHEN USED WITH ANTICOAGULANTS

Interactions with Angelica

Drug

Anticoagulants (heparin, warfarin): Many *Angelica* spp. increase prothrombin time and prolong bleeding when taken with anticoagulants. Avoid the concurrent use of angelica with all anticoagulants.

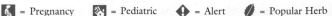

= Pregnancy   = Pediatric   = Alert   = Popular Herb

A

Interactions with Angelica—cont'd

Drug—cont'd

Doxazosin: May increase the effect of doxazosin.

Tolbutamide: Angelica dahurica may delay elimination of tolbutamide (Ishibara, 2000). Avoid the concurrent use of angelica with tolbutamide.

Food	Herb
None known	None known

Lab Test

Plasma partial thromboplastin time (PTT): Angelica may increase PTT in clients taking warfarin concurrently.

Prothrombin time (PT) and plasma International Normalized Ratio (INR): Angelica may increase test values in clients taking warfarin concurrently.

Client Considerations

Assess

- Assess for diabetes, bleeding disorders, or use of anticoagulants (see Interactions). Angelica should be used cautiously by clients with these conditions.

Administer

- Instruct the client to take angelica PO as a tincture or fluid extract, or in whole herb form. Many products require dilution. Tinctures should be taken with liquids. Essential oil requires dilution before use.

Teach Client/Family

- Advise the client not to use angelica during pregnancy. *Angelica archangelica* may be given to children.
- Inform the client that sunburn may occur, to use sunscreen protective clothing to prevent burns (Blumenthal, 2000).

Pharmacology

Pharmacokinetics

Pharmacokinetics and pharmacodynamics are unknown.

Primary Chemical Components of *Angelica* Species and Their Possible Actions

Chemical Class	Individual Component	Possible Action
Coumarin	Osthol; Xanthotoxin	Antiinflammatory; analgesic; photosensitivity
	Xanthotoxol Angelicin; Bergapten; Imperatorin; Oreoselone; Oxypeucedanin; Umbelliferone; Xanthotoxol; Angelol I, H, Methoxycoumarin, Scopoletin (Kwon, 2002); Decursinol; Peucedanone, (Kang, 2001)	
Angelica archangelica *contains:*		
Terpene hydrocarbon		
Alcohol		
Ester		
Lactone	Alpha-angelica	Increases Ca^{++} binding
Aliphatic carbonyl		
Polysaccharide		
Flavonoid		
Palmitic acid		
Volatile oil	Alpha-phellandrene; beta-phellandrene	Flavor/scent; inhibits contraction of ileal muscles

Actions

Several possible actions dealing primarily with the calcium channel blocking action and antibacterial action of the *Angelica* spp. have been researched.

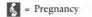 = Pregnancy  = Pediatric   = Alert 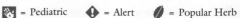 = Popular Herb

Calcium Channel Blocking Action

All coumarins in *A. archangelica* exhibit significant calcium antagonist activity, and folk medicine supports this use. According to one study, these coumarins include archangelicin, bergapten, imperatorin, isoimperatorin, isopimpinellin, osthol, ostrathol, oxypeucedanin, phellopterin, and xanthotoxin (Harmala, 1991, 1992). This study used 20 solvents to measure the inhibition of depolarized increased calcium uptake in rat pituitary cells. Significant hypotensive action occurred (Hikino, 1985; Yoshiro, 1985), as did negative inotropic and antiarrhythmic action (Hikino, 1985).

Sedative Action

In order to assess the sedative/tranquilizing effect of angelica and its antiadrenergic activity, a study was performed in which xanthotoxol was isolated from the dried root of *A. archangelica*. In all species studied (dogs, cats, rats, mice, and hamsters), a significant degree of muscle relaxation occurred while the level of consciousness remained intact. This is a critical point of difference between sedative/hypnotic agents and sedative/tranquilizing effects (Jacobsen, 1964; Turner, 1965). Thus there is real potential for the use of angelica as a sedative or minor tranquilizer (Sethi, 1992). Both Japanese and Chinese angelica (see dong quai, page 355) have shown pain-relieving and mild tranquilizing effects in animals (Hikino, 1985; Yoshiro, 1985; Tanka, 1977).

Antibacterial Action

Chinese angelica has exhibited antibacterial action against both gram-negative and gram-positive bacteria. However, Japanese angelica does not possess antibacterial action (Yoshiro, 1985). The difference may be due to varying concentrations of essential oils in the two species. The oil of *A. archangelica* has shown significant antifungal but no antibacterial activity (Leung, 1980).

References

Blumenthal M, editor: *The complete German Commission E monographs: therapeutic guide to herbal medicines,* Austin, Tex, American Botanical Council; Boston, Integrative Medicine Communication, 1998.

Duke J: *CRC handbook of medicinal herbs,* Boca Raton, Fla, 1985, CRC Press.

Harmala P et al: Isolation and testing of the calcium blocking activity of furanocoumarins from *Angelica archangelica, Planta Med* 57:A58-A59, 1991.

Harmala P et al: Choice of solvent in the extraction of *Angelica archangelica* roots with reference to calcium blocking activity, *Planta Med* 58:176-183, 1992.

Hikino H: Recent research on oriental medicinal plants, *Economic Med Plant Res* 1:53-85, 1985.

Ishihara, K et al: Interactions of drugs and Chinese herbs: Pharmacokinetic changes of tolbutamide and diazepam caused by extract of *Angelica dahuria*, *J Pharm Pharmacol* 52(8):1023-1029, 2000.

Jacobsen E: Tranquilizers and sedatives. In Laurence DR, Bacharach AL, editors: *Evaluation of drug activities, vol I, pharmacometrics,* New York, 1964, Academic Press, pp 215-237.

Kang SY et al: Coumarins isolated from *Angelica gigas* inhibits acetylcholinesterase: structure-activity relationships, *J Nat Prod* 64(5):683-685, 2001.

Kwon YS et al: A new coumarin from the stem of *Angelica dahurica*, *Arch Pharm Res* 25(1):53-56, 2002.

Leung AY: *Encyclopedia of common natural ingredients used in food, drugs, and cosmetics,* New York, 1980, John Wiley & Sons, pp 28-29.

Moore M: *Materia medica,* Bisbee, Ariz, 1995, Author.

Pizzorno J, Murray M: *Textbook of natural medicine,* Edinburgh, 1999, Churchill Livingstone.

Sethi OP et al: Evaluation of xanthotoxol for central nervous system activity, *J Ethnopharmacol* 36:239-247, 1992.

Tanka S et al: Effects of "toki" (*Angelica acutiloba* Kitawaga) extracts on writhing and capillary permeability in mice (analgesic and antiinflammatory effects), *Yakugaku Zassh* 91:1098-1104, 1977.

Turner RA: *Screening methods in pharmacology,* vol 1, New York, 1965, Academic Press.

Yoshiro K: The physiological actions of tang-kuei and cnidium, *Bull Oriental Healing Arts Institute USA* 10:269-278, 1985.

Anise
(a′nus)

Scientific name: *Pimpinella anisum*

Other common names: Aniseed, sweet cumin

Origin: Anise is an annual grown throughout the world.

Uses

Reported Uses

Anise is used internally as an expectorant to treat bronchiectasis, bronchitis, emphysema, and whooping cough. It is also used internally as an antibacterial, an antispasmodic, an abortifacient,

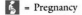 = Pregnancy  = Pediatric   = Alert 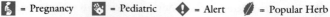 = Popular Herb

a diaphoretic, a diuretic, a stimulant, and a tonic. It can be used by steam inhalation with tea tree, pine, and chamomile to treat acute and chronic sinusitis. It is used externally to treat catarrhs of the respiratory system (asthma, bronchitis). Other reported uses include treatment for cancer, cholera, colic, dysmenorrhea, epilepsy, indigestion, insomnia, lice, migraine, nausea, neuralgia, rash, and scabies (Duke, 1985). It is used as a fragrance and flavoring in food. Anise may be given to children to reduce gas, colic, and respiratory symptoms (Romm, 2000).

Product Availability and Dosages
Available Forms
Essential oil; toothpaste; whole herb

Plant Parts Used: Fruit (ripe and dried)

Dosages and Routes
Adult
- PO essential oil: 1-5 drops diluted prn (Moore, 1995)
- PO whole herb: 3 g (Blumenthal, 1998)
- Topical: 5%-10% concentration essential oil, applied prn; spirit of anise 0.25-0.50 tsp (1:10 dilution in alcohol), diluted (Moore, 1995)

Child
- PO tea: ½-3 cups qd (Romm, 2000)

Precautionary Information
Contraindications
Anise is not recommended for therapeutic use during pregnancy. It should not be used by persons with hypersensitivity to anise or anethole. The essential oil should never be given to children.

Side Effects/Adverse Reactions
Central Nervous System: SEIZURES (essential oil)
Ear, Eye, Nose, and Throat: Stomatitis (toothpaste)
Endocrine: Hypermineralocorticism
Gastrointestinal: Nausea, vomiting, anorexia
Integumentary: Hypersensitivity, contact dermatitis
Respiratory: PULMONARY EDEMA (essential oil)

Interactions with Anise

Drug

Iron: Anise may increase the action of iron; do not use concurrently.

Warfarin: Anise may increase the action of warfarin, do not use concurrently (Heck, 2000).

Food	Herb	Lab Test
None known	None known	None known

Client Considerations

Assess

- Assess the client for hypersensitivity reactions and contact dermatitis. If these are present, discontinue use of anise and institute antihistamines or another appropriate therapy.
- Assess for the use of iron supplements, warfarin (see Interactions).
- Assess the client's fluid and electrolyte balance. Weigh the client weekly to determine water and sodium retention.

Administer

 • Instruct the client to take anise PO using the whole herb or essential oil; however, the essential oil should be used under an herbalist's supervision only. Toxicity can occur.

Teach Client/Family

 • Caution the client not to use anise therapeutically during pregnancy. Anise tea is often used to treat children's respiratory conditions, but the essential oil should never be given to children.
- Caution the client not to use anise essential oil without an herbalist's supervision; toxicity is common. Both seizures and pulmonary edema can result.
- Caution the client that *Illicium anisatum* L. is poisonous and that it can easily be confused with *Illicium verum* (Small, 1996).

Pharmacology

Pharmacokinetics

Pharmacokinetics and pharmacodynamics are unknown.

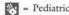 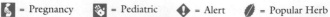

Primary Chemical Components of Anise and Their Possible Actions		
Chemical Class	**Individual Component**	**Possible Action**
Volatile oil	Anethole	Antimicrobial
Alpha-pinene		
Coumarin	Bergapten	Photosensitivity
	Umbelliprenine; Umbelliferone; Scopoletin	
Lipid/fatty acid		
Flavonoid	Quercetin	Antiinflammatory
	Rutin; Luteolin; Isoorientin; Isovitexin; Apigenin	
Sitosterol		
Linalool		
Anisaldehyde		

Actions

Of the scant research that is available, most studies have focused on the use of anise as a flavoring or spice.

Antibacterial Action

One study identifies the inhibition of gram-positive and gram-negative organisms. Another shows the inhibition of the mycotoxin of *Aspergillus*.

Other Actions

Anise is also used for a variety of purposes. It has been used topically (bergapten, one of the chemical components, has been isolated) in conjunction with ultraviolet light to treat psoriasis (Newell, 1996). Anise oil mixed with sassafras oil is used as an insect repellent (Chandler, 1984), and anise oil may be applied topically to treat lice and scabies (Chevallier, 1996). In addition, one study has shown that the essential oil of *Pimpinella anisum* exerts an anticonvulsant effect in mice. In this study the essential oil not only suppressed induced tonic convulsions, but it also increased the threshold of clonic convulsions (Pourgholami, 1999). Anise also acts as a catecholamine similar to adrenalin and possesses estrogenic properties (Albert-Puleo, 1980). A recent study has shown the ability of this herb to block inflammation, carcinogenesis, possibly due to TNF-mediated signaling (Chainy, 2000). Another study (Boskabady, 2001) has identified the relaxant effects of *Pimpinella anisum,* including bronchodilation.

References

Albert-Puleo M J: Fennel and anise as estrogenic agents, *J Ethnopharmacol* 2:337-344, 1980.

Blumenthal M, editor: *The complete German Commission E monographs: therapeutic guide to herbal medicines,* Austin, Tex, American Botanical Council; Boston, Integrative Medicine Communication, 1998.

Boskabady, MH et al: Relaxant effect of *Pimpinella anisum* on isolated guinea pig tracheal chains and its possible mechanism, *J Ethnopharmacol* 74(1):83-88, 2001.

Chainy, GB et al: Anethole blocks both early and late cellular responses transduced by tumor necrosis factor: effect on NF-kappa B, AP-1, JNK, MAPKK and apoptosis, *Oncogene* 19(25):2943-2950, 2000.

Chandler R et al: *Can Pharm J* 117:28-29, 1984.

Chevallier A: *Encyclopedia of medicinal plants,* New York, 1996, DK, pp 246-247.

Duke J: *CRC handbook of medicinal herbs,* Boca Raton, Fla, 1985, CRC Press, pp 374-375.

Heck, AM et al: Potential interactions between alternative therapies and warfarin, *Am J Health Syst Pharm* 57(13):1221-1227, 2000.

Moore M: *Materia medica,* Bisbee, Ariz, 1995, Author.

Newell C et al: *Herbal medicines,* London, 1996, Pharmaceutical Press, pp 30-31.

Pourgholami MH et al: The fruit essential oil of *Pimpinella anisum* exerts anticonvulsant effects in mice, *J Ethnopharmacol* 66(2):211-215, 1999.

Romm A: Better Nutrition's 2000 guide to children's supplements, *Better Nutrition* pp 38-43, Oct 2000.

Small E: Confusion of common names for toxic and edible "star anise" *(Illicium)* species, *Economic Botany* 50(3):337-339, 1996.

Arginine
(ahr'juh-neen)

Scientific names: Arginine hydrochloride, L-arginine

Other common names: None

Origin: Synthetic

Uses

Reported Uses

Arginine is a supplement used for congestive heart failure, erectile dysfunction, peripheral vascular disease, angina, interstitial

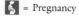 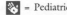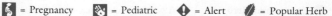

cystitis, and chronic renal failure. Other uses may include upper respiratory infections, diabetes, and AIDS.

Product Availability and Dosages

Available Forms

Tablets, capsules

Dosages and Routes

Adult
- PO: 2-3 g/day; may increase to 15 g/day in cardiac disease
- Very little information is available on dosages.

Precautionary Information

Contraindications

Until more research is completed, avoid use in pregnancy, in lactation, or for young children. Avoid use in severe hepatic disease.

Side Effects/Adverse Reactions

Gastrointestinal: Nausea, vomiting, anorexia
Metabolic (IV use): Increased BUN, hyperkalemia

Interactions with Arginine

Drug
ACE inhibitors: ACE inhibitors taken with arginine (IV) may lead to fatal hypokalemia (theoretical).
Alcohol: Alcohol taken with arginine may cause gastric irritation.
NSAIDs: NSAIDs taken with arginine may cause gastric irritation.
Potassium-sparing diuretics: Potassium-sparing diuretics taken with arginine (IV) may lead to fatal hypokalemia (theoretical).
Platelet inhibitors: Platelet inhibitors taken with arginine may cause gastric irritation.
Salicylates: Salicylates taken with arginine may cause gastric irritation.

Food	Herb	Lab Test
None known	None known	None known

 Endangered Herb   Adverse effects: **BOLD** = life-threatening

Client Considerations

Assess

- Assess reason for use.
- Assess for severe hepatic disease. Avoid giving arginine in severe hepatic disease.
- Identify medications taken such as ACE inhibitors, alcohol, NSAIDs, potassium-sparing diuretics, platelet inhibitors, salicylates. Avoid use of arginine with these medications.

Administer

- Arginine IV should be given only by a qualified herbalist or other expert. Severe hypokalemia and increased BUN may occur.

Teach Client/Family

- Advise the client not to use in pregnancy, in lactation, or for young children. Research is lacking in these populations.

Pharmacology

Pharmacokinetics

Pharmacokinetics and pharmacodynamics are unknown.

Primary Chemical Components of Arginine and Their Possible Actions		
Chemical Class	**Individual Component**	**Possible Action**
N/A	N/A	N/A

Actions

Cardiovascular Action

Several studies have identified the cardiovascular actions of arginine. Hambrecht et al (2000) showed a corrective action on endothelial dysfunction in chronic congestive heart failure. In another study (Rector et al, 1996) patients showed a considerable improvement in congestive heart failure when arginine was given for 4-6 weeks. The effect on angina patients was similar. Three studies (Bednarz et al, 2000; Blum et al, 1999; Maxwell et al, 2002) showed consistent improvement in the

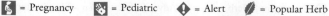

EKG and symptoms of angina when arginine was added at the dose of 6 g/day.

Erectile Dysfunction

The use in erectile dysfunction showed contradictory results. One study (Chen et al, 1999) showed considerable improvement in erectile dysfunction after the addition of 5 g/day for 6 weeks. Another study (Moody et al, 1997) showed no improvement when 1.5 g/day was administered for 17 days.

Other Actions

Other actions that have been studied include peripheral vascular disease, intercystitis, chronic renal failure, diabetes, and upper respiratory infections. Most of these conditions have only one study each, with very limited results.

References

Bednarz B et al: Effects of oral L-arginine supplementation on exercise-induced QT dispersion and exercise tolerance in stable angina pectoris, *Int J Cardiol,* 75:205-210, 2000.

Blum A et al: Clinical and inflammatory effects of dietary L-arginine in patients with intractable angina pectoris, *Am J Cardiol* 83:1488-1490, 1999.

Chen J et al: Effect of oral administration of high-dose nitric oxide donor L-arginine in men with organic erectile dysfunction: results of a double-blind randomized placebo-controlled study, *BJU Int* 83:269-273, 1999.

Hambrecht R et al: Correction of endothelial dysfunction in chronic heart failure: additional effects of exercise training and oral L-arginine supplementation, *J Am Coll Cardiol* 35:706-713, 2000.

Maxwell A et al: Nutritional therapy for peripheral arterial disease: a double-blind study, placebo-controlled, randomized trial of HeartBar, *Vas Med* 5(1):11-19, 2000.

Moody J et al: Effects of long-term administration of L-arginine on the rat erectile response, *J Urol* 158:942-947, 1997.

Rector T et al: Randomized, double-blind, placebo-controlled study of supplement oral L-arginine in patients with heart failure, *Circulation* 93:2135-2141, 1996.

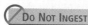 Do Not Ingest

Arnica
(ahr'ni-kuh)

Scientific name: *Arnica montana* L.; may also include *A. chamissonis less.*, *A. cordifolia hook*, *A. fulgens pursh*, *A. soronia greene*

Other common names: Leopard's bane, common arnica, sneezewort, mountain snuff, mountain tobacco, wolf's bane

Origin: Arnica grows wild in the mountains of Europe and Russia. Some species can be found in the western United States.

Uses

Reported Uses

Arnica is used topically to decrease inflammation in bruises, sprains, wounds, acne, boils, rashes. It may be used if supervised by an expert in cardiovascular problems to decrease cholesterol. Arnica should never be used internally except under the supervision of a qualified herbalist.

Product Availability and Dosages

Available Forms

Topical: spray, cream, salve, ointment; oral: tablets, tea, tincture, sublingual

Plants Part Used: Dried flower heads, rhizome

Dosages and Routes

Adult
- Topically: Apply to affected area as needed
- Very little information is available on dosages.

Precautionary Information

Contraindications

Because arnica is considered poisonous, injection is contraindicated; death can occur. Internal use is contraindicated unless supervised by an expert; serious kidney and liver damage can occur. Arnica is not to be used in pregnancy; uterine stimulation can occur. Do not use full-strength tincture on broken skin; contact dermatitis can occur. Do not use for prolonged periods.

A

Precautionary Information—cont'd

Side effects/Adverse Reactions

Integumentary: Rash, contact dermatitis

If taken internally (contraindicated)

Cardiovascular: CARDIAC ARREST, CADIOTOXICITY, hypertension

Central Nervous System: Nervousness, restlessness, COMA, DEATH

Gastrointestinal: Abdominal pain, diarrhea, vomiting, anorexia, HEPATIC FAILURE

Hematologic: BLEEDING

Integumentary: Contact dermatitis (topical), SWEET SYNDROME

Musculoskeletal: Weakness

Respiratory: Dyspnea

Interactions with Arnica

Drug

Antihypertensives: May decrease the antihypertenisve effect if arcina is taken internally.

Food

None known; not to be taken internally unless supervised by an expert.

Herb

None known; not to be taken internally unless supervised by an expert.

Lab Test

None known

Client Considerations

Assess

- Assess the condition of the skin: broken, bruised, rashes. Arnica should not be used for prolonged periods on this type of skin.
- Assess for reason for use.
- Assess for Sweet syndrome

🌀 Endangered Herb   Adverse effects: BOLD = life-threatening

Administer

- Use only topically, unless under the supervision of a qualified herbalist.
- Do not used for prolonged periods; allergic reactions may occur.
- Do not use full-strength on broken, hypersensitive skin. Do not use on open wounds or abrasions.

Teach Client/Family

- Teach the client not to use internally unless supervised by a competent herbalist. Serious liver and kidney toxicity can occur.
- Advise the client not to use during pregnancy; uterine stimulation can occur.
- Instruct the client not to use for extended periods on broken or bruised skin; contact dermatitis can occur.
- Keep out of reach of children; ingestion of flowers or roots can lead to death.

Pharmacology

Pharmacokinetics

Pharmacokinetics and pharmacodynamics are unknown.

Primary Chemical Components of Arnica and Their Possible Actions		
Chemical Class	**Individual Component**	**Possible Action**
Polysaccharide	Galacturonic acid	Inhibits complement; increases immune response
Sesquiterpenes	Phenolic compound Helenalin;11-Alpha; 13-Dihydrohelenalin	Cardiotoxic; inhibits platelet aggregation; cytotoxicity (Willuhn et al, 1994)

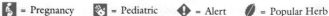

Actions

Antiinflammatory Action

Two studies have identified antiinflammatory properties of arnica. One study (Lussignol et al, 1999) found that inflammation was decreased in rat paw edema, possibly due to a decrease in interleukin-6. Another study (Schaffener, 1997) showed the antiinflammatory effect of Helenalin, one of the chemical components of arnica.

Cytotoxic Action

One study (Willuhn et al, 1994) showed low cytotoxicity when compared with other antineoplastics. Helenalin showed the greatest cytotoxic effect.

References

Lussignoli S et al: Effect on Traumel S, a homoeopathic formulation, on blood induced inflammation in rats, *Complement Ther Med* 7(4):225-230, 1999.

Schaffener W: Granny's remedy explained at the molecular level: helenalin inhibits NF-kappa B, *Biol Chem* 378:935, 1997.

Willuhn G et al: Cytotoxicity of flavoinoids and sequiterpene lactones from *Arnica* species against GLC4 and COLO 320 cell lines, *Planta Med* 60:434-r37, 1994.

Artichoke

(ahr'tuh-chowk)

Scientific name: *Cynara scolymus asteraceae*

Other common names: Alcachofra, garden artichoke, globe artichoke

Origin: Artichoke is cultivated in central Europe and the Mediterranean.

Uses

Reported Uses

Artichoke is used to lower cholesterol levels, to increase appetite, to aid digestion, and for indigestion in the upper gastrointestinal tract. It also has antioxidant and hepatoprotective properties.

Product Availability and Dosages
Available forms
Standardized extract (2.5%-15% caffeylquinic acid), tincture (5:1 dilution)

Plant Parts Used: Leaf

Dosages and Routes
Adult
- PO: Standardized extract 1-2 (320 mg) caps tid (McCaleb et al, 2000)
- Tincture (5:1 dilution): 15-30 drops in a small amount of water tid (McCaleb et al, 2000)
- Dried herb: 6 g in three divided doses (Blumenthal, 2000)

Precautionary Information
Contraindications
Artichoke should not be used by those with bile duct blockage, gallstones, or hypersensitivity to artichoke or Asteraceae family herbs such as arnica or chrysanthemums. Until further research is completed, medicinal artichoke should be avoided in pregnancy, lactation, and children. At present there is a lack of research in these populations. Use cautiously in hepatic or renal disease.

Side effects/Adverse Reactions
Gastrointestinal: Hunger
Musculoskeletal: Weakness

Interactions with Artichoke

Drug
Iron salts: Artichoke tea may interfere with the absorption of iron salts.

Food	Herb	Lab Test
None known	None known	None known

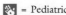 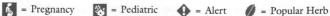

Client Considerations

Assess

- Assess client for the presence of gallstones, bile duct blockage, or past hypersensitivity to artichoke or plants in the Asteraceae family.
- Identify if the client is using iron salts, since artichoke in a tea may interfere with iron salts absorption.

Hyperlipidemia

- Obtain cholesterol testing on a regular basis if client is using for hyperlipidemia.
- Obtain a diet history to identify high-cholesterol foods that may need to be eliminated.

Administer

- Using tincture or fluid extract mixed in a small amount of water.

Teach Client/Family

- Advise the client to avoid use in pregnancy, lactation, or children until more research is complete.

Pharmacology

Pharmacokinetics

Pharmacokinetics and pharmacodynamics are unknown.

Primary Chemical Components of Artichoke and Their Possible Actions		
Chemical Class	**Individual Component**	**Possible Action**
Acid	Caffeic acid; Caffeylquinic acids; Chlorogenic acid	
	Cynarin	Antilipidemic
	Cynaroside	
	Luteolin	Antilipidemic
	Scolymoside	

Actions

There are very few studies for any use or action. However, artichoke is being marketed for its possible antilipidemic, hepatoprotective, and digestant properties.

 Endangered Herb   Adverse effects: BOLD = life-threatening

Antilipidemic Action

The studies relating to the antilipidemic action of artichoke are minimal. In one study (Petrowicz et al, 1997) artichoke leaf was administered to 44 individuals with no change in cholesterol levels. However, a more recent study (English et al, 2000) saw a drop in cholesterol and LDL/HDL ratios that was statistically significant. The drop in cholesterol levels may be due to cynarin and luteolin, two chemical components in artichoke. These components may interfere with cholesterol synthesis.

Other Actions

Two other actions are included in beginning research. These include the hepatoprotective effects of artichoke and the reduction in gastrointestinal symptoms, including dyspepsia.

Artichoke leaf may protect the liver from harmful effects (Kraft, 1997).

References

Blumenthal M, editor: *The complete German E monographs: therapeutic guide to herbal medicines,* Austin, Tex, American Botanical Council; Boston, 1998, Integrative Medicine Communications.

English W et al: Efficacy of artichoke dry extract in clients with hyperlipoproteinemia, *Arzneimittelforschung* 50:260-265, 2000.

Kraft K: Artichoke leaf extract: recent findings reflecting effects on lipid metabolism, liver and gastrointestinal tracts, *Phytomedicine* 4:369-378, 1997.

McCaleb R et al: *The encyclopedia of popular herbs: your complete guide to medicinal plants,* Roseville, Calif, 2000, Prima Health.

Petrowicz O et al: Effects of artichoke leaf on lipoprotein metabolism in vitro and in vivo. *Athersclerosis* 56:129-147, 1997.

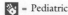 = Pregnancy    = Pediatric   ◆ = Alert   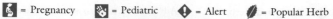 = Popular Herb

A

Ash

Scientific names: *Fraxinus americana, Fraxinus atrovirens, Fraxinus excelsior, Fraxinus heterophylla, Fraxinus jaspida, Fraxinus polemoniipolia, Fraxinus simplifolia, Fraxinus verticillata*

Other common names: Bird's tongue, common ash, European ash, weeping ash, white ash (not the same as prickly ash)   **Class 1 (Bark)**

Origin: Ash is a tree found in regions of North America.

Uses

Reported Uses

Ash has been used traditionally as a diuretic and tonic.

Investigational Uses

Ash is being investigated as an antiinflammatory for rheumatic and arthritic conditions. Some reports identify ash to be as good an antiinflammatory as nonsteroidal antiinflammatories.

Product Availability and Dosages

Available Forms

Liquid extract (no standardized extract is available)

Plant Parts Used: Leaves, bark

Dosage and Routes

Adult

• PO 20-40 drops tid-qid, use in water or other fluids

Precautionary Information

Contraindications

Ash should not be used in pregnancy, lactation, or children until more research is available. In clients with hypersensitivity to this product or salicylates, ash is contraindicated.

Side Effects/Adverse Reactions

Gastrointestinal: Slight nausea

 Endangered Herb   Adverse effects: BOLD = life-threatening

Interactions with Ash			
Drug	Food	Herb	Lab Test
None known	None known	None known	None known

Client Considerations

Assess

- Identify the reason the client is taking ash.
- Assess mobility and decrease in inflammation if using for arthritic conditions. Monitor ROM, swelling, and heat of joints.

Administer

- Give fluid extract in a small amount of water or other fluids.

Teach Client/Family

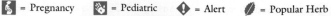

- Advise the client to keep ash away from children and pets. The FDA considers this herb unsafe and poisonous.

Pharmacology

Pharmacokinetics

Pharmacokinetics and pharmacodynamics are unknown.

Primary Chemical Components of Ash and Their Possible Actions		
Chemical Class	**Individual Component**	**Possible Action**
Flavonoids	Rutin	
Iridoide monoterpenes		
Mannitol		
Tannins		
Triterpenes		
Phenolic acids		
Phytosterols		
Mucilages		
Hydroxycoumarins	Fraxin; Isofraxidin; Aesculin	

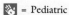

Actions

Very little research has been done on ash. A few studies have focused on the antiinflammatory properties of ash. One study (el-Ghazaly et al, 1992) compared ash with diclofenac. The results from both were similar.

References

El-Ghazaly M et al: Study of anti-inflammatory activity of *Populus tremula, solidago virgaurea* and *Fraxinus execelsior, Arzneimittelforschung,* 42(3):333-336, 1992.

Astragalus
(as'tri-guh-lus)

Scientific names: *Astragalus gummifer, Astragalus membranaceus*

Other common names: Huang-qi, tragacanth, Milk Vetch, Yellow Leader   Class 1

Origin: Astragalus is available throughout the world. The most common species are grown in China, Japan, and Korea.

Uses

Reported Uses

Astragalus is used to treat bronchitis, chronic obstructive pulmonary disease, colds, flu, gastrointestinal conditions, weakness, fatigue, chronic hepatitis, ulcers, hypertension, and (by injection) viral myocarditis (Chang, 1987). This herb is used in contemporary Chinese medicine and other models to improve immune system health. It is thought to be an aphrodisiac and may improve sperm motility.

Investigational Uses

Researchers are experimenting with the use of astragalus to treat cancer and to increase immunity in HIV/AIDS. It is also commonly used to decrease the toxic effects of radiation or chemotherapy. It may be used in combination with other herbs.

Product Availability and Dosages

Available Forms

Capsules, decoction, fluid extract, solid (dry) extract, tincture

Plant Parts Used: Roots

Dosages and Routes

Adult

All dosages listed are PO.
- Capsules: 400-500 mg 8-9 times/day (Foster, 1998), up to 8-15 g/day
- Decoction: 10-30 g dried root/day (Mills, 2000), boil for 1-2 hrs, drain
- Fluid extract: 4-8 ml/day in divided doses (1:2 dilution) (Mills, 2000) or 2-4 ml tid (1:1 dilution) (Murray, 1998)
- Solid (dry) extract: 100-150 mg tid (0.5% 4-hydroxy-3-methoxy isoflavone) (Murray, 1998)

Precautionary Information

Contraindications

Astragalus should not be used during pregnancy and lactation, and it should not be used by persons with acute infections, in the presence of fever, or inflammation. Astragalus may be given to children. Class 1 herb.

Side Effects/Adverse Reactions

Integumentary: Allergic reactions (rare)

Interactions with Astragalus

Drug

Antihypertensives: Astragalus may decrease or increase the action of antihypertensives, avoid concurrent use.

Interleukin-2: Astragalus may increase the effect of drugs such as interleukin-2 (IL-2) (Chu, 1988). In contrast, other studies have shown that the effects of IL-2 can be decreased when combined with astragalus. Research is inconclusive at this time.

Interferon: The combination of interferon and astragalus has been shown to prevent or shorten the duration of upper respiratory infections (Yunde, 1987).

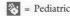 = Pregnancy   = Pediatric   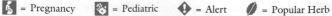 = Alert   = Popular Herb

Interactions with Astragalus—cont'd	
Food	**Herb**
None known	None known

Lab Test
Semen specimen analysis: Astragalus may increase sperm motility in vitro

Client Considerations

Assess
- Assess for allergic reactions; if present, discontinue use of this herb and administer antihistamine or other appropriate therapy.
- Assess for the use of other medications, including IL-2, the action of which may be increased (see Interactions).
- Assess for infections, fever, inflammation. Astragalus should not be used in infection, fever, or inflammation.

Administer
- Instruct the client to take astragalus PO as a tincture, decoction, fluid extract, or in capsule form.
- Inform the client that astragalus injections, which are used to treat viral myocarditis, are to be given by naturopaths only.

Teach Client/Family

- Caution the client not to use astragalus during pregnancy and lactation. However, it may be given to children.
- Caution the client not to use astragalus if experiencing acute infections or inflammation.
- Inform client that this herb is generally considered safe.

Pharmacology

Pharmacokinetics
Pharmacokinetics and pharmacodynamics are unknown.

Primary Chemical Components of Astragalus and Their Possible Actions		
Chemical Class	**Individual Component**	**Possible Action**
Glycosides	Astragalan I, II, III; Bassorin; Tragacanthin	Increased immunity
Saponin	Astramembrannin I, II	Increased immunity
Betaine		
Beta-sitosterol choline		
Polysaccharides	Astroglucans A, B, C	
Vitamin A		

Actions

Stimulation of Immunity and Anticancer Action

Studies have shown that astragalus improves immune function in a number of ways. It increases the numbers of both macrophages (Kajimura, 1996) and white blood cells. Another study has shown an increase in immunoglobulins A, G, and M and a concurrent decrease in upper respiratory infections. Astragalus also increases the functioning of B-cells (Kajimura, 1997) and T-cells (Mavligit, 1979). Astragalus may intensify phagocytosis, stimulate pituitary-adrenal activity, and stimulate production of interferon. These research studies provide evidence for the use of astragalus to treat cancer and other conditions with decreased immune response such as HIV/AIDS.

References

Chang HM et al: *Pharmacology and applications of Chinese materia medica, vol 2,* Hong Kong, 1987, World Scientific.

Chu DT et al: Fractioned extract of *Astragalus membranaceus,* a Chinese medicinal herb, potenates LAK cell cytotoxicity generated by a dose of recombinant interleukin-2, *J Clin Lab Immunol* 26:183-187, 1988.

Foster S: *101 medicinal herbs,* Loveland, Colo, 1998, Interweave Press.

Kajimura K et al: Protective effect of astragali radix by intraperitoneal injection against Japanese encephalitis virus infection in mice, *Biol Pharm Bull* 19(6):855-859, 1996.

Kajimura K et al: Polysaccharide os astragali radix enhances IgM antibody production in aged mice, *Biol Pharm Bull* 20(11):1178-1182, 1997.

Mavligit G et al: Local xenogeneic graft-vs-host reaction: a practical

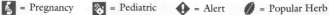 = Pregnancy   = Pediatric ◆ = Alert ✦ = Popular Herb

assessment of T-cell function among cancer patients, *J Immunol* 123(5):2185-2188, 1979.

Mills S, Bone K: *Principles and practice of phytotherapy*, Edinburgh, 2000, Churchill Livingstone.

Murray M, Pizzarno J: *The encyclopedia of natural medicine*, 2 ed (revised), Roseville, Calif, 1998, Prima.

Yunde H et al: Effect of radix astragali seu hedysari on the interferon system, *Chin Med J* 94(1):35-40, 1987.

Avens
(a'vunz)

Scientific name: *Geum urbanum*

Other common names: Benedict's herb, bennet's root, blessed herb, city avens, clove root, colewort, geum, goldy star, herb bennet, way bennet, wild rye, wood avens

Origin: Avens is a member of the rose family found in Europe.

Uses

Reported Uses

Avens has traditionally been used internally to treat diarrhea, sore throat, fever, headache, and gastric inflammation. It has also been used as an astringent, antiinflammatory, and antiseptic. Topically, avens has been used to treat wounds and hemorrhoids. It is rarely used today.

Product Availability and Dosages

Available Forms

Fluid extract, powder, tea, tincture

Plant Parts Used: Dried plant, rhizome, roots

Dosages and Routes

Many different dosages are reported.

Adult

Wound Healing
• Topical: apply prn

Other
• PO fluid extract of herb: 1 dram
• PO fluid extract of root: ½-1 dram
• PO powdered root/herb: 15-30 grains as a tonic

Precautionary Information

Contraindications

Until more research is available, avens should not be used during pregnancy and lactation and it should not be given to children.

Side Effects/Adverse Reactions

Gastrointestinal: Nausea, anorexia, dyspepsia

Interactions with Avens			
Drug	Food	Herb	Lab Test
None known	None known	None known	None known

Client Considerations

Assess

Antiinflammatory
- Assess the client for pain: location, intensity, duration. Determine what alleviates and aggravates the condition.
- Assess for the use of prescription and over-the-counter medications to treat pain and inflammation.

Administer
- Instruct the client to take avens PO as an extract, or as a powder made from the herb or its roots.

Teach Client/Family
- Until more research is available, caution the client not to use avens during pregnancy and lactation and not to give it to children.
- Instruct the client to report any changes in the symptoms or characteristics of the condition.
- Because research on the use, side effects, and toxicity of avens is rare, advise the client to use this herb with caution or under the supervision of a qualified herbalist.

Pharmacology

Pharmacokinetics

All pharmacokinetics and pharmacodynamics are unknown.

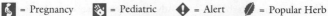

Primary Chemical Components of Avens and Their Possible Actions		
Chemical Class	**Individual Component**	**Possible Action**
Volatile oil	Eugenol	Antiinflammatory; antioxidant
Tannin		Wound healing; antiinflammatory
Gum		
Resin		
Roots Also Contain		
Acid	Gallic acid; Caffeic acid; Chlorogenic acid	

Actions

Research studies of the effects of avens on humans are nonexistent, and animal studies are rare. Most reported uses for this herb are anecdotal. Few avens products are available in the United States.

Antiinflammatory Action

The antiinflammatory action of avens may result from its ability to produce prostaglandins and decrease cyclooxygenase (Tunon, 1995). Avens is thought to possess antiinflammatory action equal to that of NSAIDs; however, no research is available to either confirm or disprove this action.

References

Tunon H et al: Evaluation of anti-inflammatory activity of some Swedish medicinal plants: inhibition of prostaglandin biosynthesis and PAF-induced exocytosis, *J Ethnopharmacol* 48:61-76, 1995.

🌓 Endangered Herb   Adverse effects: BOLD = life-threatening

Balsam of Peru
(bawl'sum uv Peh'rew)

Scientific names: *Myroxylon balsamum, Myroxylon pereirae*

Other common names: Balsam of tolu, balsam tree,
opobalsam, Peruvian balsam, resina tolutana, resin
tolu, Thomas balsam   Class 2d

Origin: Balsam of Peru is a tree found in Central and South
America.

Uses
Reported Uses
Balsam of Peru in suppository form is used to treat hemorrhoids. This herb is used internally to treat postextraction alveo-
litis, cough, bronchitis, colds, burns, fever, lowered immunity,
and parasites (scabies). Topically, it is used to heal wounds,
promote local circulation, and ease joint and arthritic complaints. Use of balsam of Peru is uncommon.

Product Availability and Dosages
Available Forms
Cream, feminine hygiene products, lotion, ointment, other
commercial products, shampoo

Plant Parts Used: Bark (oleo resin)

Dosages and Routes
Adult
Hemorrhoids
• Suppositories: 1.8-3 mg prn
Wound Healing
• Topical: 5%-20% concentration ointment, used for no longer
  than 7 days

Precautionary Information
Contraindications
Use topically for no longer than 7 days. Persons with kidney
irritation or febrile illnesses should avoid the use of balsam
of Peru. Class 2d herb.

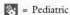

 = Pregnancy   = Pediatric   = Alert   = Popular Herb

B

Side Effects/Adverse Reactions
Genitourinary: ALBUMINURIA, PYELITIS, NECROSIS OF THE
KIDNEY (if taken internally)
Integumentary: Contact dermatitis, photodermatitis

Interactions with Balsam of Peru			
Drug	Food	Herb	Lab Test
None known	None known	None known	None known

Client Considerations

Assess

- Assess the client for contact dermatitis and photodermatitis
  after prolonged use. Discontinue use of this herb if these
  conditions are present.

Administer

- Instruct the client to use as a topical or suppository. May be
  used PO if under the direction of a qualified herbalist.

Pharmacology

Pharmacokinetics

Pharmacokinetics and pharmacodynamics are unknown.

Primary Chemical Components of Balsam of Peru and Their Possible Actions		
Chemical Class	Individual Component	Possible Action
Ester mixture	Cinnamein	Antiseptic; antibacterial
Resin	Cinnamic acid ester	Antiseptic; antibacterial
Benzoic acid		Wound healing
Volatile oil		

Actions

Balsam of Peru is not used to exert any particular pharmacologic action. Its primary use is for generalized wound healing. Because it is an oleoresin and tends to be a warming herb, it is used to improve circulation and relieve congestion.

Barberry
(bahr′beh-ree)

Scientific name: *Berberis aquifolium* Pursh

Other common names: Berberry, jaundice berry, pepperridge bush, pipperidge, sour-spine, sowberry, trailing mahonia, wood sour

Class 2b

Origin: Barberry is a shrub found in Europe and North America.

Uses

Reported Uses

Barberry has been used as an antimicrobial against a wide variety of bacteria, fungi, viruses, helminths, and chlamydia. It is primarily used for bacterial diarrhea, intestinal parasite infection, and ocular trachoma infections. It antagonizes the effects of cholera and *Escherichia coli,* decreases ventricular tachyarrhythmias, decreases inflammation, and increases platelets in thrombocytopenia. Barberry can lower heart rate and enhance the flow of bile through liver function. It may be used topically to treat dry, scaly skin.

Product Availability and Dosages

Available Forms

Fluid extract tablets, tea, tincture,

Plant Parts Used: Fruit (rarely used), root bark

Dosages and Routes

Adult

All dosages listed are PO.

- Decoction: 1.5-3 g/day (Mills, 2000)
- Fruits: 1-2 tsp whole or mashed barberries in 150 ml boiling water, steeped 10-15 min and strained (berberidis fructus)
- Fluid extract: 7-14 ml/day (1:5 dilution) (Mills, 2000)

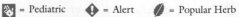

 = Pregnancy   = Pediatric   = Alert   = Popular Herb

- Tablets: 200 mg bid-qid
- Tincture: 3-6 ml/day (1:2 dilution) (Mills, 2000)

Precautionary Information
Contraindications
Because it can cause spontaneous abortion, barberry should not be used during pregnancy or if trying to become pregnant. Class 2b herb.

Side Effects/Adverse Reactions
Calcium channel blockers: Barberry may increase the effect of calcium channel blockers.
Cardiovascular: Hypotension, CARDIAC DAMAGE
Central Nervous System: Confusion, disorientation
Gastrointestinal: Diarrhea, gastrointestinal discomfort, HEPATOTOXICITY
Genitourinary: NEPHRITIS, SPONTANEOUS ABORTION
Respiratory: Dyspnea

Interactions with Barberry

Drug
Antihypertensives: Barberry may increase the antihypertensive action; use cautiously.
Calcium channel blockers: Barberry may increase the effect of calcium channel blockers.

Food	Herb
None known	None known

Lab Test
AST/ALT: Barberry may increase test values.
Total bilirubin: Barberry may increase test values.
Urine bilirubin: Barberry may increase test values.

Client Considerations
Assess
- Assess the client for hypersensitivity reactions and toxicity. Discontinue use of this herb if these are present.
- Assess for possible or confirmed pregnancy.

- Assess cardiac status (blood pressure; ECG; pulse; heart rate, rhythm, and character) in clients who are using barberry to treat ventricular tachyarrhythmias.
- Assess for confusion and disorientation, diarrhea, nephritis. Discontinue use of this herb if these conditions are present.

Administer

- Instruct the client to take barberry PO as the whole herb, commercial tablets, or tincture. It is bitter and should be taken in small doses. Large doses may cause nausea, vomiting, and a drop in blood pressure.

Teach Client/Family

- Because it can cause spontaneous abortion, caution the client not to use barberry during pregnancy.
- Inform the client that medications are available that are more effective than barberry for controlling ventricular tachyarrhythmias.

Pharmacology

Pharmacokinetics

Pharmacokinetics and pharmacodynamics are unknown.

Primary Chemical Components of Barberry and Their Possible Actions		
Chemical Class	**Individual Component**	**Possible Action**
Alkaloid, isoquinoline	Berberine	Decreased blood pressure
	Oxyacanthine	K+ channel blocking
	Isochinoline	Uterine stimulant
	Berbamine	
	Bervulcine	
	Jatorrhizine	
	Magnoflorine	
	Aporphine	
Anthocyan		
Chlorogenic acid		
Phenol	Syringaresinol	Antiinflammatory

Actions

Barberry has been used for more than 3000 years in Chinese and Ayurvedic medicine.

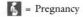 = Pregnancy  = Pediatric   = Alert 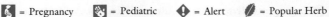 = Popular Herb

Antimicrobial Action

Several studies have demonstrated the effectiveness of barberry against a wide variety of fungi, protozoans, helminths, viruses, and bacteria, including *Chlamydia* spp. (Altern, 2000; Amin, 1969; Nakamoto, 1990; Subbaiah, 1967; Gupte, 1975). Sensitivity screens were performed on 54 different microorganisms using berberine, one of the alkaloids of barberry. Antimicrobial effects were found against gram-positive and gram-negative organisms, as well as protozoa. Barberry was found to be effective against *Bacillus cereus, Bacillus pumilus, Bacillus subtilis, Candida albicans, Candida glabrata, Candida tropicalis, Candida utilis, Corynebacterium diphtheriae, E. coli, Entamoeba histolytica, Giardia lamblia, Klebsiella pneumoniae, Leishmaniasis* spp., *Mycobacterium tuberculosis, Shigella boydii, Sporotrichum schenkii, Staphylococcus albus, Staphylococcus aureus, Streptococcus pyogenes, Trichophyton mentagrophytes, Trichomonas vaginalis,* and *Vibrio cholerae* (Amin, 1969). Barberry may also be effective against HIV-1 by inhibiting HIV-1 reverse transcriptase (Gudima, 1994).

Cardiovascular Action

In one study using cats, barberry demonstrated both positive and negative inotropic and antihypertensive effects. In a human study of 12 patients with refractory congestive heart failure, participants were studied before and after intravenous administration of berberine. Low doses produced no circulatory changes, whereas higher doses caused a significant reduction in pulmonary vascular resistance and a decrease in left ventricular end-diastolic pressure. Measurable increases occurred in stroke index, ventricular injection fraction, and left ventricular ejection fraction (Marin-Neto, 1988). Another study of 100 individuals with ventricular tachyarrhythmias reported that berberine suppressed premature ventricular contractions without serious side effects (Huang, 1990). Several methods of action have been proposed for the cardiovascular actions of berberine, including calcium channel blocking (Zhou, 1995), potassium channel blocking (Hua, 1994), and inhibition of catecholamine synthesis (Lee, 1996).

References

Amin AH et al: Berberine sulfate: antimicrobial activity, bioassay and mode of action, *Can J Microbiol* 15:1067-1076, 1969.
Berberine, *Altern Med Rev* 5(2):175-177, 2000.

Gudima SO et al: Kinetic analysis of interaction of human immunodeficiency virus reverse transcriptase with alkaloids, *Mol Biol* 28(6):1308-1314.

Gupte S: Use of berberine in treatment of giardiasis, *Am J Dis Child* 129:866, 1975.

Hua Z et al: Inhibitory effects of berberine on potassium channels in guinea pig ventricular myocytes, *Yao Hsueh Hsueh Pao* 29:576-580, 1994.

Huang W et al: Ventricular tachyarrhythmias treated with berberine, *Chung Hua Hsin Hsueh Kuan Ping Tsa Chih* 18:155-156, 190, 1990.

Lee MK et al: Inhibitory effects of protoberberine alkaloids from the roots of *Coptis japonica* on catecholamine biosynthesis in PC12 cells, *Planta Med* 62:31-34, 1996.

Marin-Neto JA et al: Cardiovascular effects of berberine in patients with severe congestive heart failure, *Clin Cardiol* 11:253-260, 1988.

Mills S, Bone K: *Principles and practice of phytotherapy*, London, 2000, Churchill Livingstone.

Nakamoto K et al: Effects of crude drugs and berberine hydrochloride on the activities of fungi, *J Prosthet Dent* 64:691-694, 1990.

Subbaiah TV et al: Effect of berberin sulphate on *Entamoeba histolytica*, *Nature* 215:527-528, 1967.

Zhou Z et al: Effects of berberine on single Ca^{2+} channel current in cultured embryoic chick ventricular monocytes, *Hua Hsi I Ko Ta Hsueh Hsueh Pao* 26:287-290.

Barley
(bahr'lee)

Scientific names: *Hordeum distichon, Hordeum irregulare, Hordeum jubalum, Hordeum leporinum, Hordeum vulgare*

Other common names: Barley grass, foxtail grass, hare barley, milled barley, pearl barley, scotch barley, wild barley

Origin: Barley grows wild in Asia and parts of Ethiopia. It is cultivated in many parts of the world.

Uses

Reported Uses

Barley has been used traditionally for irritable bowel syndrome, diarrhea, and gastritis, and to decrease cholesterol, for control of diabetes, and for prevention of cancer.

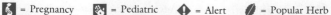

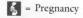 = Pregnancy    = Pediatric   = Alert   = Popular Herb

Product Availability and Dosages
Available Forms
Contained in food; no specific forms are available

Plant Parts Used: Grain

Dosages and Routes
No published dosages are available.

Precautionary Information
Contraindications
Barley should not be used medicinally in pregnancy.

Side Effects/Adverse Reactions
None known

Interactions with Barley

Drug	Food	Herb	Lab Test
None known	None known	None known	None known

Client Considerations
Assess
• Determine the reason client is using barley medicinally.

Administer
• Administer after receiving diagnosis of gastrointestinal symptoms.
• Instruct the client to store barley in a cool, dry place, away from moisture.

Teach Client/Family
• Until more research is available, caution the client that barley should not be used medicinally in pregnancy.

Pharmacology
Pharmacokinetics
Pharmacokinetics and pharmacodynamics are unknown.

🌀 Endangered Herb   Adverse effects: BOLD = life-threatening

Primary Chemical Components of Barley and Their Possible Actions

Chemical Class	Individual Component	Possible Action
Fatty oils	Linoleic acid; Oleic acid	Demulcent
Hydroxycoumarins	Aesculetin; Gramine; Herniarin;	
	Hordenine	Sympathomimetic
	Scopotetin; Tyramine Umbelliferone	
Oligosaccharides	Glucodifructose; Glucose; Fructose; Raffinose; Saccharose	
Polysaccharides	Starch; Fructans	
Vitamins	B_2; B_6; E; Folic acid; Nicotinic acid; Panothenic acid	
Proteins	Albumin; Globulin; Glutelines; Prolamines	

Actions

Most studies using barley focus on the intestinal actions. One study (Gruenwald et al, 1998) identified barley as a demulcent and reported healing of the gastrointestinal tract. Another study (Mitsyama et al, 1998) identified the barley in food as having a healing effect and improving damage in the gastrointestinal tract in animals. The juice contains many vitamins, including B_1, B_2, B_6, B_{12}, panothenic acid, folic acid, and beta carotene and many minerals, including potassium, calcium, magnesium, and phosphorous.

References

Gruenwald J et al: *PDR for herbal medicines,* Montvale, NJ, 1998, Medical Economics.

Mitsyama K et al: Treatment of ulcerative colitis with germinating barley foodstuff feeding: a pilot study, *Aliment Pharmacol Ther* 12(12):1225-1230, 1998.

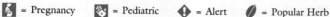

B

Basil
(ba'zul)

Scientific names: *Ocimum basilicum, Ocimum sanctum*

Other common names: Common basil, sweet basil, holy basil, St. Josephwort

Class 2b/2c/2d

Origin: Basil is a member of the mint family found throughout the world.

Uses

Reported Uses

Basil is used as an antiseptic, antidiabetic, antiinflammatory, and immunostimulant. It is also used to treat ulcers, arthritis, and joint edema. Contemporary uses include treatment for flatulence, anxiety, and coughs.

Investigational Uses

Researchers are studying the immunostimulant properties and the performance enhancement properties (Maity, 2000) of *Ocimum sanctum.*

Product Availability and Dosages

Available Forms

Leaves (chopped and powdered), tea, tincture

Plant Parts Used: Leaves (fresh and dried)

Dosages and Routes

Adult
- PO dried leaves: 2.5 g in ½ cup water, strained, qd or bid
- PO tincture: 1-2 ml 3-5 times/day (1:5 dilution) (Smith, 1999)

Precautionary Information

Contraindications

Basil is not recommended for therapeutic use during pregnancy and lactation and should not be given therapeutically to infants or toddlers. Basil should be used cautiously by persons with diabetes and those who use this herb for extended periods. Class 2b/2c/2d herb.

Continued

 Endangered Herb   Adverse effects: BOLD = life-threatening

> **Precautionary Information—cont'd**
> **Side Effects/Adverse Reactions**
> *Endocrine:* Hypoglycemia
> *Gastrointestinal:* LIVER CARCINOMA

Interactions with Basil

Drug

Insulin: Basil may increase the hypoglycemic effects of insulin; do not use concurrently.

Oral antidiabetics: Basil may increase the hypoglycemic effects of oral antidiabetics; do not use concurrently.

Food	Herb	Lab Test
None known	None known	None known

Client Considerations

Assess

- Assess diabetic clients for the use of oral antidiabetic agents or insulin (see Interactions).
- Assess diabetic clients for symptoms of hypoglycemia and hyperglycemia.

Administer

- Instruct the client to take basil PO either fresh or as a powder. Only the leaves should be used.

Teach Client/Family

- Caution the client not to use basil therapeutically during pregnancy and lactation and not to give it therapeutically to infants or toddlers. One of the chemical components of basil, estragole, can produce mutagenic effects when taken in high levels during pregnancy.
- Caution the client not to use basil for extended periods of time; it is a known mutagen.
- Caution the client not to use basil concurrently with oral antidiabetic agents or insulin; hypoglycemia may occur.

Pharmacology

Pharmacokinetics

Pharmacokinetics and pharmacodynamics are unknown.

 = Pregnancy    = Pediatric   = Alert   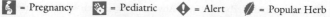 = Popular Herb

Primary Chemical Components of Basil and Their Possible Actions

Chemical Class	Individual Component	Possible Action
Sesquiterpenes Volatile oil	Linalool	Analgesic
	Estragole	Increased immunity; mutagenic (DeVincenzi, 2000)
	Eugenol; Methyleugenol	Antioxidant
	Triterpene	
Flavonoid Phenylpropanes Caffeic acid		Antiulcer
Monoterpenes	Cineol; Geraniol; Camphor; Ocimene	

Actions

Research has focused on the hypoglycemic, antiinflammatory, and immunostimulant properties of basil.

Hypoglycemic Action

One recent study of 62 patients with type 2 diabetes demonstrated the ability of basil to lower blood glucose levels (Reichart, 1997). All of the participants underwent a 10-hour fasting blood glucose test after discontinuing any other hypoglycemics 1 week before the test. In addition, all patients completed a 5-day washout period to clear all other agents from their systems before the study began. Results showed that fasting blood glucose levels decreased 17% with the use of basil as compared with the use of a placebo. Both cholesterol and urinary glucose levels also decreased, but not significantly.

Antiinflammatory Action

A 1996 study by Singh used fixed *O. sanctum* to treat rats with inflamed paws. Basil exerted significant activity as an antiarthritic and antiinflammatory. The study also demonstrated the antiinflammatory and analgesic effects of basil when given intraperitoneally (Singh, 1996).

Immunostimulant Action

To identify its immunoregulatory profile in sheep erythrocytes, basil was tested against *Salmonella typhosa*. The results showed an increased antibody titer and may indicate that basil could be used as an immunostimulant (Godhwani, 1988). In Ayurvedic medicine, basil has been used to increase immunity and metabolic function and to treat respiratory problems.

Other Actions

Ocimum Sanctum root extract was found to increase swimming performance in mice. This study suggests that this effect may be due to a central nervous system stimulant and/or antistress activity (Maity, 2000).

References

DeVincenzi M et al: Constituents of aromatic plants: II. Estragole, *Fitoterapia* 71(6):725-729, 2000.

Godhwani S et al: *Ocimum sanctum:* a preliminary study evaluating its immunoregulatory profile of albino rats, *J Ethnopharmacol* 24:193-198, 1988.

Maity TK et al: Effect of *Ocimum Sanctum* roots extract on swimming performance in mice, *Phytother Res* 14(2):120-121, 2000.

Reichart R: Holy basil leaves and type II diabetes, *Q Rev Nat Med* pp 267-268, Winter 1997.

Singh S et al: Effect of fixed oil of *Ocimum sanctum* against experimentally induced arthritis and joint edema in laboratory animals, *Int J Pharmacognosy* 34(3):218-222,1996.

Smith E: *Therapeutic herb manual,* Williams, Ore, 1999, Author.

Bay
(bay)

Scientific name: *Laurus nobilis*

Other common names: Bay laurel, bay leaf, bay tree, laurel, sweet bay, Roman laurel

Class 1

Origin: Bay is found in Mediterranean areas.

Uses

Reported Uses

Bay is used as a rubefacient and as a treatment for rheumatic disorders, gastric ulcers, amenorrhea, colic, polyps, and spasms. Bay fruits are used in the treatment of uterine fibroids, cirrhosis, and joint pain (Duke, 1985). Bay has been used as a re-

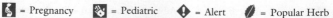

🔆 = Pregnancy   🐾 = Pediatric   ◆ = Alert   🖋 = Popular Herb

pellent for cockroaches (Verma, 1981), and it is used as a cooling herb. Therapeutic use of bay is uncommon.

Product Availability and Dosages
Available Forms
Creams (essential oil), extract, fruit, leaves (typically used as a spice), lotions (essential oil), soaps (essential oil)

Plant Parts Used: Berries, leaves, oil

Dosages and Routes
Adult
• Topical: apply creams, lotions, and soaps as desired

Precautionary Information
Contraindications
Until more research is available, bay should not be used therapeutically during pregnancy and lactation and should not be given therapeutically to children. Class 1 herb.

Side Effects/Adverse Reactions
Gastrointestinal: IMPACTION, PERFORATION OF GASTROINTESTINAL TRACT, SEVERE GASTROINTESTINAL BLEEDING
Integumentary: Contact dermatitis
Respiratory: ASTHMA, dyspnea

Interactions with Bay

Drug
Insulin: Bay may increase the hypoglycemic effects of insulin; do not use concurrently.
Oral antidiabetics: Bay may increase the hypoglycemic effects of oral antidiabetic agents; do not use concurrently.

Food	Herb	Lab Test
None known	None known	None known

Client Considerations
Assess
• Assess diabetic clients' use of insulin or oral antidiabetic agents; monitor blood glucose levels (see Interactions).
• Assess for symptoms of hypoglycemia or hyperglycemia.

 Endangered Herb   Adverse effects: BOLD = life-threatening

Administer

- Instruct the client to take bay PO with a diabetic diet to enhance hypoglycemia.

Teach Client/Family

- Until more research is available, caution the client not to use bay during pregnancy and lactation and not to give to children.
- Advise the client not to use bay concurrently with oral antidiabetic agents or insulin; hypoglycemia may occur.

Pharmacology

Pharmacokinetics

Pharmacokinetics and pharmacodynamics are unknown.

Primary Chemical Components of Bay and Their Possible Actions		
Chemical Class	**Individual Component**	**Possible Action**
Volatile oil	Eugenol	Antistress; anti-inflammatory; antioxidant
	Linalool	Analgesic
	Alpha-pinene; Sabinene; Limonene; Piperidine; Cineole; Camphene; Phenylhydrazine; Geraniol	
Nandergine		
Lactone	Costunolide; Laurenobiolide	
Catechin		
Proanthocyanidin		
Launobine		
Boldine		
Alkaloid	Reticulin	
Isodomesticine		
Neolitsine		

Actions

Antiulcerogenic Action

When researchers administered bay to rats with induced gastric ulcers, results indicated antiulcerogenic activity for bay ex-

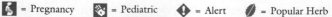

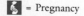 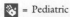

tracts at 20% and 40% and an oily fraction of the seeds. Acute toxicity studies also found bay to be safe when used in this manner.

Antidiabetic Action

Bay has been shown to both stimulate and decrease the actions of glucose. Hypoglycemic activity has been reported for bay leaf extracts (Ashaeva, 1984).

Other Actions

The volatile oil of bay leaves has been shown to possess bactericidal and fungicidal activity (MacGregor, 1975).

References

Ashaeva LA et al: The study of sugar decreasing action of *Laurus nobilis* leaves, *Farmatsiya* 33:49-51, 1984.

Duke JA: *CRC handbook of medicinal herbs,* CRC Press, Boca Raton, Fla, 1985, p 271.

MacGregor JT et al: California bay oil II: biological effects of constituents. *J Agric Food Chem* 22:777-780, 1975.

Verma M et al: A natural cockroach repellent in bay leaves, *Am Laboratories* 13:66-69, 1981.

Bayberry
(bay'beh-ree)

Scientific name: *Myrica cerifera*

Other common names: Candleberry, myrica, wax myrtle, spicebush, sweet oak, tallow shrub, vegetable tallow, waxberry, wax myrtle

Class 1

Origin: Bayberry is a shrub found in the southern and eastern regions of the United States.

Uses

Reported Uses

Traditionally, bayberry has been used internally to treat diarrhea, jaundice, coughs, and colds, as well as to induce emesis for uterine bleeding. Topically, it is used to treat skin conditions (such as varicose veins, hemorrhoids) and ulcers and to promote wound healing. It is also used as a douche for treatment of leukorrhea. Bayberry may be used as a gargle to relieve sore

🐢 Endangered Herb   Adverse effects: BOLD = life-threatening throats and gums. Contemporary use is eclectic. Bayberry is mostly used as an adjunct in formulas.

Product Availability and Dosages

Available Forms

Capsules: 450, 475 mg; fluid extract; tea

Plant Parts Used: Dried root bark, flowers

Dosages and Routes

Adult

Skin Conditions

• Topical: apply prn as a wash made by decoction

Sore Throat

• Gargle: use diluted in water (Smith, 1999), up to 3×/day

Other

• PO cold infusion: 2-4 oz tid (Moore, 1995)
• PO fluid extract: 1-3 ml tid (either 1:2 or 1:5 dilution) (Moore, 1995)
• PO capsules 1 cap up to 3×/day

Precautionary Information

Contraindications

Until further research is available, bayberry is not recommended for internal use during pregnancy and lactation and should not be given to children. Plant parts should not be consumed; hepatotoxicity can occur. Class 1 herb.

Side Effects/Adverse Reactions

Cardiovascular: Hypertension, weight gain, hypernatremia

Gastrointestinal: Nausea, vomiting, anorexia, gastric irritation, **hepatotoxicity**

Systemic: Allergic rhinitis, hypersensitivity, POSSIBLE MALIG-NANCIES (injectable form)

Interactions with Bayberry

Drug	Food	Herb	Lab Test
None known	None known	None known	None known

 = Pregnancy   = Pediatric    = Alert   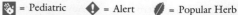 = Popular Herb

Client Considerations

Assess

- Assess for cardiovascular disease (hypertension, tachycardia); monitor blood pressure, pulse, and weight weekly; monitor electrolytes.
- Assess client's weight and for edema; mineralocorticoid effect may occur.

Administer

- Instruct the client to take bayberry fluid extract PO.
- Instruct the client to apply topically as needed. A hot compress can be made by pouring hot bayberry tea on a towel.

Teach Client/Family

- Until more research is available, caution the client not to use bayberry during pregnancy and lactation and not to give it to children.
- Advise the client that excessive use in large doses can cause nausea and vomiting.

Pharmacology

Pharmacokinetics

Pharmacokinetics and pharmacodynamics are unknown.

Primary Chemical Components of Bayberry and Their Possible Actions*

Chemical Class	Individual Component	Possible Action
Tannin		Astringent; wound healing; anti-inflammatory
Flavonoid glycoside	Myricitrin	Bile stimulant
Triterpene	Myricadiol	Mineralocorticoid; antibacterial
	Myricalactone	
	Myrica acid (Nagai, 2000)	
	Taraxerol; Taraxerone	
	Palmitic acid; Lauric acid	
Gum		
Starch		
Volatile oil		

*The constituents have not been reported to any great extent in primary research.

🌀 Endangered Herb   Adverse effects: BOLD = life-threatening

Actions

Almost no primary research is available on bayberry. Its possible actions include antipyretic and antibacterial effects (Paul, 1974). It is a stimulating, warming astringent with action similar to that of cinnamon. Choleretic activity and mineralocorticoid effects have also been reported (Duke, 1985).

After bioassay *Myrica cerifera* showed increased antithrombin activity (Chistokhodova, 2002).

References

Chistokhodova N et al: Antithrombin activity of medicinal plants from central Florida, *J Ethnopharmacol* 81(2):277-280, 2002.
Duke JA: *Handbook of medicinal herbs,* Boca Raton, Fla, 1985, CRC Press.
Moore M: *Materia medica,* Bisbee, Ariz, 1995, Author.
Nagai M et al: Oleanane acid from *Myrica cerifera, Chem Pharm Bull* 48(10):1427-1428, 2000.
Paul BD: Isolation of myricadiol, myriciatrin, taraxerol, and taxerone from *Myrica cerifera* root bark, *J Pharm Sci* 63:958-959, 1974.
Smith E: *Therapeutic herb manual,* Williams, Ore, 1999, Author.

Bearberry
(behr'beh-ree)

Scientific names: *Arctostaphylos uva-ursi, Arctostaphylos coactylis, Arctostaphylos adenotricha*

Other common names: arctostaphylos, bear's grape, crowberry, foxberry, hogberry, kinnikinnick, manzanita, mountain box, rockberry, uva-ursi   **Class 2b/2d**

Origin: Bearberry is an evergreen found in rocky, mountainous regions.

Uses

Reported Uses

Bearberry exerts antimicrobial effects against *Escherichia coli, Proteus vulgaris, Enterobacter aerogenes, Streptococcus faecalis, Staphylococcus aureus, Salmonella typhi,* and *Candida albicans.* Bearberry traditionally has been used as a diuretic (it is especially effective in cases of highly acidic urine), an antiinflammatory, and an astringent. Contemporarily it is used as a decoc-

⬟ = Pregnancy   **⬚** = Pediatric   **◆** = Alert   **✿** = Popular Herb

tion to treat urinary tract infections. Bearberry may be useful in premenstrual bloating.

B

Product Availability and Dosages

Available Forms

Dried leaves, drops, fluid extract, powdered extract, tablets, tea

Plant Parts Used: Dried leaves

Dosages and Routes

Adult

All dosages listed are PO.

- Fluid extract: 1-2 ml of a 1:1 dilution tid
- Freeze dried leaves: 500-1000 mg tid
- Infusion: 1.5-4 g (1-2 tsp), infuse in cold water to decrease tannin extraction, take 1 cup tid
- Powdered solid extract: 250-500 mg (expressed as 10% arbutin, one of the chemical components of bearberry) tid
- Tincture: 1-1.5 ml of a 1:5 dilution, tid (Moore, 1995)

Precautionary Information

Contraindications

Bearberry is not recommended for use during pregnancy and should not be given to children younger than 12 years of age. Hepatotoxicity may occur in pediatric patients. Bearberry should be used cautiously by persons with electrolyte imbalances, renal disease, acidic urine, and disorders involving gastrointestinal irritation. It is not intended for prolonged use unless used under the direction of an experienced herbalist. Class 2b/2d herb.

Side Effects/Adverse Reactions

In very high doses only.

Gastrointestinal: Nausea, vomiting, anorexia, HEPATO-TOXICITY

Genitourinary: Discolored urine (dark green)

Integumentary: Cyanosis

Toxicity: TINNITUS, VOMITING, SEIZURES, CARDIOVASCULAR COLLAPSE, DELIRIUM, SHORTNESS OF BREATH, FEELING OF SUFFOCATION

Interactions with Bearberry

Drug
Diuretics: Concurrent use of bearberry and diuretics can lead to electrolyte loss, primarily hypokalemia.
NSAIDs: Bearberry may increase the effect of NSAIDs.
Urine acidifiers: Urine acidifiers may inactivate bearberry; do not use concurrently.

Food	**Herb**	**Lab Test**
None known	None known	None known

Client Considerations

Assess

- Determine the reason the client is using bearberry.
- Assess for the use of urinary acidifiers and diuretics. If the client is using diuretics, monitor electrolytes (see Interactions).
- Assess urine alkalinity. Urine may need to be alkaline in order for bearberry to be effective.

 - Assess for signs and symptoms of toxicity: tinnitus, vomiting, seizures, change in cardiovascular status, hepatotoxicity.

Administer

- Instruct the client to take dried leaves PO. The berries should not be used.

Teach Client/Family

 - Until more research is available, caution the client not to use bearberry during pregnancy and not to give this herb to children younger than 12 years of age.

Pharmacology

Pharmacokinetics

Very little is known about the pharmacokinetics in humans. In one study examining the pharmacokinetics of the chemical components of bearberry, six healthy clients drank a tea made from uva-ursi and their urine was subsequently analyzed. After 3 hours, 53% of the arbutin equivalents were recovered in the urine, and after 3 to 6 hours, another 14% of the other hydroquinones were excreted (Paper, 1993).

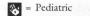 = Pregnancy   = Pediatric   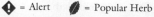 = Alert   = Popular Herb

Primary Chemical Components of Bearberry and Their Possible Actions

Chemical Class	Individual Component	Possible Action
Hydroquinone	Arbutin	Antiseptic; astringent; anti-inflammatory; antibacterial
	Corilagin Monoglucoside; Methylarbutin	Antibacterial
Tannin	Gallo; Ellgic; Condensed	
Triterpene		Diuretic
Iridoid monoterpene	Monotropein	
Piceoside		
Phenol carboxylic acid	Gallic acid	
Flavonoid	Quercitrin Myricitrin; Hyperoside	Antiinflammatory
Volatile oil		

Actions

Little primary research is available detailing the mode of action of bearberry.

Antiseptic/Diuretic Action

The diuretic effect of bearberry results from both its triterpene chemical components and arbutin, a hydroquinone. These components stimulate diuresis.

Antiinflammatory Action

One of the flavonoid components of bearberry, quercitrin, is responsible for decreased inflammation. Arbutin and urosolic acid may also be responsible for its antiinflammatory effects (Jahodar, 1985).

Antimicrobial Action

Research on the antimicrobial effect of bearberry has focused on arbutin. Arbutin has been reported to be effective as a diuretic and as a urinary antiseptic in moderate doses, but only if the urine is alkaline. Use of the whole plant is most effective because of the combined effects of arbutin and gallic acid, another chemical component (Leung, 1996; Constantine, 1966). Urosolic acid has been found to be effective against gram-positive and gram-negative bacteria and yeast (Kowalewski, 1976; Zaletova, 1986). *Arctostaphylos uva-ursi* has been shown to be effective against methicillin-resistant *Staphylococcus aureus* (Shimizu, 2001).

References

Constantine GH et al: Chromatographic study of the alkaloids of *Aquilegia formosa, J Pharm Sci* 559:982-984, 1966.

Jahodar L et al: *Cesk Farm* 34:174, 1985.

Kowalewski Z et al: Antibiotic action of beta-urosolic acid, *Arch Immunol Ther Exp* 24:115, 1976.

Leung A, Foster S: *Encyclopedia of common natural ingredients used in food, drugs and cosmetics,* ed 2, New York, 1996, Wiley & Sons.

Moore M: *Materia medica,* Bisbee, Ariz, 1995, Author.

Paper DH et al: *Planta Med* 59(suppl):A589, 1993.

Shimizu M et al: Marked potentiation of activity of beta-lactams against methicillin-resistant *Staphylococcus aureus* by Corilagin, *Antimicrob Agents Chemother,* 45(11):3198-3201, 2001.

Zaletova NI et al: *Khim-Farm Zh* 20:568, 1986.

Bee Pollen
(bee pah'lun)

Scientific name: *Apis mellifera* (source organism)

Other common names: Buckwheat pollen, maize pollen, pine pollen, pollen pini, puhuang, rape pollen, royal jelly, songhuafen, typha pollen

Origin: Bee pollen is available throughout the world.

Uses

Reported Uses

Bee pollen is used to treat asthma, prostatitis, impotence, bleeding gastric ulcers, and high altitude sickness; to desensitize allergies; to increase appetite; to increase immunogenic effects, and to increase energy level thereby combating fatigue and depression.

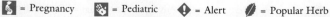

= Pregnancy   = Pediatric   = Alert   = Popular Herb

Investigational Uses
Studies are underway to determine the effectiveness of bee pollen in treating cancer, hypercholesteremia, and heart disease.

B

Product Availability and Dosages
Available Forms
Bars; capsules: 500, 1000 mg; granules: 300 mg; liquid; tablets: 500, 1000 mg; wafers

Source
Bee pollen is a combination of flower pollen, nectar, and the digestive juices of the worker honeybee *Apis mellifera*.

Dosages and Routes
Adult
- PO: 500-1000 mg tid ½ hr before meals

Precautionary Information
Contraindications
Bee pollen should not be used by persons with pollen allergy or diabetes. Persons with known pollen allergy should be tested for allergic reaction before using bee pollen products.

Side Effects/Adverse Reactions
Gastrointestinal: Nausea, diarrhea, vomiting, anorexia
Integumentary: Rash, allergic reactions, hypersensitivity
Systemic: ANAPHYLAXIS

Interactions with Bee Pollen

Drug
Insulin: Bee pollen decreases the effectiveness of insulin and increases hyperglycemia; do not use concurrently.
Oral antidiabetics: Bee pollen decreases the effectiveness of oral antidiabetics and increases hyperglycemia; avoid concurrent use.

Food	Herb	Lab Test
None known	None known	None known

🌐 Endangered Herb　　　　Adverse effects: BOLD = life-threatening

Client Considerations

Assess

- Assess for allergies to bee pollen before using; anaphylaxis may occur. Client should be tested for an allergic reaction to the particular bee pollen to be used.
- Assess patient for use of antidiabetics or insulin; bee pollen may decrease the effectiveness of these products (see Interactions).

Administer

- Instruct the client to take bee pollen PO before meals.
- Instruct the client to store bee pollen in a cool, dry place, away from heat and moisture.

Teach Client/Family

- Inform the client that bee pollen may be used during pregnancy and lactation and may be given to children.
- Caution the client that allergic reactions can be severe in individuals with sensitivity to bee pollen.
- Instruct clients taking oral antidiabetics or insulin to monitor blood glucose often.

Pharmacology

Pharmacokinetics

Pharmacokinetics and pharmacodynamics are unknown.

Primary Chemical Components of Bee Pollen and Their Possible Actions		
Chemical Class	**Individual Component**	**Possible Action**
Protein		
Carbohydrate	Glucose; Fructose	
Mineral		
Fatty acid	Alpha-linolenic acid; Linolenic acid	
Vitamin	B complex; C	
Flavonoid		
Phytosterin		
Nicotinic acid		
Riboflavin		
Ash		

Actions

Bee pollen has been used for many years as a food source in times of scarcity. Its high nutrient content can sustain people and animals when food is not available.

Gastric Protective Action

In a study of patients with bleeding gastric ulcers (Georgieva, 1971), 40 patients were given 250 mg of bee pollen bid. The patients exhibited a positive response, with ulcers showing signs of healing.

Altitude Sickness Prevention

Chinese research has investigated the use of bee pollen to prevent altitude sickness by testing rats and mice exposed to low partial-pressure oxygen to simulate 12,000 masl. Some rats and mice were given no bee pollen, while others were fed various bee pollen species. Those fed bee pollen proved to have a higher survival rate than those not fed bee pollen. In another 2-year study using humans (Peng, 1990), some participants were given bee pollen over a period of 3 to 7 days before a change in altitude to more than 5000 meters above masl. As compared with individuals who received no bee pollen, these individuals showed either no adverse reaction or a greatly lessened reaction to the rise in altitude. Thus bee pollen appears to increase the ability to adapt to a high-altitude environment.

Antiallergy Action

In folk medicine, bee pollen is sometimes given to individuals with allergies to stimulate desensitization.

References

Georgieva E et al: Symposium on use of bee products in human and veterinary medicine, International Beekeeping Congress 23, 1971.

Peng H et al: The effect of pollen in enhancing tolerance to hypoxia and promoting adaptation to highlands, *J Chin Med* 70:77-81, 1990.

DO NOT INGEST

Benzoin
(behn'zuh-wun)

Scientific names: *Styrax benzoin, Styrax paralleloneurus, Styrax tonkinesis*

Other common names: Benjamin tree, benzoe, benzoin tree, gum benjamin, Siam benzoin, Sumatra benzoin

Class 1

Origin: Benzoin is a resin from the trees of genus *Styrax*.

Uses
Reported Uses
Benzoin is used topically to promote wound healing and as an antiseptic, a mucosal protectant, and an adhesive. It is also used as an expectorant and as an inhalant for bronchial disorders.

Product Availability and Dosages
Available Forms
Cream, lotion, ointment, tincture

Plant Parts Used: Bark gum resin

Dosages and Routes
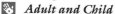 *Adult and Child*
- Inhalant: 5 ml benzoin gum/1 pt water; breathe vapors
- Topical: may be applied to the affected area q2h-q4h; test a small area before applying to larger area

Precautionary Information
Contraindications
Benzoin should not be used by those with hypersensitivity to this herb. It should not be used internally. Class 1 herb.

Side Effects/Adverse Reactions
Gastrointestinal: Gastritis, GASTROINTESTINAL HEMORRHAGE (ingestion) (Arys, 1987)
Integumentary: Rash, allergic reactions, hypersensitivity, contact dermatitis
Respiratory: Asthma (inhalation)
Systemic: ANAPHYLAXIS

 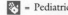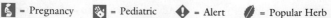

Interactions with Benzoin			
Drug	Food	Herb	Lab Test
None known	None known	None known	None known

Client Considerations

Assess

- Assess for hypersensitivity reactions, including anaphylaxis. Benzoin use should be discontinued if any hypersensitivity reactions occur.
- Assess for GI bleeding: dark tarry stools, frank blood, gastritis, abdominal pain; do not use internally.

Administer

- Instruct the client to use benzoin as a topical or an inhalant only; skin may become discolored.

Teach Client/Family

- Caution the client that gastritis and gastrointestinal hemorrhage can occur if benzoin is taken internally.

Pharmacology

Pharmacokinetics

Pharmacokinetics and pharmacodynamics are unknown.

Primary Chemical Components of Benzoin and Their Possible Actions		
Chemical Class	Individual Component	Possible Action
Acid	Benzoic acid Cinnamic acid	Antiseptic; protectant

Actions

Benzoin has been used topically for many years as an antiseptic and a skin protectant. However, many other products are just as effective.

References

Arys TVS et al: Severe GI hemorrhage following accidental ingestion of tincture of benzoi compound, *J Assoc Phys India* 35:805, 1987.

Betel Palm
(bee'tul pahlm)

Scientific name: *Areca catechu*

Other common names: Areca nut, betal, chavica betal, hmarg, maag, paan, pan masala, pan parag, pinang, supai

Origin: Betel palm is a palm found in China, India, the Philippines, and the tropical regions of Africa.

Uses
Reported Uses
Betel palm is used to treat depression, respiratory conditions, cough, and sore throat. It is also used as a psychostimulant.

Product Availability and Dosages
Available Forms
Leaves, nut, pressed juice

Plant Parts Used: Leaves, nut

Dosages and Routes
Adult
Sore Throat
• Gargle: use prn
Other
• PO: 2 g fresh nut, chew for 15 min or more and spit out
• PO: roll leaves and place between teeth and gums/lips

Precautionary Information
Contraindications

Betel palm should not be used during pregnancy and lactation and should not be given to children. Clients with oral or esophageal cancers, ulcers, esophagitis, or renal disease should avoid its use. Do not confuse betel palm with betel nut, *Piper betel* L.

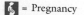 = Pregnancy    = Pediatric   = Alert   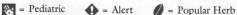 = Popular Herb

Precautionary Information—cont'd

Side Effects/Adverse Reactions

Cardiovascular: Palpitations, TACHYCARDIA OR BRADYCARDIA

Central Nervous System: Stimulation, facial flushing, fever, dizziness, SEIZURES, acute psychosis, anxiety, insomnia, restlessness

Ear, Eye, Nose, and Throat: Red stains on teeth, oral leukoplakia, oral submucosal fibrosis, ORAL CARCINOGENESIS (chewing) (Chen, 1999; Norton, 1998), blurred vision

Gastrointestinal: Nausea, vomiting, diarrhea or constipation, red feces, abdominal cramping/pain; INTESTINAL EPITHELIAL CELL LINING ALTERATION (Kumar, 2000)

Respiratory: Increased asthma symptoms

Interactions with Betel Palm

Drug

Alcohol: Betel palm increases the effects of alcohol; do not use concurrently.

Antiglaucoma agents: Betel palm decreases the action of antiglaucoma agents; do not use concurrently.

Beta-blockers: Betel palm increases the action of beta-blockers; do not use concurrently.

Calcium channel blockers: Betel palm increases the action of calcium channel blockers; do not use concurrently.

Cardiac glycosides (digoxin): Betel palm increases the action of cardiac glycosides; do not use concurrently.

MAO inhibitors: Betel palm may increase chance of hypertensive crisis.

Neuroleptics: Extrapyramidal symptoms can occur when betel palm is combined with neuroleptics; do not use concurrently (Fugh-Berman, 2000).

Food

Tyramine foods: May increase the chance of hypertensive crisis.

Herb	Lab Test
None known	None known

Client Considerations

Assess

- Check the client's mouth for changes such as leukoplakia and fibrosis.
- Assess for cardiac arrhythmias, milk-alkali syndrome, and central nervous system changes.
- Assess for medications used by the client: antiglaucoma agents, beta-blockers, calcium channel blockers, cardiac glycosides, MAOIs, neuroleptics (see Interactions).
- Assess for alcohol use.

Administer

- Instruct the client to take betel palm PO using either the fresh nut, which is chewed or used as a gargle, or the leaves.

Teach Client/Family

- Caution the client not to use betel palm during pregnancy and lactation and not to give it to children.
- Caution the client that chewing the root over long periods of time can lead to mouth fibrosis and oral carcinoma.

Pharmacology

Pharmacokinetics

Pharmacokinetics and pharmacodynamics are unknown.

Primary Chemical Components of Betel Palm and Their Possible Actions		
Chemical Class	Individual Component	Possible Action
Alkaloid	Arecoline	Parasympathomimetic; sympathomimetic; monoamine oxidase inhibitor
	Arecaidine; Arecaine; Arecolidine; Guvacine; Guvacoline	
Phenol		
Volatile oil	Chavicol; Chaibetol; Cadinene; Allylpyrocatechol	
Tannin	Catechin type	Wound healing; antiinflammatory

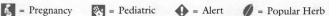

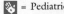 = Pregnancy   = Pediatric   ◆ = Alert   ∦ = Popular Herb

Actions

Psychiatric Action

Betel has been used for centuries in Asia as a psychostimulant. However, recent studies of the rat brain have shown that betel inhibits monoamine oxidase (MAO). The aqueous fraction is the most potent inhibitor of MAO-A. Several other older studies have also demonstrated the antidepressant action of betel palm (Dar, 1997; Van der Hyden, 1987). Betel chewing is shown to decrease symptomatology in schizophrenia (Sullivan, 2000).

Parasympathetic Nervous System Action

Betel palm has been shown to increase muscarinic action, salivation, and central nervous system stimulation in mice. When chewed, betel palm also lowers heart rate and induces euphoria.

Thyroid Function Action

A study of mice given betel leaf extract demonstrated a dual role on thyroid function (Panda, 1998). At high doses, the leaf extract increased T4 (thyroxine) and decreased T3 (triiodothyronine), while at lower doses the opposite was true. High doses also increased lipid peroxidation. Thus, betel leaf has been shown to produce both inhibitory and stimulatory effects on thyroid function.

References

Chen CL et al: Safrole-like DNA adducts in oral tissue from oral cancer patients with a betel quid chewing history, *Carcinogenesis* 20(12): 2331-2334, 1999.

Dar A et al: Anti-depressant activities of *Areca catechu* fruit extract, *Phytomedicine* 4(1):41-45, 1997.

Fugh-Berman A: Herb-drug interactions, *Lancet* 355(9198):134-138, 2000.

Kumar M et al: Effect of betel/areca nut *(Areca catechu)* extracts on intestinal epithelial cell lining, *Vet Hum Toxicol* 42(5):257-260, 2000.

Norton SA: Betel: consumption and consequences, *J Am Acad Dermatol* 38(1):81-88, 1998.

Panda S et al: Dual role of betel leaf extract on thyroid function in male mice, *Pharmacol Res* 38(6):493-496, 1998.

Sullivan RJ et al: Effects of chewing betel nut *(Areca catechu)* on the symptoms of people with schizophrenia in Palau, Micronesia, *Br J Psychiatry* 177:174-178, 2000.

Van der Hyden JAM et al: Strain differences in response to drugs in the tail suspension test for anti-depressant activity, *Psychopharmacology* 92:127-130, 1987.

Beth Root
(bayth rewt)

Scientific names: *Trillium erectum, Trillium grandiflorum*

Other common names: Birthroot, cough root, ground lily, Indian balm, Indian shamrock, Jew's harp, purple trillium, rattlesnake root, snake bite, squaw root, stinking benjamin, three-leafed trillium, trillium pendulum, wake-robin   **Class 2b**

Origin: Beth root is a member of the lily family found in Canada and parts of the United States.

Uses

Reported Uses

Beth root is used externally to treat insect bites, hemorrhoids, hematoma, varicose veins, and ulcers. It is used as a douche to treat leukorrhea. Internally, it is used to relieve pain. Traditionally, beth root has been used as an expectorant and to treat bleeding, snake bites, and skin irritation. This plant is on the endangered species list in many states and therefore should not be harvested from the wild.

Product Availability and Dosages

Available Forms

Extract, powder, powdered root

Plant Parts Used: Leaves, rhizome, roots

Dosages and Routes

Adult

Astringent/Expectorant
• Fluid extract: 30 minims
Bleeding
• Tincture: 1-3 ml q 15 min, up to 4 doses daily
Other
• PO powder: 1 tsp powder/1 pt water prn

Precautionary Information

Contraindications

Because it can cause uterine stimulation, beth root should not be used during pregnancy. Until more research is avail-

---

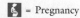 = Pregnancy    = Pediatric    = Alert   = Popular Herb

Precautionary Information—cont'd

Contraindications—cont'd

able, this herb should not be used during lactation and it should not be given to children. Class 2b herb.

Side Effects/Adverse Reactions

Cardiovascular: CARDIOTOXICITY—CHANGE IN BLOOD PRESSURE, PULSE, ECG

Gastrointestinal: Nausea, vomiting, anorexia, gastrointestinal irritation, abdominal cramping

Hematologic: Constriction of blood vessels

Interactions with Beth Root

Drug

Cardiac glycosides (digoxin): Beth root may decrease the effects of cardiac glycosides; use together cautiously.

Food	Herb	Lab Test
None known	None known	None known

Client Considerations

Assess

- Assess for cardiotoxicity: monitor blood pressure, pulse, and changes in cardiac status.
- Assess for use of cardiac glycosides (see Interactions).
- Assess for change in respiratory status (expectorant use) or decrease in surface bleeding.

Administer

- Instruct the client to take beth root PO as a tincture or an expectorant.
- Store beth root in a cool, dry place, away from heat and moisture.

Teach Client/Family

- Caution the client not to use beth root during pregnancy because it can induce labor. Until more research is available, caution the client not to use this herb during lactation and not to give it to children.

Pharmacology

Pharmacokinetics

Pharmacokinetics and pharmacodynamics are unknown.

Primary Chemical Components of Beth Root and Their Possible Actions		
Chemical Class	Individual Component	Possible Action
Saponin	Trillin; Trillarin; Kryptogenin; Chlorogenin; Nologenin	Astringent; expectorant
Glycoside	Convallamerin-like	Cardiotoxicity

Actions

Very little research is available for beth root.

Astringent Action

The astringent activity of beth root may account for its ability to control bleeding by constricting the blood vessels (Duke, 1985).

Antifungal Action

The saponins in beth root are believed to exert significant antifungal effects (Duke, 1985).

References

Duke J: *Handbook of medicinal herbs,* Boca Raton, Fla, 1985, CRC Press.

Betony
(beht'nee)

Scientific name: *Stachys officinalis* L. (Trevisan)

Other common names: Bishopswort, wood betony

Class 1

Origin: Betony is a member of the mint family found in the southern and western regions of Europe and Siberia.

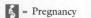 = Pregnancy  = Pediatric   = Alert 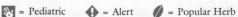 = Popular Herb

B

Uses
Reported Uses
Betony is used to treat seizures, palpitations, diarrhea, asthma, bronchitis, wounds, renal stones, and hypertension.

Product Availability and Dosages
Available Forms
Capsules, tea, tincture

Plant Parts Used: Flowers, leaves

Dosages and Routes
Adult
- PO as a tea, infusion, or gargle, or smoked
- Tincture: 2-4 ml bid-tid

Precautionary Information
Contraindications
Because uterine stimulation can occur, betony should not be used during pregnancy (Chevallier, 1996). Until more research is available, avoid its use during lactation, and avoid giving it to children. Class 1 herb.

Side Effects/Adverse Reactions
Gastrointestinal: HEPATOTOXICITY, gastrointestinal irritation, nausea, anorexia

---

Interactions with Betony

Drug
Antihypertensives: The hypotensive effects of betony may increase the action of antihypertensives; avoid concurrent use.

Food	Herb	Lab Test
None known	None known	None known

Client Considerations
Assess
- Assess the client's use of antihypertensives; monitor blood pressure, pulse, and character (see Interactions).
- Assess liver function test results (AST, ALT, bilirubin) to iden-

 Endangered Herb   Adverse effects: BOLD = life-threatening

tify liver damage. If liver function levels are increased, discontinue use of this herb.

Administer

- Instruct the client to take betony PO as a tea, tincture, or infusion.
- Instruct the client to store betony in a cool, dry place, away from heat and moisture.

Teach Client/Family

- Because it can stimulate the uterus, caution the client not to use betony during pregnancy (Chevallier, 1996). Until more research is available, advise the client to avoid the use of this herb during lactation and to avoid giving it to children.

Pharmacology

Pharmacokinetics

Pharmacokinetics and pharmacodynamics are unknown.

Primary Chemical Components of Betony and Their Possible Actions		
Chemical Class	**Individual Component**	**Possible Action**
Tannin		Astringent; anti-diarrheal; wound healing; anti-inflammatory
Flavonoid Glycoside	Stachydrine Betaine; Betonicide; Acetoside; Campneoside; Forsythoside B	Systolic depressant
Leucosceptoside B		

Actions

Very little research exists to verify any of the uses of betony.

Antihypertensive Action

The antihypertensive effect of betony may result from glycosides present in the herb. Stachydrine, one of the chemical components in this herb, is a systolic depressant.

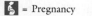 = Pregnancy = Pediatric = Alert 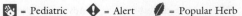 = Popular Herb

Other Actions

The astringent and antidiarrheal actions of betony are a result of its high tannin content.

B

References

Chevallier A: *Encyclopedia of medicinal plants,* New York, 1996, DK, p 270.

Bilberry
(bil'beh-ree)

Scientific name: *Vaccinium myrtillus*

Other common names: Airelle, bilberry, black whortle, bleaberry, bog bilberry, European blueberry, huckleberry, trackleberry, whinberry, whortleberry   Class 4

Origin: Bilberry is found in the central, northern, and south-eastern regions of Europe.

Uses

Reported Uses

Bilberry has been used to improve night vision; to prevent cataracts, macular degeneration, and glaucoma; to treat varicose veins and hemorrhoids; to prevent hemorrhage after surgery; and to prevent and treat diabetic retinopathy and myopia. Other uses for bilberry include decreasing diarrhea, dyspepsia in adults or children, controlling insulin levels, as a diuretic and as a urinary antiseptic.

Product Availability and Dosages

Available Forms

Capsules: 60, 80, 120, 450 mg; fluid extract; fresh berries, dried berries; liquid; tincture; dried roots, dried leaves

Plant Parts Used: Berries, roots, leaves

Dosages and Routes

Adult

Cataracts

- PO extract: 40-80 mg standardized to 25% anthocyanosides (anthocyanadin) tid (Murray, 1998)

🌀 Endangered Herb   Adverse effects: BOLD = life-threatening

Diabetes Mellitus
- PO extract: 80-160 mg standardized to 25% anthocyanosides tid (Murray, 1998)

Glaucoma
- PO extract: 80 mg standardized to 25% anthocyanosides tid (Murray, 1998)

Other
- PO fresh berries: 55-115 g tid
- Topical decoction: ⅛-¼ ounce (5-8 g) of crushed dried fruit in 150 ml of water, boil 10 min, strain, use warm
- Gargle/mouthwash: prepare decoction 10%, rinse or gargle

Precautionary Information

Contraindications

Until more research is available, bilberry should not be used during pregnancy and lactation. Bilberry has been used traditionally to help stop lactation (Blumenthal, 2000). Class 4 herb.

Side Effects/Adverse Reactions

Gastrointestinal: Constipation (large consumption of dried fruits)

Interactions with Bilberry

Drug

Anticoagulants (heparin, warfarin): Bilberry may increase the action of anticoagulants; use caution if taking concurrently.

Antiplatelet agents: Bilberry may cause antiaggregation of platelets; use caution if taking concurrently with antiplatelet agents.

Aspirin: Bilberry may increase the anticoagulation action of aspirin; use caution if taking concurrently.

Insulin: Bilberry leaves may significantly decrease blood sugar levels; monitor carefully (Brinter, 1998).

Iron: Bilberry interferes with iron absorption, avoid concurrent use.

NSAIDs: Bilberry may increase the action of NSAIDs; use caution if taking concurrently.

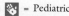 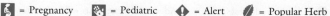

| Interactions with Bilberry—cont'd | | |

Drug—cont'd
Oral antidiabetics: Bilberry may increase hypoglycemia; use caution if taking concurrently with oral antidiabetics.

Food	Herb	Lab Test
None known	None known	None known

Client Considerations

Assess

- Assess whether the client is taking anticoagulants, antidiabetics, or antiplatelet agents. Bilberry is known to induce hypoglycemia, anticoagulation, and antiplatelet aggregation (see Interactions).
- Monitor improvement in vision if using to treat cataracts or glaucoma
- Monitor blood glucose if using to treat diabetes mellitus.

Administer

- Instruct the client to take bilberry PO in the form of tincture, capsules, fluid extract, or fresh berries.

Teach Client/Family

- Until more research is available, advise the client to avoid the use of this herb during pregnancy and lactation.
- Advise the client to notify the herbalist if diarrhea persists for more than 4 days.
- Advise the client that use of higher-than-recommended doses or use of this herb for extended periods will result in toxicity, and may result in death (leaves).

Pharmacology

Pharmacokinetics

Peak 15 minutes; eliminated via bile.

Primary Chemical Components of Bilberry and Their Possible Actions

Chemical Class	Individual Component	Possible Action
Tannin		Astringent; anti-inflammatory
Flavonoid	Cinnamic acid;	
Acid	Benzoic acid	
Pectin		
Anthocyanosides		Antioxidant; increased circulation; anti-aggregation of platelets
Rutin		Lowered intraocular pressure

Actions

Research is more extensive for bilberry than for many other commonly used herbs. Areas of research include the use of bilberry for treating circulatory disorders, glaucoma, cataracts, macular degeneration, poor night vision, and diabetic/hypertensive retinopathy. Studies have also focused on its use as an antilipemic.

Ophthalmologic Action

Studies indicate that night vision improved significantly when individuals were given bilberry (Sala, 1979; Caselli, 1985). Participants experienced improved night visual acuity, improved adjustment to darkness, and restoration of acuity after glare. Further research has confirmed the findings of the previous studies (Muth, 2000). These actions may be due to the affinity of bilberry for the retina. In addition, bilberry may be useful for the prevention and treatment of glaucoma, cataracts, and macular degeneration of the eye (Bravetti, 1989). Chemical components in bilberry may alter the collagen structure of the eye and decrease intraocular pressure. The collagen-stabilizing effects of *Vaccinium* may offer protection against glaucoma and the development of cataracts and macular degeneration of the eye (Gabor, 1972; Paulter, 1984).

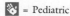 = Pregnancy = Pediatric = Alert = Popular Herb

B

Antidiabetic Action

The anthocyanoside components of bilberry have been shown to decrease hyperglycemia in dogs (Bever, 1979). Their effect is somewhat weaker than that of insulin; however, a single dose has an extended duration of up to several weeks (Bever, 1979).

Other Actions

Some of the other proposed actions of bilberry include its lipid-lowering effect and its ability to treat inflammatory joint disease, microscopic hematuria, and varicose veins. Studies in rats have shown that the anthocyanosides promote collagen synthesis and inhibit collagen loss (Rao, 1981).

References

Bever B et al: Plants with oral hypoglycemic action *Q J Crude Drugs Res* 17:139-196, 1979.

Bravetti G: Preventative medical treatment of senile cataracts with vitamin E and anthocyanosides: clinical evaluation, *Ann Ottalmol Clin Ocul* 115:109, 1989.

Caselli L: Clinical and electroretinographic study on activity of anthocyanosides on photoreceptors: cytoenzymatic aspects, *Ann Histochem* 14:237-256, 1985.

Gabor M: Pharmacologic effects of flavonoids on blood vessels, *Angiologia* 9:355-374, 1972.

Murray M, Pizzorno J: *Encyclopedia of natural medicine,* 2 ed (revised), Roseville, Calif, 1998, Prima.

Muth ER et al: The effect of bilberry nutritional supplementation on night visual acuity and contrast sensitivity (in process citation), *Altern Med Rev* 5(2):164-173, 2000.

Paulter EL et al: The effect of diet on inherited retinal dystrophy in the rat, *Curr Eye Res* 3:1221-1234, 1984.

Rao CN et al: Influence of bioflavonoids on the collagen metabolism in rats with adjuvant induced arthritis, *Ital J Biochem* 30:1771-1776, 1981.

Sala D et al: Effect of anthocyanosides on visual performances at low illumination, *Minerva Oftalmol* 21:283-285, 1979.

Birch
(burch)

Scientific names: *Betula alba, Betula pendula, Betula verrucosa, Betula pubescens, Betula lenta*

Other common names: Birch tar oil, birch wood oil, black birch, cherry birch, sweet birch oil, white birch

Class 1

Origin: Birch is found in Russia, throughout Europe, and in the eastern region of the United States.

Uses

Reported Uses

Birch is used internally as an analgesic and to treat urinary stones and gout and as a diuretic. It is also used as a topical treatment for arthritic joints, aching muscles, and muscle spasms. Birch can also be applied externally for sores and boils.

Investigational Uses

Studies are underway to determine the effectiveness of birch as an antioxidant used to decrease free radicals.

Product Availability and Dosages

Available Forms

Decoction, dried bark, essential oil, tea

Plant Parts Used: Bark, leaves, twigs

Dosages and Routes

Adult

- PO tea: boil 2-3 g (Blumenthal, 1998) bark and twigs for 1 hr, strain, use tid
- Topical: apply only to area to be treated; to prevent contact dermatitis, do not apply essential oil to broken skin

Precautionary Information

Contraindications

Until more research is available, birch should not be used internally by persons who are pregnant or lactating and should not be given to children. Birch should not be used by persons with hypersensitivity to it or with other allergic con-

---

 = Pregnancy    = Pediatric   ◆ = Alert   = Popular Herb

Precautionary Information—cont'd
Contraindications—cont'd
ditions, or by persons with congestive heart failure or severe kidney disease. Class 1 herb.

Side Effects/Adverse Reactions
Systemic: Allergic reactions

Interactions with Birch		
Food	Herb	Lab Test
None known	None known	None known
Herb		
Celery: Birch used with celery may cause cross-sensitization.		

Client Considerations
Assess
- Assess for allergic reactions, rash, wheezing, and chest tightness. If present, administer antihistamine or other appropriate therapy.

Administer
- Instruct the client to take birch PO as a tea or infusion, or apply topically.

Teach Client/Family
- Until more research is available, caution the client not to use birch internally during pregnancy and lactation and not to give it to children.
- Because contact dermatitis may occur, advise the client to avoid direct skin contact with birch by using a carrier oil, to avoid use on broken skin, and to first test the oil on a small area.
- Keep sweet birch essential oil away from children, may result in fatal reaction when applied to the skin.

Pharmacology
Pharmacokinetics
Pharmacokinetics and pharmacodynamics are unknown.

Primary Chemical Components of Birch and Their Possible Actions		
Chemical Class	**Individual Component**	**Possible Action**
Flavonoid	Quercetin	Antioxidant; anti-inflammatory
	Hyperoside; Avicularin	
Birch tar oil		
Turpentine oil		
Creosol		
Betulin		Antitumor action

Actions

Almost no research is available on birch. Existing information on its uses comes from anecdotal evidence taken from traditional herbal medicine. However, birch is thought to possess significant antioxidant activity (Matsuda, 1998), and one study has investigated its diuretic effects (Bisset, 1994).

References

Bisset NG: *Herbal drugs and phytopharmaceuticals,* Boca Raton, Fla, 1994, CRC Press.

Blumenthal M, editor: *The complete German Commission E monographs: therapeutic guide to herbal medicines,* Austin, Tex, American Botanical Council; Boston, Integrative Medicine Communication, 1998.

Matsuda H: Hepatoprotective, superoxide scavenging, and antioxidative activities of aromatic constituents from the bark of *Betula platyphylla* var. japonica, *Bioorg Med Chem Lett* 8(21):2939-2944, 1998.

 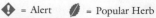

Bistort
(bis-tawrt´)

Scientific name: *Polygonum bistorta*

Other common names: Adderwort, common bistort, Easter ledges, Easter mangiant, knotweed, oderwort, osterick, patience dock, snakeroot, snakeweed, twice writhen

Class 1

B

Origin: Bistort is found in Europe and is cultivated in North America.

Uses

Reported Uses

Bistort is used externally to treat bites, stings, burns, snakebites, and hemorrhoids. It is used internally to treat peptic ulcers, irritable bowel syndrome, ulcerative colitis, and diarrhea.

Investigational Uses

Research is ongoing into the potential use of bistort as an antiviral to induce interferon-like activity.

Product Availability and Dosages

Available Forms

Powder, roots (cut and dried), tea

Plant Parts Used: Leaves, rhizome, roots

Dosages and Routes

Adult
- PO: 1 tsp powdered root in 1 cup boiling water, take as often as tid
- Topical: use powder and water to make a poultice, apply to area prn

Precautionary Information

Contraindications

Until more research is available, bistort should not be used during pregnancy and lactation. Class 1 herb.

Side Effects/Adverse Reactions

Gastrointestinal: Gastrointestinal irritation, HEPATOTOXICITY

Interactions with Bistort			
Drug	Food	Herb	Lab Test
None known	None known	None known	None known

Client Considerations

Assess

- Assess the client's gastrointestinal symptoms (cramping, diarrhea, bleeding).
- 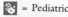 Assess liver function test results; hepatotoxicity can occur.

Administer

- Instruct the client to take bistort PO no more often than tid.
- Instruct the client use bistort topically as a poultice to decrease inflammation.

Teach Client/Family

- Until more research is available, caution the client not to use bistort during pregnancy and lactation.

Pharmacology

Pharmacokinetics

Pharmacokinetics and pharmacodynamics are unknown.

Primary Chemical Components of Bistort and Their Possible Actions		
Chemical Class	**Individual Component**	**Possible Action**
Leaves Contain		
Tannin		Wound healing; antiinflammatory
Phenol		
Roots Contain		
Flavonoids		
Starch		
Gallic acid		
Phlobaphene		
Anthranoide	Emodin	Laxative

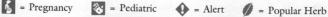

Actions

In traditional herbal medicine, bistort has been used both internally and externally to treat a variety of conditions. Currently, research is focused on the antiviral and interferon activity of the *Polygonum* species. One study focused on the antiinflammatory action of bistort (Duwiejua, 1999). In this study, two compounds with significant antiinflammatory properties were isolated. Another study has shown a substance that is able to induce interferon-like activity (Smolarz, 1999).

References

Duwiejua M et al: The anti-inflammatory compounds of *Polygonum bistorta:* isolation and characterization, *Planta Med* 65(4):371-374, 1999.

Smolarz HD et al: The investigations into the interferon-like activity of *Polygonum* L. genus, *Acta Pol Pharm* 56(6):459-462, 1999.

Bitter Melon
(bi'tur meh'lun)

Scientific name: *Momordica charantia* L.

Other common names: Balsam apple, balsam pear, bitter cucumber, bitter gourd, bitter pear, carilla cundeamor, karolla

Origin: Bitter melon is an annual and is cultivated in Africa, India, South America, and parts of Asia.

Uses

Reported Uses

Bitter melon is used as an antipyretic, an anthelmintic, and a laxative.

Investigational Uses

Researchers are experimenting with the use of bitter melon as an antifungal and androgenic, as well as its use as a treatment for HIV and other viral infections, malaria, *Helicobacter pylori,* diabetes, and infertility.

Product Availability and Dosages
Available Forms
Aqueous extract, juice, tincture, fruit

Plant Parts Used: Fruit, leaves, seed oil, seeds

Dosages and Routes
Adult
- PO aqueous extract: 15 g/day (Murray, 1998)
- PO juice: 2 oz/day (Murray, 1998)

Precautionary Information
Contraindications
Because it may cause uterine contractions and bleeding, bitter melon should not be used during pregnancy. Bitter melon also should not be used during lactation or by persons with hypersensitivity to it. When taken internally, the seeds are toxic to children.

Side Effects/Adverse Reactions
Gastrointestinal: HEPATOTOXICITY, nausea, vomiting, anorexia

Interactions with Bitter Melon

Drug
Oral hypoglycemics: Bitter melon may increase the effects of oral hypoglycemics; use together cautiously.

Food
None known

Herb
None known

Lab Test
Blood glucose: Bitter melon may decrease test values (if taken with chlorpropamide)

Client Considerations
Assess
- Assess blood glucose (both fasting and postprandial) while the client is taking this herb.
- Assess all medications taken by diabetic clients (see Interactions).

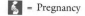 = Pregnancy    = Pediatric   = Alert   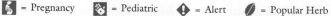 = Popular Herb

- Assess for gastrointestinal symptoms: nausea, vomiting, anorexia; if these occur, discontinue bitter melon.

Administer

- Instruct the client not to use the red arils (outer coverings) around the seeds if taking PO.

Teach Client/Family

- Caution the client not to use bitter melon during pregnancy; uterine stimulation and bleeding can occur. This herb should be avoided during lactation, and the seeds should not be given to children.

Pharmacology

Pharmacokinetics

Pharmacokinetics and pharmacodynamics are unknown.

Primary Chemical Components of Bitter Melon and Their Possible Actions		
Chemical Class	**Individual Component**	**Possible Action**
Triterpenoid Steroid glycoside	Momordincines Momordin Charantin	Antifungal Hypoglycemia
Polypeptide Vicine Proteins Serine protease inhibitors	Alpha, Beta-Momordarin BGIA, BGTI	Hypoglycemia Toxicity

Actions

Antidiabetic Action

Several studies have focused on the hypoglycemic effects of bitter melon. One study of 100 participants with moderated non–insulin-dependent diabetes showed a significant reduction in fasting and postprandial blood glucose levels with the use of bitter melon (Ahmed, 1999). The diabetic action of this herb is thought to result from its ability to increase the functioning of beta cells in the pancreas (Ahmed, 1998). Another study demonstrated that the mechanism of action of this herb could be attributed in part to the increased glucose utilization of the liver, rather than an insulin secretion effect (Sarkar, 1996).

Antiinfective Action

One study noted a marked inhibition of HIV-1 replication in participants with T-lymphocytes that were acutely but not chronically infected with HIV-1 (Zheng, 1999). Another study focused on the antimalarial effects of *M. charantia*. A total of 46 different plant species were studied in vitro for their antimalarial activity on *Plasmodium falciparum* chloroquine-resistant malaria. *M. charantia* was shown to be moderately effective, as were other species. However, another study showed no antimalarial effects for bitter melon (Ueno, 1996).

References

Ahmed I et al: Effects of *Momordica charantia* fruit juice on islet morphology in the pancreas of the streptozotocin-diabetic rat, *Diabetes Res Clin Pract* 40(3):145-151, 1998.

Ahmed N et al: Effect of *Momordica charantia* (Karolla) extracts on fasting and postprandial serum glucose levels in NIDDM patients, *Bangladesh Med Res Counc Bull* 25(1):11-13, 1999.

Murray M, Pizzorno J: *Encyclopedia of natural medicine,* 2 ed (revised), Roseville, Calif, 1998, Prima.

Sarkar S et al: Demonstration of the hypoglycemic action of *Momordica charantia* in a validated animal model of diabetes, *Pharmacol Res* 33(1):1-4, 1996.

Ueno HM et al: Effect of *Momordica charantia* L. in mice infected with *Plasmodium berghei, Rev Soc Bras Med Trop* 29(5):455-460, 1996.

Zheng YT et al: Alpha-momorcharin inhibits HIV-1 replication in acutely but not chronically infected T-lymphocytes, *Chung Kuo Yao Li Hsueh Pao* 20(3):239-243, 1999.

Bitter Orange
(bit'uhr owr'uhj)

Scientific name: *Citrus aurantium*

Other common names: Bigarade orange, nerol, Seville orange, sour orange

Origin: Bitter orange is grown Asia and parts of the Mediterranean.

 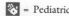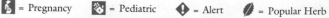

Uses

Reported Uses

Bitter orange has been used traditionally as a sedative and as an insecticide for mosquitos.

Investigational Uses

Studies are underway for the use of bitter orange as a topical antifungal agent.

Product Availability and Dosages

Available Forms

Fluid extract, tincture, tea

Plant Parts Used: Fruit

Dosage and Routes

No published dosages are available

Precautionary Information

Contraindications

Bitter orange should not be used medicinally in pregnancy, lactation, peptic ulcer disease, children, or individuals using tanning beds or other ultraviolet light.

Side Effects/Adverse Reactions

Central Nervous System: Anxiety, restlessness, nervousness, headache
Gastrointestinal: Anorexia, gastrointestinal upset, nausea
Eye, Ear, Nose, and Throat: Sore throat
Integumentary: Photosensitivity, skin redness, edema
Musculoskeletal: Gout

Interactions with Bitter Orange

Drug	Food	Herb	Lab Test
None known	None known	None known	None known

🌀 Endangered Herb   Adverse effects: BOLD = life-threatening

Client Considerations

Assess

- Determine the reason the client is using bitter orange.
- Assess if the client is pregnant or lactating or has been diagnosed with peptic ulcer disease.

Administer

- Advise client to keep bitter orange in a cool, dry place.

Teach Client/Family

- Teach the client that bitter orange should not be used medicinally in pregnancy, in lactation, or for children until more research is available.
- Inform the client that gastrointestinal symptoms (nausea, anorexia, gastrointestinal upset) are common.
- Advise the client to use sunscreen and protective clothing or stay out of the sun to prevent burns. Caution the client not to use tanning beds while taking this herb.

Pharmacology

Pharmacokinetics

Pharmacokinetics and pharmacodynamics are unknown.

Primary Chemical Components of Bitter Orange and Their Possible Actions		
Chemical Class	**Individual Component**	**Possible Action**
Neohesperidin Hesperidin Oxypeucedanin		Antifungal Phototoxicity (Naganuma et al, 1985)

Actions

Antifungal Action

One study is available identifying bitter orange's possible topical antifungal action (Ramadan et al, 1996). The research available deals with topical fungal infections such as tinea corporis, tinea cruis, and tinea pedis. There was a cure rate of 80% in the

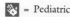 = Pregnancy   = Pediatric   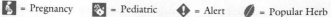 = Alert   = Popular Herb

group treated with bitter orange oil. Very little research other than this study is available for the action of bitter orange.

References

Naganuma M et al: A study of the phototoxicity of lemon oil, *Arch Dermatol Res* 278(1):31-36, 1985.

Ramadan W et al: Oil of bitter orange: new topical antifungal agent, *Int J Dermatol* 35(6):448-449, 1996.

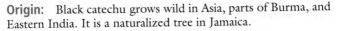

Black Catechu
(blak cat'uh-shoo)

Scientific name: *Acacia catechu*

Other common names: Catechu wood extract

Origin: Black catechu grows wild in Asia, parts of Burma, and Eastern India. It is a naturalized tree in Jamaica.

Uses

Reported Uses

Black catechu has been used traditionally for diabetes and hypertension and topically for mouth ulcers such as stomatitis. Since it is an astringent and an antiseptic with a high tannin content, it is used for diarrhea, irritable bowel syndrome, and other gastrointestinal disorders. It is also used as a contraceptive.

Product Availability and Dosages

Available Forms

Dried extract, tea/infusion, tincture

Plant Parts Used: Heartwood of the tree

Dosages and Routes

Adult

- Dried extract: PO 0.3-2 g tid or a single dose of 0.5 g
- Tea/infusion: 0.3-2 g of dried extract prepared as a tea or infusion in 8 oz of water
- Tincture: 2.5-5 ml of a 1:5 dilution in 45% alcohol added to a small amount of liquid
- Topical: Use tincture as a mouthwash or paint on mucous membranes

Precautionary Information

Contraindications

Black catechu should not be used in pregnancy, in lactation, for children, or in immunosuppressive conditions. Do not use for long-term treatment because of high tannin content.

Side Effects/Adverse Reactions

Cardiovascular: Hypotension
Endocrine: Hypoglycemia
Gastrointestinal: Constipation

Interactions with Black Catechu

Drug

Antidiabetics: Black catechu may increase hypoglycemia (theoretical).
Anticholinergics: Increased constipation may occur when black catechu is used with anticholinergics.
Antihypertensives: Black catechu may increase hypotension when used with antihypertensives.
Captopril: Black catechu may increase hypotension when used with antihypertensives.
Iron salts: Black catechu combined with iron salts form an insoluble complex; do not use together.
Zinc: Black catechu combined with zinc form an insoluble complex, do not use together.

Food	Herb	Lab Test
None known	None known	None known

Client Considerations

Assess

- Assess the reason client is using black catechu.
- Assess gastrointestinal system if using for gastrointestinal symptoms: diarrhea, constipation, abdominal pain, flatulence.
- Assess cardiac status in cardiac clients: heart rate, B/P; hypotension may occur.
- Monitor blood glucose in diabetic clients; hypoglycemia may occur.

 = Pregnancy    = Pediatric   = Alert   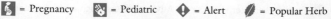 = Popular Herb

Administer
- PO: Use dried extract, tea, infusion or tincture

Teach Client/Family
- Teach the client that black catechu should not be used in pregnancy, in lactation, or for children until more research is completed with these populations.
- Inform the client that constipation may occur.

Pharmacology

Pharmacokinetics

Pharmacokinetics and pharmacodynamics are unknown.

Primary Chemical Components of Black Catechu and Their Possible Actions		
Chemical Class	**Individual Component**	**Possible Action**
Flavonoids	Catechu-red Galactopyranosyl (Yadava et al, 2002)	Decreases gastrointestinal inflammation
Catechu tannic acid Acacatechin Quercetin Gum		

Actions

Very little research is available on the actions of black catechu. A few animal studies are available, but most information comes from anecdotal reports.

Antidiabetic Action

One study identified the hypoglycemic action of black catechu using animals (Singh, 1976).

Cardiovascular Action

One small study (Sham, 1984) identified the hypotensive action of this herb.

Other Actions

The other actions studied include contraception (Azad et al, 1984) and antineoplastic effect (Agrawal et al, 1990). The antineoplastic effect was tested on leukemic cells, including chronic myeloid, acute myeloblastic, acute lymphoblastic, and chronic lymphocytic. All types showed a marked reduction in leukemic cells.

References

Agrawal S et al: Preliminary observations on leukaemic specific agglutinins from seeds, *Indian J Med Res* 92:38-42, 1990.

Azad AK et al: Antifertility activity of a traditional contraceptive pill comprising *Acacia catechu, A. arabica,* and *Tragia involuceria, Indian J Med Res* 80:372-374, 1984.

Sham JS et al: Hypertensive action of *Acacia catechu, Planta Med* 50:177-180, 1984.

Singh KN et al: Hypotensive action of *Acacia catechu, Planta Med* 50:177-180, 1976.

Yadava RN et al: A new flavone glycoside from the stem of *Acacia.* 2000.

Black Cohosh
(blak koe'hahsh)

Scientific names: *Actaea racemosa, Cimicifuga racemosa*

Other common names: Black snakeroot, bugbane, bugwort, cimicifuga, fairy candles, rattleroot, rattleweed, squaw root

Class 2b/2c

Origin: Black cohosh is a perennial that grows in the eastern region of the United States and in parts of Canada.

Uses

Reported Uses

Black cohosh is used as a smooth-muscle relaxant, an antispasmodic, an antitussive, an astringent, a diuretic, an antidiarrheal, an antiarthritic, and a hormone balancer in perimenopausal women. It is also used to decrease uterine spasms in the first trimester of pregnancy, as an antiabortion agent, and as a treatment for dysmenorrhea. For children it is used as an antiasthmatic, for measles, and for chicken pox.

Investigational Uses

Investigation is ongoing into the use of black cohosh to treat menopausal symptoms.

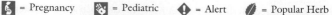

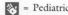 = Pregnancy   = Pediatric   ◆ = Alert   ✔ = Popular Herb

Product Availability and Dosages
Available Forms
Caplets: 40, 400, 420 mg; capsules: 25, 525 mg; fluid extract; powdered rhizome; solid (dry) powdered extract; tincture

Plant Parts Used: Rhizome (dried and fresh); roots

Dosages and Routes
Adult
All dosages listed are PO.
- Caplets/capsules: 500-600 mg tid standardized to 1 mg triterpenes (27-deoxyactein) per caplet/capsule
- Extract: 3-4 ml tid (1:1)
- Powdered rhizome: 1-2 g
- Solid dry powdered extract: 250-500 mg (4:1)
- Tincture: 4-6 ml (1:5) bid-tid; or 0.4 ml qd (1:10) (Blumenthal, 1998)
- Decoction 1.5-9 g qd

Precautionary Information
Contraindications
Because uterine stimulation can occur, black cohosh should not be used during pregnancy. However, it can be used in the first trimester of pregnancy to decrease uterine spasms and as an antiabortion agent. Black cohosh should not be used during lactation and should not be given to children except under the supervision of a qualified herbalist. Black cohosh should not be used in patients with a history of estrogen receptor–positive breast cancer. Class 2b/2c herb.

Side Effects/Adverse Reactions
Cardiovascular: Hypotension, slow heart rate
Endocrine: Uterine stimulation, miscarriage
Gastrointestinal: Nausea, vomiting, anorexia

Interactions with Black Cohosh

Drug

Antihypertensives: Black cohosh increases the action of anti-hypertensives; avoid concurrent use.

Hormone replacement therapy: Black cohosh may alter the effects of other hormone replacement therapies; use together cautiously.

Oral Contraceptives: Black cohosh may increase the effects; avoid concurrent use.

Sedatives/Hypnotics: Black cohosh may increase the hypotension; avoid concurrent use.

Food	Herb	Lab Test
None known	None known	None known

Client Considerations

Assess

- Assess for menopausal and menstrual irregularities: length of cycle, amount of flow, spotting, pain, and hot flashes.
- Assess for the presence of ovarian cysts or fibroids.
- Assess for the use of other hormonal products: estrogen, progesterone, oral contraceptives, thyroid products, steroids, and androgens. Concurrent use requires caution (see Interactions).

Administer

- Instruct the client to take black cohosh PO using standardized products.

Teach Client/Family

- Caution the client not to use black cohosh during pregnancy and lactation unless under the supervision of a qualified herbalist and not to give it to children.

Pharmacology

Pharmacokinetics

Pharmacokinetics and pharmacodynamics are unknown.

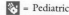 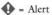

Primary Chemical Components of Black Cohosh and Their Possible Actions

Chemical Class	Individual Component	Possible Action
Acid	Caffeic acid; Fukinolic acid; Cimicifugic acids (A, B, E, F)	Inhibits neutrophil elastase
	Ferulic acid Isoferulic acid Salicylic acid	Antiinflammatory
Triterpene glycoside	Actein; 27-Deoxyactein; Cimicifugoside; Cimicifugoside (B, M)	
Actacaepoxide		
Cycloartane glycoside		
Flavonoid	Formononetin	Phytoestrogenic
Caffeic acid derivative	Isoferulic acid	
Tannins		
Saponins		

Actions

Black cohosh has been researched extensively in the past few years, primarily for its effects when used to treat menopausal symptoms.

Estrogenic Action

In a very large study involving more than 100 physicians and more than 600 female patients, cimicifuga extract was given. Within 6 to 8 weeks, both physical and psychological menopausal symptoms improved significantly. Most improved within 4 weeks (Stolze, 1982). Another double-blind study included 60 female patients who received cimicifuga extract, conjugated estrogens, or diazepam for 12 weeks. Patients using cimicifuga extract showed a significant improvement compared with patients using the two drugs (Warnecke, 1985). In a third study (also double blind), 80 female patients received cimicifuga extract, conjugated estrogens, or a placebo for 12 weeks. Those taking cimicifuga showed better results on the Kupperman

Menopausal Index than the other patients (Stoll, 1987). These studies and others provide adequate evidence to support the use of black cohosh as an alternative to estrogen therapy in menopausal women. Unlike estrogens, black cohosh does not affect the secretion of prolactin, follicle-stimulating hormone, luteinizing hormone (Freudenstein, 2002). A new study (Zierau, 2002) identified contradictory results from previous studies. In this study antiestrogen results occurred when estradiol activities were antagonized.

Bone Resorption Action

No long-term studies have provided information on the role of black cohosh in the prevention of osteoporosis. However, epidemiological studies have shown that black cohosh prevents osteoporosis in postmenopausal women.

References

Blumenthal M (ed): The complete German Commission E monographs: therapeutic guide to herbal medicines, Austin, TX, American Botanical Council; Boston, Integrative Medical Communications, 1998.

Freudenstein J et al: Lack of promotion of estrogen-dependent mammary gland tumors in vivo by an isopropanitic *Cimicifuga racemosa* extract, *Cancer Res* 62(12):3448-3452, 2002.

Stoll W: Phytopharmacon influences atrophic vaginal epithelium: double-blind study—cimicifuga vs. estrogenic substances, *Therapeuticum* 1:23-31, 1987.

Stolze H: An alternative to treatment menopausal complaints, *Gynecol* 3:14-16, 1982.

Warnecke G: Influencing menopausal symptoms with a phytotherapeutic agent, *Med Walt* 36:871-874, 1985.

Zierau O et al: Antiestrogenic activities of Cimicifuga racemosa extracts, *J Steroid Biochem Mol Biol* 80(1):125-130, 2000.

Black Haw
(blak haw)

Scientific names: *Viburnum prunifolium; Viburnum opulus*

Other common names: American sloe, cramp bark, guelder-rose, may rose, nannyberry, sheepberry, shonny, silver bells, sloe, stagbush, sweet haw, sweet viburnum

Class 2d

Origin: Black haw is found in the eastern region of the United States.

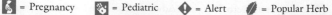

🜂 = Pregnancy   🐾 = Pediatric   ❗ = Alert   🌿 = Popular Herb

Uses

Reported Uses

Black haw is used as a diuretic; an antispasmodic; a sedative; for headaches, arthritis, fever, and other pains; as a uterine relaxant; and to treat dysmenorrhea and cardiovascular conditions such as hypertension.

Product Availability and Dosages

Available Forms

Capsules, extract, tablets

Plant Parts Used: Bark of the roots, stem, or trunk

Dosages and Routes

Adult

- PO decoction: may be taken tid; may also be used with other herbs (peppermint, chamomile, cramp bark, false unicorn root)

Precautionary Information

Contraindications

Persons with kidney stones should use this herb cautiously. Do not use black haw in pregnancy or lactation (Jarobe, 1966). Class 2d herb.

Side Effects/Adverse Reactions

Gastrointestinal: Gastrointestinal upset, irritation

Interactions with Black Haw

Drug

Anticoagulants (aspirin, heparin, warfarin): Black haw increases the action of anticoagulants; do not use concurrently.

Food	Herb	Lab Test
None known	None known	None known

Client Considerations

Assess

- Assess for allergic reactions such as rash, chest tightness, and trouble breathing. If present, administer antihistamine or other appropriate therapy.

🍂 Endangered Herb   Adverse effects: BOLD = life-threatening

- Assess for bleeding; check for the use of aspirin, NSAIDs, and anticoagulants (see Interactions).
- Assess for menstrual discomfort and relief after using this herb.

Administer

- Instruct the client to take black haw as an infusion or tea.

Teach Client/Family

- Because uterine relaxation occurs, caution the client to use black haw during pregnancy, lactation only under the supervision of a qualified herbalist. May be given to children as an antispasmodic.

Pharmacology

Pharmacokinetics

Pharmacokinetics and pharmacodynamics are unknown.

Primary Chemical Components of Black Haw and Their Possible Actions		
Chemical Component	**Individual Component**	**Possible Action**
Coumarin	Scopoletin	Antispasmodic
	Scoplin; aesculetin	
Phenol acid	Salicin; Salicylic acids	
Flavonoid	Amentoflavon	
Oxalate		
Volatile oil		
Tannin		
Resin		
Triterpenoids	Virgatic acid; Vibsanin B; 3-Hydroxyvibsanin E; Oleanadien (Fukuyama, 2002)	

Actions

The only major action of black haw that has been studied is its ability to reduce uterine excitability in laboratory animals (Reynolds, 1996). However, preliminary studies have shown cardiovascular activity of the iridoid glucosides of *Viburnum prunifolium* (Cometa, 1998). One other study showed a digitalis-like activity on frogs and guinea pigs (Vlad, 1977).

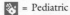

= Pregnancy   = Pediatric   ◆ = Alert   ∕∕ = Popular Herb

References

Cometa MF et al: Preliminary studies on cardiovascular activity of *Viburnum prunifolium* L. and its iridoid glucosides, *Fitoterapia* suppl: (5):23, 1998.

Fukuyama Y et al: Triterpenoids from *Viburnum* suspension, *Phytochemistry* 60(8):765-768, 2002.

Jarobe CH et al: Uterine relaxant properties of *Viburnum*, *Nature* 50(64):837, 1966.

Reynolds JEF, editor: *Martindale: the extra pharmacopoeia*, ed 31, London, 1996, Royal Pharmaceutical Society, p 1555.

Vlad L et al: Digitalis-type cardiotonic action of *Viburnum* species extracts, *Planta Med* (31):228, 1977.

Black Hellebore
(blak heh-luh-bowr)

Scientific name: *Helleborus niger*

Other common names: Christe herbe, Christmas rose, Easter rose, melampode

Origin: Black hellebore is a perennial ornamental plant.

Uses

Reported Uses

Black hellebore traditionally has been used as an anthelmintic, antianxiety, and antipsychotic; as a treatment for restlessness; and for its laxative effect. It has also been used to induce abortion and to treat pregnancy-induced hypertension, amenorrhea, and central nervous system conditions such as seizure disorders, meningitis, and encephalitis.

Investigational Uses

Investigation is ongoing into the use of black hellebore as an immunostimulant for cancer patients.

Product Availability and Dosages

Available Forms

Fluid extract, powdered root, solid extract

Plant Parts Used: Rhizome (dried), root

🌐 Endangered Herb   Adverse effects: BOLD = life-threatening

Dosages and Routes
Adult
All dosages listed are PO.
Laxative
- Fluid extract: 1-10 drops prn
- Powder: 10-20 grains prn
- Solid extract: 1-2 grains prn

No other dosage information is available.

Precautionary Information

Contraindications

Because it can cause abortion, black hellebore should not be used during pregnancy. Until more research is available, this herb should not be used during lactation and should not be given to children. Persons with hypersensitivity to black hellebore should not use it. This plant is considered poisonous; therefore its use is discouraged.

Side Effects/Adverse Reactions

Cardiovascular: Hypertension, hypotension, BRADYCARDIA, ARRHYTHMIAS

Central Nervous System: Dizziness, paresthesia, SEIZURES

Gastrointestinal: Nausea, vomiting, anorexia, diarrhea, abdominal cramps, burning in throat

Integumentary: HYPERSENSITIVITY REACTIONS, dermatitis

Respiratory: Shortness of breath, RESPIRATORY FAILURE RELATED TO CONTAMINATION OF THE HERB

Toxicity: NAUSEA, VOMITING, DIARRHEA, ABDOMINAL PAIN, CHANGE IN VISION, BURNING THROAT, COMA, PARALYSIS

Interactions with Black Hellebore

Drug	Food	Lab Test
None known	None known	None known

Herb

Hypokalemia can result from the use of buckthorn or cascara sagrada with *Helleborus* spp.; avoid concurrent use.

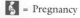 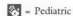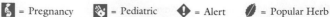

Client Considerations

Assess

- Assess for hypersensitivity reactions. If present, discontinue use of this herb and administer antihistamine or other appropriate therapy.
- Determine the reason the client is using black hellebore and suggest safer, more conventional alternatives. This herb is rarely used because its toxic and therapeutic levels are so close.

Administer

- Instruct the client to store black hellebore in a cool, dry place, away from heat and moisture.

Teach Client/Family

- Because it can cause abortion, caution the client not to use black hellebore during pregnancy. Until more research is available, caution the client not to use this herb during lactation and not to give it to children.
- Advise the client that this plant is considered poisonous and should not be used. Black hellebore is commonly contaminated with other *Helleborus* spp., which yields a more poisonous plant.

Pharmacology

Pharmacokinetics

Pharmacokinetics and pharmacodynamics are unknown.

Primary Chemical Components of Black Hellebore and Their Possible Actions		
Chemical Class	**Individual Components**	**Possible Action**
Agylcone Glycosides	Hellebrin Helleborin; Helleborcin; Bufadienole	Toxicity
Saponosides **Resin** **Ranunculosides**		

Actions

Black hellebore is considered poisonous. Most herbal practitioners do not use it because of the potential for toxic reactions. Its only identified therapeutic actions are its possible antifungal and antineoplastic properties. Very little research has been done on this herb because it is so toxic.

Reference

Bussing A et al: Effects of phytopreparation from *Helleborus niger* on immunocompetent cells in vitro, *J Ethnopharmacol* 59:139-146, 1998.

Black Pepper
(blak peh'pur)

Scientific name: *Piper nigrum*

Other common names: Biber, filfil, hu-chiao, kosho, krishnadi, lada, pepe, peper, pfeffer, phi noi, pimenta, pjerets, poivre, the king of spices, the master spice

Class 1 (Fruit)

Origin: Black pepper is found in the Spice Islands.

Uses

Reported Uses

Black pepper traditionally has been used internally to treat gastrointestinal symptoms such as flatus, anorexia, indigestion, heartburn, peptic ulcers, abdominal pain, cramps, colic, diarrhea, and constipation. It has also been used to treat joint and respiratory disorders and to stimulate mental processes. It is used externally to treat neuralgia and scabies.

Product Availability and Dosages

Available Forms

Powder

Plant Parts Used: Fruit

Dosages and Routes

No published dosages are available.

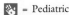 = Pregnancy   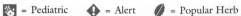 = Pediatric   ◆ = Alert   ✐ = Popular Herb

B

Precautionary Information

Contraindications

Until more research is available, black pepper should not be used therapeutically during pregnancy and lactation and should not be given therapeutically to children. Black pepper should not be used therapeutically by persons with hypersensitivity to it. Class 1 herb (fruit).

Side Effects/Adverse Reactions

Integumentary: Hypersensitivity reactions
Respiratory: **Apnea** (large amounts in children)
Miscellaneous: Weak carcinogenic action

Interactions with Black Pepper

Drug
Concurrent use of black pepper with drugs metabolized by cytochrome P-450 should be avoided.

Food	Herb	Lab Test
None known	None known	None known

Client Considerations

Assess

- Assess for hypersensitivity reactions. If these are present, discontinue use of black pepper and administer antihistamine or other appropriate therapy.
- Assess for the use of drugs metabolized by cytochrome P-450 (see Interactions).

Administer

- Instruct the client to store black pepper in a cool, dry place, away from heat and moisture.

Teach Client/Family

- Until more research is available, caution the client not to use black pepper therapeutically during pregnancy and lactation and not to give it therapeutically to children.

 Endangered Herb   Adverse effects: BOLD = life-threatening

Pharmacology

Pharmacokinetics

Pharmacokinetics and pharmacodynamics are unknown.

Primary Chemical Components of Black Pepper and Their Possible Actions		
Chemical Class	**Individual Component**	**Possible Action**
Alkaloid	Piperine	Melanocyte proliferation (Lin, 1999); hepatoprotective (Koul, 1993); antiinflammatory (Mujumdar, 1990)
	Piperyline; Piperlongumine; Piperidine; Piperettine; Piperanine; Chavicin	
Essential oil	Sabinene; Carvone; Myrcene; Limonene; Borneol; Carvacrol; Linalool; Alpha-pinene; Beta-pinene; Humelene; Bisabolone; Caryophyllene; Limonene	Aromatic
Safrole		Weak carcinogen
Eugenol		
Myristicin		
Tannic acid		Weak carcinogen
Amide	Feruperine	Antioxidant (Nakatani, 1986)

Actions

Black pepper has been researched for its melanocyte proliferation, antibacterial and antioxidant actions, and chemoprotective/carcinogenic action.

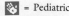 = Pregnancy   = Pediatric   = Alert   = Popular Herb

Melanocyte Proliferation

One recent study undertaken to identify repigmenting agents (Lin, 1999) identified the ability of black pepper to promote melanocyte proliferation. Black pepper was found to stimulate melanocyte growth. This was also true of piperine, one of the alkaloids of black pepper.

Antibacterial and Antioxidant Actions

Two studies have identified the antibacterial properties of black pepper (Dorman, 2000). One study focused on several herbs possessing powerful antibacterial effects. The other study demonstrated the antibacterial effect of black pepper against *Staphylococcus aureus* growth. *Piper nigrum* was also found to act as an antioxidant when it was studied to determine its potential application in food preservation (Nakatani, 1986).

Chemoprotective/Carcinogenic Action

Several studies have focused on the carcinogenic properties of black pepper. Most of these studies used laboratory animals that were force-fed black pepper in large amounts. These laboratory animals developed various tumors, depending on the study (El-Mofty, 1988, 1991; Shwaireb, 1990). Other studies have shown a chemoprotective effect in the colon. This effect may be due to the reduction of toxins (Nalini, 1998).

References

Dorman HJ et al: Antimicrobial agents from plants: antibacterial activity of plant volatile oils, *J Appl Microbiol* 88(2):308-316, 2000.

El-Mofty MM et al: Carcinogenicity testing of black pepper *(Piper nigrum)* using the Egyptian toad *(Bufo regularis)* as a quick biological test animal, *Oncology* 43(3):247-252, 1988.

El-Mofty MM et al: Carinogenic effect of force-feeding an extract of black pepper *(Piper nigrum)* in Egyptian toads *(Bufo regularis)*, *Oncology* 48(4):347-350, 1991.

Koul IB et al: Evaluation of the liver protective potential of piperine, an active principle of black and long peppers, *Planta Med* 59(5):413-417, 1993.

Lin Z et al: Stimulation of mouse melanocyte proliferation by *Piper nigrum* fruit extract and its main alkaloid, piperine, *Planta Med* 65(7):600-603, 1999.

Mujumdar AM et al: Anti-inflammatory activity of piperine, *Jpn J Med Sci Biol* 43(3):91-100, 1990.

Nakatani K et al: Chemical constituents of peppers *(Piper* sp.) and application to food preservation: naturally occurring antioxidative compounds, *Environ Health Perspect* 67:135-142, 1986.

Nalini N et al: Influence of spices on the bacterial activity in experimental colon cancer, *J Ethnopharmacol* 62:15-24, 1998.

Shwaireb MH et al: Carcinogenesis induced by black pepper *(Piper nigrum)* and modulated by vitamin A, *Exp Pathol* 40(4):233-238, 1990.

Black Root
(blak rewt)

Scientific names: *Veronicastrum virginicum, Leptandra virginica, Veronica virginica*

Other common names: Bowman root, brinton root, Culver's physic, Culver's root, high veronica, hini, leptandra, physic root, quitel, tall speed-well, Veronica

Class 1 (Dried Root)
Class 2b/2d (Fresh Root)

Origin: Black root is found in the United States and Canada.

Uses
Reported Uses
Black root is used as an emetic, a diuretic, and an astringent, as well as to relieve jaundice. This herb is rarely used today.

Product Availability and Dosages
Available Forms
Root (dried and fresh), tincture

Plant Parts Used: Rhizome, roots

Dosages and Routes
Adult
- PO tea: 1-2 tsp dried root, mixed in cold water, then boiled and steeped for 15 min
- PO tincture: 1-2 ml tid

Precautionary Information
Contraindications
Black root should not be used during pregnancy and lactation and should not be given to children. Class 1 herb (dried root); class 2b/2d herb (fresh root).

Side Effects/Adverse Reactions
Central Nervous System: Headache, drowsiness

 = Pregnancy    = Pediatric   = Alert   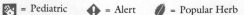 = Popular Herb

Precautionary Information—cont'd
Side Effects/Adverse Reactions—cont'd
Gastrointestinal: Nausea, vomiting, anorexia, abdominal cramps, stool color change; HEPATOTOXICITY (large amounts of dried leaves)

Interactions with Black Root

Drug
Atropine: Black root forms an insoluble complex with atropine; do not use concurrently.
Cardiac glycosides: Black root forms an insoluble complex with cardiac glycosides; do not use concurrently.
Hepatotoxic agents: Avoid the concurrent use of black root with any hepatotoxic agents.
Scopolamine: Black root forms an insoluble complex with scopolamine; do not use concurrently.

Food	Herb	Lab Test
None known	None known	None known

Client Considerations
Assess

- Assess liver function test results (AST, ALT); monitor for hepatotoxicity, including jaundice, fever, and increases in liver function levels. If increased levels are present, discontinue use of this herb.

Administer

- Caution the client to avoid the consumption of dried leaves; hepatotoxicity can occur.

Teach Client/Family

- Until more research is available, caution the client not to use black root during pregnancy and lactation and not to give it to children.

Pharmacology
Pharmacokinetics
Pharmacokinetics and pharmacodynamics are unknown.

Primary Chemical Components of Black Root and Their Possible Actions

Chemical Class	Individual Component	Possible Action
Volatile oil	Verosterol	
Tannic acid		Astringent; wound healing
Leptandrin		
Acid	Cinnamic acid; Parameth-oxycinnamic acid	
Resin		
Gum		
Mannite		Diuretic
D-Mannitol		

Actions

Very little primary research is available for black root. In traditional herbal medicine, black root has been used for the astringent properties of its tannic acid component and the diuretic effect of d-mannitol/mannite.

Blessed Thistle
(bleh'suhd thi'sul)

Scientific names: *Carbenia benedicta, Cnicus benedictus, Carduus benedictus*

Other common names: Cardo santo, chardon benit, holy thistle, kardobenediktenkraut, spotted thistle, St. Benedict thistle

Class 2b

Origin: Blessed thistle is an annual found in Europe and Asia.

Uses

Reported Uses

Blessed thistle is used to treat anorexia, gastrointestinal discomfort, to improve digestion, to improve memory, for liver

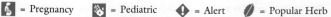

disorders such as jaundice, hepatitis, myrroghia, and dyspepsia, as well as to stimulate lactation.

Product Availability and Dosages
Available Forms
Capsules, dried herb, tea, tincture

Plant Parts Used: Dried leaves, upper stems, seeds

Dosages and Routes
Adult
• PO: 4-6 g herb qd (Blumenthal, 1998)

Precautionary Information
Contraindications
Blessed thistle should not be used during pregnancy and should not be given to children. It should not be used by persons with hypersensitivity to this herb. Class 2b herb.

Side Effects/Adverse Reactions
Gastrointestinal: Nausea, vomiting, anorexia
Integumentary: Contact dermatitis
Systemic: Hypersensitivity

Interactions with Blessed Thistle

Drug	Food
None known	None known

Herb
Asteraceae species (arnica, boneset, burdock, bullerbur, carlile thistle, chamomile, chicory, colts' foot daisy, dandelion, echinacea, elecampane, feverfew, goldenrod, lutein, marigold, milk thistle, mugwort, ragwort, safflower, santonica, saw palmetto, southern wood, stevia, tansy, wild lettuce, wormwood, yarrow): May cause cross sensitivity.

Lab Test
None known

 Endangered Herb   Adverse effects: BOLD = life-threatening

Client Considerations

Assess

- Assess for allergic reactions and contact dermatitis; if these are present, discontinue use of this herb.

Administer

- Instruct the client to store blessed thistle in a cool, dry place, away from heat and moisture.

Teach Client/Family

- Until more research is available, caution the client not to use blessed thistle during pregnancy and not to give it to children.
- Inform the client that research on this herb is lacking.

Pharmacology

Pharmacokinetics

Pharmacokinetics and pharmacodynamics are unknown.

Primary Chemical Components of Blessed Thistle and Their Possible Actions		
Chemical Class	**Individual Component**	**Possible Action**
Lactone	Cnicin Salonitenolide	Weak cytotoxic

Actions

Blessed thistle has primarily been used to stimulate the appetite and increase gastric secretion. However, some reports indicate that this herb may possess antiinfective properties.

References

Blumenthal M, editor: *The complete German Commission E monographs: therapeutic guide to herbal medicines,* Austin, Tex, American Botanical Council; Boston, Integrative Medicine Communication, 1998.

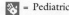 = Pregnancy   = Pediatric   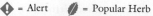 ◆ = Alert   ⬦ = Popular Herb

B

Bloodroot
(bluhd'rewt)

Scientific name: *Sanguinaria canadensis* L.

Other common names: Coon root, Indian paint, paucon, pauson, red puccoon, redroot, sweet slumber, tetterwort

Class 2b/2d

Origin: Bloodroot is a perennial found in Canada and the southern region of the United States.

Uses

Reported Uses

Bloodroot has been used for its expectorant, antimicrobial, antiinflammatory, antiplaque, and antifungal properties; as a topical treatment for skin, ear, and nose cancer; and as a treatment for nasal polyps.

Product Availability and Dosages

Available Forms

Extract, tincture

Plant Parts Used: Rhizome

Dosages and Routes

Adult
- PO extract: 0.06-0.3 ml tid (1:1 in 60% alcohol)
- PO tincture: 0.3-2 ml tid

Precautionary Information

Contraindications

Bloodroot should not be used during pregnancy and lactation, and it should not be given to children. It should not be used to treat deep wounds. The FDA classifies this herb as unsafe; therefore this herb should be used only under the supervision of a qualified herbalist. Handling the fresh root without gloves can cause skin irritation. Class 2b/2d herb.

Side Effects/Adverse Reactions

Cardiovascular: HYPOTENSION, SHOCK, COMA (excessive doses)

Continued

Precautionary Information—cont'd
Side Effects/Adverse Reactions—cont'd
Central Nervous System: Headache, CENTRAL NERVOUS SYSTEM DEPRESSION, LOSS OF CONSCIOUSNESS
Gastrointestinal: Nausea, vomiting, anorexia

Interactions with Bloodroot

Drug
Antihypertensives: Bloodroot may increase the hypotensive effects of antihypertensives.

Food	Herb	Lab Test
None known	None known	None known

Client Considerations

Assess

- Assess the client's cardiovascular status (blood pressure; pulse, including character) and level of consciousness. Hypotension, shock, and coma may occur with increased doses.
- Determine the quantity of the herb ingested.

Administer

- Caution the client to take only carefully calculated doses of bloodroot. Higher doses can lead to coma.
- Caution the client to not take orally the juice or powdered rhizome of bloodroot; may cause toxicity.

Teach Client/Family

- Until more research is available, caution the client not to use bloodroot during pregnancy and lactation and to not give it to children.
- Caution the client to use bloodroot only under the direction of a competent herbalist. Bloodroot is considered unsafe by the FDA.

Pharmacology

Pharmacokinetics

Pharmacokinetics and pharmacodynamics are unknown.

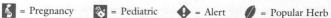

 = Pregnancy　　 = Pediatric　　◆ = Alert　　✦ = Popular Herb

Primary Chemical Components of Bloodroot and Their Possible Actions		
Chemical Class	**Individual Component**	**Possible Action**
Alkaloid	Sanguinarine	Hypotensive, dental antiplaque, central nervous system depressant, antimicrobial, antimycobacterial
	Homochelidonine; Sanguidimerine; Chelirubine; Sanguilutine; Allocryptopine	
	Chelerythrine	Antimycobacterial (Newton, 2002)
	Protopine; Oxysanguinarine; Berberine; Coptisine	
Resin		

B

Actions

The use of bloodroot is considered to be obsolete because of its toxicity. However, its various actions account for its continued use.

Analgesic Action

The analgesic action of bloodroot occurs via mechanisms similar to those of opioids, with paralysis of the nerve endings leading to lessened pain.

Antiplaque Action

The antiplaque action of bloodroot is well documented in the literature. Some toothpaste and mouthwash manufacturers include bloodroot as an ingredient to help limit oral plaque. The alkaloid sanguinarine is effective against various oral bacteria (Dzink, 1985; Godowski, 1989). This action appears to be due to an alkaloid present in the herb.

Topical Action

Bloodroot has been found to corrode and destroy topical cancers and topical fungal infections (Phelan, 1963). In cancers of the nose and ears, bloodroot has been shown to destroy these lesions.

References

Dzink JL et al: Comparative in vitro activity of sanguinarine against oral microbial isolates, *Antimicrob Agents Chemother* 27:663, 1985.

Godowski KC: Antimicrobial action of sanguinarine, *J Clin Dent* 1:96-101, 1989.

Newton SM et al: The evaluation of forty-three plant species for in vitro antimycobacterial activities; isolation of active constituents from *Psoralea corylifolia* and *Sanguineria canadensis, J Ethnopharmacol* 79(1): 57-67, 2002.

Phelan JT et al: *Surgery* 53:310, 1963.

Blue Cohosh
(blew koe'hahsh)

Scientific name: *Caulophyllum thalictroides*

Other common names: Blue ginseng, papoose root, squaw root, yellow ginseng

Class 2b

Origin: Blue cohosh is a perennial found in the midwestern and eastern regions of the United States.

Uses
Reported Uses

Blue cohosh is used as an anticonvulsant and antispasmodic, to induce labor, to treat rheumatism, and to increase menstrual flow.

Product Availability and Dosages
Available Forms

Capsules: 500 mg; dried root; powder; tablets; tea; tincture

Plant Parts Used: Aerial parts, rhizome, roots

Dosages and Routes
Adult

- PO dried root/rhizome: 0.3-1 g tid
- PO extract: 0.5-1 ml tid (1:1 in 70% alcohol)

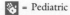

Precautionary Information

Contraindications

Because blue cohosh is a uterine stimulant, it should not be used during pregnancy. Until more research is available, this herb should not be used during lactation and should not be given to children; the seeds are poisonous to children. Persons with cardiac disease should not use blue cohosh. Class 2b herb.

Side Effects/Adverse Reactions

Cardiovascular: Chest pain, hypertension
Endocrine: Hyperglycemia
Gastrointestinal: Gastrointestinal irritation, cramps, diarrhea, mucous membrane irritation
Reproductive: EMBRYOTOXIC
Systemic: Nicotinic toxicity (Rao, 2002)

Interactions with Blue Cohosh

Drug

Antianginals: Blue cohosh may decrease the action of antianginals, causing chest pain; do not use concurrently.
Antidiabetics: Blue cohosh may decrease the action of antidiabetics; avoid concurrent use.
Antihypertensives: When used with antihypertensives, blue cohosh will decrease their action and increase blood pressure; do not use concurrently.
Nicotine: Blue cohosh will increase the effects of nicotine and may cause toxicity; do not use concurrently.

Food	Herb	Lab Test
None known	None known	None known

Client Considerations

Assess

- Assess cardiac status (blood pressure; pulse, including character, rate, and rhythm). Assess for the use of antianginals, antihypertensives, and nicotine, which may affect the cardiovascular status (see Interactions).
- Assess diabetic clients for hypoglycemia; check glucose levels.

 Endangered Herb   Adverse effects: BOLD = life-threatening

• Assess for toxicity; look for signs similar to those of nicotine poisoning (tachycardia, diaphoresis, abdominal pain, vomiting, muscle weakness, fasciculations).

Administer

• Ensure that commercial preparations are taken in the correct dosage.

Teach Client/Family

• Because uterine stimulation can occur, caution the client not to use blue cohosh during pregnancy. (Herbalists use blue cohosh to induce labor.) Until more research is available, caution the client to avoid the use of this herb during lactation and not to give it to children.

• Caution the client to keep blue cohosh products out of the reach of children; seeds are poisonous to children.

• Advise the client not to use nicotine products while using blue cohosh. The effects of nicotine will be increased.

Pharmacology

Pharmacokinetics

Pharmacokinetics and pharmacodynamics are unknown.

Primary Chemical Components of Blue Cohosh and Their Possible Actions		
Chemical Class	**Individual Component**	**Possible Action**
Alkaloid	Methylcystine	Central nervous system stimulant; nicotinic toxicity (Rao, 2002)
	Taspine	Embryotoxicity (Kennelly, 1999)
	Magnoflorine; Anagyrine; Baptifoline; Ubiquitous Thalictroidine; Lupanine; Sparteine	Uterine stimulant
Saponin	Caulosaponin; Cauloside	
Phosphoric acid		
Phytosterol		

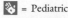 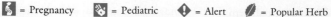

Actions

Embryotoxic Action

Blue cohosh is known to contain embryotoxic alkaloids (Jones, 1998). Both blue and black cohosh have been used for centuries to stimulate uterine contractions. However, studies have only recently confirmed the embryotoxic nature of blue cohosh. Two studies have shown significant embryotoxicity when a mother ingested blue cohosh to stimulate uterine contractions. In one case, the infant was born with acute myocardial infarction associated with congestive heart failure and shock (Jones, 1998).

Uterine Stimulant Action

Four of the alkaloids present in blue cohosh—baptifoline, anagyrine, ubiquitous, and magnoflorine—were tested to determine their uterine stimulant actions. Research revealed that the four are effective only when present together. When tested individually, each exhibited marginal uterotonic activity but showed no uterine stimulant activity. Saponins of the root and rhizome exert a definite oxytocic action, increasing the tone and rate of contractions (Brinker, 1995).

References

Brinker FJ: *Eclectic dispensatory of botanical therapeutics,* vol 2, Sandy, Ore, 1995, Eclectic.

Jones TK et al: Profound neonatal congestive heart failure caused by maternal consumption of blue cohosh herbal medication, *J Pediatr* 132(3 pt 1):550-552, 1998.

Kennelly EF et al: Detecting potential teratogenic alkaloids from blue cohosh rhizomes using an in vitro rat embryo culture, *J Nat Prod* 62(10):1385-1389, 1999.

Rao RB et al: Nicotinic toxicity from tincture of blue cohosh *(Caulophyllum thalictroides)* used as an abortifacient, *Vet Hum Toxicol* 44(4):221-222, 2002.

Blue Flag
(blew flag)

Scientific name: *Iris versicolor*

Other common names: Dagger flower, dragon flower, flag lily, fleur-de-lis, flower-de-luce, liver lily, poison flag, snake lily, water flag, wild iris   **Class 2b/2d**

Origin: Blue flag is a perennial found in the wetlands of the United States.

Uses

Reported Uses

Blue flag is used primarily for its antimicrobial effects. It is also used for its laxative side effect and its emetic and diuretic properties. Blue flag is used topically to treat sores, bites, and bruises.

Product Availability and Dosages

Available Forms

Extract: 0.5-1 fluid drams (2.5-5 ml); powdered root: 20 grains (1300 mg); solid extract: 10-15 grains (650-975 mg); tincture: 1-3 fluid drams (5-15 ml)

Plant Parts Used: Rhizome with roots

Dosages and Routes

Adult

Laxative
- PO powdered root: 10-20 grains one-time dose
- PO tincture: ½-3 fluid drams one-time dose

Other
- Topical powdered root: make poultice, apply prn

Precautionary Information

Contraindications

Until more research is available, blue flag should not be used during pregnancy and lactation, and it should not be given to children. Class 2b/2d herb.

Side Effects/Adverse Reactions

Central Nervous System: Headache

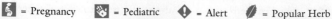

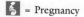 = Pregnancy   = Pediatric   = Alert   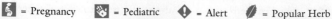 = Popular Herb

Precautionary Information—cont'd

Side Effects/Adverse Reactions—cont'd

Ear, Eye, Nose, and Throat: Mucous membrane irritation, soreness

Gastrointestinal: Nausea, vomiting, anorexia, **hepatotoxicity**

Systemic: DEATH BY POISONING

Interactions with Blue Flag			
Drug	Food	Herb	Lab Test
None known	None known	None known	None known

Client Considerations

Assess

- Assess for severe nausea and vomiting.
- Assess for irritation or soreness of the mucous membranes.
 • Assess for toxicity.

Administer

- Instruct the client to take blue flag PO to treat constipation. Dosages for other uses are not documented.

Teach Client/Family

 • Until more research is available, caution the client not to use blue flag during pregnancy and lactation and not to give it to children.
- Advise the client not to use blue flag internally except under the direction of a competent herbalist and not to use it topically near mucous membranes.

Pharmacology

Pharmacokinetics

Pharmacokinetics and pharmacodynamics are unknown.

Primary Chemical Components of Blue Flag and Their Possible Actions

Chemical Class	Individual Component	Possible Action
Volatile oil	Furfural	
Triterpene	Irigermanal	
Isoflavonoid	Irilon; Irisolone	Laxative
Xanthone	Irigenin; Tectoridine	
Flavonoid		
Starch		
Tannin		Wound healing; antiinflammatory
Gum		

Actions

Most of the information available on the actions of blue flag is based on anecdotal evidence rather than primary research. The anecdotal evidence focuses on the use of this herb as a laxative and an antiinflammatory.

Because of the toxicity of this herb, the unsupervised internal use of blue flag is not recommended.

Bogbean
(bahg'been)

Scientific name: *Menyanthes trifoliata*

Other common names: Buckbean, marsh trefoil, water shamrock

Class 2d

Origin: Bogbean is found in the wetlands of the United States and Europe.

Uses

Reported Uses

Bogbean is used as an antiinflammatory and to treat anorexia and gastrointestinal distress.

 = Pregnancy   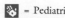 = Pediatric   ◆ = Alert   = Popular Herb

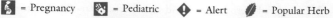

Product Availability and Dosages

Available Forms
Dried leaf, fluid extract, tincture

Plant Parts Used: Leaves

Dosages and Routes

Adult
- PO dried leaf: 1.5-3 g (Blumenthal, 1998) prepared as tea, used as often as tid
- PO fluid extract: 1-2 ml (1:1 dilution) tid with 8 oz water

Precautionary Information

Contraindications
Because uterine stimulation can occur, bogbean should not be used during pregnancy. Until more research is available, this herb should not be used during lactation and should not be given to children. Class 2d herb.

Side Effects/Adverse Reactions
Gastrointestinal: Nausea, vomiting, anorexia
Systemic: BLEEDING, HEMOLYSIS (if taken with anticoagulants, NSAIDs, antiplatelets)

Interactions with Bogbean

Drug
Anticoagulants, antiplatelets, aspirin, NSAIDS: Use of bogbean with anticoagulants, antiplatelets, aspirin, and NSAIDs may increase the risk of bleeding; do not use concurrently.

Food	Herb	Lab Test
None known	None known	None known

Client Considerations

Assess
- Assess for bleeding. Determine whether the client is also taking aspirin, NSAIDs, anticoagulants, or antiplatelets, all of which will increase the risk of bleeding.
- Assess for pain and inflammation. Determine whether the client is taking bogbean to treat these conditions.

 Endangered Herb   Adverse effects: BOLD = life-threatening

Administer

- Instruct the client to store bogbean in a cool, dry place, away from heat and moisture.

Teach Client/Family

- Because uterine stimulation can occur, caution the client not to use bogbean during pregnancy. Until more research is available, caution the client not to use bogbean during lactation and not to give it to children.
- Advise the client to avoid using bogbean with other medications that can cause bleeding: aspirin, anticoagulants, antiplatelets, NSAIDs.

Pharmacology

Pharmacokinetics

Pharmacokinetics and pharmacodynamics are unknown.

Primary Chemical Components of Bogbean and Their Possible Actions		
Chemical Class	**Individual Component**	**Possible Action**
Acid	Caffeic acid; Ferulic acid Chlorogenic acid; Salicylic acid; Vanillic acid; Folic acid; Palmitic acid	Bile stimulant
Alkaloid	Gentianin; Gentianidine; Choline	
Flavonoid	Quercetin Rutin Hyperin; Kaempferol; Trifolioside	Antiinflammatory Antioxidant
Coumarin Scopoletin Iridoid Carotene Ceryl alcohol		

Actions

Very limited primary research exists on bogbean. One study researched its analgesic effect, postulating that bogbean decreases prostaglandin synthesis (Huang, 1995). Two chemical components of bogbean, caffeic acid and ferulic acid, have been identified as bile stimulants. Antiinfective properties have also been identified (Bishop, 1951). In addition, anecdotal information suggests that bogbean stimulates the appetite and gastric juices.

References

Bishop CJ et al: A survey of higher plants for antibacterial substances, *Botany* 15:231-259, 1951.

Blumenthal M, editor: *The complete German Commission E monographs: therapeutic guide to herbal medicines,* Austin, Tex, American Botanical Council; Boston, Integrative Medicine Communication, 1998.

Huang C et al: Antiinflammatory compounds isolated from *Menyanthes trifoliata* L., *Yao Hsueh Hsueh Pao* 30:621-626, 1995.

Boldo
(bole'doe)

Scientific names: *Boldea boldus, Peumus boldus*

Other common names: Boldea, boldine, boldo-do-Chile, boldus

Class 2d

Origin: Boldo is an evergreen found in Chile, Peru, and Morocco.

Uses

Reported Uses

Boldo is used as a laxative, liver tonic, and sedative. It is also used to treat spastic conditions of the gastrointestinal tract, flatulence, gout, dysmenorrhea, colds, gout, and weakness.

Investigational Uses

Research is ongoing into the use of boldo as a treatment for gallstones.

Product Availability and Dosages

Available Forms

Extract, tea, tincture

Plant Parts Used: Leaves

🌀 Endangered Herb   Adverse effects: BOLD = life-threatening

Dosages and Routes
Adult
• PO: 3 g leaves qd (Blumenthal, 1998)

> **Precautionary Information**
> **Contraindications**
> Until more research is available, boldo should not be used during pregnancy and lactation, and it should not be given to children. Persons with neurologic or respiratory disease, obstruction of the bile duct, or severe hepatic disease should avoid the use of this herb. Persons with gallstones should use this herb cautiously. Class 2d herb.
>
> **Side Effects/Adverse Reactions**
> *Central Nervous System:* PARALYSIS, EXAGGERATED REFLEXES, CONVULSIONS, COMA, DEATH
> *Respiratory:* RESPIRATORY DEPRESSION

Interactions with Boldo			
Drug	Food	Herb	Lab Test
None known	None known	None known	None known

Client Considerations
Assess
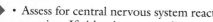
• Assess for central nervous system reactions and respiratory depression. If either is present, discontinue use of this herb.

Administer
• Instruct the client to store boldo in a cool, dry place, away from heat and moisture.

Teach Client/Family

• Until more research is available, caution the client not to use boldo during pregnancy and lactation and not to give it to children.
• Caution the client to keep boldo products out of the reach of children. This herb is toxic in high doses.

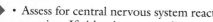 = Pregnancy   = Pediatric   = Alert   ∥ = Popular Herb

- Advise the client to avoid the use of boldo if central nervous system disorder, respiratory disorder, or severe hepatic disease is present.

Pharmacology

Pharmacokinetics

Pharmacokinetics and pharmacodynamics are unknown.

Primary Chemical Components of Boldo and Their Possible Actions		
Chemical Class	Individual Component	Possible Action
Alkaloid	Boldine; Isoboldine; Reticuline	Antispasmodic; diuretic; antiinflammatory; antipyretic; antioxidant
Flavonoid		
Volatile oil	Ascaridole	Anthelmintic
Coumarin		
Resin		
Tannin		Wound healing; antiinflammatory

Actions

Although boldo has been used to treat various conditions in many parts of the world, its actions are not well researched. Boldo is thought to possess diuretic, anthelmintic, and hepatoprotective actions. However, very little primary research is available to confirm these actions.

Diuretic Action

Boldo has been shown to possess diuretic effects. In a study of dogs given boldo, urine excretion increased by 50% (Speisky, 1994).

Anthelmintic Action

One of the chemical components of boldo, the volatile oil ascaridole, exhibits anthelmintic activity (Johnson, 1984).

Other Actions

Boldo may exert antioxidant, hepatoprotective, and antiinflammatory activity. However, little research currently exists to confirm these possible actions. Boldo has shown uterine stimulant effects and teratogenic effects in rats (Almedia, 2000). Only one study (Lanhers, 1991) could be found to confirm these effects. This study used an in vitro technique in mice. Boldine, the main alkaloid, appears to possess a hepatoprotective action but does not possess antiinflammatory action.

References

Almedia ER: Toxicological evaluation of the hydro-alcohol extract of the dry leaves of *Peumus boldus* and *Boldine* in rats, *Phytother Res* 14(2):99-102, 2000.

Blumenthal M, editor: *The complete German Commission E monographs: therapeutic guide to herbal medicines,* Austin, Tex, American Botanical Council; Boston, Integrative Medicine Communication, 1998.

Johnson MA et al: Biosynthesis of ascaridole: iodid peroxidase-catalyzed synthesis of a monoterpene endoperoxide in soluble extracts of *Chenopodium ambrosioides* fruit, *Arch Biochem Biophys* 235(1):254, 1984.

Lanhers MC et al: Hepatoprotective and antiinflammatory effects of a traditional medicinal plant of Chile, *Peumus boldus, Planta Med* 57(2):110-115, 1991.

Speisky H et al: Boldo and boldine: an emerging case of natural drug development, *Pharmacol Res* 29:1-12, 1994.

Boneset
(bown'seht)

Scientific name: *Eupatorium perfoliatum*

Other common names: Agueweed, crosswort, eupatorium, feverwort, Indian sage, Joe-pye-weed, sweating plant, thoroughwort, vegetable antimony

Class 4

Origin: Boneset is a perennial found in the wetlands of the United States and Canada.

Uses

Reported Uses

Boneset is used to treat fever, bronchitis, and influenza. It is also used as a sedative, as a laxative and an expectorant.

Investigational Uses:

Beginning research has shown antiinflammatory, immunostimulant, and wound-healing properties of boneset. Also, it has the

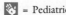 = Pregnancy   = Pediatric   ◆ = Alert   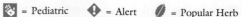 = Popular Herb

possibility of a weak antibacterial action against gram-positive organisms and a cytotoxic response.

Product Availability and Dosages

Available Forms

Extract, tea

Plant Parts Used: Dried leaves, flowers, whole herb

Dosages and Routes

Adult

- PO extract: 10-40 drops mixed in a small amount of liquid, tid
- PO tea: 2-6 tsp dried leaves (crushed) or flowers in ≥8 oz water, boiled then steeped for 15 min, tid

Precautionary Information

Contraindications

Because uterine stimulation can occur, boneset should not be used during pregnancy. Until more research is available, this herb should not be used during lactation. Persons with hypersensitivity to boneset should not use this herb, and persons with hepatic disorders should avoid the use of this herb. Avoid long-term use; toxicity can occur. Class 4 herb.

Side Effects/Adverse Reactions

Gastrointestinal: Nausea, vomiting, anorexia, diarrhea, HEPATOTOXICITY
Systemic: Hypersensitivity

Interactions with Boneset

Drug	Food	Herb	Lab Test
None known	None known	None known	None known

Client Considerations

Assess

- Assess for hepatotoxicity (jaundice, increased liver function test levels, clay-colored stools, right upper-quadrant pain). If these symptoms occur, use of this herb should be discontinued.

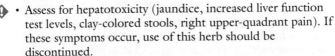

🐢 Endangered Herb   Adverse effects: BOLD = life-threatening

- Assess for gastrointestinal symptoms, nausea, vomiting, diarrhea; if these symptoms occur, use of herb should be discontinued.
- Assess for hypersensitivity reactions; if present, discontinue use of this herb.

Administer

- Instruct the client to take boneset PO as a tea or extract.
- Instruct the client to store boneset in a cool, dry place, away from heat and moisture.
- Inform the client that boneset may be given to children in small doses.

Teach Client/Family

- Because uterine stimulation can occur, caution the client not to use boneset during pregnancy. Until more research is available, advise the client not to use this herb during lactation.

Pharmacology

Pharmacokinetics

Pharmacokinetics and pharmacodynamics are unknown.

Primary Chemical Components of Boneset and Their Possible Actions		
Chemical Class	**Individual Component**	**Possible Action**
Volatile oil **Triterpenes** **Flavonoid** **Glycoside**	Kaempferol; Quercetin; Astragalin; Rutin Eupatorin	Wound healing; antiinflammatory

Actions

Immunostimulant Action

One study has demonstrated that the chemical components of boneset increase both granulocytes and macrophages (Wagner, 1985). Another study showed an increase in phagocytosis when boneset was combined with *Echinacea angustifolia*, *Baptisia tinctoria*, and *Arnica montana*. This increase in phagocytosis was much more pronounced when boneset was used in combination with the three other species than when it was used alone (Wagner, 1991).

Other Actions

Boneset has been shown to possess emetic, antiinflammatory, and antimalarial properties (Hall, 1974). A study focused on the possible effects of boneset on the common cold and showed no changes in the cold as a result of the use of this herb (Gassinger, 1981). Habtemariam (2000) discovered a weak antibacterial effect (gram-positive organisms *[Staphylococcus aureus, Bacillus megaterium]*) and a potent cytotoxic effect when compared with chlorambucil.

References

Gassinger CA et al: A controlled clinical trial for testing the efficacy of the homeopathic drug *Eupatorium perfoliatum* D2 in the treatment of the common cold, *Arzneimittelforschung* 31(4):732-736, 1981.

Habtemariam S et al: Cytotoxicity and antibacterial activity of ethanol extract from leaves of a herbal drug, boneset *(Eupatorium perfoliatum)*, *Phytother Res* 14(7):575-577, 2000.

Hall TB Jr: *Eupatorium perfoliatum:* a plant with a history, *Mo Med* 71(9):527-528, 1974.

Wagner H et al: Immunostimulating polysaccharides of higher plants, *Arzneimittelforschung* 35:1069, 1985.

Wagner H et al: Immunologic studies of plant combination preparations: in-vitro and in-vivo studies on the stimulation of phagocytosis, *Arzneimittelforschung* 41(10):1072-1076, 1991.

Borage
(baw'rij)

Scientific name: *Borage officinalis*

Other common names: Beebread, common borage, common bugloss, cool tankard, ox's tongue, starflower

Class 2a/2b/2c

Origin: Borage is an annual found in North America and Europe.

Uses

Reported Uses

Borage is used to treat arthritis, hypertension, the common cold, and bronchitis. It has been used primarily as a galactagogue but should not be used during lactation until research confirms or denies the presence of pyrrolizidine alkaloids.

Endangered Herb   Adverse effects: **BOLD** = life-threatening

Investigational Uses:
Borage may decrease body fat accumulation.

Product Availability and Dosages
Available Forms
Capsules: 240, 500, 1300 mg; seed oil

Plant Parts Used: Leaves, seeds, stems

Dosages and Routes
Adult
Joint Inflammation
- PO seed oil: 1.1-1.4 g gamma-linolenic acid qd (Pullman-Mooar, 1990; Leventhal, 1993)

Precautionary Information
Contraindications
Until more research is available, borage should not be used during pregnancy and lactation because of the possible presence of pyrrolizidine alkaloids, and it should not be given to children. Class 2a/2b/2c herb.

Side Effects/Adverse Reactions
Gastrointestinal: HEPATOTOXICITY

Interactions with Borage			
Drug	Food	Herb	Lab Test
None known	None known	None known	None known

Client Considerations
Assess
- Assess for hepatotoxicity (jaundice, increased liver function test levels, clay-colored stools, right upper-quadrant pain). If these occur, use of borage should be discontinued.
- If the client is using borage to treat joint conditions, assess for pain and inflammation (location, duration, intensity), including aggravating and alleviating factors.

- Assess blood pressure and pulse if borage is being used to treat hypertension.
- Assess body weight if using to decrease body fat accumulation.

B

Administer

- Instruct the client to use borage oil that contains 20% to 26% gamma linolenic acid.

Teach Client/Family

- Until more research is available, caution the client not to use borage during pregnancy and lactation and not to give it to children.
- Caution the client that one of the chemical components of borage, an alkaloid known as amabiline, can cause hepatotoxicity. Nettle, dandelion, and marshmallow root treat the same conditions as borage and are safer herbs; therefore they may be better choices.

Pharmacology

Pharmacokinetics

Pharmacokinetics and pharmacodynamics are unknown.

Primary Chemical Components of Borage and Their Possible Actions		
Chemical Class	Individual **Component**	**Possible Action**
Mucilage		Expectorant
Acid	Malic acid	Diuretic
Tannin		Wound healing; antiinflammatory
Essential oil		
Seeds Also Contain		
Fatty acid	Gamma-linolenic acid	Antiinflammatory; antihypertensive
	Linoleic acid	
Oleic	Saturated	
Alkaloid, pyrrolizidine	Amabiline	Hepatotoxic
	Thesinine	

Actions

Antiinflammatory Action

Several studies have demonstrated the beneficial effects of borage oil for treating rheumatoid conditions. Diets high in arachidonic acid have been shown to increase the formation of prostaglandin and leukotriene with proinflammatory action (Zurier, 1996). Two studies have shown that doses of 1.1 to 1.4 g gamma-linolenic acid in borage seed oil reduces joint inflammation significantly (Pullman-Mooar, 1990; Leventhal, 1993). A study using a combination of evening primrose oil and borage oil showed positive results in rheumatologic conditions (Belch, 2000). However, not all studies have shown positive results.

Antihypertensive Action

One study has shown that the high levels of gamma-linolenic acid in borage oil are responsible for its ability to decrease hypertension. The decrease in blood pressure occurred in response to two factors: (1) a reduction in the affinity to angiotensin II receptors in cells that produce aldosterone and (2) a reduction in the aldosterone/renin ratio (Engler, 1998).

Other Actions

A borage oil study has shown a decrease in body fat accumulation in rats. Rats were fed a low-fat diet containing borage oil. The result was a decrease in body fat mass (Takahashi, 2000).

References

Belch JJ et al: Evening primrose oil and borage oil in rheumatologic conditions, *Am J Clin Nutr* 71(1 Suppl):3525-3565, 2000.

Engler M et al: Effects of dietary linolenic acid on blood pressure and adrenal angiotensin receptors in hypertensive rats, *Proc Soc Exp Biol Med* 218:234-237, 1998.

Leventhal L et al: Treatment of rheumatoid arthritis with gamma-linolenic acid, *Ann Intern Med* 119:867-873, 1993.

Pullman-Mooar S et al: Alteration of the cellular fatty acid profile and the production of eicosanoids in human monocytes by gamma-linolenic acid, *Arthritis Rheum* 33:1526-1533, 1990.

Takahashi Y et al: Dietary gamma-linolenic acid in the form of borage oil causes less body fat accumulation accompanying an increase in uncoupling protein 1 mRNA level in brown adipose tissue, *Comp Biochem Physiol B Biochem Mol Biol* 127(2):213-222, 2000.

Zurier RB et al: Gamma-linolenic acid treatment of rheumatoid arthritis: a randomized, placebo-controlled trial, *Arthritis Rheum* 39:1808-1817, 1996.

🐾 = Pregnancy   👶 = Pediatric   ❗ = Alert   🖊 = Popular Herb

Boswellia
(bahz'weh-lee-uh)

Scientific name: *Boswellia serrata*
Other common names: Indian frankincense, olibanum

Origin: Boswellia is a tree or shrub and is found in India, America, North Africa, and Arab countries.

Uses
Reported Uses
Boswellia has been used traditionally for arthritis and other inflammatory conditions. It has been used commonly for syphilis, asthma, and cancer.

Product Availability and Dosages
Available Forms
Caps, tabs, standardized fluid extract (60%-65% boswellic acids), cream, resin

Plant Parts Used: Dried resin

Dosages and Routes
Adult
Inflammation
• PO: Cap/tabs 400 mg tid
Ulcerative colitis
• PO: Cap/tabs 350-400 mg tid for 6 weeks

Precautionary Information
Contraindications
Boswellia should not be used in pregnancy, in lactation, or for children until more information is available.

Side Effects/Adverse Reactions
None known

Interactions with Boswellia			
Drug	Food	Herb	Lab Test
None known	None known	None known	None known

Client Considerations

Assess
• Assess the reason client is using boswellia medicinally.

Administer
 • Do not administer large doses; lethal doses have been identified in rodents.

Teach Client/Family
 • Teach the client that boswellia should not be used in pregnancy, in lactation, or for children until more research is completed.

Pharmacology

Pharmacokinetics
Pharmacokinetics and pharmacodynamics are unknown.

Primary Chemical Components of Boswellia and Their Possible Actions		
Chemical Class	**Individual Component**	**Possible Action**
Boswellic acids	Beta-boswellic acid; Acetyl-beta boswellic acid; 11-keto-beta boswellic acid; Acetyl 11-keto beta boswellic acid	
Volatile oils		
Terpinols		
Arabinose		
Xylose		
Beta sitosterin		

Actions
Antiinflammatory Action
Boswellia was studied in animals to determine the result on inflammatory disease. Boswellia decreases leukotriene synthesis that is responsible for maintaining inflammation and edema. Boswellia resin action in ulcerative colitis may be due to the inhibition of 5-lipoxygenase (Bruneton, 1995, Gupta et al, 1997).

References
Bruneton J: *Pharmacognosy, pytochemistry, medicinal plants.* Paris, 1995, Lavoisier.
Gupta I et al: Effects of *Boswellia serrata* gum resin in patients with ulcerative colitis. *Eur J Med Res* 2(1):37-43, 1997.

Brewers Yeast
(brew'uhrz yeest)

Scientific name: *Saccharomyces cerevisiae*

Other common names: Medicinal yeast

Origin: Brewers yeast originates from the beer brewing process.

Uses
Reported Uses
Brewers yeast has been used traditionally for irritable bowel syndrome, diarrhea, and gastritis and has been used topically for acne and contact dermatitis.

Investigational Uses
Studies are underway to confirm the antiinfective and antidiabetic uses of brewers yeast.

Product Availability and Dosages
Available Forms
Tablets, powder, liquid

Plant Parts Used: Yeast from beer brewing process

Dosage and Routes
Gastrointestinal symptoms

🌸 Endangered Herb   Adverse effects: ʙᴏʟᴅ = life-threatening

Adult
- PO: Powder 1-2 tsp tid

Precautionary Information

Contraindications

Brewers yeast should not be used in individuals with compromised immune systems.

Brewers yeast should not be used in clients with Crohn disease. These clients are likely to have developed antibodies to the yeast.

Side Effects/Adverse Reactions

Central Nervous System: Severe headache (hypersensitive reactions)
Gastrointestinal: Abdominal cramps, flatulence
Endocrine: Increased blood glucose (diabetic clients)
Systemic: Allergic reactions

Interactions with Brewers Yeast

Drug	Food	Herb	Lab Test
None known	None known	None known	None known

Client Considerations

Assess

- Determine the reason client is using brewers yeast.
- Assess for severe, migraine-like headaches that may be due to a hypersensitive reaction. Brewers yeast should be discontinued if this occurs.
- Assess diabetic client's blood glucose levels. Brewers yeast may lower blood glucose control.

Administer

- PO: Using powder.

Teach Client/Family

- Teach the client that brewers yeast should not be used in immunocompromised individuals.

Pharmacology
Pharmacokinetics
Pharmacokinetics and pharmacodynamics are unknown.

B

Primary Chemical Components of Brewers Yeast and Their Possible Actions		
Chemical Class	**Individual Component**	**Possible Action**
Unknown	Unknown	Unknown

Actions
Antiinfective Action
One study (Izachia et al, 1998) identified that brewers yeast is capable of preventing *Clostridium difficile*–associated diarrhea. The action may be due to the reduction of *C. difficile* toxin–mediated secretion. Another study (Li et al, 1998) identified the antiviral effect of polysaccharides in brewers yeast. The viruses that were inhibited were poliovirus III, adenovirus III, ECHO6 virus, enterovirus 71, vesicular stomatitis virus, herpesviruses I and II, and coxsackie A16 and B3 viruses.

Antidiabetic Action
Two studies (Holdsworth et al, 1988; Li, 1994) identified the antidiabetic effects of brewers yeast. Glucose values were lowered in both studies.

References
Holdsworth ES et al: Extracts of brewers yeast contain GABA which enhances activation of glycogen synthetase by insulin in isolated rat hepatocyte, *Biochem Int* 17(6):1107-1116, 1988.

Izachia F et al: Brewer's yeast and *Saccharomyces boulardii* both attenuate *Clostridum difficile*-induced colonic secretion in the rat. *Dig Dis Sci* 43(9):2055-2060, 1998.

Li F et al: Antivirus effect of polysaccharides of brewer yeast in vitro, *Zhongguo Zhong Yao Za Zhi* 23(3):171-173, 1998.

Li YC: Effects of brewer's yeast on glucose tolerance and serum lipids in Chinese adults, *Biol Trace Elem Res* 41(3):341-347, 1994.

Broom
(brewm)

Scientific names: *Sarothamnus scoparius*

Other common names: Bannal, broom top, genista, ginsterkraut, hogweed, Irish broom top, sarothamni herb, Scotch broom, Scotch broom top

Origin: Broom is a deciduous plant found in Europe and in the Pacific Northwest and eastern regions of the United States.

Uses

Reported Uses

Broom is used as an antiarrhythmic, a diuretic, and an emetic or uterine contactant.

Product Availability and Dosages

Available Forms

Cigarette, extract, root, tea

Plant Parts Used: Flowers, twigs

Dosages and Routes

Adult

Dosages are not clearly delineated in the literature.

Precautionary Information

Contraindications

Because it can cause spontaneous abortion, broom should not be used during pregnancy. Until more research is available, broom should not be used during lactation and should not be given to children. It should not be used by persons with hypertension, arrhythmias, or other severe cardiac conditions. The FDA considers this herb unsafe.

Side Effects/Adverse Reactions

Cardiovascular: Arrhythmias
Central Nervous System: Headache, mind-altering effect (smoking)

 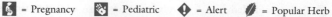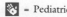

B

Precautionary Information—cont'd

Side Effects/Adverse Reactions—cont'd

Overdose: Nausea, vomiting, dizziness, confusion, tachycardia, shock

Reproductive: Uterine contractions and spasms, spontaneous abortion

---

Interactions with Broom

Drug

Antiarrhythmics, antihypertensives, cardiac glycosides: Broom may increase the effect of antiarrhythmics, antihypertensives, and cardiac glycosides; do not use concurrently.

Antidiabetics (glyburide, insulin, miglitol): Broom decreases the hypoglycemic; avoid concurrent use.

Food	Herb	Lab Test
None known	None known	None known

Client Considerations

Assess

◆ • Assess cardiac status (blood pressure; pulse, including character; rhythm). Identify any other cardiac agents (antiarrhythmics, antihypertensives, cardiac glycosides) the client is taking.

◆ • Assess for overdose symptoms such as nausea, vomiting, dizziness, confusion, tachycardia, and shock. If any of these symptoms are present, use of this herb should be discontinued immediately.

Administer

• Inform the client that there is no consensus on dosage.

Teach Client/Family

• Because broom can cause spontaneous abortion, caution the client not to use this herb during pregnancy. Until more research is available, broom should not be used during lactation and should not be given to children.

• Caution the client that the FDA considers this herb unsafe because of its hepatotoxic effects.

• Caution the client that using this herb to induce abortion is unsafe; a follow-up therapeutic abortion may be needed.

🌀 Endangered Herb   Adverse effects: BOLD = life-threatening

- Teach the client the symptoms of overdose (nausea, vomiting, dizziness, confusion, tachycardia, shock).

Pharmacology

Pharmacokinetics

Pharmacokinetics and pharmacodynamics are unknown.

Primary Chemical Components of Broom and Their Possible Actions		
Chemical Class	**Individual Component**	**Possible Action**
Alkaloid	Sparteine	Antiarrhythmic IA
Flavone glycoside	Scoparoside	Diuretic
	Kaempferol; Quercetin derivatives	Antiinflammatory
	Oxysparteine; Spiraeoside; Lupanine; Genitoside; Isoquercetin	
Isoflavone	Sarothamnoside	
Caffeic acid derivative		
Essential oil		

Actions

Antiarrhythmic Action

One of the alkaloid components of broom, sparteine, has shown antiarrhythmic activity similar to that of IA. Sparteine decreases heart rate and is considered to be similar to quinidine (Bowman, 1980). It can also inhibit sodium and potassium transport across the cell membrane in cardiac cells (Pugsley, 1995) and is used in Germany to treat cardiac disorders.

Diuretic Action

Scoparoside, one of the flavone glycosides of broom, exerts a powerful diuretic effect at high doses.

Other Actions

Sparteine has been shown to cause strong uterine contractions and for this reason should not be used during pregnancy. In many countries, broom is used to stimulate labor. In addition, many of the lectins (a type of plant-derived hemagglutinin) have

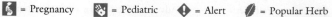 = Pregnancy　 = Pediatric　◆ = Alert　▮ = Popular Herb

been used as pharmacologic probes (Young, 1984). One study has shown that the lectins are able to bind B- and T-lymphocytes (Malin-Berdel, 1984).

References

Bowman WC et al: *Textbook of pharmacology,* London, 1980, Bowman & Blackwell.

Malin-Berdel J: Flow cytometric analysis of the binding of eleven lectin to human T- and B-cells and to human T- and B-cell lines, *Cytometry* 5(2):204-209, 1984.

Pugsley MK et al: The cardiac electrophysiological effects of sparteine and its analogue BRB-I-28 in the rat, *Eur J Pharmacol* 27:319-327, 1995.

Young NM et al: Structural differences between two lectins from *Cytisus scoparius,* both specific for D-galactose and N acetyl- D-galactosamine, *Biochem J* 222:41, 1984.

Buchu
(boo′choo)

Scientific names: *Barosma betulina (Agathosma betulina), Barosma serratifolia, Barosma crenulata*

Other common names: Agathosma, betuline, bocco

Class 2b/2d

Origin: Buchu is found in South Africa.

Uses

Reported Uses

Buchu is used as a diuretic; an antiseptic; and a treatment for urinary tract infections, including cystitis; the common cold, stomachache, rheumatism (Simpson, 1998), gout, leukorrhea, and yeast infection. Buchu is also used in combination with uva-ursi for benign prostatic hyperplasia.

Product Availability and Dosages

Available Forms

Decoction, dried leaves, fluid extract, tablets, tincture

Plant Parts Used: Leaves

Dosages and Routes

Adult

All dosages listed are PO.

• Infusion: 3-6 g dried leaves/day (Mills, 2000)

🌱 Endangered Herb   Adverse effects: BOLD = life-threatening

- Fluid extract: 2-4 ml/day (1:2 dilution) (Mills, 2000)
- Tincture: 5-10 ml/day (1:5 dilution) (Mills, 2000)

Precautionary Information
Contraindications
Because it can cause spontaneous abortion, buchu should not be used during pregnancy. Until more research is available, this herb should not be used during lactation and should not be given to children. It should not be used by persons with severe liver or kidney disease. Class 2b/2d herb.

Side Effects/Adverse Reactions
Gastrointestinal: Nausea, vomiting, anorexia, diarrhea, HEPATOTOXICITY
Genitourinary: Increased menstrual flow, SPONTANEOUS ABORTION, NEPHRITIS

Interactions with Buchu

Drug
Anticoagulants (heparin, warfarin): Buchu can increase the action of anticoagulants, causing bleeding; do not use concurrently.
Antidiabetics (glyburide, insulin, miglitol): Buchu decreases the hypoglycemic effect; avoid concurrent use.

Food	Herb	Lab Test
None known	None known	None known

Client Considerations
Assess
- Assess liver function test results (ALT, AST, bilirubin); buchu can cause hepatotoxicity. Watch for jaundice, right upper-quadrant pain, and clay-colored stools. If symptoms occur, use of this herb should be discontinued.
- Assess for use of anticoagulants (see Interactions).

Diuretic Use
- Assess urinary status (intake and output, bladder distension, pain, burning during urination); watch for beginning nephritis. If these symptoms occur, use of this herb should be discontinued.

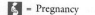 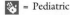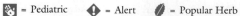

Administer

- Instruct the client to take PO as dried leaves, infusion, fluid extract, or tincture. Buchu should not be boiled; boiling robs the herb of its healing properties.
- Instruct the client to store buchu in a cool, dry place, away from heat and moisture.

Teach Client/Family

- Because buchu can cause spontaneous abortion, caution the client not to use it during pregnancy. Until more research is available, this herb should not be used during lactation and should not be given to children.
- Advise the client to report changes in urinary status, jaundice, and stool color.

Pharmacology

Pharmacokinetics

Pharmacokinetics and pharmacodynamics are unknown.

Primary Chemical Components of Buchu and Their Possible Actions		
Chemical Class	**Individual Component**	**Possible Action**
Flavonoid	Diosphenol	Antibacterial; diuretic
	Quercetin	Antiinflammatory
	Diosmin; Rutin; Diosmetin	
Volatile oil	Pulegone	Hepatotoxicity; abortifacient
Terpene-4-ol		Diuretic
Mucilage		
Resin		
Coumarin		

Actions

No substantial information exists to document any of the actions or uses of this herb.

Diuretic Action

One of the flavonoid components of buchu, diosphenol, may be responsible for its diuretic action. However, diosphenol is not considered to be a more powerful diuretic than caffeine or any other xanthane product (Simpson, 1998).

Antibacterial Action

A douche made from an infusion of buchu leaves may be used as an antibacterial treatment for yeast infections and leukorrhea. Diosphenol may be responsible for the antibacterial effect (Chevallier, 1996). A recent study suggests there is little potential for buchu to be used as an antimicrobial (Lis-Balchin, 2001).

References

Chevallier A: *Encyclopedia of medicinal plants,* New York, 1996, DK.

Lis-Balchin M et al: Buchu essential oils: their pharmacological action on guinea-pig ileum and antimicrobial activity on microorganisms, *J Pharm Pharmacol* 53(4):579-582, 2001.

Mills S, Bone K: *Principles and practice of phytotherapy,* London, 2000, Churchill Livingstone.

Simpson D: Buchu: South Africa's amazing herbal remedy, *Scott Med J* 43(6):189-191, 1998.

Buckthorn
(buhk'thawrn)

Scientific name: *Rhamnus cathartica*

Other common names: Common buckthorn, hartsthorn, purging buckthorn, waythorn   **Class 2b/2c/2d**

Origin: Buckthorn is found in Canada, Europe, and the United States.

Uses

Reported Uses

Buckthorn is used as a powerful laxative.

Product Availability and Dosages

Available Forms

Crushed herb, syrup

Plant Parts Used: Bark, fruit

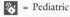 = Pregnancy    = Pediatric   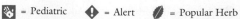 = Alert   = Popular Herb

B

Dosages and Routes
Adult
- PO: 20-30 mg hydroxyanthracene derivative (glucofrangulin A) (Blumenthal, 1998)

Precautionary Information
Contraindications
Buckthorn should not be used during pregnancy and lactation and should not be given to children younger than 12 years of age. This herb should not be used by elderly persons or persons with the following disorders: colitis, irritable bowel syndrome, Crohn's disease, gastrointestinal obstruction, unknown abdominal pain, appendicitis, gastrointestinal bleeding, hepatic disease. Dehydration and electrolyte loss will occur if buckthorn is used for more than 8 to 10 days. Class 2b/2c/2d herb.

Side Effects/Adverse Reactions
Central Nervous System: Nervousness, tremors
Gastrointestinal: Nausea, vomiting, diarrhea, anorexia, abdominal cramps; possible hepatotoxicity (Lichtensteiger, 1997)
Metabolic: Dehydration, fluid and electrolyte imbalances (with increased dose or increased duration)
Respiratory: Decreased respirations

Interactions with Buckthorn

Drug
Antacids: Antacids may decrease the action of buckthorn if taken within 1 hour of the herb.
Antiarrhythmics: Chronic buckthorn use can cause hypokalemia and enhance the effects of antiarrhythmics; do not use concurrently.
Cardiac glycosides (digoxin): Chronic buckthorn use can cause hypokalemia and enhance the effects of cardiac glycosides; do not use concurrently.
Corticosteroids: Hypokalemia can result from use of buckthorn with corticosteroids; do not use concurrently.

Continued

 Endangered Herb   Adverse effects: BOLD = life-threatening

Interactions with Buckthorn—cont'd

Drug—cont'd

Thiazide diuretics: Hypokalemia can result from the use of buckthorn with thiazide diuretics; do not use concurrently.

Food

Milk: Milk may decrease the action of buckthorn; avoid concurrent use.

Herb

Jimsonweed: The action of jimsonweed is increased in cases of chronic abuse of buckthorn.

Other herbs: Hypokalemia can result from the use of buckthorn with adonis, convallaria, helleborus, licorice root, and strophanthus; avoid concurrent use (Brinker, 1998).

Lab Test

None known

Client Considerations

Assess

- Assess blood and urine electrolytes if the client uses this herb often.
- Assess the cause of constipation; identify whether bulk, fluids, or exercise is lacking.
- Assess for cramping, rectal bleeding, nausea, and vomiting. If these symptoms occur, buckthorn use should be discontinued.
- Assess for medications and herbs used (see Interactions).

Administer

- Instruct the client not to take buckthorn within 1 hour of other drugs, antacids, or milk. This herb should be taken with other herbs to buffer its effects and prevent griping.

Teach Client/Family

- Caution the client not to use buckthorn during pregnancy and lactation and not to give it to children younger than 12 years of age.
- Advise the client to avoid long-term use of buckthorn, which can result in the loss of bowel tone.

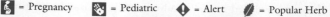

- Instruct the client to notify the provider if constipation is unrelieved or if symptoms of electrolyte imbalance occur (muscle cramps, pain, weakness, dizziness).

Pharmacology

Pharmacokinetics

Pharmacokinetics and pharmacodynamics are unknown.

Primary Chemical Components of Buckthorn and Their Possible Actions		
Chemical Class	Individual Component	Possible Action
Anthranoid	Emodin	Laxative

Actions

Laxative Action

The laxative action of the anthranoid components of buckthorn is well documented in the mainstream pharmacological literature. This action results from direct chemical irritation of the colon, which increases the rate at which stool is propelled through the bowel. A similar laxative herb is cascara sagrada.

References

Blumenthal M, editor: *The complete German Commission E monographs: therapeutic guide to herbal medicines,* Austin, Tex, American Botanical Council; Boston, Integrative Medicine Communication, 1998.

Brinker F: *Herb contraindications and drug interactions,* Sandy, Ore, 1998, Eclectic.

Lichtensteiger CA et al: *Rhamnus cathartica* (buckthorn) hepatocellular toxicity in mice, *Toxicol Pathol* 25(5):449-452, 1997.

Bugleweed
(byew'guhl-weed)

Scientific names: *Lycopus virginicus, Lycopus europaeus*

Other common names: Carpenter's herb, common bugle,
Egyptian's herb, farasyon maiy, gypsy-weed, gypsy-wort,
lycopi herba, menta de lobo, middle comfrey, Paul's betony,
sicklewort, su ferasyunu, water bugle, water
horehound   Class 2b/2c/2d

Origin: Bugleweed is a member of the mint family found in
Europe and the United States.

Uses

Reported Uses

Bugleweed is used as an astringent; an analgesic; and a treatment for Graves' disease, fever, tachycardia, and mastodynia.
Mild forms of hyperthyroidism can be successfully treated with
bugleweed.

Product Availability and Dosages

Available Forms

Dried herb, fluid extract, tincture

Plant Parts Used: Flowers, leaves (dried and fresh), roots,
stems

The leaf extract contains a much higher concentration of the
active components than does the root extract.

Dosages and Routes

Adult

All dosages listed are PO.
- Dried herb: 1-3 g tid
- Fluid extract: 1-3 ml (1:1 dilution in 25% alcohol) tid
- Infusion: 1-3 g dried herb, infused, tid
- Tincture: 2-6 ml (1:5 dilution in 45% alcohol) tid (British
Herbal Pharmacopoeia, 1983)

Precautionary Information

Contraindications

Until more research is available, bugleweed should not be
used during pregnancy and lactation, and it should not be

 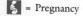 = Pregnancy    = Pediatric    = Alert   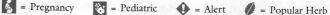 = Popular Herb

B

Precautionary Information—cont'd

Contraindications—cont'd

given to children. Persons with thyroid tumors, hypopituitarism, pituitary adenoma, hypogonadism, congestive heart failure, or hypothyroidism should avoid the use of this herb. Class 2b/2c/2d herb.

Side Effects/Adverse Reactions

Endocrine: Hypothyroidism, enlarged thyroid gland (high doses)

Interactions with Bugleweed

Drug

Radioactive isotopes: Bugleweed can interfere with the action of radioactive isotopes; do not use concurrently.
Thyroid preparations: Bugleweed can interfere with the action of thyroid preparations; do not use concurrently.

Food	Herb	Lab Test
None known	None known	None known

Client Considerations

Assess

Treatment of Graves' Disease

- Assess the client's thyroid panel (T3, T4, T7, TSH levels). Bugleweed should not be used in place of antithyroid agents.
- Assess for use of antithyroid agents. Bugleweed should not be used with other thyroid medications but may be used with other antithyroid herbs (see Interactions).
- Assess for nervousness, excitability, and irritability.
- Check the client's weight, blood pressure, and pulse weekly. Check for puffiness of the periorbits, hands, and feet, which may indicate hypothyroidism.

Administer

- Instruct the client to take this herb at the same time each day to maintain blood levels.
- Instruct the client to store bugleweed in a cool, dry place, away from heat and moisture.

Teach Client/Family

- Until more research is available, caution the client not to use bugleweed during pregnancy and lactation and not to give it to children.
- Caution the client not to use bugleweed with thyroid products or radioisotopes.
- Teach the client how to keep a graph of weight, pulse, and mood.
- Teach the client the symptoms of continuing hyperthyroidism: diarrhea, fever, irritability, sleeplessness, intolerance to heat, and tachycardia.
- Instruct the client to inform all other health care providers of herbs taken.

Pharmacology

Pharmacokinetics

Pharmacokinetics and pharmacodynamics are unknown.

Primary Chemical Components of Bugleweed and Their Possible Actions		
Chemical Class	**Individual Component**	**Possible Action**
Phenol	Lithospermic acid; Rosmarinic acid	Antithyroid; antigonadotropic
	Chlorogenic acid; Caffeic acid; Ellagic acid; Ursolic acid; Sinapinic acid; Hydrocinnamic acid	
Flavone	Luteolin-7-glucoside	
Amino acid		
Mineral		
Sugar		
Tannin		Wound healing; antiinflammatory

Actions

Antithyroid Action

Bugleweed has been shown to inhibit thyroid stimulating hormone (TSH), Graves' immunoglobulin, and iodothyronine deiodinase (Brinker, 1990; Winterhoff, 1994). One study

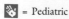 = Pregnancy   = Pediatric    = Alert   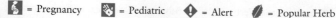 = Popular Herb

demonstrated pronounced antithyroid activity, pronounced peripheral T4 conversion, and decreased thyroid secretion independent of TSH activation (Auf'mkolk, 1984). These actions differ from those of the traditional antithyroid agents.

B

Other Actions

Bugleweed has shown antigonadotropic actions and an ability to decrease prolactin. A significant decrease occurred in both luteinizing hormone (LH) and testosterone levels when *Lycopus europaeus* extract was given orally. Bugleweed has been shown to decrease the binding of human chorionic gonadotropin (HCG) to rat testes (Auf'mkolk, 1984). This research indicates that bugleweed may also exert contraceptive effects.

References

Auf'mkolk M et al: Antihormonal effects of plant extracts: iodothyronine deiodinase of rat liver is inhibited by extracts and secondary metabolites of plants, *Horm Metab Res* 16(4):188-192, 1984.

Brinker F: Inhibition of endocrine function by botanical agents, *J Nat Med* 1(1), 1990.

British Herbal Medicine Association: *British herbal pharmacopoeia,* Cowling, England, 1983, Author, p 136.

Winterhoff H et al: Endocrine effects of *Lycopus europaeus* L. following oral application, *Arzneimittelforschung* 44(1):41-45, 1994.

Burdock
(buhr´dahk)

Scientific names: *Arctium lappa, Arctium minus*

Other common names: Bardane, beggar's buttons, clotbur, cockle buttons, cuckold, edible burdock, fox's clote, gobo, great bur, great burdock, happy major, hardock, lappa, love leaves, personata, Philanthropium, thorny burr, wild gobo

Class 1

Origin: Burdock is a perennial found in China, Europe, and the United States.

Uses

Reported Uses

Burdock seeds are used for their hypotensive, myodepressant, and renotropic properties. Burdock roots are used for their hypoglycemic, antiseptic, toxicopectic, and antitumor actions.

Burdock is used for skin disorders such as psoriasis, eczema, poison ivy, boils, canker sores. Burdock compresses can soothe the swelling of arthritis, rheumatism, and hemorrhoids.

Product Availability and Dosages

Available Forms

Capsules: 425, 475 mg; cream; salve; fluid extract; root; tea; tincture

Plant Parts Used: Dried roots, leaves, seeds

Dosages and Routes

Adult

- PO decoction: 1 cup tid-qid
- PO fluid extract: 1-3 ml bid
- PO tincture of root: 3-5 ml bid-qid
- Topical: apply as compress or as a cream prn

Precautionary Information

Contraindications

Burdock should not be used by persons who are hypersensitive to this plant. It should be used cautiously by persons with diabetes or cardiac disorders. Class 1 herb.

Side Effects/Adverse Reactions

Cardiovascular: Hypotension
Endocrine: Hypoglycemia

Interactions with Burdock

Drug

Antidiabetics (glyburide, insulin, miglitol): An increased hypoglycemic effect can occur when burdock is taken with antidiabetics; avoid concurrent use.
Antihypertensives: Burdock may possibly increase the hypotensive effect of antihypertensives; avoid concurrent use.
Calcium channel blockers: Burdock may possibly increase the hypotensive effect of calcium channel blockers; avoid concurrent use.

Food	Herb	Lab Test
None known	None known	None known

= Pregnancy   = Pediatric   = Alert   = Popular Herb

Client Considerations

Assess
- Determine the reason the client is taking burdock.
- Monitor blood pressure and blood glucose levels while the client is taking this herb.
- Assess for the use of antidiabetics, antihypertensives, and calcium channel blockers (see Interactions).

Administer
- Instruct the client to store burdock in a tight container away from sunlight and moisture.

Teach Client/Family

- Inform the client that burdock may be used during pregnancy and lactation and may be given to children.

Pharmacology

Pharmacokinetics
Pharmacokinetics and pharmacodynamics are unknown.

Primary Chemical Components of Burdock and Their Possible Actions		
Chemical Class	Individual Component	Possible Action
Carbohydrate		
Insulin		Hypoglycemia
Tannin		Wound healing; antiinflammatory
Polyphenolic acid		
Volatile acid		
Nonhydroxy acid		
Polyacetylene		
Glycoside	Anthroquinones	
Gamma-guanidino-*n*-butyric acid		
Lactone glycoside	Arctiin	Antinephrotic; central nervous system stimulant; hypotensive
Lignan	A; B; C; D; E; F; Neoarctin	Calcium antagonist; hypotensive

Continued

Primary Chemical Components of Burdock and Their Possible Actions—cont'd		
Chemical Class	**Individual Component**	**Possible Action**
Daucosterol Matairesinol Lappaol Arctigenin Xyloglucan		

Actions

Hypoglycemic Action

The inulin content of burdock root makes up approximately 60% of its weight. When used to treat diabetes in rats, *Arctium lappa* extract caused a long-lasting reduction in blood sugar and an increased tolerance of carbohydrate (Lapinina, 1964).

Antibacterial Action

The roots of *Arctium* spp. have demonstrated antibacterial activity against *Staphylococcus* spp., and two compounds present in the fresh root have been found to possess antifungal and antibacterial properties. *Arctium* was active in vitro against the gram-negative organisms *Escherichia coli* and *Pseudomonas aeruginosa;* against the gram-positive organism *Staphylococcus aureus;* and against the fungi *Microsporum gypseum, Trichophyton* spp., and *Epidermophyton floccosum* (Reisch, 1967). These actions were lost when the roots were dried.

Antitumor Action

A polymer from burdock root may assist in the prevention of cancer by decreasing mutagens, possibly by adsorption (Morita, 1984, 1985). An extract of *A. lappa* root also decreased tumor growth (Foldeak, 1964).

Other actions

One study identified a hepatoprotective effect of burdock. Mice were injected with carbon tetrachloride or acetaminophen. *A. lappa* was able to reverse hepatic effects (Lin, 2000; Lin, 2002).

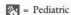 = Pregnancy   = Pediatric   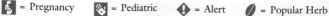 = Alert   = Popular Herb

References

Foldeak S et al: Aceta univ szeged, *Acta Phys Chem* 10:91, 1964.

Lapinina LO et al: *Farmatsevt Zh* 19:52, 1964.

Lin SC et al: Hepatoprotective effects of *Arctium lappa* Linne on liver injuries induced by chronic ethanol consumption and potentiated by carbon tetrachloride, *J Biomed Sci* 9(5):401-409, 2002.

Lin SC et al: Hepatoprotective effects of *Arctium lappa* on carbon tetrachloride- and acetaminophen-induced liver damage, *Am J Chin Med* 28(2):163-173, 2000.

Morita K et al: A desmutagenic factor isolated from burdock (*Arctium lappa* Linne), *Mutat Res* 129:25, 1984.

Morita K et al: *Agric Biol Chem* 49:925, 1985.

Reisch J et al: *Arzneimittelforschung* 17:816, 1967.

Butcher's Broom
(bu'chuhrz brewm)

Scientific name: *Ruscus aculeatus*

Other common names: Box holly, knee holly, pettigree, sweet broom

Class 1

Origin: Butcher's broom is an evergreen found in the Mediterranean and the southern region of the United States.

Uses

Reported Uses

Other Actions

Butcher's broom has been used to treat varicose veins, peripheral vascular disease, arthritis, hemorrhoids, and leg edema. It has also been used as a laxative, as a diuretic, to treat diabetic retinopathy, to relieve inflammation, and to treat carpal tunnel syndrome.

Investigational Uses

Butcher's broom may be used for orthostatic hypotension.

Product Availability and Dosages

Available Forms

Capsules: 75, 100, 150, 400, 470, 475 mg; fluid extract; ointment; suppositories (available in Europe); tablets; tea

Plant Parts Used: Dried rhizome, dried roots, leaves

🜨 Endangered Herb   Adverse effects: BOLD = life-threatening

Dosages and Routes
Adult
- PO: 7-11 mg total ruscogenin (Blumenthal, 1998)
- PO tea: 1 heaping tsp/1 cup water
- Topical Ointment: apply to area as needed

Other dosages are not consistently delineated in the literature.

Precautionary Information
Contraindications

Until more research is available, butcher's broom should not be used during pregnancy and lactation and should not be given to children. Persons with benign prostatic hypertrophy (BPH) and hypertension should avoid the use of this herb. Class 1 herb.

Side Effects/Adverse Reactions

Gastrointestinal: Nausea, vomiting, anorexia, gastritis (rare)

Interactions with Butcher's Broom

Drug

Alpha-adrenergic blockers: Butcher's broom may decrease the action of alpha-adrenergic blockers; avoid concurrent use.

MAOIs: Butcher's broom may increase the action of MAOIs and precipitate a hypertensive crisis; do not use concurrently.

Food	Herb	Lab Test
None known	None known	None known

Client Considerations
Assess

- Determine whether the client is using butcher's broom to treat venous insufficiency. If so, assess for symptoms (pain, swelling of legs when standing or sitting). If symptoms are present, check for constrictive clothing before administering herb.
- Assess for hypertension or benign prostatic hypertrophy. Avoid administering this herb to clients with these conditions.

 = Pregnancy    = Pediatric    = Alert   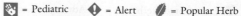 = Popular Herb

- Assess for the use of MAOIs. These drugs should not be used concurrently with butcher's broom; hypertensive crisis may occur as a result of tyramine content of herb.

Administer
- Instruct the client to take as a tea, in capsule form, or as a fluid extract.
- Instruct the client to store butcher's broom in a cool, dry place, away from moisture and heat.

Teach Client/Family
- Until more research is available, caution the client not to use butcher's broom during pregnancy and lactation and not to give it to children.

Pharmacology

Pharmacokinetics

Pharmacokinetics and pharmacodynamics are unknown.

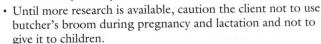

Primary Chemical Components of Butcher's Broom and Their Possible Actions		
Chemical Class	**Individual Component**	**Possible Action**
Steroidal saponin	Phytosterol; Glucopyranosyl (Mimaki, 1999)	
Flavonoid	Ruscogenin; Neoruscogenin	
Coumarin		
Sparteine		
Tyramine		Increased vasopressor effect
Glycolic acid		
Anthraquinone		Laxative
Euparone		
Ethanol		
Fatty acid		

Actions

Venous Action

Several research studies have focused on the use of butcher's broom to treat varicose veins. In fact, when *Ruscus aculeatus*

 Endangered Herb   Adverse effects: BOLD = life-threatening

was given with ascorbic acid and hesperidin to 40 patients with chronic phlebopathy of the lower limbs, an immediate and significant positive change (improvement of the varicose veins) occurred (Cappelli, 1988). Another study investigated the antielastase and antihyaluronidase effect of two chemical components present in *R. aculeatus,* the saponins and sapogenins. This study demonstrated a remarkable antielastase activity that could help improve venous insufficiency (Facino, 1995). The peripheral vascular effects of butcher's broom appear to be mediated selectively by calcium channels and alpha-1 adrenergic receptors (Bouskela, 1994). A recent study (Vanscheidt, 2002) confirms older studies in the use of butcher's broom for chronic venous insufficiency.

Antimicrobial Action

One study tested the use of 20 Palestinian plant species used in folk medicine, including *R. aculeatus.* The research tested these 20 herbs against *Staphylococcus aureus, Escherichia coli, Klebsiella pneumoniae, Proteus vulgaris, Pseudomonas aeruginosa,* and *Candida albicans.* Of the 20 plants tested, *R. aculeatus* was the least effective against *Candida albicans* and demonstrated limited activity against the other organisms (Ali-Shtayeh, 1998).

Other Actions

One study (Redman, 2000) identified the positive effect of butcher's broom in orthostatic hypotension. Butcher's broom is an alpha-adrenergic agonist.

References

Ali-Shtayeh MS et al: Antimicrobial activity of 20 plants used in folkloric medicine in the Palestinian area, *J Ethnopharmacol* 60(3):265-271, 1998.

Blumenthal M, editor: *The complete German Commission E monographs: therapeutic guide to herbal medicines,* Austin, Tex, American Botanical Council; Boston, Integrative Medicine Communication, 1998.

Bouskela E et al: Possible mechanisms for the inhibitory effect of *Ruscus* extract on increased microvascular permeability induced by histamine in hamster check pouch, *J Cardiovasc Pharmacol* 24:165-170, 1994.

Cappelli R et al: Use of extract of *Ruscus aculeatus* in venous disease in the lower limbs, *Drugs Exp Clin Res* 14(4):277-283, 1988.

Facino RM et al: Anti-elastase and anti-hyaluronidase activities of saponins and sapogenins from Hedera helix, *Aesculus hippocastanum,* and *Ruscus aculeatus:* factors contributing to their efficacy in the treatment of venous insufficiency, *Arch Pharm (Weinheim)* 328(10):720-724, 1995.

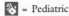 = Pregnancy   = Pediatric   = Alert   = Popular Herb

Mimaki Y et al: A spirostanol saponin from the underground parts of *Ruscus aculeatus, Phytochemistry* 51(5):689-692, 1999.

Redman DA: *Ruscus aculeatus* (butcher's broom) as a potential treatment for orthostatic hypotension, with a case report. *J Altern Complement Med* 6(6):539-549, 2000.

Vanscheidt W et al: Efficacy and safety of a butcher's broom preparation (*Ruscus aculeatus L.* extract) compared to placebo in patients suffering from chronic venous insufficiency, *Arzneimitte/forschung* 52(4):243-250, 2002.

B

Butterbur
(buh′tuhr-buhr)

Scientific names: *Petasites hybridus, Petasites officinalis, Tussilago petasites*

Other common names: Blatterdock, bog rhubarb, bogshorns, European pestroot, flapperdock, langwort, sweet coltsfoot, umbrella leaves, western coltsfoot

Origin: Butterbur is a perennial found in Europe and Asia.

Uses
Reported Uses
Butterbur is used to treat respiratory conditions such as asthma, whooping cough, and coughs resulting from other respiratory illnesses. It is used as a diuretic, sedative, and treatment for irritable bowel syndrome and arthritis. Use in the United States is uncommon.

Investigational Uses
Researchers are experimenting with the use of butterbur to treat migraine headaches, urinary tract spasms resulting from calculosis, prevention of gastric ulcers; and seasonal allergic rhinitis (Schapowal, 2002; Thome, 2002).

Product Availability and Dosages
Available Forms
Capsules: 25 mg; cigarette; extract; fluid extract; fresh leaves

Plant Parts Used: Flowers, leaves, roots, stems

🝚 Endangered Herb   Adverse effects: BOLD = life-threatening

Dosages and Routes
Adult
- PO infusion: pour boiling water over 1.2-2 g of herb, steep 10 min, strain, drink 2-4 oz as often as qid (Moore, 1995)
- PO fluid extract: 1-3 ml tid (1:2 dilution) (Moore, 1995)
- Topical: apply fresh leaves as a poultice prn

Precautionary Information

Contraindications
Butterbur should not be used during pregnancy and lactation and should not be given to children. Persons with decreased gastrointestinal or genitourinary motility should avoid the use of this herb; symptoms may worsen. The pyrrolizidine alkaloids in this herb can cause irreversible liver damage.

Side Effects/Adverse Reactions
Ear, Eye, Nose, and Throat: Color change of sclera
Gastrointestinal: Nausea, vomiting, anorexia, abdominal pain, color change of stools, constipation, HEPATOTOXICITY
Genitourinary: Difficulty in urination
Integumentary: Color change of skin
Respiratory: Dyspnea, shortness of breath
Systemic: **Carcinogenesis** (resulting from high levels of pyrrolizidine alkaloids)

Interactions with Butterbur

Drug
Anticholinergics: The effects of anticholinergics may be enhanced by the use of butterbur; avoid concurrent use.
Antimigraine agents: The effects of antimigraine agents may be enhanced by the use of butterbur; avoid concurrent use.
Beta-blockers: The effects of beta-blockers may be enhanced by the use of butterbur; avoid concurrent use.

Food	Herb	Lab Test
None known	None known	None known

 = Pregnancy   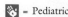 = Pediatric   ◆ = Alert   = Popular Herb

Client Considerations

Assess

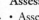

- Assess for hepatotoxicity: increased liver function test results (AST, ALT, bilirubin), clay-colored stools, and upper-quadrant pain. If symptoms are present, discontinue use of butterbur immediately.
- Assess for medications used (see Interactions).

Administer

- Instruct the client to take PO, use topically, or smoke.
- Instruct the client to store butterbur in a cool, dry place, away from heat and moisture.

Teach Client/Family

- Until more research is available, caution the client not to use butterbur during pregnancy and lactation and not to give it to children.
- Caution the client not to use excessive doses of this herb; carcinogens are present in the pyrrolizidine alkaloids.
- Caution the client not to confuse the leaves of butterbur with those of other *Petasites* spp.

Pharmacology

Pharmacokinetics

Pharmacokinetics and pharmacodynamics are unknown.

Primary Chemical Components of Butterbur and Their Possible Actions		
Chemical Class	**Individual Component**	**Possible Action**
Alkaloid	Petasin; Isopetasin	Antispasmodic; antiinflammatory
	Pyrrolizidine alkaloids Oxopetasin esters; Senecionine; Integerrimine; Senkirkine	Carcinogenesis
Volatile oil Sesquiterpene hydrocarbons	Pethybrene; Petasitene (Saritas, 2002)	

Actions

Antimigraine Action

One study showed that a group of migraine sufferers who received butterbur experienced a 56% reduction in the number of migraine headaches. In addition, the headaches experienced by this group were of shorter duration than those experienced by participants who received a placebo (Eaton, 1998).

Antispasmodic Action

The active chemical components petasin and isopetasin may be responsible for the antispasmodic action of butterbur, which includes reduction of spontaneous activity and spasm in the smooth muscle system. Butterbur thus may have the potential for treating urinary tract spasms resulting from calculosis (Eaton, 1998).

Carcinogenesis Action

The butterbur root contains pyrrolizidine alkaloids, which in animal studies have been linked to the development of cancer and hepatotoxicity. The recommendation is that human daily intake of pyrrolizidine alkaloids not exceed 1 µg (Reglin, 1998). New formulas of butterbur are available in which the pyrrolizidine alkaloid content is well below this recommended level (pyrrolizidine alkaloid–free *Petasites* sp.).

Other Actions

Studies have shown that butterbur may be used for seasonal allergic rhinitis, without sedative effects of traditional antihistamines (Schapowal, 2002; Thome, 2002).

References

Eaton J: Butterbur: herbal help for migraine, *Natr Pharmacy* 10(10):23-24, 1998.

Moore M: *Materia medica,* Bisbee, Ariz, 1995, Author.

Reglin F et al: Butterbur root, a pain reliever with wide-range application possibilities, *Praxis-Telegram* 1:13-14, 1998.

Saritas Y et al: Sesquiterpene constituents in *Petasites hybridus, Phytochemistry* 59(8):795-803, 2002.

Schapowal A: Randomised controlled trial of butterbur and cetrizine for treating seasonal allergic rhinitis, *BMJ* 324(7330):144-146, 2002.

Thome OA et al: Antiinflammatory activity of an extract of *Petasites hybridus* in allergic rhinitis, *Int Immunopharmacol* 2(7):997-1006, 2002.

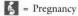 = Pregnancy    = Pediatric   = Alert   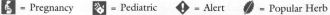 = Popular Herb

Cacao Tree
(kuh-kau' tree)

Scientific name: *Theobroma cacao*

Other common names: Cacao, chocolate, cocoa, cocoa butter

Origin: The cacao tree is found in Mexico and is cultivated in other parts of the world.

Uses

Reported Uses

Cacao is used extensively in food and drink. The flavonoids in cacao are potent diuretics, mild central nervous system stimulants, and cardiac stimulants. Cacao is not used therapeutically by herbalists or naturopaths.

Product Availability and Dosages

Available Forms

Butter, extract, powder, syrup

Plant Parts Used: Seeds

Dosages and Routes

Adult

Dosages are not clearly delineated in the literature.

Precautionary Information

Contraindications

Until more research is available, consumption of cacao should be avoided by persons with hypersensitivity to this herb, persons with irritable bowel syndrome or colitis, pregnant or lactating women, and children. Consumption of cacao in large amounts may cause death in animals.

Side Effects/Adverse Reactions

Cacao is generally well tolerated, although it may cause hypersensitivity in some individuals.

 Endangered Herb   Adverse effects: BOLD = life-threatening

Interactions with Cacao Tree

Drug

MAOIs: The tyramine content in cacao may increase the vasopressor effect of MAOIs; do not use concurrently.

Theophylline: Cacao may decrease the metabolism of xanthines such as theophylline; do not use concurrently.

Food

Coffee, tea, cola: Cacao may increase central nervous system stimulation when used with caffeinated foods and drinks.

Herb	Lab Test
None known	None known

Client Considerations

Assess

- Assess for hypersensitivity to chocolate. Individuals with this hypersensitivity should not use cacao.
- Assess for cardiovascular disease, colitis, and irritable bowel syndrome. Individuals with these conditions should not use cacao.
- Assess for the use of MAOIs and theophylline (see Interactions).

Administer

- Instruct the client to store cacao in a cool, dry place, away from heat and moisture.

Teach Client/Family

- Until more research is available, caution the client not to use cacao during pregnancy and lactation and not to give it to children.
- Caution the client to keep cacao-containing products away from pets.

Pharmacology

Pharmacokinetics

Pharmacodynamics and pharmacokinetics are unknown.

 = Pregnancy = Pediatric 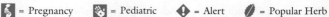 = Alert = Popular Herb

Primary Chemical Components of Cacao and Their Possible Actions

Chemical Class	Individual Component	Possible Action
Flavonoid	Catechin	Antioxidant
	Epicatechin	
Alkaloid	Theobromine	Central nervous system stimulant; diuretic
	Caffeine	Cardiac stimulant
	Tyramine	Increased vasopressor effect
	Trigonelline	
	Polysaccharides (Redgwell, 2000)	

Actions

Cacao has been used for centuries as a food and as a flavoring for food and drink.

Antioxidant Action

Cacao may exert significant antioxidant effects because of one of its chemical components, catechin, a flavonoid also found in black tea. Catechin has been shown to increase immune response and decrease mutagenesis (Waterhouse, 1996).

Stimulant Action

Since cacao contains xanthines, which are also present in coffee and tea, it acts as a mild central nervous system stimulant. It also acts as a cardiac stimulant and produces a mild diuretic effect. Theobromine, a chemical component of cacao, is one of the weakest xanthines.

References

Redgwell RJ et al: Isolation and characteristics of cell wall polysaccharides from cocoa *(Theobroma cacao L.)* beans, *Planta* 210(5):823-830, 2000.
Waterhouse AL et al: Antioxidants in chocolate, *Lancet* 348:834, 1996.

Calumba
(kal-um'ba)

Scientific names: *Jateorrhiza calumba, Jateorrhiza palmata*
Other common names: *Cocculus palmatus,* columbo root

Origin: Calumba is found only in Madagascar and
Mozambique.

Uses
Reported Uses
Calumba has traditionally been used to treat diarrhea and flatulence. It is an old, eclectic herb from South Africa whose use
is uncommon in the United States.

Product Availability and Dosages
Available Forms
Capsules, tincture

Plant Parts Used: Roots

Dosages and Routes
Adult
- PO infusion: 1-2 oz tid (Moore, 1995)
- PO tincture: 1-2 ml ac (1:5 dilution) (Moore, 1995)

Precautionary Information
Contraindications
Until more research is available, calumba should not be used
during pregnancy and lactation and should not be given to
children.

Side Effects/Adverse Reactions
None known

Interactions with Calumba

Drug	Food	Herb	Lab Test
None known	None known	None known	None known

 = Pregnancy   = Pediatric   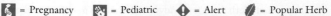 = Alert   🖊 = Popular Herb

Client Considerations

Assess

- Determine the reason the client is using calumba.

Administer

- Instruct the client to store calumba in a tightly sealed container.

Teach Client/Family

- Until more research is available, caution the client not to use calumba during pregnancy and lactation and not to give it to children.

Pharmacology

Pharmacokinetics

Pharmacokinetics and pharmacodynamics are unknown.

Primary Chemical Components of Calumba and Their Possible Actions		
Chemical Class	Individual Component	Possible Action
Columbamine Jateorhizine Palmatine Alkaloid Columbin		

Actions

Very little research is available documenting any uses or actions of calumba. There are no human studies for any use, and for that reason the use of this herb is not recommended. Calumba has been used in Africa as a dye for clothing and a flavoring for food.

References

Moore M: *Materia medica,* Bisbee, Ariz, 1995, Author.

Capsicum Peppers
(kap′si-kuhm peh′puhrz)

Scientific names: *Capsicum frutescens, Capsicum annum*

Other common names: Capsaicin, cayenne pepper, chili pepper, hot pepper, paprika, pimiento, red pepper, tabasco pepper

Class 1 (Internal Use)
Class 2d (External Use)

Origin: Capsicum peppers are found in tropical areas of the Americas.

Uses

Reported Uses

Capsicum peppers are used topically to treat diabetic neuropathy, psoriasis, postmastectomy pain, Raynaud's disease, and herpes zoster. They are used internally to promote cardiovascular health; as a gastroprotective agent in peptic ulcer disease; and to treat the common cold, flu, and vascular congestive conditions. Capsicum peppers be used topically to treat arthritic, muscular pain and poor peripheral circulation. The are commonly used by herbalists in the United States as an adjunct where vasodilation or warmth is needed.

Product Availability and Dosages

Available Forms

Capsules, tablets: 400, 500 mg; cream: 0.025%, 0.075%, 0.25% concentrations; gel: 0.025% concentration; lotion: 0.025%, 0.075% concentrations; spice; spray: 5%, 10% concentrations; tincture

Plant Parts Used: Dried fruit

Dosages and Routes

Adult

Pain Relief

- Topical: apply cream (0.025%-0.075% concentration) for at least 2 wk for beginning pain relief; may use up to qid

Other

- PO capsules/tablets: 400-500 mg qd tid
- PO tincture: 5-15 drops in water qid (1:5 dilution) (Moore, 1995).

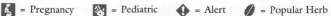

= Pregnancy   = Pediatric   = Alert   = Popular Herb

Precautionary Information

Contraindications

Until more research is available, capsicum peppers should not be used during pregnancy and lactation, should not be used by persons with hypersensitivity, and should not be given to children. This herb should not be used on open wounds or abrasions, or near the eyes. It is extremely vesicant in undiluted form. Class 1 herb (internal use); class 2d herb (external use).

Side Effects/Adverse Reactions

Gastrointestinal: Gastrointestinal cramping, pain, diarrhea (internal use)
Integumentary: Severe burning, itching, and stinging that lessen with each application; painful irritation of mucous membranes (all topical use)

Interactions with Capsicum Peppers

Drug
Alpha-adrenergic blockers: Capsicum peppers may decrease the action of alpha-adrenergic blockers; avoid concurrent use.
Clonidine: Capsicum peppers may decrease the antihypertensive effects of clonidine; avoid concurrent use.
MAOIs: Capsicum peppers may precipitate hypertensive crisis when used with MAOIs; do not use concurrently.
Methyldopa: Capsicum peppers may decrease the antihypertensive effects of methyldopa; avoid concurrent use.
Topical products: There are no known drug interactions of topical capsicum preparations with other topical products.

Food	Herb	Lab Test
None known	None known	None known

Client Considerations

Assess

- Assess for gastrointestinal conditions such as peptic ulcer, irritable bowel syndrome, and colitis. Some recent research has identified gastroprotective effects of capsicum peppers; however, other researchers believe capsicum should not be used if the aforementioned conditions are present (see Actions).

 Endangered Herb   Adverse effects: BOLD = life-threatening

- Assess for improvement in the symptoms of diabetic neuropathy, psoriasis, or herpes zoster if the client is using capsicum for any of these conditions.
- Determine whether the client is using MAOIs or antihypertensives. Capsicum should not be used concurrently with these medications (see Interactions).

Administer

- Instruct the client to use topically as soon as pain is starting to return. The stinging and burning sensations that some people experience with topical capsicum products should subside after repeated applications.

Teach Client/Family

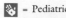 · Until more research is available, caution the client not to use capsicum during pregnancy and lactation and not to give it to children.

Pharmacology

Pharmacokinetics

Pharmacokinetics and pharmacodynamics are unknown.

Primary Chemical Components of Capsicum Peppers and Their Possible Actions		
Chemical Class	**Individual Component**	**Possible Action**
Volatile oil	Capsaicin	Pain relief; anti–*Helicobacter pylori*
Capsaicinoid	Lutein	Antioxidant
	Capsanthin; Capsorubin; Carotene; Oleoresin; Resiniferatoxin; 3,6-Epoxide (Maoka, 2001)	
Saponins	Capsicoside E, F, G	Antimicrobial (Iorizzi, 2002)
Protein		
Fat		
Vitamin	A; C	
Provitamin	E	Antioxidant
	P; B_1; B_2; B_3	

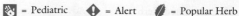

Actions

Gastroprotective Action

Capsaicin, one of the chemical components of capsicum, was found to protect against *Helicobacter pylori*–associated gastrointestinal disease. Test results have shown that doses similar to those that can be achieved in the diet are sufficient to provide the anti–*H. pylori* action (Jones, 1997).

Pain Relief Action

Topical capsicum preparations are used to relieve muscular pain and the pain associated with arthritis and a variety of other conditions (Keitel, 2001). The chemical components responsible for pain relief are the capsaicinoids. The most effective of these is capsaicin (Cordell, 1993), which can alter P-mediated pain transmission. Research has shown that capsaicin cream is an effective and safe treatment for relief of the pain associated with diabetic neuropathy (Tandan, 1992).

Possible Cardiovascular Actions

Research on rats has shown cardiovascular responses such as hypotension, decreased heart rate, and vasodilation that may be due to the tachykinins in capsaicin. Capsaicin acts on the vanilloid receptors found in many tissues (Cuprian, 1998).

Enhanced Immunity Action

In one study, rats were divided into five groups and fed various amounts of capsaicin in their diets. The rats that were fed a medium level of capsaicin (20 ppm) showed an increase in the T-cell mitogen-induced lymphocyte proliferative response, and an increase in B-cell, immunoglobulin G (IgG), immunoglobulin M (IgM), and tissue necrosis factor-alpha (TNF-alpha) levels, suggesting an increased immune function (Yu, 1998).

References

Cordell GA et al: Capsaicin: identification, nomenclature, and pharmacotherapy, *Ann Pharmacother* 27:330-336, 1993.

Cuprian A et al: Effects of the intrathecal administration of capsaicin on the cardiac rhythm in anaesthetized rats, *J Pharm Pharmacol* 50(suppl): 212, 1998.

Iorizzi M et al: Antimicrobial furostanol saponins from the seeds of *Capsicum annuum L.* var. *acuminatum, J Agric Food Chem* 50(15): 4310-4316, 2002.

Jones N et al: Capsaicin as an inhibitor of the growth of the gastric pathogen *Helicobacter pylori, FEMS Microbiol Lett* 146:223-227, 1997.

Keitel W et al: Capsicum pain plaster in chronic non-specific low back pain *Arzheimittel forschung* 51(11):896-903, 2001.

Maoka T et al: Capsanthose 3,6-epoxide, a new carotenoid from the fruits of the red paprika *Capsicum annuum L., J Agric Food Chem* 49(8): 3965-3968, 2001.

Moore M: *Materia medica,* Bisbee, Ariz, 1995, Author.

Tandan R et al: Topical capsaicin in painful diabetic neuropathy: a controlled study with long-term follow-up, *Diabetes Care* 15:8-14, 1992.

Yu R et al: Modulation of select immune responses by dietary capsaicin, *Int J Vitam Nutr Res* 68:114-119, 1998.

Caraway
(kar'uh-way)

Scientific name: *Carum carvi* L.

Other common names: Kummel, kummelol, oleum cari, oleum carvi

Class 1 Herb

Origin: Caraway is a biennial herb grown in Europe, Siberia, the Himalayas, parts of Asia, and now in the United States.

Uses

Reported Uses

Caraway has been used traditionally for gastrointestinal disorders such as flatulence, constipation, abdominal distension, irritable bowel syndrome, dyspepsia, colic, heartburn, indigestion, and stomach ulcers, and as a gargle for laryngitis. It is also used for the common cold and bronchitis.

Investigational Uses

Studies are underway for antiinfective uses against *Bacillus, Pseudomonas, Candida,* and *Dermatomyces* and as an antineoplastic.

Product Availability and Dosages

Available Forms

Tea, capsules, oil, volatile oil, seeds, water, powder, infusion

Plant Parts Used: Seeds

Dosage and Routes

Adult

- Essential oil: PO 1-4 drops in a tsp of water or on a sugar cube before meals
- Seeds: 1.5-6g finely crushed seeds, chewed and swallowed

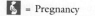 = Pregnancy = Pediatric  = Alert 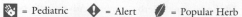 = Popular Herb

- Infusion: Use to make infusion bid-tid between meals; press 1-2 tsp of finely ground seeds, add 150 ml of hot water, let steep 10-15 min before straining and drinking

C

Precautionary Information
Contraindications
Caraway should not be used in hypersensitivity or gastro-esophageal reflux disease or during pregnancy (uterine relaxation may occur) (theoretical). Class 1 Herb.

Side Effects/Adverse Reactions
Gastrointestinal: Anorexia, diarrhea, hepatic dysfunction
Genitourinary: Renal dysfunction
Integumentary: Redness, irritation, contact dermatitis

Interactions with Caraway			
Drug	Food	Herb	Lab Test
None known	None known	None known	None known

Client Considerations
Administer
- Protect from light and moisture; place in metal or glass containers.

Teach Client/Family

- Teach the client that caraway should not be used medicinally in pregnancy (uterine relaxation may occur), in lactation, or for children until more research is available.

Pharmacology
Pharmacokinetics
Pharmacokinetics and pharmacodynamics are unknown.

Primary Chemical Components of Caraway and Their Possible Actions		
Chemical Class	**Individual Component**	**Possible Action**
Glucosides (Matsumara, 2002)	Janipediol; L-Fucitol	
Monoterpenoides (Matsumara, 2002)	Terpene; D-Limonene; Ketone	Chemoprotective
Volatile oil	Ketone, D-Carvone; Terpene; D-Limonene	

Actions

Antispasmodic Action

The effects of peppermint oil used in conjunction with caraway oil are comparable with cisapride for treating dyspepsia. Both peppermint and caraway oils were well tolerated and produced a minimum of side effects. Caraway oil has been shown to be effective in treatment of *H. pylori* infections, epigastric pain, and gastric ulcers (Khayyal, 2001; Madisch, 1999, Mickelfield, 2000).

Antimicrobial Action

When tested on animals, caraway has demonstrated effectiveness against *Bacillus, Pseudomonas, Candida,* and *Dermatomyces* spp. (Hopf, 1977).

Antiulcergenic Action

In one study 32 patients with duodenal ulcers or gastroduodenitis were given several laxative herbs, including caraway. Patients with obstipation syndrome improved (Matev et al, 1981).

References

Hopf H et al: *Phytochemistry* 16:1715, 1977.

Khayyal MT et al: Antiulcerogenic effect of some gastrointesinally acting plant extracts and their combination, *Arzneimittelforschung* 51(7): 545-553, 2001.

Madisch A et al: Treatment of functional dyspepsia with a fixed peppermint oil caraway oil in combination preparation as compared to cisapride, *Arzneimittelforschung* 49(1):925-932, 1999.

Matev M et al: Use of an herbal combination with laxative action on duodenal peptic ulcer and gastroduodenitis patients with a concomitant obstipation syndrome, *Vutr Boles* 20(6):48-51, 1981.

§ = Pregnancy   � = Pediatric   ◆ = Alert   ✍ = Popular Herb

Matsumara T et al: Water-soluble constituents of caraway: carvone derivatives and their glucosides, *Chem Pharm Bull* 50(1):66-72, 2002.

Mickelfield GH et al: Effects of peppermint oil and caraway oil on gastroduodenal motility, *Phytother Res* 14(1)20-23, 2000.

C

Cardamom
(kahr'duh-muhm)

Scientific name: *Elettaria cardamomum*

Other common names: Cardamom seeds, Malabar cardamom

Class 1

Origin: Cardamom is a perennial found in India.

Uses

Reported Uses

Cardamom is an aromatic used to treat dyspepsia, colic, flatulence, irritable bowel syndrome, gallstones, viruses, the common cold, cough, bronchial congestion, and anorexia. It is most commonly used therapeutically by Ayurvedic practitioners.

Product Availability and Dosages

Available Forms

Fluid extract, powder, seeds (dried and whole), tincture

Plant Parts Used: Seeds

Dosages and Routes

Adult

Recommended dosages vary widely. All dosages listed are PO.

- Fluid extract: 10-30 drops ac
- Powder: 15-30 grains ac
- Tincture: 5-10 drops prn or ac (Moore, 1995)
- Whole seeds: 1.5 g (Blumenthal, 1998) chewed ac

Precautionary Information

Contraindications

Until more research is available, cardamom should not be used during pregnancy and lactation and should not be given to children. Persons with gastroesophageal reflux disease should avoid the use of this herb, and persons with gallstones should use it with caution. Class 1 herb.

Continued

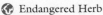

 Endangered Herb   Adverse effects: BOLD = life-threatening

Precautionary Information—cont'd

Side Effects/Adverse Reactions
Gastrointestinal: Gallstone colic
Integumentary: Contact dermatitis (rare)

Interactions with Cardamom

Drug	Food	Herb	Lab Test
None known	None known	None known	None known

Client Considerations

Assess
- Assess for contact dermatitis; if present, discontinue use of cardamom.

Administer
- Instruct the client to store cardamom away from sunlight and moisture.
- Instruct the client to take right before meals.

Teach Client/Family
- Until more research is available, caution against use during pregnancy or lactation, and not to give it to children.
- Advise the client not to exceed the recommended dosage.

Pharmacology

Pharmacokinetics
Pharmacokinetics and pharmacodynamics are unknown.

Primary Chemical Components of Cardamom and Their Possible Actions

Chemical Class	Individual Component	Possible Action
Volatile oil		
Linalyl acetate		
Linalool		
Alpha-terpineol		Analgesic
Alpha-pinene		
Limonene		
Myrcene		

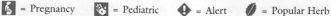

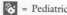 = Pregnancy   = Pediatric   = Alert   = Popular Herb

Actions
Enhanced Skin Permeation
One study showed that cardamom oil enhances skin permeation for indomethacin. Pretreating the skin with cardamom oil for 5 minutes greatly enhanced the permeation of indomethacin (Huang, 1999). Much research is underway to identify which crude herb extracts increase permeation.

References
Blumenthal M, editor: *The complete German Commission E monographs: therapeutic guide to herbal medicines,* Austin, Tex, American Botanical Council; Boston, Integrative Medicine Communication, 1998.

Huang Y et al: Cyclic monoterpene extract from cardamom oil as a skin permeation enhancer for indomethacin: in vitro and in vivo studies, *Biol Pharm Bull* 22(6):642-646, 1999.

Moore M: *Materia medica,* Bisbee, Ariz, 1995, Author.

Carline Thistle
(kahr′luhn thi′suhl)

Scientific name: *Carlina acaulis*

Other common names: Dwarf carline, felon herb, ground thistle, southernwood root, stemless carline root

Origin: Carline thistle is found in Europe.

Uses
Reported Uses
When used internally, carline thistle is a treatment for gallbladder disease, a mild diuretic, a diaphoretic, a spasmolytic, and an antimicrobial against *Staphylococcus aureus*. It is used topically to treat dermatosis, wounds, ulcers, and cancer of the tongue (Tamuki, 1994).

Product Availability and Dosages
Available Forms
Liquid, tea, tincture

Plant Parts Used: Leaves, roots, seeds

Dosages and Routes
Adult
• PO decoction: 3 g herb in 150 ml water, boil 5 min, 1 cup tid

🌀 Endangered Herb   Adverse effects: **BOLD** = life-threatening

- PO infusion: 2 tbl herb in 8 oz water, boil 15 min and let stand ½ hr; 1 cup tid between meals
- PO tincture: 20 g chopped herb in 80 g ethanol (60%), let stand 10 days, 40 drops qid
- Topical liquid: may be applied prn

Precautionary Information
Contraindications
Until more research is available, carline thistle should not be used during pregnancy and lactation and should not be given to children.

Side Effects/Adverse Reactions
Central Nervous System: PAIN, SPASMS, SEIZURES (overdose)

Interactions with Carline Thistle

Drug	Food	Herb	Lab Test
None known	None known	None known	None known

Client Considerations
Assess
- Assess for symptoms of overdose: pain, spasms, seizures. If these symptoms occur, use of carline thistle should be discontinued.

Administer
- Instruct the client to store carline thistle in a sealed container away from sunlight and moisture.

Teach Client/Family
- Until more research is available, caution the client not to use carline thistle during pregnancy and lactation and not to give it to children.
- Inform the client that very little scientific research is available to support claims for the therapeutic use of carline thistle.
- Advise the client not to confuse carline thistle with other *Carlina* spp.

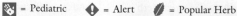

Pharmacology

Pharmacokinetics

Pharmacokinetics and pharmacodynamics are unknown.

C

Primary Chemical Components of Carline Thistle and Their Possible Actions		
Chemical Class	**Individual Component**	**Possible Action**
Volatile oil		
Inulin		Hypoglycemia
Tannin		Wound healing; antiinflammatory

Actions

Very little research exists on carline thistle. Most of the available information is anecdotal.

References

Tamuki A et al: Clinical trial of SY skin care series containing mugwort extract, *Skin Res* 36:369-378, 1994.

Carnitine

(kahr'nuh-teen)

Scientific names: L-Carnitine

Other common names: LPT, LAT, ALC

Origin: Synthetic

Uses

Reported Uses

Carnitine is used post myocardial infarction, for angina, and for congestive heart failure; to improve athletic performance; and for Alzheimer's disease and other types of dementia.

Product Availability and Dosages

Available Forms

Tablets

🌐 Endangered Herb   Adverse effects: BOLD = life-threatening

Plant Parts Used: N/A

Dosage and Routes
Adult
PO: 1500-6000 mg tid

Precautionary Information

Contraindications

The effects of carnitine are not known in severe hepatic or renal disease. Recommended amounts are not known in pregnancy, in lactation, or for children.

Side Effects/Adverse Reactions

Endocrine: Myasthenia gravis–like symptoms
Gastrointestinal: Anorexia, nausea, vomiting, diarrhea, abdominal pain

---

Interactions with Carnitine

Drug

Thyroid hormones: Carnitine may inhibit the effects of thyroid hormone replacement therapy; avoid concurrent use.

Food	Herb	Lab Test
None known	None known	None known

Client Considerations

Assess

- Assess the reason client is using carnitine.
- Monitor cardiac status, if client is using as a supplement in angina, post myocardial infarction, or congestive heart failure.
- Monitor mental status if client is using carnitine for dementia.

Administer

- Keep carnitine in a cool, dry area, away from excessive light.

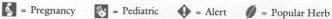

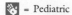 = Pregnancy   = Pediatric   ◆ = Alert   ⫻ = Popular Herb

Teach Client/Family

- Teach the client that it is not known how much carnitine is needed in pregnancy, in lactation, or for children.

Pharmacology

Pharmacokinetics

Pharmacokinetics and pharmacodynamics are unknown.

Actions

Carnitine is needed in the body for the transport of fatty acids into the cell.

Cardiovascular Action

Several studies have identified the positive results of carnitine in post myocardial infarction recovery, intermittent claudication, angina, and congestive heart failure. All studies point to the improvement in ventricular hypertrophy, decreased angina attacks, and decreased mortality (Davini, 1992; Illicento, 1995; Singh, 1996). Significant improvement in walking distance was reported in those diagnosed with intermittent claudication (Bolognesi, 1996; Brevett, 1995).

Other Actions

Carnitine has also shown positive results in Alzheimer's disease and other dementias (Bonavita, 1986; Calvani, 1992). Beginning research has shown carnitine to be beneficial in decreasing the harmful effects from antiretrioviral therapy in HIV (Semino-Mora, 1994).

References

Bolognesi M et al: Effect of 8 day therapy on propionyl-L-carnitine on muscular and subcutaneous blood flow of the limbs in patients with peripheral arterial disease, *Clin Physiol* 15:417-423, 1995.

Bonavita E: Study of the efficacy and tolerability of L-acetylcarnitine therapy in the senile brain, *Int J Clin Pharmacol Ther Toxicol* 24:511-516, 1986.

Brevett D et al: European multicenter study on propionyl-L-carnitine in intermittent claudication, *J Am Coll Cardiol* 34:1618-1624, 1999.

Calvani M et al: Action of acetyl-L-carnitine in neurodegeneration and Alzheimer's disease, *Ann NY Acad Sci* 663:483-486, 1992.

Davini P et al: Controlled study on L-carnitine therapeutic efficacy in post-infarction, *Drugs Exp Clin Res* 18:355-365, 1992.

Illicento S et al: Effects of L-carnitine administration on left ventricular remodeling after acute anterior myocardial infarction, *J Am Coll Cardiol* 26:380-387, 1995.

Semino-Mora MC et al: Effect of L-carnitine on zidovudine-induced destruction of human myotublesm. I, *Lab Invest* 71:102-112, 1994.

Singh RB et al: A randomized, double-blind, placebo-controlled trial of L-carnitine in suspected acute myocardial infarction, *Postgrad Med J* 72:45-50, 1996.

Cascara Sagrada
(ka-skar'uh suh-grah'duh)

Scientific name: *Rhamnus purshiana*

Other common names: Californian buckthorn, sacred bark

Class 2b/2c/2d

Origin: Cascara sagrada is found along the coast in the Pacific Northwest region of the United States.

Uses

Reported Uses

Cascara sagrada is used as a laxative.

Product Availability and Dosages

Available Forms

Capsules, fluid extract, tea, tincture

Plant Parts Used: Dried aged bark

Dosages and Routes

Laxative

Adult

- PO: 20-30 mg hydroxyanthracene (cascaroside A), one-time dose (Blumenthal, 1998)
- PO tincture: 1-2 tsp (5-10 ml) (1:5 dilution), one-time dose (Moore, 1995)

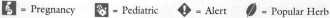

⑤ = Pregnancy   **🐾** = Pediatric   **❶** = Alert   **✒** = Popular Herb

Precautionary Information

Contraindications

Until more research is available, cascara should not be used during pregnancy and lactation, and it should not be given to children. Use of this herb is contraindicated when gastrointestinal bleeding, obstruction, abdominal pain, nausea, vomiting, appendicitis, and Crohn's disease are present. Cascara should not be used by those who are hypersensitive to this product. Class 2b/2c/2d herb.

Side Effects/Adverse Reactions

Gastrointestinal: Nausea, vomiting, diarrhea, abdominal cramps, laxative dependency

Genitourinary: Urine discoloration; hematuria, albuminuria (high doses, extended use)

Musculoskeletal: Osteomalacia

Systemic: Vitamin and mineral deficiencies, fluid and electrolyte imbalances (high doses, extended use)

Interactions with Cascara Sagrada

Drug

Antacids: Antacids may decrease the action of cascara if taken within 1 hour of the herb.

Antiarrhythmics: Chronic cascara use can cause hypokalemia and enhance the effects of antiarrhythmics; do not use concurrently.

Cardiac glycosides: Chronic cascara use can cause hypokalemia and enhance the effects of cardiac glycosides; do not use concurrently.

Corticosteroids: Hypokalemia can result from use of cascara with corticosteroids; avoid concurrent use.

Thiazide diuretics: Hypokalemia can result from the use of cascara with thiazide diuretics; avoid concurrent use.

Food

Milk: Milk may decrease the action of cascara; avoid concurrent use.

Continued

🐾 Endangered Herb   Adverse effects: BOLD = life-threatening

> **Interactions with Cascara Sagrada—cont'd**
>
> **Herb**
>
> Hypokalemia can result from the use of cascara with adonis, convallaria, helleborus, licorice root, and strophanthus; avoid concurrent use. The action of jimsonweed is increased in cases of chronic use or abuse of cascara.
>
> **Lab Test**
>
> *Serum and 24-hour urine estrogens:* Cascara Sagrada may increase or decrease test values.

Client Considerations

Assess

- Assess blood and urine electrolytes if the client uses this herb often.
- Assess the cause of constipation: determine whether bulk, fluids, or exercise is missing from the client's lifestyle.
- Assess for cramping, rectal bleeding, nausea, and vomiting; if these symptoms occur, discontinue use of cascara.
- Assess for all medications and herbs taken by client; evaluate if drug interactions could occur (see Interactions).

Administer

- Instruct the client not to take cascara within 1 hour of other drugs, antacids, or milk. This herb should be taken with a carminative to prevent griping.

Teach Client/Family

- Until more research is available, caution the client not to use cascara during pregnancy and lactation and not to give it to children.
- Advise the client to avoid long-term use of cascara because it can cause loss of bowel tone.
- Instruct the client to notify the provider if constipation is unrelieved or if symptoms of electrolyte imbalance occur (muscle cramps, pain, weakness, dizziness).

Pharmacology

Pharmacokinetics

Pharmacokinetics and pharmacodynamics are unknown.

 = Pregnancy  = Pediatric 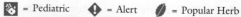 = Alert 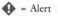 = Popular Herb

Primary Chemical Components of Cascara Sagrada and Their Possible Actions		
Chemical Class	**Individual Component**	**Possible Action**
Anthraglycoside	Cascarosides A, B, C, D Barbaloin; Deoxybarbaloin; Chrysaloin	Laxative
Emodin glycoside		Laxative

Actions

Laxative Action

The laxative action of the anthraglycosides in cascara is well documented in the mainstream pharmacological literature. This action results from direct chemical irritation in the colon, which increases the propulsion of stool through the bowel.

References

Blumenthal M, editor: *The complete German Commission E monographs: therapeutic guide to herbal medicines,* Austin, Tex, American Botanical Council; Boston, Integrative Medicine Communication, 1998.
Moore M: *Materia medica,* Bisbee, Ariz, 1995, Author.
Skidmore-Roth L: *Mosby's nursing drug reference,* St Louis, 2001, Mosby.

Castor
(kas′tuhr)

Scientific name: *Ricinum communis*

Other common names: African coffee bean, bofareira, castor bean, castor oil plant, Mexico seed, Mexico weed, palma Christi, tangantangan oil plant, wonder tree, wunderbaum

Class 2b/2d

Origin: Castor is a perennial found in India and Africa.

Uses

Reported Uses

Castor oil is used internally as a laxative, an emetic, a gastroin-

🌱 Endangered Herb   Adverse effects: BOLD = life-threatening

testinal antiinflammatory, and an anthelmintic. It is also used to treat leprosy and syphilis (Scarpa, 1982). Externally, it is used to treat boils, abscesses, carbuncles, tumors, inflammation of the middle ear, and migraine headache. It may also be used topically to stimulate the resolving of toughened tissue and wound healing.

Investigational Uses

Studies are ongoing to determine the effectiveness of castor as a contraceptive.

Product Availability and Dosages

Available Forms

Oil emulsion in concentrations of 36.4%, 60%, 67%, and 95%; oil liquid in 100% concentration; purge in 95% concentration

Plant Parts Used: Seeds

Dosages and Routes

Adult
- PO: 15-60 ml qd
- Topical oil pack: apply prn bid for up to 2 wk

Precautionary Information

Contraindications

Castor should not be used during pregnancy and lactation and it should not be given to children. Persons with hypersensitivity to castor or with gastrointestinal disorders such as obstruction or bleeding should avoid the use of this herb. Class 2b/2d herb.

Side Effects/Adverse Reactions

Gastrointestinal: Nausea, vomiting, abdominal cramps
Metabolic: Fluid and electrolyte imbalances (chronic use)
Systemic: Allergic reactions

Interactions with Castor

Drug

Antacids and other drugs: To prevent decreased absorption of castor, do not take within 1 hour of antacids and other drugs.

 = Pregnancy    = Pediatric    = Alert   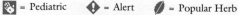 = Popular Herb

Interactions with Castor—cont'd

Food
Milk: To prevent decreased absorption of castor, do not take within 1 hour of milk.

Herb	Lab Test
None known	None known

Client Considerations

Assess
- Assess blood and urine electrolytes if the client uses this herb often.
- Assess for the cause of constipation: determine whether bulk, fluids, or exercise are missing from the client's lifestyle.
- Assess for cramping, nausea, and vomiting. If these symptoms occur, discontinue use of castor.

Administer
- Instruct the client to take castor alone for better absorption. It should not be taken within 1 hour of other drugs, antacids, or milk.

Teach Client/Family
- Caution the client not to use castor during pregnancy and lactation and not to give it to children.
- Advise the client to avoid the long-term use of castor because it can cause loss of bowel tone, as well as severe nutrient depletion and electrolyte loss.
- Instruct the client to notify the provider if constipation is unrelieved or if symptoms of electrolyte imbalance occur (muscle cramps, pain, weakness, dizziness).

Pharmacology

Pharmacokinetics
Pharmacokinetics and pharmacodynamics are unknown.

Primary Chemical Components of Castor and Their Possible Actions		
Chemical Class	**Individual Component**	**Possible Action**
Fatty oil		
Lectin	Ricin D	Toxic
Pyridine alkaloid		
Triglyceride	Ricinoleic acid; oleic acid	
Tocopherol		

Actions

Laxative Action

The laxative action of castor occurs as a result of its ability to increase fluid in the colon and stimulate peristalsis, which results in increased propulsion of stool through the colon. Castor can be used to empty the colon completely of stool, as is necessary to expel worms.

Contraceptive Action

Reports confirm that women in Korea, India, Algiers, and Egypt have used castor beans in some form to prevent pregnancy. Some Egyptians believe that pregnancy will be prevented for at least 9 months if a woman consumes one castor seed after her baby is born). (NOTE: This practice could be extremely toxic.) One recent study evaluated the contraceptive action of castor beans in female rabbits. The rabbits were treated with 7.5 mg/kg of castor for 10 days, then mated with proven male rabbits. The treated rabbits showed a 4.3-fold decrease in pregnancy (Salhab, 1997).

References

Salhab AS et al: On the contraceptive effect of castor beans, *Int J Pharmacognosy* 35(1):63-65, 1997.

Scarpa A et al: Various uses of the castor oil plant: a review, *J Ethnopharmacol* 5(2):117, 1982.

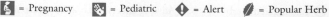 = Pregnancy   = Pediatric   = Alert   = Popular Herb

Catnip
(kat'nip)

Scientific name: *Nepeta cataria*

Other common names: Cataria, catmint, catnep, cat's play, catwort, field balm, nip

Class 2b

Origin: Catnip is a perennial found in the United States.

Uses

Reported Uses

Catnip is used internally to treat migraine, anxiety, colic, the common cold, digestive disorders, and influenzae. It is used externally to treat arthritis and hemorrhoids. Catnip is commonly used only to treat mild conditions, and it may be given to infants and children.

Investigational Uses

Catnip may be used to inhibit infections of *Staphylococcus aureus* (Nostro, 2001).

Product Availability and Dosages

Available Forms

Capsules: 360 mg; dried leaves; elixir; liquid; tea; tincture

Plant Parts Used: Dried leaves, flowers

Dosages and Routes

Adult

- PO infusion: 10 tsp dried leaves in 1 L water, cover while steeping, allow to stand 10 min; 2-6 oz tid (Moore, 1995)
- PO tincture: 1-5 ml tid (Moore, 1995)

Precautionary Information

Contraindications

Catnip should not be used during pregnancy because of its mild uterine stimulant action. Class 2b herb.

Side Effects/Adverse Reactions

Central Nervous System: Headache, malaise
Gastrointestinal: Nausea, vomiting, anorexia

Interactions with Catnip		
Drug		
Alcohol: The effects of alcohol may be enhanced when used with catnip.		
Sedatives: The effects of sedatives may be enhanced when used with catnip.		
Food	Herb	Lab Test
None known	None known	None known

Client Considerations

Assess

- Assess for possible pregnancy. Because of its uterine stimulant action, catnip should not be used during pregnancy.
- Assess for menstrual irregularities such as increased flow and pain.
- Assess for the use of alcohol and sedatives (see Interactions).

Administer

- Instruct the client to take catnip internally as an infusion or use topically.

Teach Client/Family

- Because it is a mild uterine stimulant, caution the client not to use catnip during pregnancy.
- Advise the client that catnip may be given to infants and children.

Pharmacology

Pharmacokinetics

Pharmacokinetics and pharmacodynamics are unknown.

 = Pregnancy   = Pediatric   = Alert   = Popular Herb

Primary Chemical Components of Catnip and Their Possible Actions

Chemical Class	Individual Component	Possible Action
Volatile oil	Nepetalactone Camphor; Epinepetalactone; caryophyllene; Thymol; Carvacrol	Sedative
Tannin		Wound healing; antiinflammatory
Terpene		

Actions

Very little research is available on the actions of catnip. Most reports are anecdotal.

Sedative Action

One of the chemical components of catnip, nepetalactone (a volatile oil), may be responsible for the sedative, calming effect of catnip. These effects are similar to those of valerian. Catnip is best known for the reaction cats have to it and the euphoria that results (Hatch, 1972). Its calming effects on humans make *Nepeta cataria* useful for treating anxiety and digestive disorders and colic (Chevallier, 1996).

Antiinflammatory Action

Anecdotal reports are available that document the topical use of catnip to improve the inflammation seen in arthritis and joint conditions (Chevallier, 1996). Currently, no primary research studies are available to substantiate these claims.

Antimicrobial Action

An extract of *N. cataria* was tested on 44 *Staphylococcus aureus* strains. There was significant inhibition of these organisms (Nostro, 2001).

References

Chevallier A: *Encyclopedia of medicinal plants,* New York, 1996, DK.
Hatch RC: Effects of other drugs on catnip-induced pleasure behavior in cats, *Am J Vet Res* 33:143-155, 1972.

Endangered Herb   Adverse effects: BOLD = life-threatening

Moore M: *Materia medica*, Bisbee, Ariz, 1995, Author.

Nostro A et al: The effect of *Nepeta cataria* extract on adherence and enzyme production of *Staphylococcus aureus, Int J Antimicrob Agents* 18(6):583-585, 2001.

Cat's Claw
(kats klaw)

Scientific names: *Uncaria tomentosa, Uncaria guianensis*

Other common names: Life-giving vine of Peru, samento, una de gato

Class 4

Origin: Cat's claw is a member of the madder family and is found in South America and Southeast Asia.

Uses
Reported Uses
Cat's claw is used today as an immune system stimulant, an antiinflammatory, and a contraceptive. It is used to treat arthritis, irritable bowel syndrome, colitis, and Crohn's disease.

Product Availability and Dosages
Available Forms
Capsules: 500, 600 mg; root (powdered and raw); tablets (standardized extract): 25, 150, 175, 300, 350 mg

Plant Parts Used: Leaves, roots, stem bark

Dosages and Routes
Adult
All dosages listed are PO.
- Bark (traditional Peruvian dose): 20-30 g finely chopped, then boiled in 1 L water ½ hr and allowed to stand until it reaches room temperature, tid
- Capsules/tablets: may be taken in amounts up to 5400 mg/ day in divided doses
- Decoction: 1 tbl powdered root in 1 qt water, simmered 45 min; 1 tsp in hot water qAM, ac
- Tincture: 20-40 drops up to qid; tincture may be standardized to contain 3% total oxindole alkaloids and 15% total polyphenol

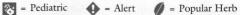

🜪 = Pregnancy   = Pediatric   ❶ = Alert   ✎ = Popular Herb

Precautionary Information

Contraindications

Until more research is available, cat's claw should not be used during pregnancy and lactation and should not be given to children younger than 3 years of age. Persons with multiple sclerosis, tuberculosis, AIDS, or hemophilia, and those who have had organ transplants, should not use this herb. Class 4 herb.

Side Effects/Adverse Reactions

Cardiovascular: Hypotension
Gastrointestinal: Diarrhea

Interactions with Cat's Claw

Drug

Antihypertensives: Cat's claw may increase the hypotensive effects of antihypertensives; avoid concurrent use.

Hormones, animal: Cat's claw may interact with hormones made from animal products (Foster, 1995); avoid concurrent use.

Immunostimulants: Do not use cat's claw with other immunostimulants (Jones, 1995).

Insulin: Cat's claw may interact with insulin (Foster, 1995); avoid concurrent use.

Plasma, fresh: Cat's claw may interact with fresh plasma (Foster, 1995); avoid concurrent use.

Vaccines, passive: Cat's claw may interact with passive vaccines composed of animal sera (Foster, 1995); avoid concurrent use.

Food	Herb	Lab Test
None known	None known	None known

Client Considerations

Assess

• Assess for decreasing blood pressure. If the decrease is significant, discontinue use of cat's claw. Determine whether the client is using antihypertensives, which will lower blood pressure further.

 Endangered Herb   Adverse effects: BOLD = life-threatening

- Assess for recent use of vaccines, hormones, insulin, or fresh plasma, all of which may contraindicate the use of this herb. In Europe, use of these drugs is considered a contraindication to the use of cat's claw (see Interactions).

Administer

- Instruct the client to use only standardized cat's claw products if possible.

Teach Client/Family

- Until more research is available, caution the client not to use cat's claw during pregnancy and lactation and not to give it to children.
- Instruct the client to have blood pressure checked regularly while taking this herb.

Pharmacology

Pharmacokinetics

Pharmacokinetics and pharmacodynamics are unknown.

Primary Chemical Components of Cat's Claw and Their Possible Actions		
Chemical Class	**Individual Component**	**Possible Action**
Oxindole alkaloid	Isopteropodine; Pteropodine; Isomitraphylline	Immune stimulant
	Rhynchophylline	Decrease hypertension, heart rate, cholesterol
	Mytraphylline	Diuretic
	Hirsutine	Bladder contractions
	Gambirine	Cardiovascular
	Isorynchophylline; Uncarine F	
Indole alkaloid	Glucosides; Cadambine; 3-Dihydro-cadambine; 3-Isodihydro-cadambine	

Primary Chemical Components of Cat's Claw and Their Possible Actions—cont'd		
Chemical Class	**Individual Component**	**Possible Action**
Quinovic acid glycoside		Antiviral; antiinflammatory
Tannin		Wound healing; antiinflammatory
Proanthocyanidin		
Polyphenol		
Catechin		
Beta sitosterol		
Indole alkaloid	Carboxystrictosidine	

Actions

Cat's claw is used widely in traditional Peruvian medicine. However, little is known about this herb from a purely scientific standpoint.

Immunostimulant Action

In Europe, cat's claw is used in combination with antiviral drugs to treat AIDS patients. However, no scientific research confirms this use. The immunostimulant action of cat's claw may be due to the combined actions of several of its chemical components, but no research confirms that possibility. In one limited study, cat's claw bark was shown to inhibit the growth of leukemia cells in humans without damaging normal healthy bone marrow (Stuppner, 1993). Another study demonstrated the ability of cat's claw to increase phagocytosis, thereby increasing the immune system (Wagner, 1985). Cat's claw shows enhancement of DNA repair, mitogenic response, and leukocyte recovery after chemotherapy-induced DNA-damage in human volunteers (Sheng, 2001). This study confirms another study using laboratory animals (Sheng, 2000).

References

Foster S: Cat's claw, *Health Food Bus* June 24, 1995.
Jones K: *Cat's claw: healing vine of Peru,* Seattle, 1995, Sylvan.
Sheng Y et al: DNA repair enhancement of aqueous extracts of *Uncaria tomentosa* in a human volunteer study, *Phytomedicine* 8(4):275-282, 2001.

🌀 Endangered Herb   Adverse effects: BOLD = life-threatening

Sheng Y et al: Treatment of chemotherapy-induced leukopenia in a rat model with aqueous extract from *Uncaria tomentosa*, *Phytomedicine* 7(2):137-143, 2000.

Stuppner H et al: A differential sensitivity of oxindole alkaloids to normal and leukemic cell lines, *Planta Medica* 59(suppl):A583, 1993.

Wagner H et al: Alkaloids of *Uncaria tomentosa* and their phagocytosis enhancement activity, *Planta Medica* 51:419-423, 1985.

Celandine
(seh'luhn-deen)

Scientific name: *Chelidonium majus*

Other common names: Celandine poppy, common celandine, felonwort, garden celandine, greater celandine, rock poppy, swallow wort, tetter wort, wart wort

Class 2b/2d

Origin: Celandine is a member of the poppy family found in Asia, North America, and Europe.

Uses

Reported Uses

Celandine is used to treat spastic conditions of the gastrointestinal tract. It is also used as a liver and gallbladder tonic, to stimulate digestion, and to decrease inflammation.

Investigational Uses

Researchers are experimenting with the use of celandine to strengthen the immune system and to treat cancer and AIDS.

Product Availability and Dosages

Available Forms

Extract, tea, tincture

Plant Parts Used: Flowers, leaves, roots

Dosages and Routes

Adult
- PO: 2-5 g herb (12-30 mg total alkaloids as chelidonine) qd (Blumenthal, 1998)
- PO tincture: 10-25 drops, up to 1 ml (1:2 dilution) tid (Moore, 1995)
- Topical extract: apply to warts and corns full strength

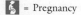 = Pregnancy　　 = Pediatric　　 = Alert　　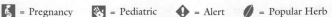 = Popular Herb

C

Precautionary Information

Contraindications

Celandine should not be used during pregnancy and lactation, and it should not be given to children. If used alone, this herb is for short-term use only; if used in a formula, it can be used long-term (Moore, 1995). Class 2b/2d herb.

Side Effects/Adverse Reactions

Cardiovascular: Hypotension
Central Nervous System: Dizziness, drowsiness, fatigue, lethargy, insomnia, restlessness
Gastrointestinal: Nausea, HEPATOTOXICITY (mild to severe)
Genitourinary: Polyuria, polydipsia
Integumentary: Stabbing or itching sensation at lesion

Interactions with Celandine			
Drug	Food	Herb	Lab Test
None known	None known	None known	None known

Client Considerations

Assess

- Assess for hepatotoxicity (increased liver function test results, clay-colored stools, right upper-quadrant pain, jaundice). If present, discontinue use of celandine.

Administer

- Instruct the client to store celandine in a cool, dry place, away from heat and moisture.

Teach Client/Family

- Until more research is available, caution the client not to use celandine during pregnancy and lactation and not to give it to children.
- Teach the client to recognize the symptoms of hepatotoxicity: clay-colored stools, jaundice, and right upper-quadrant pain.

Pharmacology
Pharmacokinetics
Pharmacokinetics and pharmacodynamics are unknown.

Primary Chemical Components of Celandine and Their Possible Actions		
Chemical Class	**Individual Component**	**Possible Action**
Alkaloid	Chelidonine	Reverse T-helper cell deficiency
	Chelerythrine; Sanguinarine; Lectin	Antimicrobial

Actions
Antispasmodic Action
In studies using frogs and mice, a celandine extract reduced gastralgia and pain from gastric ulcers. Chelidonium has been shown to stimulate bile flow when tested in guinea pigs (Rentz, 1948). It also has also been shown to relieve histamine-induced spasms in guinea pigs (Kustrak, 1982).

Nonspecific Immune Stimulation
Celandine may act as a chemoprotective agent for stomach cancer in humans. One study using 6-week-old rats showed that celandine inhibited glandular stomach carcinogenesis (Kim, 1997). One celandine product that is used in Europe but is not approved in the United States is Ukrain, which is reported to be an antitumor product that acts by inhibiting RNA and DNA replication (Ukranian Anticancer Institute, 1997).

Antimicrobial Action
Several research articles have discussed the powerful antimicrobial effects of celandine. Its effectiveness has been demonstrated against *Candida pseudotropicalis, Microsporum gypseum, Microsporum canis, Trichophyton mentagrophytes,* and *Epidermophyton floccosum* using herbs gathered during the fall harvest (Vukusic, 1991). The strength of the herb varies depending on the season of harvest.

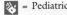 = Pregnancy   = Pediatric   ◆ = Alert   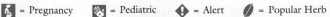 = Popular Herb

References

Blumenthal M, editor: *The complete German Commission E monographs: therapeutic guide to herbal medicines,* Austin, Tex, American Botanical Council; Boston, Integrative Medicine Communication, 1998.

Kim DJ et al: Potential preventive effects of *Chelidonium majis* L. (Papaveraceae) herb extract on glandular stomach tumor development in rats treated N-methyl-N'-nitro-N-nitrosoguanidine (MNNG) and hypertonic sodium chloride, *Cancer Lett* 112:203-208, 1997.

Kustrak D et al: *Acta Pharm Jugosl* 32:225, 1982.

Moore M: *Materia medica,* Bisbee, Ariz, 1995, Author.

Rentz E: *Arch Exptl Path Pharmakol* 205:332, 1948.

Ukrainian Anticancer Institute: *Ukrain information for physicians,* Vienna, Sept 1997, Nowicky Pharma.

Vukusic I et al: *Planta Med* 57(suppl 2):A46, 1991.

C

Celery
(seh'luh-ree)

Scientific name: *Apium graveolens*

Other common names: Apium, celery seed, celery seed oil, marsh parsley, smallage, wild cherry   Class 2b/2d

Origin: Celery is a biennial found worldwide.

Uses

Reported Uses

Celery seeds are used to treat hypertension and seizure disorders and to stimulate labor. Celery juice is used to treat edema, hypertension, joint inflammation, anxiety, and headache. Therapeutic use in the United States is uncommon.

Product Availability and Dosages

Available Forms

Capsules: 450, 505 mg; seeds; tincture

Plant Parts Used: Seeds, whole plant

Dosages and Routes

Adult
- PO: ½-1 tsp seeds in 1 cup hot water tid (Moore, 1995)
- PO: 1-2 ml 2-5 times/day (Smith, 1999)

🍀 Endangered Herb   Adverse effects: BOLD = life-threatening

Precautionary Information

Contraindications

Because they can stimulate the uterus, celery seeds should not be used during pregnancy. Until more research is available, except as a food source, celery seeds should not be used during lactation and should not be given to children. Persons with allergies to birch or mugwort, and those with kidney inflammation, should never use celery products. Class 2b/2d herb.

Side Effects/Adverse Reactions

Central Nervous System: CENTRAL NERVOUS SYSTEM DEPRESSION
Genitourinary: Uterine stimulation
Integumentary: Dermatitis, PHOTOTOXIC BULLOUS LESIONS (BIRCH-CELERY SYNDROME)
Systemic: HYPERSENSITIVITY REACTIONS, ANAPHYLAXIS, ANGIOEDEMA

Interactions with Celery			
Drug	Food	Herb	Lab Test
None known	None known	None known	None known

Client Considerations

Assess

- Assess for hypersensitivity reactions, including birch-celery syndrome and anaphylaxis.
- Assess the client's level of consciousness; central nervous system depression can occur.

Administer

- Instruct the client that celery seeds and juice are used to treat different conditions.

Teach Client/Family

- Because celery is a known uterine stimulant, caution the client not to use celery products, except as a food source, during pregnancy. Until more research is available, caution the client

 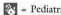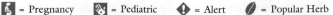

not to use celery products during lactation and not to give them to children, except as a food source.
- Warn clients with allergies to birch or mugwort, and those with kidney inflammation, never to use celery products.
- Advise the client to stay out of the sun or to wear protective clothing when using celery products. Psoralen, one of the chemical components of celery, may cause a phototoxic rash.

Pharmacology

Pharmacokinetics

Pharmacokinetics and pharmacodynamics are unknown.

Primary Chemical Components of Celery and Their Possible Actions

Chemical Class	Individual Component	Possible Action
Mineral	Sodium	Maintain electrolyte balance
	Chlorine	
D-Limonene		
Selinene		
Phthalide		Hypotensive
Flavonoid	Luteolin	Antiinflammatory
	Apigenin	Antiplatelet; histamine inhibitor
Nitrate		
Alkaloid		Anticonvulsant
Furanocoumarins	Xanthotoxin; Bergapten (Lombaert, 2001)	

Actions

Antihypertensive/Anticholesterol Action

Studies using dogs have shown that celery products lower the levels of circulating dopamine, norepinephrine, and epinephrine. This action is believed to result from the ability of celery to inhibit tyrosine hydroxylase. These findings support the traditional use of celery as an antihypertensive (Le Ot, 1992). Drinking aqueous celery extract for 8 weeks caused a significant reduction in serum total cholesterol in rats. The action was due to increased bile acid excretion (Tsi, 2000).

Anticonvulsant Action

One of the chemical components of celery, an alkaloid, has been shown to be an effective anticonvulsant (Yu, 1984). In one study, celery seeds were able to protect rats and mice from seizures initiated by chemical, audio, and electric means. The seeds contain an alkaloid that exerts both anticonvulsant and central nervous system depressant actions (Kulshrestha, 1970).

Other Actions

Studies have shown that apigenin, one of the chemical components of celery, exerts a strong antiplatelet effect and also inhibits the formation of thromboxane B (Teng, 1988). Information has also become available regarding the antifungal effects of celery (Jain, 1973). In addition, the oil may possess hypoglycemic and antitumor effects.

References

Jain SR et al: Effect of some common essential oils on pathogenic fungi, *Planta Medica* 24(2):127, 1973.

Kulshrestha VK et al: A study of central pharmacological activity of alkaloid fraction of *Apium graveolens* Linn, *Indian J Med Res* 58:99, 1970.

Le Ot et al: *Clin Res* 40:326A, 1992.

Lombaert GA et al: Furano-coumarins in celery and parsnips: method and multiyear Canadian survey, *J AOAC Int* 84(4):1135-1143, 2001.

Moore M: *Materia medica,* Bisbee, Ariz, 1995, Author.

Smith E: *Therapeutic herb manual,* Williams, Ore, 1999, Author.

Teng CM et al: *Asia Pac J Pharmacol* 3:85, 1988.

Tsi D et al: The mechanism underlying the hypocholesterolaemic activity of aqueous celery extracts, its butanol and aqueous fractions in genetically hypercholesterolaemic RICO rats, *Life Sci* 66(8):755-767, 2000.

Yu S et al: The anticonvulsant action of 3-n-butylphthalide (Ag-1) and 3-n-butyl-4, 5-dihydrophthalide (Ag-2), *Yao Hsueh Hsueh Pao* 19:566, 1984.

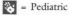 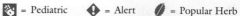

Centaury
(sen'taw-ree)

Scientific names: *Centaurium erythraea, Centaurium umbellatum, Centaurium minus*

Other common names: Bitter clover, bitter herb, bitterbloom, centaurea, common centaury, European centaury, eyebright, feverwort, filwort, lesser centaury, minor centaury

Class 1

Origin: Centaury is an annual or biennial member of the Gentian family found in Europe.

Uses

Reported Uses

Centaury is used to treat dyspepsia, lack of gastric secretions, and loss of appetite. In traditional herbal medicine, centaury is used as an anthelmintic, an antidiabetic, an antihypertensive, and a treatment for kidney stones. No scientific evidence supports any of these uses or actions. Centaury may be given to infants and children to treat anxiety, insomnia, tension, colic, irritable bowel syndrome, and topical inflammation. It may also be used to treat symptoms of attention deficit hyperactivity disorder (ADHD) (Romm, 2000). Centaury is commonly used in the United Kingdom and Australia; its use is less common in the United States.

Product Availability and Dosages

Available Forms

Fluid extract, powder, whole herb

Plant Parts Used: Flowers, leaves, stem

Dosages and Routes

Adult

All dosages listed are PO.

- Fluid extract: 1-3 ml taken before meals (1:5 dilution) (Hobbs, 1995)
- Cold infusion: 1-2 oz tid (Moore, 1995)
- Powder: 1 g taken tid with honey on a cracker
- Tincture: 0.5-1ml taken before meals (1:2 dilution) (Moore, 1995)
- Whole herb: 1-2 g taken qd

🌀 Endangered Herb   Adverse effects: **BOLD** = life-threatening

Precautionary Information

Contraindications

Until more research is available, centaury should not be used during pregnancy and lactation. Persons with gastric or peptic ulcers should not use this herb. Class 1 herb.

Side Effects/Adverse Reactions

Gastrointestinal: Anorexia

Interactions with Centaury			
Drug	Food	Herb	Lab Test
None known	None known	None known	None known

Client Considerations

Assess

• Determine the reasons the client is using centaury.

Administer

• Instruct the client to store centaury away from light and moisture.

Teach Client/Family

• Until more research is available, caution the client not to use centaury during pregnancy and lactation.
• Caution the client not to confuse the three *Centaurium* spp. listed in the Scientific names section with other *Centaurium* spp. They are different herbs.
• Inform the client that no supporting research is available to document any uses for or actions of this herb.

Pharmacology

Pharmacokinetics

Pharmacokinetics and pharmacodynamics are unknown.

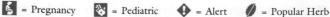

 = Pregnancy   = Pediatric   ◆ = Alert   🖊 = Popular Herb

Primary Chemical Components of Centaury and Their Possible Actions

Chemical Class	Individual Component	Possible Action
Alkaloid	Gentianine; Gentianidine; Gentioflavine	
Monoterpenoid	Iridoids; Gentiopicroside; Centapicrin; Gentioflavoside; Sweroside; Swertiamarin	
Triterpenoid	Alpha-amyrin; Beta-amyrin; Erythrodiol; Crataegolic acid; Oleanolic acid; Oleanolic lactone; Sitosterol; Stigmasterol; Campesterol; Brassicasterol	
Phenolic acid		
Flavonoid		
Xanthone	Eustomin; Demethyleustomin	Antioxidant
Fatty acid	Palmitic acid; Stearic acid	

Actions

No supporting evidence exists to document any actions of this herb. However, initial studies have suggested that the xanthone chemical components in centaury may show promise as antioxidants and that they may possess some antiinflammatory properties, although these are thought to be weak.

References

Hobbs C: *Handbook for healing: a concise guide to herbal products,* 1995, Botanica Press.

Moore M: *Materia medica,* Bisbee, Ariz, 1995, Author.

Romm A: Children's supplement guide, *Better Nutrition* (suppl):38-43, Oct 2000.

Endangered Herb   Adverse effects: BOLD = life-threatening

Chamomile
(ka'muh-meel)

Scientific names: *Matricaria chamomilla, Matricaria recutita, Chamaemelum nobile, Anthemis nobile*

Other common names: Common chamomile, English chamomile, German chamomile, Hungarian chamomile, Roman chamomile, sweet false chamomile, true chamomile, wild chamomile

Class 2b

Origin: Chamomile is a perennial found in Europe.

Uses

Reported Uses

Chamomile is used as an antiinflammatory and to treat insomnia, anxiety, and spasms. It is commonly used to treat digestive conditions such as irritable bowel syndrome, indigestion, colitis, and Crohn's disease, and as a topical treatment to promote wound healing.

Investigational Uses

Studies are underway to determine the effectiveness of chamomile as an antioxidant and as a treatment for menopausal symptoms.

Product Availability and Dosages

Available Forms

Capsules: 360 mg; cream; fluid extract; lotion; shampoo and conditioner; tea; tincture; various cosmetics

Plant Parts Used: Dried flowers

Dosages and Routes

Adult

- PO capsules: 300-400 mg, standardized to 1% apigenin and 0.5 % essential oil, as often as 6 times/day, (Foster, 1998)
- PO fluid extract: 1-2 ml tid (1:1, 45% ethanol) (Smith, 1999)
- PO tea: 2-4 oz prn (Moore, 1995)

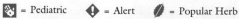

🔥 = Pregnancy   🐾 = Pediatric   ❗ = Alert   🌿 = Popular Herb

- PO tincture: 3-10 ml tid (1:5, 45% ethanol) (Bradley, 1992)
- Topical: 1½ cups water mixed with 2 tsp dried flowers, cover, let stand 10-15 min, strain, apply as a compress

Child

- PO tea: ½-4 cups qd (Romm, 2000)
- PO tincture: ¼-1 tsp as often as qid (Romm, 2000)
- Topical: as a wash or cream, apply prn to treat inflammation (Romm, 2000)

Precautionary Information

Contraindications

Chamomile *(Chamaemelum nobile)* is a known abortifacient and should not be used during pregnancy and lactation, but it may be given to children. Persons with asthma should not use this herb. Cross-hypersensitivity may result from allergy to sunflowers, ragweed, or members of the aster family (echinacea, feverfew, milk thistle). Class 2b herb.

Side Effects/Adverse Reactions

Ear, Eye, Nose, and Throat: Burning of the face, eyes, mucous membranes (topical)
Systemic: Hypersensitivity

Interactions with Chamomile

Drug

Alcohol: Chamomile may increase the effects of alcohol (theoretical).
Anticoagulants: Chamomile *(C. nobile)* may interfere with the actions of anticoagulants; avoid concurrent use.
Sedatives: Chamomile may increase the effects of other sedatives; avoid concurrent use.

Food	Herb	Lab Test
None known	None known	None known

Client Considerations

Assess

- Determine whether the client is using chamomile for insomnia.

- Assess the client's sleeping patterns: ability to fall asleep and stay asleep, hours of sleep.
- Assess for the use of alcohol, anticoagulants, and sedatives (see Interactions).

Administer

- Instruct the client to store chamomile in a cool, dry place, away from heat and moisture.

Teach Client/Family

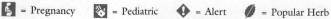

- Caution the client not to use *C. nobile* during pregnancy; it is a known abortifacient.
- Instruct the client to avoid using chamomile concurrently with other sedatives or alcohol; chamomile may increase their effects.

Pharmacology

Pharmacokinetics

Pharmacokinetics and pharmacodynamics are unknown.

Primary Chemical Components of Chamomile and Their Possible Actions		
Chemical Class	**Individual Component**	**Possible Action**
Flavonoid	Apigenin	Anxiolytic/phytoestrogen
	Glucoside; Chamaemeloside	Hypoglycemia
	Luteolin	
Volatile oil	Chamazulene	Antiallergy
	Bisabolol; Bisabololo-sides A, B; Azulenes	Antiinflammatory; antispasmodic
Acid	Angelic acid; Tiglic acid	
Farnesol		
Nerolidol		
Germacranolide		
Alcohol	Amyl alcohol; Isobutyl alcohol	
Coumarin		
Glycoside		
Heniarin		
Umbelliferone		
Fatty acid		

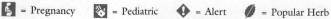 = Pregnancy   = Pediatric   = Alert   = Popular Herb

C

Actions

Antianxiety Action

One of the flavonoid components of chamomile, apigenin, has shown an affinity for benzodiazepine receptors, which accounts for the antianxiety and sedative qualities of this herb (Viola, 1995; Medina, 1998). Two other studies have shown a mild hypnotic effect in laboratory animals as a result of the flavonoid component (Berry, 1995; Mills, 1991). Multiple studies have documented the ability of chamomile to decrease anxiety and promote relaxation and sleep.

Antidiabetic Action

Recent evidence has demonstrated that two flavonoids in chamomile, glucoside and chamaemeloside, produce hypoglycemic effects (Konig, 1998). However, the current recommended dose for humans of 0.05% to 0.1% is too low to have any significant effect on glucose levels.

Phytoestrogen Action

A recent study evaluated the efficacy of 13 isoflavonoids, flavonoids, and lignans, plus several phytoestrogens, in the treatment of estrogen-dependent tumors. Apigenin, a flavonoid present in chamomile, exerted a significant effect on DNA synthesis in estrogen-dependent and estrogen-independent human breast cancer cells (Wang, 1997). Further studies are necessary to clarify the possible cancer preventative effects of these chemical components.

Antispasmodic Action in the Gastrointestinal Tract

Studies have shown the antispasmodic action of chamomile on the gastrointestinal tract. In one study, infant colic was significantly reduced when chamomile tea was given to 69 infants with colic symptoms (Weizman, 1993). However, this was a study of short duration (7 days).

References

Berry M: The chamomiles, *Pharmacol J* 254:191-193, 1995.

Bradley PR, editor: *British herbal compendium, vol 1,* London, 1992, British Herbal Medicine Assoc.

Foster S: *101 medicinal herbs,* Loveland, Colo, 1998, Interweave.

Medina JH et al: Neuroactive flavonoids: new ligands for benzodiazepine receptors, *Phytomedicine* 5(2):235-243, 1998.

Mills S, Bones K: *The essential book of herbal medicine,* ed 2, London, 1991, Penguin, p 677.

Moore M: *Materia medica,* Bisbee, Ariz, 1995, Author.

Konig G et al: Hypoglycaemic activity on an HMG-containing flavonoid glucoside, chamaemeloside, from *Chamaemelum nobile, Planta Med* 64:612-614, 1998.

Romm A: Children's supplement guide, *Better Nutrition* (suppl):38-43, Oct 2000.

Smith E: *Therapeutic herb manual,* Williams, Ore, 1999, Author.

Viola H et al: Apigenin, a component of *Matricaria recutita* flowers, is a central benzodiazepine receptors-ligand with anxiolytic effects, *Planta Med* 81:213-216, 1995.

Wang C et al: Phytoestrogen concentration determines effects on DNA synthesis in human breast cancer cells, *Nutr Cancer* 28(3):236-247, 1997.

Weizman Z et al: Efficacy of herbal tea preparation in infant colic, *J Pediatr* 122:650-652, 1993.

Chaparral
(sha-puh-rehl')

Scientific names: *Larrea tridentata, Larrea divaricata*

Other common names: Creosote bush, greasewood, *Hediondilla*

Class 2d

Origin: Chaparral is a shrub found in Mexico and the southwestern region of the United States.

Uses

Reported Uses

Chaparral has traditionally been used to treat bronchitis, fever, joint inflammation, cancer, and diabetes.

Investigational Uses

Studies are underway to determine the efficacy of chaparral as an antitumor agent; as an antimicrobial (Verastegui, 1996); and as an anti-HIV-1 agent (Ghabre, 1996).

Product Availability and Dosages

Available Forms

Capsules, tablets, tea, tincture

Plant Parts Used: Leaves

Dosages and Routes

Adult

• PO capsules: 2-4/day (Moore, 1995)

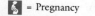 = Pregnancy   = Pediatric   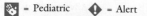 = Alert    = Popular Herb

- PO tincture: 1-3 ml (1:5 dilution) tid (Moore, 1995)
- Topical: apply strong decoction tid (Moore, 1995)

C

Precautionary Information
Contraindications

Until more research is available, chaparral should not be used during pregnancy and lactation and should not be given to children. Persons with liver or renal disease should avoid the use of this herb. The American Herbal Product Association has recommended that chaparral products not be sold until the hepatotoxicity question has been answered. Class 2d herb.

Side Effects/Adverse Reactions
Gastrointestinal: HEPATOTOXICITY (Sheikh, 1997; Stickel, 2000), HEPATIC FAILURE
Integumentary: Contact dermatitis

Interactions with Chaparral

Drug	Food	Herb
None known	None known	None known

Lab Test
Chaparral may increase ALT, AST, total bilirubin, and urine bilirubin.

Client Considerations
Assess

- Assess for hepatotoxicity (increasing AST and ALT test results, clay-colored stools, right upper-quadrant pain). If symptoms are present, use of this herb should be discontinued immediately.
- Assess for contact dermatitis. If it is present, use of this herb should be discontinued.

Administer

- Instruct the client to store chaparral away from moisture and sunlight.

Teach Client/Family

- Until more research is available, caution the client not to use chaparral during pregnancy and lactation and not to give it to children.
- Because chaparral can cause serious liver damage, advise the client to avoid its use. The FDA considers chaparral an unsafe herb.

Pharmacology

Pharmacokinetics

Pharmacokinetics and pharmacodynamics are unknown.

Primary Chemical Components of Chaparral and Their Possible Actions		
Chemical Class	**Individual Component**	**Possible Action**
Phenolic compound	Nordihydroguaiaretic acid	Hepatotoxicity
	Lignans	Anti-HIV
	Dihydroguaiaretic acid; Nor-Isoguaiasin	

Actions

Hypoglycemic Action

One study evaluated the glucose-lowering ability of chaparral in mice with type 2 diabetes. Blood glucose decreased significantly, a finding that suggests the need for further study of the hypoglycemic effect of this herb (Luo, 1998). It is a well-documented fact that the Pima Indians have treated diabetes with chaparral for centuries.

Antitumor Action

Chaparral may represent a new class of HIV-responsive agents with clinical significance. Lignans isolated from chaparral have shown anti–HIV-1 activity (Gnabre, 1997). Factors used to evaluate tumors were survival time and the percentages of tumors that decreased in size, remained static, or increased in size. Results showed that the antitumor effects were better in vivo (Anesini, 1998). Previous studies demonstrated the

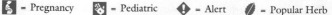

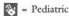

antiproliferative activity of chaparral on T lymphoma cells in culture (Anesini, 1996).

Other Actions

One study (Verastegui, 1996) showed good antimicrobial activity against growth of yeasts, molds, bacteria. More research needs to be completed to confirm these results. Another study (Gnabre, 1996) showed anti–HIV-1 activity. This activity may be due to two tricyclic ligans.

References

Anesini C et al: "In vivo" and "in vitro" antitumoral action of *Larrea divaricata* Cav., *Acta Physiol Pharmacol Ther Latinoam* 46(1):33-40, 1996.

Anesini C et al "In vivo" antitumor activity of *Larrea divaricata* C.: comparison of two routes of administration, *Phytomedicine* 5(1):41-45, 1998.

Gnabre JN et al: Isolation of anti-HIV-1 lignans from *Larrea tridentata* by counter-current chromatography, *J Chromatrogr A* 19(2):353-364, 1996.

Gnabre JN et al: Chaparral revisited: with a dash of linseed, *Mediherb Monitor* 23:1-2, 1997.

Luo J et al: Masoprocol (nordihydroguaiaretic acid): a new antihyperglycemic agent isolated from the creosote bush *(Larrea tridentata)*, *Eur J Pharmacol* 346:77-79, 1998.

Moore M: *Materia medica*, Bisbee, Ariz, 1995, Author.

Sheikh NM et al: Chaparral-associated hepatotoxicity, *Arch Intern Med* 157:913-919, 1997.

Stickel F et al: Hepatotoxicity of botanicals, *Public Health Nutr* 3(2):113-124, 2000.

Verastegui: MA et al: Antimicrobial activity of extracts of three major plants from the chihuahuan desert, *J Ethnopharmacol* 52(3):175-177, 1996.

Chaste Tree
(chayst tree)

Scientific name: *Vitex agnus castus*

Other common names: Chasteberry, gatillier, hemp tree, keuschbaum, monk's pepper

Class 2b/2d

Origin: Chaste tree is a shrub found in the Mediterranean and Europe.

🍃 Endangered Herb   Adverse effects: BOLD = life-threatening

Uses

Reported Uses

Chaste tree is used to treat PMS symptoms, mastodynia, uterine bleeding, impotence, spermatorrhea, prostatitis, and infertility in women. *Vitex* is thought to enhance the natural production of progesterone and luteinizing hormone and diminish the release of follicle-stimulating hormone.

Product Availability and Dosages

Available Forms

Aqueous-alcoholic extract, capsules, fluid extract, powder, solid extract, tea, tincture

Plant Parts Used: Ripe, dried fruit

Dosages and Routes

Adult

All dosages listed are PO.

Impotence
• Extract: 350-500 mg qd (Murray, 1998)

Menopause
• Dry powdered extract: 250-500 mg tid (4:1 dilution) (Murray, 1998)
• Fluid extract: 4 ml (1 tsp) tid (1:1 dilution) (Murray, 1998)
• Powdered berries or tea: 1-2 g tid (Murray, 1998)

Premenstrual Syndrome
• Fluid extract: 2 ml (Murray, 1998)
• Dry powdered extract: 175-225 mg (0.5% agnuside content) (Murray, 1998)

Other
• Capsules: 20 mg qd
• Fluid extract: 30-40 mg qd (Blumenthal, 1998)
• Tincture: 1-2 ml bid-tid (Smith, 1999)

Precautionary Information

Contraindications

Chaste tree should not be used during pregnancy except under the strict supervision of an herbalist. Until more research is completed, this herb should not be used during lactation and should not be given to children. Class 2b/2d herb.

C

Precautionary Information—cont'd

Side Effects/Adverse Reactions

Central Nervous System: Headache
Gastrointestinal: Diarrhea, abdominal cramps, anorexia
Integumentary: Rash, itching
Psychological: SEVERE DEPRESSION, SUICIDAL IDEATION

Interactions with Chaste Tree

Drug
Oral contraceptives: Chaste tree may interfere with the action; avoid concurrent use.

Food	Herb
None known	None known

Lab Test
Chaste tree may decrease serum prolactin

Client Considerations

Assess

- Determine the condition for which the client is using chaste tree.
- Assess for menstrual irregularities and whether the client is using chaste tree to treat conditions such as PMS, uterine bleeding, or increased menstrual flow. Discontinue use of herb if nausea, diarrhea, or abnormal changes in menses occurs (Smith, 1999).
- Assess for increasing depression to suicidal proportions as a result of estrogen deficiency.

Administer

- Instruct the client to store chaste tree in a cool, dry place, away from heat and moisture.

Teach Client/Family

- Caution the client not to use chaste tree during pregnancy unless under the strict supervision of an herbalist, and then only to prevent miscarriage as a result of progesterone deficiency. Until more research is available, caution the client not to use this herb during lactation and not to give it to children.

 Endangered Herb   Adverse effects: BOLD = life-threatening

- Inform the client that few scientific studies confirm any of the claims made for chaste tree.
- Advise the client to notify the prescriber immediately if depression occurs.

Pharmacology

Pharmacokinetics

Pharmacokinetics and pharmacodynamics are unknown.

Primary Chemical Components of Chaste Tree and Their Possible Actions		
Chemical Class	**Individual Component**	**Possible Action**
Essential oil	Sesquiterpenoids; Alpha-pinene; Beta-pinene; Castine; Eucalyptol; Limonene; Cineole	
Flavonoid		
Iridoid glycoside		
Progesterone		Hormonal
Hydroxyprogesterone		Hormonal
Testosterone		Hormonal

Actions

Scientific studies to support any of the uses for or actions of chaste tree are lacking.

Antiprolactin Secretion

The few studies that have been published focus on the hypoprolactinemic effect of chaste tree. In concentrations of 3.3 mg/ml, the extract significantly inhibited thyrotropin-releasing hormone (TRH)-stimulated prolactin release (Jarry, 1991). Another study confirms the inhibition of prolactin secretion (Sliutz, 1993). These studies suggest that chaste tree may produce beneficial effects in all conditions that relate to luteal phase defects.

Premenstrual Syndrome Action

One study using the PMTS (premenstrual tension syndrome) scale has shown that chaste tree significantly reduces PMS

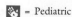 = Pregnancy   = Pediatric   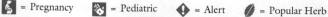 = Alert   = Popular Herb

symptoms. Participants reported decreased incidence of breast tenderness, headache, constipation, edema, and tension (Lauritzen, 1997). Two other studies confirm the results of the 1997 study (Berger, 2000; Loch, 2000).

Other Actions

Dopaminergic action via opioid receptors was identified (Meier, 2000). This is the first study suggesting this action.

References

Berger D et al: Efficacy of *Vitex agnus castus L.* extract Ze 440 in patients with pre-menstrual syndrome (PMS), *Arch Gynecol Obstet* 264(3):150-153, 2000.

Blumenthal M, editor: *The complete German Commission E monographs: therapeutic guide to herbal medicines,* Austin, Tex, American Botanical Council; Boston, Integrative Medicine Communication, 1998.

Jarry H et al: *Agnus castus* as a dopaminergic active principle, *Phtotherapie* 12:77-82, 1991.

Loch EG et al: Treatment of premenstrual syndrome with a phytopharmaceutical formulation containing *Vitex agnus castus, J Women's Health Gend Based Med* 9(3):315-320, 2000.

Meir B et al: Pharmacological activities of *Vitex agnus castus* extracts in vitro, *Phytomedicine* 7(5):373-381, 2000.

Lauritzen CH et al: Treatment of premenstrual tension syndrome with *Vitex agnus castus* controlled, double-bind study versus pyridoxine, *Phytomedicine* 4(3):183-189, 1997.

Murray M, Pizzorno J: *Encyclopedia of natural medicine,* Roseville, Calif, 1998, Prima.

Sliutz G et al: *Agnus castus* extracts inhibit prolactin secretion of rat pituitary cell, *Horm Metab Res* 25:253-255, 1993.

Smith E: *Therapeutic herb manual,* Williams, Ore, 1999, Author.

Chaulmoogra Oil
(chawl-mew'gruh)

Scientific names: *Hydnocarpus wightiana, Hydnocarpus anthelmintica, Taraktogenos kurzii*

Other common names: Gynocardia oil, hydnocarpus oil, krabao's tree seed

Origin: Chaulmoogra oil is found in India and China.

Uses

Reported Uses

In traditional herbal medicine, chaulmoogra oil (in an injectable, subcutaneous form) has been used to treat leprosy, eczema, and psoriasis. Traditional Chinese medicine practitioners use the seeds in a decoction for external use only to treat scabies, trichomoniasis, tinea, and yeast infections *(Hydnocarpus da fengzi)*.

Investigational Uses

Beginning research shows positive results using *Hydnocarpus* oil to treat wounds in leprosy (Oommen, 1999).

Product Availability and Dosages

Available Forms

Oil, injectable (subcutaneous); oil, topical; topical

Plant Parts Used: Seeds

Dosages and Routes

Adult

• Subcutaneous oil: 15 ml injected twice weekly until remission

Precautionary Information

Contraindications

Until more research is available, chaulmoogra oil should not be used during pregnancy and lactation and should not be given to children.

Side Effects/Adverse Reactions

Gastrointestinal: Gastrointestinal upset, irritation (subcutaneous)

 = Pregnancy   = Pediatric   = Alert   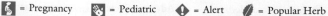 = Popular Herb

Precautionary Information—cont'd
Side Effects/Adverse Reactions—cont'd
Integumentary: Precipitation under skin (subcutaneous), pain at injection site

C

Interactions with Chaulmoogra Oil			
Drug	Food	Herb	Lab Test
None known	None known	None known	None known

Client Considerations
Assess
- Assess for eczema and psoriasis before and after treatment with this product.
- Determine whether the client is using chaulmoogra oil to treat possible leprosy. Inform the client that safer, better-tested treatments exist.

Administer
- Instruct the client to store chaulmoogra oil in a cool, dry place, away from heat and moisture.

Teach Client/Family
- Until more research is available, caution the client not to use chaulmoogra oil during pregnancy and lactation and not to give it to children.
- Inform the client that mainstream medications are more effective than chaulmoogra oil for the treatment of leprosy.
- Advise the client that only an experienced health care provider should diagnose leprosy.

Pharmacology
Pharmacokinetics
Pharmacokinetics and pharmacodynamics are unknown.

Primary Chemical Components of Chaulmoogra Oil and Their Possible Actions		
Chemical Class	**Individual Component**	**Possible Action**
Cyanogenic glycoside Fatty acid	Palmitic acid; Oleic acid	
Acid	Chaulmoogric acid; Hypnocarpic acid; Gorlic acid	
Flavolignan Protein		

Actions

Antileprotic Action

Several research studies have confirmed the efficacy of chaulmoogra oil against *Mycobacterium leprae* (Levy, 1975; Noordeen, 1991). However, many more effective treatments are available via traditional pharmacology. Since the 1940s, practitioners in developed countries have rarely used chaulmoogra oil to treat leprosy. Another study (Oommen, 1999) showed more positive wound healing than with traditional chemotherapeutic agents for leprosy. The rats tested showed an increase in weight and strength of scar tissue.

References

Levy L: The activity of chaulmoogra acids against *Mycobacterium leprae*, *Am Rev Respir Dis* 111:703-705, 1975.

Noordeen SK: A look at world leprosy, *Lepr Rev* 62:72-86, 1991.

Oommen ST et al: Effect of oil of *Hydnocarpus* on wound healing, *Int J Lepr Other Mycobact Dis* 67(2):154-158, 1999.

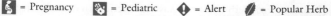

Chickweed
(chik'weed)

Scientific name: *Stellaria media*

Other common names: Mouse-ear, satinflower, star chickweed, starweed, stitchwort, tongue grass, white bird's eye, winterweed

Class 1

Origin: Chickweed is an annual found in Europe and North America.

Uses

Reported Uses

Chickweed is used internally as an antitussive, an expectorant, a demulcent, and as a treatment for sore throat, peptic ulcer, gastroesophageal reflux disease, and dyspepsia. Externally, chickweed is used to treat boils, abscesses, burns, rashes, psoriasis, eczema, pruritus and insect bites, and also to promote wound healing.

Investigational Uses

Chickweed may be useful as an antihepatoma agent (Lin, 2002) and as an antioxidant (Pieroni, 2002).

Product Availability and Dosages

Available Forms

Capsules, crude herb, fluid extract, oil, ointment, tea, tincture

Plant Parts Used: Flowers, leaves, stems

Dosages and Routes

Adult

Skin Conditions

• Topical ointment: apply prn
• Topical poultice: apply prn

Other

• PO capsules: 3 capsules tid
• PO fluid extract: 15-30 drops diluted, as often as tid
• PO tea: take qid prn
• PO tincture: take prn

Precautionary Information

Contraindications

Until more research is available, chickweed should not be used during pregnancy and lactation and it should not be given to children. High doses of chickweed can be toxic (Duke, 1985). Class 1 herb.

Side Effects/Adverse Reactions

Central Nervous System: Headache, dizziness
Systemic: NITRATE TOXICITY, PARALYSIS (high doses)

Interactions with Chickweed			
Drug	Food	Herb	Lab Test
None known	None known	None known	None known

Client Considerations

Assess

- Assess for toxicity.
- Determine the reason the client is using chickweed.

Administer

- Inform the client that, because of the potential for nitrate toxicity, only qualified herbalists should administer this herb (Duke 1985).

Teach Client/Family

- Until more research is available, caution the client not to use chickweed during pregnancy and lactation and not to give it to children.
- Instruct the client not to use this herb unless under the supervision of a qualified herbalist. No scientific studies exist to document any of its actions or uses. Nitrate toxicity and paralysis can occur.

Pharmacology

Pharmacokinetics

Pharmacokinetics and pharmacodynamics are unknown.

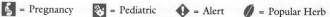
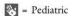

Primary Chemical Components of Chickweed and Their Possible Actions

Chemical Class	Individual Component	Possible Action
Saponin		Nitrate toxicity
Vitamin	A; B complex; C (375 mg/100 g)	
Coumarin		
Hydroxycoumarin		
Flavonoid	Rutin	Antioxidant
Nitrate salt		
Mineral	Calcium	
	Iron	

Actions

Scientific studies of the medicinal uses of chickweed are lacking. Human cases of nitrate toxicity and paralysis have been reported. The available literature supports the use of chickweed as a weed killer.

Other Actions

Antioxidant activity was identified. 27 extracts of weedy vegetables were tested for antioxidant effect. *Stellaria media* along with two other herbs showed strong in vitro inhibition of *Xanthine Oxidase* (Pieroni, 2002).

15 crude drugs including *Stellaria media* were tested for in vitro antihepatoma activity on five human liver cancer cell lines. *Stellaria media* was not as effective as *Coptis groenlandica* (Lin, 2002).

References

Duke JA: *Handbook of medicinal herbs,* Boca Raton, Fla, 1985, CRC Press.

Lin LT et al: In vitro anti-hepatoma activity of fifteen natural medicines from Canada, *Phytother Res* 16(5):440-444, 2002.

Pieroni A et al: In vitro antioxidant activity of non-cultivated vegetables of ethnic Albanians in southern Italy, *Phytother Res* 16(5):467-473, 2002.

Chicory
(chik'o-ree)

Scientific name: *Cichorium intybus*

Other common names: Blue sailors, garden
endive, succory, wild succory

Class 1

Origin: Chicory is a perennial found in Egypt, India, and the
United States.

Uses
Reported Uses

Chicory is used as a diuretic and laxative, a coffee substitute, a
sedative, an appetite stimulant, and a treatment for cancer. It
can be found in many tea product formulas. Chicory is a very
mild herb used for its bitter properties, mostly as a tonic.

Product Availability and Dosages
Available Forms

Crude herb, extract, root (roasted and raw)

Plant Parts Used: Leaves, roots

Dosages and Routes
Adult
- PO crude herb: 3 g qd (Blumenthal, 1998) (NOTE: dosages
  vary widely)
- PO decoction: 3-6 oz prn

Precautionary Information
Contraindications

Chicory should not be used during pregnancy and lactation
and should not be given to children. Persons who have cardiovascular disease or are hypersensitive to chicory or
Asteraceae/Compositae herbs should avoid its use. Persons
with gallstones should use chicory only under the supervision of an herbalist. Class 1 herb.

Side Effects/Adverse Reactions

Integumentary: Contact dermatitis, other allergic skin
rashes

 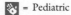

Interactions with Chicory			
Drug	Food	Herb	Lab Test
None known	None known	None known	None known

C

Client Considerations

Assess

- Assess for allergic reactions (rash, itching, contact dermatitis); discontinue use if any of these symptoms are present and administer antihistamine or other appropirate therapy.

Administer

- Instruct the client to store chicory away from moisture and light.

Teach Client/Family

- Caution the client not to use chicory during pregnancy and lactation and not to give it to children.
- Advise clients with cardiovascular disease not to use chicory; advise clients with gallstones to use this herb only with caution and under the supervision of a qualified herbalist.

Pharmacology

Pharmacokinetics

Pharmacokinetics and pharmacodynamics are unknown.

Primary Chemical Components of Chicory and Their Possible Actions		
Chemical Class	Individual Component	Possible Action
Guaianolides (Kisiel, 2001) Polysaccharide	Inulin Lactucin; Lactucopicrin	Increased probiotic
Chicoric acid Glycoside Carbohydrate Sterol		

Continued

 Endangered Herb   Adverse effects: BOLD = life-threatening

Primary Chemical Components of Chicory and Their Possible Actions—cont'd		
Chemical Class	**Individual Component**	**Possible Action**
Triterpenoid		
Lactone		
Tartaric acid		
Acetophenone		Aromatic
Phenolic coumarin	Esculetin	Hepatoprotective
Flowers: Anthocyanins	Delphinidin (Norbaek, 2002)	

Actions

Very few studies are available for chicory. This herb is thought to possess sedative, laxative, and antiarrhythmic properties, but no studies have proven any of these claims.

Hepatoprotective Action

One of the chemical components of chicory, esculetin (a phenolic coumarin), has been found to exert hepatoprotective effects (Zafar, 1998). In one study, rats were given paracetamol, a chemical that causes liver damage, followed by esculetin. Esculetin reduced mortality rates and prevented a rise in liver function enzymes (Gilani, 1998).

Other Actions

Mast cell–mediated allergic reactions were inhibited in vivo and in vitro by *Cichorium intybus* (Kim, 1999).

References

Blumenthal M, editor: *The complete German Commission E monographs: therapeutic guide to herbal medicines,* Austin, Tex, American Botanical Council; Boston, Integrative Medicine Communication, 1998.

Gilani AH et al: Esculetin prevents liver damage induced by paracetamol and CCL 4, *Pharmacol Res* 37:31-35, 1998.

Kim HM et al: Inhibitory effect of mast cell-mediated immediate-type allergic reactions by *Cichorium intybus, Pharmacol Res* 40(1):61–65, 1999.

Kisiel W et al: Guaianolides from *Cichorium intybus* and structure revision of *Chichorium* sesquiterpene lactones, *Phytochemistry* 57(4):523-527, 2001.

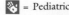 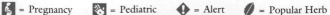

Norbaek R et al: Anthocyanins from flowers of *Cichorium intybus,* *Phytochemistry* 60(4):357-379, 2002.

Zafar R et al: Anti-hepatotoxic effects of root and root callus extracts of *Cichorium intybus* L., *J Ethnopharmacol* 63:227-231, 1998.

C

Chinese Cucumber
(chy-neez' kyew'kuhm-buhr)

Scientific name: *Trichosanthes kirilowii*

Other common names: Chinese snake gourd, gua-lou, tia-hua-fen

Class 1

Origin: Chinese cucumber is a member of the gourd family found in China.

Uses
Reported Uses
Chinese cucumber is used to treat HIV/AIDS, cancer, inflammation, ulcers, and diabetes. It is also used to induce abortion. Not a commonly used herb, gua lou ren (the seed) is primarily used in traditional Chinese medicine as a respiratory sedative, demulcent, and expectorant.

Product Availability and Dosages
Available Forms
Juice

Plant Parts Used: Fruit, rind of fruit, seed

Dosages and Routes
Adult
Dosages are not clearly delineated in the literature. Chinese cucumber juice is used to induce abortion.

Precautionary Information
Contraindications
Because Chinese cucumber is a powerful abortifacient, it should not be used during pregnancy. Until more research is available, this herb should not be used during lactation, and

Continued

Precautionary Information—cont'd

Contraindications—cont'd

it should not be given to children. Persons with seizure disorders or diarrhea should not use this herb. Class 1 herb.

Side Effects/Adverse Reactions

Central Nervous System: Fever, SEIZURES

Reproductive: ABORTION

Systemic: Hypersensitivity, FLUID IN THE LUNGS AND BRAIN, HEART DAMAGE, DEATH

Interactions with Chinese Cucumber			
Drug	Food	Herb	Lab Test
None known	None known	None known	None known

Client Considerations

Assess

- Assess for the presence of seizure disorders. If present, do not use Chinese cucumber.

Administer

- To induce abortion, apply Chinese cucumber juice to a sponge and insert into vagina. Under the supervision of a competent herbalist, this herb can be injected intramuscularly or extraamniotically to induce first-trimester abortions.

Teach Client/Family

- Because it is an abortifacient, caution the client not to use Chinese cucumber during pregnancy. Until more research is available, caution the client not to use this herb during lactation and not to give it to children.

Pharmacology

Pharmacokinetics

Pharmacokinetics and pharmacodynamics are unknown.

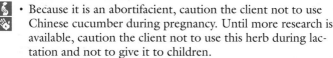

Primary Chemical Components of Chinese Cucumber and Their Possible Actions

Chemical Class	Individual Component	Possible Action
Trichobitacin		Anti–HIV-1 (Zheung, 2000)
Trichosanthin	Alpha-trichosanthin; Beta-trichosanthin	
Trichokirin		Ribosome inactivator
Karasurin		Abortifacient
Sterol		Antiinflammatory
Palmitic acid		
Galactose		
Galactonic acid gamma-lactone (Chao, 1999)		

Actions

Uterine Stimulation

Trichokirin inhibits protein synthesis and also acts as an aborti-facient. This action is believed to be mediated by the ribosome inactivation (Nie, 1998).

Antitumor Action

Trichokirin has exhibited anti-HIV activity (Nie, 1998). The antitumor action may be due to modulation of programmed cell death and arrested proliferation. Other medicinal plants with this action are soy, garlic, ginger, and green tea (Thatte, 2000). Another study (Akihisa, 2001) identified compounds from the seeds of *Trichosanthes kirilowii*. The compounds tested showed inhibition of Epstein-Barr virus, early antigen (EBV-EA).

References

Akihisa T et al: Antitumor promoting effects of mutiflorane type triterpenoids and cytoxic activity of Karounidiol against human cancer cell lines, *Cancer Lett* 173(1):9-14, 2001.

Chao Z et al: Studies on chemical constituents from fruits of *Trichosanthes kirilowii*, *Zhongguo Zhong Yao Za Zhi* 24(10):612-613, 638, 1999.

Nie H et al: Position 120-123: a potential active site of trichosanthin, *Life Sci* 62(6):491-500, 1998.

Thatte U et al: Modulation of programmed cell death by medicinal plants, *Cell Mol Biol* (Noisy-le-grand) 46(1):199-214, 2000.
Zheng YT et al: Anti-HIV-1 activity of trichobitacin, a novel ribosome-inactivating protein, *Aceta Pharmacol Sin* 21(2):179-182, 2000.

Chinese Rhubarb
(chy-neez' rew'bahrb)

Scientific name: *Rheum palmatum*

Other common names: Himalayan rhubarb, medicinal rhubarb, rhei radix, rhei rhizoma, rubarbo, Turkish rhubarb

Class 2b/2c/2d

Origin: Chinese rhubarb is a perennial found in China and Tibet.

Uses

Reported Uses
Chinese rhubarb is used as a laxative and as an antidiarrheal. It is commonly found in "neutralizing cordial" formulas today, which were also very popular from the 1800s through the 1940s. Short-term use is recommended. Chinese rhubarb may be used as part of a detoxifying regimen. This herb is not the same as garden rhubarb.

Product Availability and Dosages

Available Forms
Extract, powder, syrup, tablets, tincture

Plant Parts Used: Bark, dried root, dried underground parts

Dosages and Routes
Adult
All dosages listed are PO.
Diarrhea
- Decoction or tincture: 1 tsp qd
- Neutralizing cordial: 1-4 ml, dilute in water, q ½-2 hr according to urgency of symptoms (Smith, 1999)
Gastrointestinal Bleeding
- Powder or tablets: 3 g bid-qid

 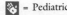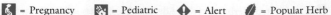

Laxative
- Decoction: 1-2 tsp qd; may be taken with evening meal
- Tincture: ½-1 tsp qd; may be taken with evening meal

Precautionary Information
Contraindications
Until more research is available, Chinese rhubarb should not be used by persons with hypersensitivity to this herb or by pregnant and lactating women, and it should not be given to children. It should not be used by persons with gastrointestinal bleeding or obstruction, abdominal pain, nausea, vomiting, appendicitis, or Crohn's disease. Use of this herb should be short-term, unless under the supervision of a qualified herbalist. Class 2b/2c/2d herb.

Side Effects/Adverse Reactions
Gastrointestinal: Nausea, vomiting, diarrhea, abdominal cramps, laxative dependency
Genitourinary: Urine discoloration, hematuria, albuminuria (high doses, long-term use)
Systemic: Vitamin and mineral deficiencies, fluid and electrolyte imbalances (high doses, long-term use)

Interactions with Chinese Rhubarb

Drug
Antacids: Antacids may decrease the effectiveness of Chinese rhubarb if taken within 1 hour of the herb.
Antiarrhythmics: Chronic use of Chinese rhubarb can cause hypokalemia and enhance the effects of antiarrhythmics.
Cardiac glycosides: Chronic use of Chinese rhubarb can cause hypokalemia and enhance the effects of cardiac glycosides.
Corticosteroids: Chronic use of Chinese rhubarb can cause hypokalemia and enhance the effects of corticosteroids.
Thiazide diuretics: Chronic use of Chinese rhubarb can cause hypokalemia and enhance the effects of thiazide diuretics; avoid concurrent use.

Food
Milk: The effectiveness of Chinese rhubarb may be decreased when taken concurrently with milk.

Continued

 Endangered Herb   Adverse effects: BOLD = life-threatening

Interactions with Chinese Rhubarb—cont'd

Herb

Jimsonweed: The action of jimsonweed is increased in cases of chronic use or abuse of Chinese rhubarb.

Licorice root: Hypokalemia can result from the use of Chinese rhubarb with licorice root; avoid concurrent use.

Lab Test

None known

Client Considerations

Assess

- Assess blood and urine electrolytes if the client uses this herb often.
- Determine the cause of constipation, identifying whether bulk, fluids, or exercise is missing from the client's lifestyle.
- Assess for cramping, nausea, and vomiting; if these symptoms occur, discontinue use of this herb.
- Assess for medications used (see Interactions).

Administer

- Instruct the client to take Chinese with other herbs to prevent griping. For best absorption, this herb should not be taken within 1 hour of other drugs, antacids, or milk.

Teach Client/Family

- Until more research is available, caution the client not to use Chinese rhubarb during pregnancy and lactation and not to give it to children.
- Caution the client to avoid long-term use of this herb, which can cause loss of bowel tone.
- Instruct the client to notify the provider if Chinese rhubarb does not relieve constipation or if symptoms of electrolyte imbalance occur (muscle cramps, pain, weakness, dizziness).

Pharmacology

Pharmacokinetics

Pharmacokinetics and pharmacodynamics are unknown.

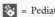 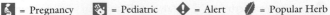

Primary Chemical Components of Chinese Rhubarb and Their Possible Actions		
Chemical Class	**Individual Component**	**Possible Action**
Anthraquinone	Rhein; Senosides (A, B, C)	Laxative
	Emodin	Decreased mitochondrial activity, energy production
	Chrysophanol; Aloe emodin	
Tannin	Gallo	Wound healing; antiinflammatory
	Galloy-1-glucose; Galloy-1-saccharose; Lindleyine; Isolindleyine	
Stilbene		
Phenolic	Glucogallin; Gallic acid; Catechin	
Polyketide synthase	Benzalacetone synthase (Abe, 2001)	

Actions

Laxative and Antidiarrheal Actions

The laxative action of anthranoids is well documented in the mainstream pharmacological literature. This action is a result of direct chemical irritation of the colon, which increases the propulsion of the stool through the bowel. The anthraquinones possess purgative properties, and the tannins and bitters possess antidiarrheal properties. Small doses have a tightening, drying effect; larger doses cause a laxative or purgative effect (Weiss, 1988; Yim, 1999).

Renal Action

In one study in which Chinese rhubarb was combined with an angiotensin-converting enzyme (ACE) inhibitor and capto-pril, an antiarrhythmic, renal failure was slowed. The use of the herb together with the two drugs produced much better results than did either the drugs or the herb alone (Zhang, 1990).

🜨 Endangered Herb   Adverse effects: **BOLD** = life-threatening

Another study (Song, 2000) identified decreasing urinary inter-
leukin 6 (IL-6) and lowered immune inflammation after *Rheum
palmatum* was given. Determination of urinary IL-6 level is
useful in studying the severity of immune inflammation of
chronic renal failure.

References

Abe I et al: Benzalacetone synthase: a novel polyketide synthase that plays
  a crucial role in the biosynthesis of phenylbutanones in *Rheum
  palmatum, Eur J Biochem* 268(1):3354-3359, 2001.
Smith E: *Therapeutic herb manual,* Williams, Ore, 1999, Author.
Song H et al: Investigation of urinary interleukin-6 level in chronic renal
  failure patients and the influence of *Rheum palmatum* in treating it,
  Zhongguo Zhong Xi Yi Jie He Za Zhi 20(2):107-109, 2000.
Weiss RF: *Herbal medicine,* England, 1988, Beaconsfield.
Yim H et al: Emodin, an anthraguinone derivative isolated from the
  rhizomes of *Rheum palmatum* selectively inhibits the activity of Casein
  kinase II as a competitive inhibitor, *Planta Med* 65(1):9-13, 1999.
Zhang JH: Clinical effects of *Rheum* and captopril on preventing
  progression of chronic renal failure, *Chin Med J* 103:788-793, 1990.

Chitosan
(kie'tuh-san)

Scientific name: N/A

Other common names: Chitosan ascorbate, deacetylated
chitin, *N*-acetylchitosan

Origin: Chitosan comes from the shell of marine crustaceans.

Uses

Reported Uses

Chitosan is used orally for weight loss, to control blood pressure, and to decrease cholesterol, and topically for periodontitis
and tissue healing.

Investigational Uses

New studies are underway for chitosan's use in chronic renal
failure, as a hemostatic, for drug delivery systems, and for assistance in nerve regeneration.

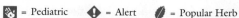

Product Availability and Dosages

Available Forms
Powder, tablets

Plant Parts Used: N/A

Dosage and Routes
Adult
- PO: Take for 2-3 days
- Can be applied topically to stop bleeding or for assistance in nerve regeneration.

Precautionary Information

Contraindications
Chitosan should not be used in hypersensitivity to shellfish, in pregnancy, in lactation, for children, or in osteoporosis or Paget's disease.

Side Effects/Adverse Reactions
Gastrointestinal: Constipation, flatulence, steatorrhea, weight loss
Cardiovascular: Hypotension

Interactions with Chitosan

Drug
Fat-soluble vitamins or minerals: Chitosan may decrease the absorption of fat-soluble vitamins, or minerals, separate by 2 hours or more.

Food	Herb	Lab Test
None known	None known	None known

Client Considerations

Assess
- Assess the reason client is using chitosan.
- Assess the gastrointestinal system for constipation, flatulence, steatorrhea; if severe, chitosan may need to be discontinued.

Administer
- Keep chitosan in a dry area, away from excessive heat or moisture.

 Endangered Herb   Adverse effects: ʙᴏʟᴅ = life-threatening

Teach Client/Family

- Teach the client that chitosan should not be used in pregnancy, in lactation, or for children until more research is completed with these populations.

Pharmacology

Pharmacokinetics

Pharmacokinetics and pharmacodynamics are unknown.

Primary Chemical Components of Chitosan and Their Possible Actions		
Chemical Class	**Individual Component**	**Possible Action**
N/A	N/A	N/A

Actions

Weight Loss Action

One study using 50 obese women studied the effects of chitosan on body weight (Zahorska et al, 2002). Significantly more weight was lost in the chitosan group. Another study (Kobayashi et al, 2002) had results that were similar. Fat deposition and lipase activity decreased significantly in chickens when chitosan was added to the diet.

Other Actions

Chitosan is able to absorb protein and adhere to nerve cells, promoting nerve regeneration (Yang, 2001).

References

Kobayasji S et al: Effects of dietary chitosan on fat deposition and lipase activity in digesta in broiler chickens, *Br Poult Sci* 43(2):270-273, 2002.

Yang Y et al: The outlook using chitosan related materials in nerve regeneration, *Sheng Wu Yi Xue Gong Cheng Xue Za Zhi* 18(3):444-447, 2001.

Zahorska B et al: Effect of chitosan in complex management of obesity, *Pol Merkuriusz Lek* 13(74):129-132, 2002.

Chondroitin
(kahn-droe'uh-tuhn)

Scientific names: Chondroitin sulfate, chondroitin sulfuric acid, chonsurid

Other common names: CAS, Chondroitin Sulfate, Chondroitin C

Origin: Chondroitin is obtained from bovine tracheal cartilage.

Uses

Reported Uses

Chondroitin is used in combination with glucosamine to treat joint conditions such as arthritis. It is also used as an antithrombotic, an extravasation therapy agent, and as a treatment for ischemic heart disease and hyperlipidemia.

Product Availability and Dosages

Available Forms

Capsules: 200, 400 mg

Source

Cartilage of the bovine trachea

Dosages and Routes

Adult

- Weight <120 pounds: 1000 mg glucosamine and 800 mg chondroitin
- Weight 120-200 pounds: 1500 mg glucosamine and 1200 mg chondroitin
- Weight >200 pounds: 2000 mg glucosamine and 1600 mg chondroitin (Theodosakis, 1997)

Precautionary Information

Contraindications

Until more research is available, chondroitin should not be used during pregnancy and lactation and it should not be given to children. It should not be used by persons with bleeding disorders or renal failure.

Continued

Precautionary Information—cont'd

Side Effects/Adverse Reactions
Central Nervous System: Headache, restlessness, euphoria
Gastrointestinal: Nausea, vomiting, anorexia
Systemic: Bleeding

Interactions with Chondroitin

Drug
Chondroitin used with anticoagulants, NSAIDs, or salicylates
can cause increased bleeding; do not use concurrently.

Food	**Herb**	**Lab Test**
None known	None known	None known

Client Considerations

Assess

- Assess for joint conditions: joints involved; aggravating and
  ameliorating factors; and pain location, intensity, and
  duration.
- Assess for other medications used; chondroitin should not be
  used concurrently with anticoagulants, NSAIDs, or salicylates
  because of the risk of increased bleeding.

Administer

- Instruct the client to store chondroitin in a cool, dry place,
  away from heat and moisture.

Teach Client/Family

- Until more research is available, caution the client not to use
  chondroitin during pregnancy and lactation and not to give it
  to children.

Pharmacology

Pharmacokinetics

Very little is known about the pharmacokinetics. The half-life of
this herb is extended when used by persons with renal failure.

 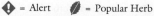

= Pregnancy   = Pediatric   ◆ = Alert   ⬥ = Popular Herb

Primary Chemical Components of Chondroitin and Their Possible Actions		
Chemical Class	Individual Component	Possible Action
Mucopolysaccharide Glycosaminoglycan (GAC) Lyases	Chondroitinase AC, B (Denholm, 2001)	Antitumor

Actions

Antiarthritic Action

Chondroitin attracts essential fluid into the joints, which acts as a shock absorber. It also attracts needed nutrients into cartilage (Benedikt, 1997). Research findings continue to conflict regarding the beneficial effects of chondroitin.

Extravasation Action

Chondroitin has been used to treat extravasation after ifosfamide therapy. One study has demonstrated its ability to decrease pain and inflammation (Mateu, 1996). The same study also used chondroitin after vindesine therapy and demonstrated that it relieved extravasation (Mateu, 1996). Similar results were obtained using chondroitin after doxorubicin therapy and vincristine therapy (Comas, 1996).

Antithrombolytic Action

Because of its ability to inhibit thrombi (Lane, 1992), chondroitin is used as an anticoagulant in hemodialysis.

References

Benedikt H: *Nat Pharmacol* 1(8):1, 22, 1997.
Comas D et al: Treatment of extravasation of both doxorubicin and vincristine administration in a Y-site infusion, *Ann Pharmacother* 30:244-246, 1996.
Denholm EM et al: Antitumor activities of chondroitinase AC and chondroitinase B: inhibition of angiogenesis, proliferation and invasion, *Eur J Pharmacol* 416(3):213-221, 2001.
Lane DA et al: Dermatan sulphate in haemodialysis, *Lancet* 8(339):334-335, 1992.
Mateu J et al: Needlestick injuries and hazardous drugs, *Am J Health Syst Pharm* 53(9):1068, 1071, 1996.
Theodosakis J: *The arthritis cure*, New York, 1997, St Martin's Press.

🦋 Endangered Herb   Adverse effects: BOLD = life-threatening

Chromium
(krow'mee-uhm)

Other common names: Chromium picolinate, chromium polynicotinate, chromium chloride

Origin: Chromium is available from dietary sources such as brewer's yeast, molasses, brown sugar, coffee, tea, and some wines and beers.

Uses

Reported Uses

Chromium is an essential trace mineral that is required for proper metabolic functioning. It may be helpful in the treatment of decreased glucose tolerance, arteriosclerosis, elevated cholesterol, glaucoma, hypoglycemia, diabetes, and obesity.

Product Availability and Dosages

Available Forms

Capsules

Dosages and Routes

All dosages listed are PO.

Adult
- 50-200 µg/day (Food and Nutritional Board, 1989)
- 200-600 µg/day (La Valle, 2001)

Child
- 0-0.5 yrs: 10-40 µg/day
- 0.5-1 yrs: 20-60 µg/day
- 1-3 yrs: 20-80 µg/day
- 4-6 yrs: 30-120 µg/day
- 7 yrs and older: 50-200 µg/day

Precautionary Information

Contraindications

Until more research is available, chromium should be given to children and used during pregnancy and lactation only in recommended dosages listed.

Side Effects/Adverse Reactions

Chromium has no known side effects or adverse reactions.

Interactions with Chromium

Drug
Antacids (calcium carbonate), calcium supplements: Calcium products reduce the absorption of chromium; separate by ≥2 hrs.

Antidiabetics (acarbose, acetohexamide, chlorpropamide, glimeperide, glipizide, insulin, metformin, miglitol, pioglitazone, tolazamide, tolbutamide, troglitazone: Chromium may reduce the action of antidiabetics.

Ascorbic acid: An increase occurs in both chromium and ascorbic acid absorption when taken together.

Iron: Absorption of chromium is decreased when taken with iron.

Zinc: Absorption of chromium is decreased when taken with zinc.

Food
Complex carbohydrates: Absorption of chromium is increased when taken with complex carbohydrates.

Herb
None known

Lab Test
Blood glucose: Chromium decreases test values.

Client Considerations

Assess
- Assess for symptoms of chromium deficiency (fasting hyperglycemia, decreased lean body mass, increased body fat, increased intraocular pressure).
- Assess for possible conditions related to chromium deficiency: stress, trauma, extreme exercise, pregnancy, infection.
- Assess for the use of ascorbic acid, iron, and zinc (see Interactions).

Administer
- Instruct the client to store chromium in a cool, dry place, away from heat and moisture.

Teach Client/Family

- Until more research is available, caution the client not to exceed recommended dosages for children or during pregnancy and lactation.

 Endangered Herb   Adverse effects: **BOLD** = life-threatening

- Instruct the client not to take chromium supplements with zinc or iron supplements; these two minerals decrease the absorption of chromium.
- Inform the client of ways to increase chromium in the diet: brewers yeast, molasses, brown sugar, coffee, tea, and some wines and beers.

Pharmacology

Pharmacokinetics

Absorption of chromium is minimal at 1% to 2% of supplement. Chromium is bound by transferrin and albumin and is transported through the circulatory system, where it is converted to an organic form and stored in tissues. Excess chromium is excreted via the kidneys.

Actions

Nutritional trivalent chromium (Cr^{+3}) is different from industrial hexavalent chromium (Cr^{+6}), which is extremely toxic. Industrial hexavalent chromium is responsible for serious pulmonary disorders and cancer in exposed workers. The population as a whole is believed to be deficient in nutritional chromium because even well-balanced diets fall short of providing the needed chromium levels (Anderson, 1985).

Improved Glucose Tolerance

Since the 1950s, at least 15 well-controlled studies have been conducted on the use of chromium to improve glucose tolerance. Chromium has been shown to increase the number of insulin receptors in peripheral tissues; to increase the binding of the insulin to receptors; to decrease tyrosine phosphatase; to terminate the receptor response; and to decrease fasting glucose, serum lipids, and HbA1c levels. Chromium may also increase HDL cholesterol (Anderson, 1998). Most of the studies showing positive results have occurred in non–insulin-dependent diabetes mellitus (NIDDM), type 2, maturity-onset. Althuia (2002) studied glucose and insulin responses to dietary chromium supplement. No changes in glucose or insulin responses were found in nondiabetic subjects.

Other Actions

Preliminary information on the ability of chromium to decrease obesity is available. Because a lack of chromium increases the percentage of body fat, supplementation in those who lack the required levels may help them lose weight. Chromium supplementation has been shown to increase muscle mass and de-

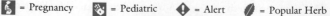

crease body fat (Kaats, 1998). Because the chromium excretion of athletes is increased, supplementation may be necessary. However, evidence supporting the need for supplementation to improve athletic performance is lacking (Clarkson, 1997). Another action may be the antithrombotic mechanism of chromium. Chromium was identified as preventing experimental venous thrombosis (Pacheco, 2000).

References

Althuis MD et al: Glucose and insulin responses to dietary chromium supplements: a meta-analysis, *Am J Clin Nutr* 76(1):148-155, 2002.

Anderson RA: Chromium intake, absorption, and excretion of subjects consuming self-selected diets, *Am J Clin Nutr* 41:1177-1183, 1985.

Anderson RA: Chromium, glucose intolerance and diabetes, *J Am Coll Nutr* 17:548-555, 1998.

Clarkson P: Effects of exercise on chromium levels: is supplementation required? *Sports Med* 23:341-349, 1997.

Food and Nutritional Board: *Recommended dietary allowances,* ed 10, Washington, DC, 1989, National Academy Press.

Kaats G et al: A randomized, double-masked, placebo-controlled study of the effects of chromium picolinate supplementation on body composition: a replication and extension of a previous study, *Curr Ther Res* 59(6):326-329, 1998.

La Valle JB et al: *Natural therapeutics pocket guide,* Hudson, Ohio, 2001, Lexi-Comp.

Pacheco RG et al: Different antithrombotic mechanisms among glycosaminoglycans revealed with a new fucosylated chrondroiten sulfate from an echinoderm, *Blood Coagul Fibrinolysis* 11(6):563-573, 2000.

Cinnamon
(si'nuh-muhn)

Scientific name: *Cinnamomum* spp.

Other common names: *Cassia, Cassia lignea,* Ceylon cinnamon, Chinese cinnamon, cinnamomom, false cinnamon, Padang cassia, Panang cinnamon, Saigon cassia, Saigon cinnamon

Class 2b/2d

Origin: Cinnamon is found in India, South America, Sri Lanka, and the West Indies.

Uses

Reported Uses

Cinnamon is used as an antifungal and analgesic and to treat diarrhea, the common cold, abdominal pain, hypertension, loss of appetite, and bronchitis. It is also used to treat passive internal bleeding, sometimes as an essential oil in combination with *Erigeron* essential oil. In contemporary use, cinnamon is rarely used alone. It is considered one of the major adjuvant herbs used in small amounts to assist in the assimilation of an herbal formula. Cinnamon is an aromatic and tends to be spicy, warming, and vasodilating, as well as cooling (see Actions).

Product Availability and Dosages

Available Forms

Dried bark, essential oil, leaves, fluid extract, powder, tincture

Plant Parts Used: Bark, leaves

Dosages and Routes

Dosages vary widely. All dosages listed are PO.

Adult

Passive Bleeding

- Essential oil: used in combination with *Erigeron* essential oil, diluted in a carrier oil such as vegetable oil; 10-30 drops (Smith, 1999)

Other

- Bark: 2-4 g qd (Blumenthal, 1998)
- Essential oil: 0.05-0.2 ml diluted in a carrier oil qd
- Infusion: 1 cup bid-tid at meals
- Fluid extract: 0.5-1 ml tid
- Tincture: 1-3 ml tid

Precautionary Information

Contraindications

Until more research is available, except as a spice or for flavoring, cinnamon should not be used during pregnancy and lactation and should not be given to children. Persons with hypersensitivity to cinnamon or balsam of Peru should not use cinnamon. Persons with intestinal or gastric ulcers or prolonged use is not recommended. Class 2b/2d herb.

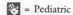

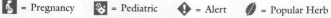

= Pregnancy   = Pediatric   = Alert   = Popular Herb

Precautionary Information—cont'd

Side Effects/Adverse Reactions

Cardiovascular: Increased heart rate
Central Nervous System: Flushing
Ear, Eye, Nose, and Throat: Stomatitis, glossitis, gingivitis
Gastrointestinal: Increased motility, anorexia, irritant
(full doses)
Respiratory: Shortness of breath
Systemic: Hypersensitivity

Interactions with Cinnamon			
Drug	Food	Herb	Lab Test
None known	None known	None known	None known

Client Considerations

Assess

- Assess for hypersensitivity (rash, wheezing); if present, discontinue use of this herb and administer antihistamine or other appropriate therapy.

Administer

- Instruct the client to store cinnamon in a cool, dry place, away from heat and moisture.
- Instruct the client to dilute cinnamon oil in a carrier oil.

Teach Client/Family

- Until more research is available, caution the client not to use cinnamon bark therapeutically during pregnancy and lactation and not to give it to children therapeutically.

Pharmacology

Pharmacokinetics

Pharmacokinetics and pharmacodynamics are unknown.

Primary Chemical Components of Cinnamon and Their Possible Actions

Chemical Class	Individual Component	Possible Action
Volatile oil	Eugenol; Cinnamaldehyde	Antimicrobial; anesthetic; antioxidant
	Weiterhin; Cinnamic acid	
O-Glucoside		Gastrointestinal protectant
Diterpene		
Mucilage		
Cyclobutane lignan	Cinbalansan (Cuong, 2001)	
Coumarin		
Cinnamyl acetate (Choi, 2001)		

Actions

Cinnamon is considered to be spicy, warming, and vasodilating due to the volatile oils; it is considered to be drying and cooling due to the tannin content. This warming and cooling combination is especially effective for the treatment of diarrhea when there is griping, and cinnamon is often added to laxative formulas for this purpose. It is an aromatic stimulant, mainly to the gastrointestinal tract; a carminative; and an astringent. Cinnamon possesses marked hemostatic power and is used to flavor unpleasant-tasting medicines.

Antimicrobial/Antifungal Action

Cinnamon bark has been shown to be effective against the following organisms that cause respiratory tract infections: *Candida albicans, Candida tropicalis, Aspergillus niger, Aspergillus fuigatis, Aspergillus midulans, Aspergillus flavus, Histoplasma,* and *Cryptococcus neoformans* (Viollon, 1994). Cinnamon extract has shown an inhibitory effect on *Helicobacter pylori* (Tabek, 1999).

Antidiabetic Action

The insulin-potentiating effect of cinnamon bark and its role in glucose metabolism have been studied (Khan, 1990). In a

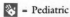 = Pregnancy   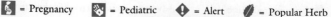 = Pediatric   = Alert   = Popular Herb

study in which streptozocin was administered long-term to induce diabetes mellitus in rats, cinnamon bark conferred some protection against diabetic conditions when administered along with the streptozocin (Onderoglu, 1999).

References

Blumenthal M, editor: *The complete German Commission E monographs: therapeutic guide to herbal medicines,* Austin, Tex, American Botanical Council; Boston, Integrative Medicine Communication, 1998.

Choi J et al: Constituents of the essential oil of the *Cinnamomum cassia* stem bark and the biological properties, *Arch Pharm Res* 24(5):418-423, 2001.

Cuong NM et al: A new cyclobutane lignan from *Cinnamomum balansae, Nat Prod Lett* 15(5):331-338, 2001.

Khan A et al: Insulin potentiating factor and chromium content of selected foods and spices, *Biol Trace Elem Res* 24:183-188, 1990.

Onderoglu S et al: The evaluation of long-term effects of cinnamon bark and olive leaf on toxicity induced by streptozotocin administration to rats, *J Pharm Pharmacol* 51:1305-1312, 1999.

Smith E: *Therapeutic herb manual,* Williams, Ore, 1999, Author.

Tabek M et al: Cinnamon extracts' inhibitory effect on *Helicobacter pylori, J Ethnopharmacol* 67(3):269-277, 1999.

Viollon C et al: Antifungal properties of essential oils and their main components upon *Cryptococcus neoformans, Mycopathologia* 128:151-153, 1994.

Clary
(kla'ree)

Scientific names: *Salvia sclarea, Euphrasia officinalis* (eyebright)

Other common names: Clary oil, clary sage, clear eye, eyebright, muscatel sage, orvale, see bright, toute-bonne

Class 1

Origin: Clary is a perennial found in Europe.

Uses

Reported Uses

Clary is used as an antiinflammatory to decrease muscle and nervous tension; an antispasmodic; a sedative; an astringent; and as a treatment for menopausal symptoms, premenstrual syndrome, decreased libido, and fatigue. It is also used to stimulate the adrenals and, in Europe, as a remedy for sore throat.

Endangered Herb   Adverse effects: BOLD = life-threatening

Product Availability and Dosages

Available Forms
Essential oil

Plant Parts Used: Essential oil of leaves and flowers

Dosages and Routes

Adult

Dosages are not clearly delineated in the literature.

Precautionary Information

Contraindications

Clary should not be used during pregnancy and lactation and should not be given to children. Persons who have estrogen-sensitive cancers, breast cysts, and uterine fibroids should not use this herb. Undiluted essential oil should not be applied topically or taken internally. Class 1 herb.

Side Effects/Adverse Reactions

Central Nervous System: Drowsiness, headache, euphoria, dizziness, nightmares, stupor (high doses)
Endocrine: Increased menstrual bleeding

Interactions with Clary

Drug

Alcohol: Clary increases the action of alcohol; do not use concurrently.
Hypnotics: Clary increases the action of hypnotics (theoretical); do not use concurrently.

Food	Herb	Lab Test
None known	None known	None known

Client Considerations

Assess
- Determine the reason the client is using clary.
- Assess for the use of alcohol and hypnotics (see Interactions).

Administer
- Instruct the client to store clary in a cool, dry place, away from heat and moisture.

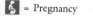 = Pregnancy    = Pediatric    = Alert   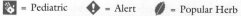 = Popular Herb

Teach Client/Family

- Until more research is available, caution the client not to use clary during pregnancy and lactation and not to give it to children.
- Advise the client not to use alcohol or hypnotics while taking this herb.

Pharmacology

Pharmacokinetics

Pharmacokinetics and pharmacodynamics are unknown.

Primary Chemical Components of Clary and Their Possible Actions

Chemical Class	Individual Component	Possible Action
Diterpene	Sclareol	Antimicrobial
	Manool; Salvipisone; Ferruginol; Microstegiol; Candidissiol	
Sesquiterpene	Caryophyllene oxide	Antimicrobial
	Spathulenol; Dehydrosalvipisone; Oxoroyleanone	
Alpha-amyrin		
Beta-sitosterol		
Flavonoid	Apigenin; Luteolin; 4-Methylapigenin	
Essential oil	Nerol	Estrogen-like
Linalyl acetate		
Linalool		
Pionene		
Lectin	SSL	Antitumor (Medeiros, 2000)

Actions

Antimicrobial Action

Several chemical components of *Salvia sclarea* have been found to possess antimicrobial properties. The diterpenoids and sesquiterpenoids were tested for antimicrobial effects against bacteria and yeast. Dehydrosalvipisone, sclareol, manool, oxoroyleanone, spathulenol, and caryophyllene were found to be active against *Staphylococcus aureus.* Dehydrosalvipisone and manool were found to be active against *Candida albicans,* and caryophyllene was found to be active against *Proteus mirabilis* (Ulubelen, 1994). Another study (Peana, 1999) demonstrated that clary exerts a weak antimicrobial effect against *S. aureus, C. albicans, Escherichia coli,* and *Staphylococcus epidermidis.* However, the antimicrobial effect increased as the microbes remained in contact with the chemical component for longer periods.

Antitumor Action

The Tn antigen, which is a specific marker in several human carcinomas, has been isolated from *Salvia sclarea.* The identification of the marker came from SSL, a lectin present in clary (Medeiros, 2000). Although still in the preliminary stages, this research on the possible antitumor action of clary shows promise.

References

Medeiros A: Biochemical and functional characterization of the Tn-specific lectin from *Salvia sclarea* seeds, *Eur J Biochem* 267(5):1434-1440, 2000.

Peana AT et al: Chemical composition and antimicrobial action of the essential oils of *Salvia desoleana* and *S. sclarea, Planta Med* 65(8):752-754, 1999.

Ulubelen A et al: Terpenoids from *Salvia sclarea, Phytochemistry* 36(4): 971-974, 1994.

Clematis
(kli-ma'tuhs)

Scientific name: *Clematis virginiana* L.

Other common names: Devil's darning needle, old man's beard, traveller's joy, vine bower, woodbine

Origin: Clematis is a perennial shrub found in Asia and North America.

Uses

Reported Uses

Clematis is used both externally and internally to treat frontal and migraine headaches. It is also used to treat skin disorders and hypertension. This herb is rarely used and is not easily found over the counter.

Product Availability and Dosages

Available Forms

Extract, juice

Plant Parts Used: Fresh leaves

Dosages and Routes

Adult

- PO extract: 0.5-2ml tid in water (Moore, 1995)
- Topical: apply prn

Precautionary Information

Contraindications

Until more research is available, clematis should not be used pregnancy and lactation and should not be given to children. Persons with vasculitis should not use this herb (Moore, 1995).

Side Effects/Adverse Reactions

Ear, Eye, Nose, and Throat: Severe mucous membrane irritation
Gastrointestinal: Irritation, colic, diarrhea
Genitourinary: Irritation
Integumentary: Severe irritation
Toxicity: DIZZINESS, SEIZURES, CONFUSION, DEATH (rare)

Interactions with Clematis

Drug
All Western medications: Avoid concurrent use with all Western medications (Moore, 1995).

Food	Herb	Lab Test
None known	None known	None known

 Endangered Herb   Adverse effects: BOLD = life-threatening

Client Considerations

Assess

- Assess for the characteristics of migraine headache: aura, halo, and blurred vision; location, intensity, and duration of pain; need for opioids in the past; alleviating, aggravating, and nutritional factors.

- Assess for toxicity.
- Assess for medication use (see Interactions).

Administer

- Instruct the client to use activated charcoal to treat overdose. Asphyxiation is the cause of death.

Teach Client/Family

- Until more research is available, caution the client not to use clematis during pregnancy and lactation and not to give it to children.
- Caution the client not to allow clematis to remain in extended contact with the skin or mucous membranes; blistering is common.

Pharmacology

Pharmacokinetics

Pharmacokinetics and pharmacodynamics are unknown.

Primary Chemical Components of Clematis and Their Possible Actions		
Chemical Class	**Individual Component**	**Possible Action**
Saponin	Anemonin	Central nervous system stimulant
	Protoanemonin	Vesicant oil

Actions

Clematis is rarely used today because of the availability of safer herbs and drugs. The fresh juice reportedly contains protoanemonin, a vesicant oil, which is a direct irritant to the skin and mucous membranes (American Herbal Products Association, 1988).

= Pregnancy   = Pediatric   = Alert   = Popular Herb

References

American Herbal Products Association, 1988.
Moore M: *Materia medica,* Bisbee, Ariz, 1995, Author.

C

Cloves
(klowvz)

Scientific names: *Syzygium aromaticum, Eugenia caryophyllata, Caryophyllus aromaticus*

Other common names: Oil of cloves, oleum caryophylli

Class 1

Origin: Cloves are found in South America, Sumatra, and Tanzania.

Uses

Reported Uses

Cloves are used mainly as an essential oil; a treatment for toothache; a topical anesthetic in dentistry; and an antiseptic, antibacterial, and antiinflammatory for the oral mucosa. They may also be used as a flavoring or antimicrobial in formulas.

Product Availability and Dosages

Available Forms

Component in cigarettes and mouthwash; essential oil; tincture

Plant Parts Used: Dried flower buds

Dosages and Routes

Adult

- Mouthwash: ≤1 oz of 1%-5% essential oil prn
- PO tincture: 5-30 drops (1:3 dilution) prn
- Topical: 1-5 drops essential oil prn

Precautionary Information

Contraindications

Until more research is available, do not use cloves during pregnancy and lactation and do not give them to children. Essential oil should be used only when diluted in a carrier oil. Class 1 herb.

Continued

🜍 Endangered Herb   Adverse effects: BOLD = life-threatening

> **Precautionary Information—cont'd**
> **Side Effects/Adverse Reactions**
> *Ear, Eye, Nose, and Throat:* Tissue irritation, airway injury
> *Integumentary:* Skin irritation
> *Respiratory:* BRONCHOSPASM, PULMONARY EDEMA

Interactions with Cloves			
Drug	Food	Herb	Lab Test
None known	None known	None known	None known

Client Considerations

Assess

- Assess for allergic reaction (bronchospasm, pulmonary edema). If allergic symptoms are present, use of the herb should be discontinued and emergency measures instituted.

Administer

- Instruct the client to store cloves in a cool, dry place, away from heat and moisture.
- Instruct the client to dilute essential oil in a carrier oil.

Teach Client/Family

- Until more research is available, caution the client not to use cloves during pregnancy and lactation and not to give them to children.

Pharmacology

Pharmacokinetics

Pharmacokinetics and pharmacodynamics are unknown.

 = Pregnancy   = Pediatric   = Alert   = Popular Herb

Primary Chemical Components of Cloves and Their Possible Actions

Chemical Class	Individual Component	Possible Action
Phenol	Eugenol; Acetyl eugenol	Antimicrobial; analgesic; antioxidant
Terpene Beta-Caryophyllene		Local anesthetic (Ghelardini, 2001)

Actions

Clove oil possesses antihistamine, spasmolytic, mildly antiseptic, anthelmintic, and larvicidal properties.

Topical Anesthetic Action

When applied topically, cloves have been found to inhibit prostaglandin synthesis, cyclooxygenase, and lipoxygenase. Eugenol, one of the chemical components of cloves, is responsible for these actions (Rasheed, 1984).

Antimicrobial Action

In underdeveloped countries where most people cannot afford the high cost of medications, cloves have been used to treat diarrheal diseases in children. In one study, the antibacterial effect of cloves was tested using a decoction of aqueous dried extract. The extract showed activity against *Salmonella* E., *Shigella* D., *Shigella* F., *Escherichia coli,* and *Enterobacter* (Tsakala, 1996). Another study investigated the efficacy of cloves against cytomegalovirus (CMV). Cloves demonstrated significant effectiveness against CMV in low concentrations in vitro (Yukawa, 1996). *Syzygium aromaticum* showed active inhibition of hepatitis C virus (HCV) when tested with 71 medicinal plant extract (Hussein, 2000). Another study (Dorman, 2000) investigated the volatile oils in several medicinal plants, including cloves. All oils exhibited significant antimicrobial effect (Dorman, 2000).

References

Dorman HJ et al: Antimicrobial agents from plants: antibacterial activity of plant volatile oils, *J Appl Microbiol* 88(2):306-318, 2000.

Ghelardini C et al: Local anaesthetic activity of beta-caryophyllene, *Farmaco* 56(5-7):387-389, 2001.

Hussein G et al: Inhibitory effects of sudanese medicinal plant extracts on hepatitis C virus (HCV) protease, *Phytother Res* 14(7):510-516, 2000.

Rasheed A et al: Eugenol and prostaglandin biosynthesis, *N Engl J Med* 310(1):50-51, 1984 (letter).

Tsakala TM et al: Screening of in vitro antibacterial activity from *Syzygium guineense* (wild) hydrosoluble dry extract, *Lab de Pharmacie Galenique, Faculte de Pharmacie* 54(6):276-279, 1996 (abstract).

Yukawa TA et al: Prophylactic treatment of cytomegalovirus infection with traditional herbs, *Antiviral Res* 32:63-70, 1996.

Coenzyme Q10
(koe-ehn'zime kyew tehn)

Scientific name: 2,3 dimethoxy-5 methyl-6-decaprenyl benzoquinone

Other common names: Co-Q10, mitoquinone, ubidecarenone, ubiquinone

Origin: Coenzyme Q10 is found in dietary sources.

Uses

Reported Uses

Coenzyme Q10 is used to treat ischemic heart disease, congestive heart failure (CHF), angina pectoris, hypertension, arrhythmias, diabetes mellitus, deafness, Bell's palsy, decreased immunity, mitral valve prolapse, periodontal disease, and infertility.

Investigational Uses

Research is underway to determine the efficacy of coenzyme Q10 in the treatment of breast cancer; migraine prevention is also being investigated as a possible use of Q10 (Rozen, 2002). Research has confirmed that coenzyme Q10 does not slow the progression of Huntington's disease (Huntington Study Group, *Neurology*, 2001) or congestive heart failure (Khatta, 2000).

Product Availability and Dosages

Available Forms

Capsules, tablets

Dosages and Routes

Dosages vary widely.

 = Pregnancy  = Pediatric = Alert 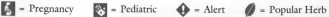 = Popular Herb

Adult
Breast Cancer, Cardiovascular Disease, Diabetes
• PO: >300mg/day (LaValle, 2001)
Other
• PO: 30-200 mg/day (LaValle, 2001)

C

Precautionary Information

Contraindications

Until more research is available, coenzyme Q10 should not be used at excessive levels during pregnancy and lactation and should not be given to children. Persons with hypersensitivity should not use this nutritional supplement.

Side Effects/Adverse Reactions

Gastrointestinal: Nausea, vomiting, anorexia, diarrhea, epigastric pain

Interactions with Coenzyme Q10

Drug

Anticoagulants (heparin, warfarin): Coenzyme Q10 may decrease the action of anticoagulants; avoid concurrent use.
Beta-blockers: Beta-blockers may decrease the action of coenzyme Q10 and deplete endogenous stores; avoid concurrent use.
HMG-CoA reductase inhibitors: HMG-CoA reductase inhibitors may decrease the action of coenzyme Q10 and deplete endogenous stores; avoid concurrent use.
Oral antidiabetics: Oral antidiabetics may decrease the action of coenzyme Q10 and deplete endogenous stores; avoid concurrent use.
Phenothiazines (chlorpromazine): Certain phenothiazines (chlorpromazine) may decrease the action of coenzyme Q10 and deplete endogenous stores; avoid concurrent use.
Tricyclic antidepressants: Tricyclic antidepressants may decrease the action of coenzyme Q10 and deplete endogenous stores; avoid concurrent use.

Food	Herb	Lab Test
None known	None known	None known

 Endangered Herb   Adverse effects: BOLD = life-threatening

Client Considerations

Assess

- If the client is using coenzyme Q10 for a cardiovascular condition, assess cardiovascular status (blood pressure; pulse rhythm, character).
- Assess medication use (see Interactions).

Administer

- Instruct the client to store coenzyme Q10 away from moisture and light.

Teach Client/Family

- Until more research is available, caution the client not to use coenzyme Q10 at increased levels during pregnancy and lactation and not to give it to children.
- Instruct the client to avoid concurrent use of coenzyme Q10 with anticoagulants, or to have lab parameters monitored carefully if used concurrently.
- Advise the client to avoid using coenzyme Q10 with phenothiazines, tricyclics, beta-blockers, and cholesterol-lowering agents.

Pharmacology

Pharmacokinetics

Supplements are absorbed at the levels of 2% to 3%. Peak occurs at approximately 6 hours.

Primary Chemical Components of Coenzyme Q10 and Their Possible Actions		
Chemical Class	**Individual Component**	**Possible Action**
Ubiquinone Benzoquinone		Antioxidant

Actions

Coenzyme Q10 is a fat-soluble vitamin-like compound known as ubiquinone. It is synthesized in humans and is involved in adenosine triphosphate (ATP) generation. Coenzyme Q10 functions as an endogenous antioxidant, protecting against free radial damage within the mitochondria.

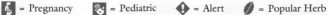

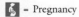 = Pregnancy    = Pediatric   = Alert   ∅ = Popular Herb

Myocardial Enhancement

Researchers have discovered lowered levels of coenzyme Q10 in patients with cardiac conditions such as ischemic heart disease (Hanaki, 1991) and dilated cardiomyopathy (Langsjoen, 1990). The greater the severity of the cardiac disease, the lower the coenzyme Q10 level (Littarru, 1972). In one study of 88 patients with cardiomyopathy who received 100 mg/day of coenzyme Q10 for up to 2 years, 75% of the patients improved significantly as noted by ejection fraction and cardiac output (Langsjoen, 1988). In another study of patients with cardiomyopathy who received coenzyme Q10 for 12 weeks, stroke volume and ejection fraction improved significantly after treatment (Langsjoen, 1985).

Adriamycin Toxicity Prevention

Coenzyme Q10 has been shown to prevent cardiac toxicity associated with adriamycin therapy. In studies using laboratory animals given adriamycin followed by coenzyme Q10, the restoration of appropriate coenzyme Q10 levels prevented changes in the heart (Ogura, 1979; Domae, 1981). Therefore, it appears that coenzyme Q10 may be used to prevent adriamycin cardiac toxicity in humans, but more research is needed to confirm this assumption.

Other Actions

Coenzyme Q10 has shown promise as a migraine preventive agent. Thirty-two patients with a history of episodic migraines were given 150 mg/day of coenzyme Q10. There was a 50% reduction in number of days with migraines (Rozen, 2000).

References

Domae N et al: Cardiomyopathy and other chronic toxic effects induced in rabbits by doxorubicin and possible prevention by coenzyme Q10, *Cancer Treat Rep* 65:79-91, 1981.

Hanaki Y et al: Ratio of low-density lipoprotein cholesterol to ubiquinone as a coronary risk factor, *N Engl J Med* 325:814-815, 1991.

Khatta M et al: The effect of coenzyme Q10 in patients with congestive heart failure, *Ann Intern Med* 132(8):636-640, 2000.

Langsjoen PH et al: Effective treatment with coenzyme Q10 of patients with chronic myocardial disease, *Drugs Exp Clin Res* 11:577-579, 1985.

Langsjoen PH et al: Effective and safe therapy with coenzyme Q10 for cardiomyopathy, *Klin Wochenschr* 66:583-590, 1988.

Langsjoen PH et al: Long-term efficacy and safety of coenzyme Q10 therapy for idiopathic dilated cardiomyopathy, *Am J Cardiol* 65:521-523, 1990.

La Valle JB et al: *Natural therapeutics pocket guide,* Hudson, Ohio, 2001, Lexi-Comp.

Littarru GP et al: Deficiency of coenzyme Q10 in human heart disease, part II, *Int J Vitam Nutr Res* 42:291-305, 1972.

Ogura R et al: The role of ubiquinone (coenzyme Q10) in preventing adriamycin-induced mitochondrial disorders in rat hearts, *J Appl Biochem* 1:325-335, 1979.

Rozen TD et al: Open label trial of coenzyme Q10 as a migraine preventive, *Cephalalgia* 22(2):137-141, 2002.

The Huntington Study Group: A randomized, placebo-controlled trial of coenzyme Q10 and remacemide in Huntington's disease, *Neurology* 57(3):397-404, 2001.

Coffee
(kaw'fee)

Scientific name: *Coffea* spp.

Other common names: Bean juice, café, espresso, java, mocha

Class 2b/2d

Origin: Coffee is found in Central and South America.

Uses

Reported Uses

Coffee is used to increase alertness and mood, to increase exercise tolerance, and to enhance bronchodilation. Historically, coffee administered by mouth or rectum was used as an antidote for opium poisoning. It is used in herbal medicine to stimulate the appetite and facilitate digestion. It promotes peristalsis and slightly accelerates circulation (Felter, 1922).

Product Availability and Dosages

Available Forms

Roasted seed (beans)

Plant Parts Used: Seeds

Dosages and Routes

Adult

• PO infusion: 2-8 oz (Felter, 1922)

NOTE: Lethal dose is approximately 100 cups of coffee

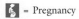 = Pregnancy    = Pediatric   = Alert   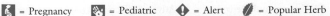 = Popular Herb

Precautionary Information
Contraindications

Until more research is available, coffee should not be used during pregnancy and lactation and should not be given to children. Coffee should also be avoided by persons with cardiovascular disease because of increased homocysteine levels, glaucoma, duodenal or gastric ulcers. Class 2b/2d herb.

Side Effects/Adverse Reactions

Cardiovascular: Palpitations, extrasystole, restlessness, increased blood pressure
Central Nervous System: Headache, insomnia, increased affect and mood, decreased seizure threshold, dizziness, irritability, depression
Gastrointestinal: Nausea, vomiting, gastroesophageal reflux disease (GERD), peptic ulcer
Genitourinary: Increased diuresis
Musculoskeletal: Tremors

Interactions with Coffee

Drug

Benzodiazepines: Caffeine reduces the benzodiazepine effect.
Beta-blockers: Caffeine increases blood pressure in those taking beta-blockers.
Bronchodilators: Large amounts of coffee increase the action of some bronchodilators.
Lithium: Levels of lithium are decreased by caffeine.
MAOIs: Large amounts of coffee should be avoided; hypertensive reactions may occur.
Xanthines (theophylline): Large amounts of coffee increase the action of xanthines such as theophylline.

Food

None known

Herb

Ephedra: Concurrent use of ephedra and coffee may increase hypertension and central nervous system stimulation; avoid concurrent use.

Continued

 Endangered Herb   Adverse effects: ʙᴏʟᴅ = life-threatening

Interactions with Coffee—cont'd

Lab Test
AST: Coffee may decrease test values in alcoholics.
Secretion provocation test: Coffee may increase test values.
Serum 2-hour postprandiol glucose: False increase if caffeine is ingested during test.
Specimen infertility screen: Heavy coffee consumption may decrease number of motile sperm.

Client Considerations

Assess

- Determine how much coffee the client consumes and its effect on mood, affect, and sleep patterns.
- Assess cardiac status of clients with cardiac disease (blood pressure, pulse, increased palpitations; hypertension and tachycardia may also be present).
- Assess for the use of bronchodilators, xanthines, and ephedra (see Interactions).

Administer

- Instruct the client to store coffee in a cool, dry place, away from heat and moisture.

Teach Client/Family

- Until more research is available, caution the client not to use coffee during pregnancy and lactation and not to give it to children.
- Inform the client that withdrawal symptoms are common after the use of coffee for extended periods.

Pharmacology

Pharmacokinetics

Half-life 3½-4½ hours.

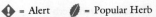

Primary Chemical Components of Coffee and Their Possible Actions

Chemical Class	Individual Component	Possible Action
Xanthine	Caffeine	Central nervous system stimulant
Diterpene		Increased cholesterol, low-density lipoproteins, triglycerides
Chlorogenic acid		
Galactomanan protein		
Free amino acid		
Polyamine		
Tannin		Wound healing; antiinflammatory
Vitamin	B	
Mineral	Niacin (trace)	
Coffee Oil Contains		
Fatty acid		
Stearic acid		
Sterol		
Tocopherol		
Cafestol		
Cahweol		
Lanosterol		

Actions

The xanthine group has been studied extensively in mainstream pharmacology research. Xanthines, of which caffeine is one, stimulate the central nervous system by binding to adenosine receptors in the brain. One study researched the effects of elevated homocysteine concentrations, which are present in unfiltered coffee. Elevated homocysteine levels are a risk factor for cardiovascular disease. Consumption of one liter of unfiltered coffee per day for 14 days significantly raised fasting homocysteine concentrations by 10% (Grubben, 2000). Another study researched the possible correlation between coffee consumption and decreased risk of gallstone disease in men. Of the 1081 subjects who had symptomatic gallstone disease,

885 required cholecystectomy. After adjusting for other factors, results showed that the men who consumed two to three cups of coffee per day showed a decrease in gallstone disease, while those who drank four or more cups of coffee per day showed an even greater decrease in the disease (Leitzmann, 1999).

References

Felter HW: *The eclectic materia medica: pharmacology and therapeutics,* Sandy, Ore, 1922, reprinted by Eclectic Medical Publications.

Grubben MA et al: Unfiltered coffee increases plasma homocysteine concentrations in healthy volunteers: a randomized trial, *Am J Clin Nutr* 71:480-484, 2000.

Leitzmann MF et al: A prospective study of coffee consumption and the risk of symptomatic gallstone disease in men, *JAMA* 281(22):2106-2111, 1999.

Cola Tree
(koe'luh tree)

Scientific names: *Cola nitida, Cola acuminata*

Other common names: Bissy nut, cola nut, guru nut, kola nut, kolatier

Class 2b/2d (Seeds)

Origin: The cola tree is an evergreen found in parts of Africa and Indonesia.

Uses

Reported Uses

Cola tree is used as an antidepressant; a diuretic; an antidiarrheal; and a treatment for heart disease, dyspnea, fatigue, morning sickness, and migraine. It may also be used topically to promote wound healing and reduce inflammation.

Product Availability and Dosages

Available Forms

Cola nut, cola wine, fluid extract, powdered herb, solid extract, tincture

Plant Parts Used: Seeds

= Pregnancy   = Pediatric   ◆ = Alert   ∥ = Popular Herb

Dosages and Routes
Adult
All dosages listed are PO.
- Cola extract: 0.25-0.75 g/day (Blumenthal, 1998)
- Cola fluid extract: 2.5-7.5 g/day (Blumenthal, 1998)
- Cola nut: 2-6 g/day (Blumenthal, 1998)
- Cola wine: 60-180 g/day (Blumenthal, 1998)
- Decoction: 1-2 tsp powder in 1 cup water, boiled 15 min
- Fluid extract: 5-40 drops bid-tid with meals, mixed in a small amount of liquid
- Solid extract: 2-8 grains tid
- Tincture: 10-30 g/day (Blumenthal, 1998)

Precautionary Information
Contraindications
Until more research is available, cola tree products should not be used during pregnancy and lactation and should not be given to children. These products should not be used by persons with hypersensitivity to chocolate or with stomach or duodenal ulcers, and persons with cardiac disease such as ischemic heart disease, hypertension, arrhythmias, or heart palpitations should avoid their use. Cola tree products should be used with caution by persons with anxiety, nervousness, or mood disorders. Avoid prolonged use. Class 2b/2d herb (seeds).

Side Effects/Adverse Reactions
Cardiovascular: Hypertension, hypotension, tachycardia, bradycardia, palpitations
Central Nervous System: Anxiety, insomnia, nervousness, irritability, restlessness, headache
Gastrointestinal: Nausea, vomiting, anorexia, abdominal distress, cramps, gastrointestinal mucosa irritation, bright yellow oral pigmentation (Ashri, 1990)
Genitourinary: Diuresis
Integumentary: Hypersensitivity reactions

Interactions with Cola Tree

Drug

Analgesics: Cola tree products may increase the effect of analgesics; avoid concurrent use.

Benzodiazepines (diazepam, clonazepam, temazepam, triazolam): Benzodiazepines may decrease the effect of cola tree products.

Beta-blockers (propranolol, metoprolol): Cola tree products may increase blood pressure when used with beta-blockers.

Furoquinolones (alatrofloxacin, ciprofloxacin, levofloxacin): Furoquinolones may increase the effect of cola tree products.

Lithium: Lithium may decrease the effect of cola tree products.

MAOIs (phenelzine, tranylcypromine): Cola tree products may increase blood pressure when used with phenelzine and tranylcypromine.

Psychoanaleptic agents: Cola tree products may increase the action of psychoanaleptic agents.

Salicylates (aspirin): Salicylates may increase the effect of cola tree products.

Xanthines: Cola tree products may increase the action of xanthines (e.g., theophylline, caffeine); avoid concurrent use.

Food

Caffeinated coffee, cola, and tea may increase the effect of cola tree products.

Herb

Ephedra: Concurrent use of ephedra and cola tree may increase hypertension and central nervous system stimulation; avoid concurrent use.

Lab Test

None known

Client Considerations

Assess

- Assess for hypersensitivity reactions. If these are present, discontinue the use of cola tree products and administer antihistamines or other appropriate therapy.

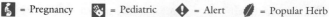

= Pregnancy   = Pediatric   = Alert   = Popular Herb

C

• Assess cardiac status in cardiac patients (blood pressure, pulse, palpitations, hypertension, tachycardia).
• Assess the client's mental status (affect, mood, euphoria).
• Assess for the use of medications, caffeinated drinks, and ephedra (see Interactions).

Administer

• Instruct the client to store cola tree products in a sealed container in a cool, dry place, away from heat and moisture.

Teach Client/Family

• Until more research is available, caution the client not to use cola tree products during pregnancy and lactation and not to give them to children.
• Instruct the client not to confuse the cola tree herb with other types of cola.

Pharmacology

Pharmacokinetics

Caffeine crosses the placenta and enters breast milk.

Primary Chemical Components of Cola Tree and Their Possible Actions		
Chemical Class	**Individual Components**	**Possible Action**
Alkaloid	Theobromine; Caffeine; Theophylline	Central nervous system stimulant
Tannin		Carcinogenic
Cardiac glycoside		
Anthraquinone		Laxative
Glucide		
Saponin		
Flavonoid		
Phenol		
Catechin		
Epicatechin		

Actions

Cola tree products have been used by people on the Ivory Coast to stimulate the central nervous system. The tribes of Hausa-Fulani in the northern part of Nigeria use *Cola nitida*

(Ibu, 1986). Because tannins, which possess carcinogenic effects, are present in the cola nut, this herb is not recommended for extended use (Morton, 1992).

Hormonal Action

In a study using rat pituitary cells, the cells first were treated for 24 hours with differing doses of cola extract, then stimulated with luteinizing hormone-releasing hormone (LH-RH). The findings indicated that cola species inhibit LH-RH. With more studies, results may point to the ability of cola tree products to regulate gonadotropin release (Benie, 1987).

Antiinfective Action

One study has identified the antiinfective action of the aqueous and alcoholic extracts of *Cola nitida* (bark) when tested against pathogenic bacteria. The results showed that the extracts inhibited beta-hemolytic streptococci, *Escherichia coli, Neisseria gonorrhoeae, Pseudomonas aeruginosa, Staphylococcus aureus, Klebsiella pneumoniae,* and *Proteus mirabilis* (Ebana, 1991). Another study (Kamagate, 2002) indicated that kola extract is not effective against bacteria at regular dose used by chewing.

Other Actions

Other actions of cola tree products include central nervous system stimulation, increased gastric acid flow, mild diuresis, and a mild positive chronotropic effect. One study identified the effects of *Cola nitida* on the locomotor activities of mice. Low doses had no effect, whereas high doses exerted a depressive effect (Ajarem, 1990).

References

Ajarem JS: Effects of fresh kola-nut extract *(Cola nitida)* on the locomotor activities of male mice, *Acta Physiol Pharmacol Bulg* 16(4): 10-15, 1990.

Ashri N et al: More unusual pigmentation of the gingiva, *Oral Surg Oral Med Oral Pathol* 70(4):445-449, 1990.

Benie T et al: Natural substances regulating fertility: effect of plant extracts in the Ivory Coast pharmacopoeia on the release of LH by hypophyseal cells in culture, *C R Seances Soc Biol Fil* 181(2):163-167, 1987.

Blumenthal M, editor: *The complete German Commission E monographs: therapeutic guide to herbal medicines,* Austin, Tex, American Botanical Council; Boston, Integrative Medicine Communication, 1998.

Duke J: *CRC handbook of medicinal herbs,* Boca Raton, Fla, 1985, CRC Press, pp 374-375.

Ebana RU et al: Microbiological exploitation of cardiac glycosides and

** ** = Pregnancy   ** ** = Pediatric   **❶** = Alert   **✇** = Popular Herb

alkaloids from *Garcinia kola, Borreria ocymoides, Kola nitida* and *Citrus aurantifolia, J Appl Bacteriol* 71(5):398-401, 1991.

Ibu JO et al: The effect of *Cola acuminata* and *Cola nitida* on gastric acid secretion, *Scand J Gastroenterol Suppl* 124:39-45, 1986.

Kamagate A et al: Etude in vitro de l' action de la kola "nitida" 5 hr les souches bacteriennes impliguees dans les caries dentaires et les maladies parodontales, *Odontostomatol Trop* 25(98):32-34, 2002.

Morton JF: Widespread tannin intake via stimulants and masticatories, especially guarana, kola nut, betel vine and accessories, *Basic Life Sci* 59:739-765, 1992.

C

Coltsfoot
(koeltz′ fut)

Scientific name: *Tussilago farfara*

Other common names: British tobacco, bullsfoot, butterbur, coughwort, donnhove, farfara, fieldhove, filius ante patrem, flower velure, foal's-foot, foalswort, hallfoot, horse-foot, horse-hoof, kuandong hua, pas díane   **Class 2b/2c/2d (Flowers)**

Origin: Coltsfoot is a perennial found in Europe; the United States; Canada; and central, western and northern Asia.

Uses

Reported Uses

Coltsfoot is used to treat respiratory conditions such as bronchitis, cough, and asthma. It is also used to treat inflammation of the oral mucosa.

Investigational Uses

Research is underway concerning coltsfoot as an antimicrobial.

Product Availability and Dosages

Available Forms

Dried herb, extract, syrup, tea, tincture

Plant Parts Used: Dried flowers, leaves, roots

Dosages and Routes

Adult

All dosages listed are PO.

• Decoction: 0.6-2.9 g dried herb
• Dried herb: 4.5-6 g/day (Blumenthal, 1998)

- Fluid extract: 0.6-2 ml tid (1:1 dilution in alcohol 25% concentration)
- Syrup: 2-8 ml tid (1:4 dilution)
- Tea: 1-3 tsp dried herb in 8 oz boiling water, let stand 10 min, strain, take tid

Precautionary Information

Contraindications

Coltsfoot should not be used during pregnancy and lactation, and it should not be given to children. It should not be used by persons with liver disease or by persons who are hypersensitive to ragweed, chamomile, or other members of the composite family. Persons with cardiac disease should use this herb cautiously. Coltsfoot should not be used for longer than 6 weeks. Pyrrolizidine alkaloid content should not exceed 10 µg. Class 2b/2c/2d herb (flowers).

Side Effects/Adverse Reactions

Cardiovascular: Hypertension
Central Nervous System: Fever
Gastrointestinal: Nausea, vomiting, anorexia, diarrhea, jaundice, HEPATOTOXICITY (rare)
Integumentary: Hypersensitivity reactions
Respiratory: Upper respiratory infection

Interactions with Coltsfoot

Drug

Coltsfoot may antagonize antiarrhythmics and antihypertensives; avoid concurrent use (theoretical).

Food	Herb	Lab Test
None known	None known	None known

Client Considerations

Assess

- Assess for hypersensitivity reactions. If these are present, discontinue the use of this herb and administer antihistamines or other appropriate therapy.
- Assess for hepatotoxicity (increased liver function tests, jaun-

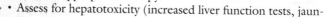

 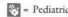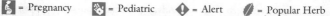

dice, clay-colored stools, right upper-quadrant pain). If these occur, herb use should be discontinued.
• Assess for the use of antiarrhythmics and antihypertensives (see Interactions).

Administer
• Instruct the client to store coltsfoot products in a cool, dry place, away from heat and moisture.
• Because of the presence of hepatotoxic pyrrolizidine alkaloids, caution the client not to use coltsfoot for longer than 6 weeks.

Teach Client/Family
• Because hepatotoxicity may occur, caution the client not to use coltsfoot during pregnancy and lactation and not to give it to children.
• Advise the client to report any side effects to the provider.
• Caution the client not to confuse peppermint with coltsfoot; they are similar in appearance.

Pharmacology
Pharmacokinetics
Pharmacokinetics and pharmacodynamics are unknown.

Primary Chemical Components of Coltsfoot and Their Possible Actions

Chemical Class	Individual Component	Possible Action
Alkaloid	Tussilagone Senkirkine Isotussilagone; Senecionine; Senecionin	Pressor effect Hepatotoxicity
Tannin		
Triterpene	Arnidiol; Faradiol; Beta-amyrin	
Sesquiterpenoid	Bisabolene; Epoxide (Ryu, 1999) Farfaratin (Wang, 1989)	Inhibition of nitric oxide synthesis
Flavonoid		
Phytosterol		
Mucilage		Demulcent

Actions

Two recent studies have demonstrated the ability of coltsfoot to inhibit nitric oxide synthesis in macrophages. The clinical significance of this finding is unknown, however (Ryu, 1999). Another study found that coltsfoot inhibits the binding of both platelet activating factor (PAF) and Ca^{2+} entry blocker to membrane vesicles (Hwang, 1987). Other studies have focused on the toxic effects of *Tussilago farfara* L. and the isolation of new chemical components (Sperl, 1995; Wang, 1989). The screening of 16 medicinal plants showed that 6 possessed significant antimicrobial action (Kokoska, 2002).

References

Blumenthal M, editor: *The complete German Commission E monographs: therapeutic guide to herbal medicines,* Austin, Tex, American Botanical Council; Boston, Integrative Medicine Communication, 1998.

Hwang SB: L-652, 469—a dual receptor antagonist of platelet activating factor and dihydropyrimidines from *Tussilago farfara* L., *Eur J Pharmacol* 141(2):269-281, 1987.

Kokoska L et al: Screening of some Siberian medicinal plants for antimicrobial activity, *J Ethnopharmacol*, 82(1):51, 2002.

Ryu JH et al: A new bisabolene epoxide from *Tussilago farfara,* and inhibition of nitric oxide synthesis in LPS-activated macrophages, *J Nat Prod* 62(10):1437-1438, 1999.

Sperl W et al: *Eur J Pediatr* 154(2):112-116, 1995.

Wang CD et al: Chemical studies of flower buds of *Tussilago farfara* L., *Yao Hsueh Hsueh Pao* 24(12):913-916, 1989.

DO NOT INGEST

Comfrey
(kuhm′free)

Scientific name: *Symphytum officinale*

Other common names: Black root, blackwort, boneset, bruisewort, consound, gum plant, healing herb, knitback, knitbone, salsifly, slippery root, wallwort

Class 2a/2b/2c
Class 3 (Leaf, Root)

Origin: Comfrey is a perennial found in the United States, Australia, and parts of Asia. It is cultivated in Japan.

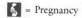 = Pregnancy    = Pediatric   = Alert    = Popular Herb

Uses

Reported Uses

Comfrey is used topically to promote wound healing and to de-crease inflammation caused by bruises and sprains. It has also been used internally for many years as a treatment for colitis and peptic ulcer disease. However, because hepatotoxicity may occur, internal use is no longer recommended.

Product Availability and Dosages

Available Forms

Capsules, extract, ointment, tea

Plant Parts Used: Leaves, roots

Dosages and Routes

Adult

NOTE: Because of the potential for hepatotoxicity, internal use of comfrey is no longer recommended.

Wound Healing

- Topical products: may be applied to wounds as needed (5%-20% dried herb present in product); use no longer than 6 weeks (Blumenthal, 1998)
- Poultice of fresh green leaves: may be applied prn to granulate wounds over broken bones

Precautionary Information

Contraindications

Until more research is available, comfrey should not be used during pregnancy and lactation, and it should not be given to children. It should not be used by persons who are hyper-sensitive to this herb. Comfrey is for external use only, and should not be used for more than 6 weeks in 1 year. Internal use may cause fatal hepatotoxicity. Do not use this herb on broken skin. Class 2a/2b/2c herb; class 3 herb (leaf, root).

Side Effects/Adverse Reactions

Integumentary: Hypersensitivity reactions (oral and topi-cal use)

Gastrointestinal: Nausea, vomiting, anorexia, abdominal pain, hepatomegaly, HEPATOTOXICITY, HEPATIC ADENOMA (all reactions from oral use)

Interactions with Comfrey		
Drug	**Food**	**Herb**
None known	None known	None known
Lab Test		

Comfrey may increase ALT, AST, total bilirubin, and urine bilirubin.

Client Considerations

Assess

- If the client is taking comfrey internally, assess for hepatotoxicity: increased liver function tests (AST, ALT, bilirubin), jaundice, clay-colored stools. If these symptoms are present, use of the herb should be discontinued.
- If the client is using comfrey topically to promote wound healing, assess the wound for temperature, redness, swelling, bleeding, and purulent drainage.

Administer

- Instruct the client to store comfrey products in a cool, dry place, away from heat and moisture.
- Instruct the client not to use comfrey for more than 6 weeks in 1 year.

Teach Client/Family

- Until more research is available, caution the client not to use comfrey during pregnancy and lactation and not to give it to children.
- Because hepatotoxicity may occur, caution the client not to take comfrey internally.
- Advise client not to use comfrey on broken skin. Absorption of pyrrolizidine alkaloids may occur.

Pharmacology

Pharmacokinetics

Pharmacokinetics and pharmacodynamics are unknown.

Primary Chemical Components of Comfrey and Their Possible Actions

Chemical Class	Individual Component	Possible Action
Pyrrolizidine Alkaloids	Lasiocarpine; Symlandine; Symphytine; Echimidine (Kim, 2001)	Hepatotoxic
Triterpenoid	Symphytoxide A	Hypotensive
Asparagine		
Tannin		Astringent
Allantoin		Wound healing
Mucilage		Demulcent
Polysaccharides		

Actions

In the past, comfrey was used internally to treat many conditions, including gastrointestinal complaints. However, because its pyrrolizidine alkaloids can cause hepatotoxicity, comfrey is now recommended for topical use only. Comfrey should be applied once the wound has begun to heal; the allantoin stimulates cell division.

Several studies have focused on the toxic results of the internal use of comfrey (Garrett, 1982; Couet, 1996). Another study found comfrey to be carcinogenic (Hirono, 1978). Plantain *(Plantago major)* can be used in place of comfrey, both internally for its healing properties and topically on open wounds.

References

Blumenthal M, editor: *The complete German Commission E monographs: therapeutic guide to herbal medicines,* Austin, Tex, American Botanical Council; Boston, Integrative Medicine Communication, 1998.

Couet CE et al: Analysis, separation, and bioassay of pyrrolizidine alkaloids from comfrey *(Symphytum officinale),* Nat Toxins 4(4):163-167, 1996.

Garrett BJ et al: Consumption of poisonous plants *(Senecio jacobaea, Symphytum officinale, Pteridium aquilinum, Hypericum perforatum)* by rats: chronic toxicity, mineral metabolism, and hepatic drug-metabolizing enzymes, *Toxicol Lett* 10(2-3):183-188, 1982.

Hirono I et al: Carcinogenic activity of *Symphytum officinale, J Natl Cancer Inst* 61(3):865-869, 1978.

Kim NC et al: Isolation of symlandine from the roots of common comfrey
(Symphytum officinale) using countercurrent chromatography, *J Nat Prod* 64(2):251-253, 2001.

Stickel F et al: The efficacy and safety of comfrey, *Pub Health Nutr* 3(4A):501-508, 2000.

Condurango
(kohn-du-rahn′go)

Scientific name: *Marsedenia condurango*

Other common names: Condor-vine bark, condurango bark, condurango blanco, eagle vine, gonolobus, condurango triana, marsedenia condurango

Origin: Condurango is found in South America.

Uses

Reported Uses

In traditional herbal medicine, condurango is used as an astringent and as a treatment for anorexia and syphilis.

Investigational Use

Research is underway to determine the efficacy of condurango as a cancer treatment.

Product Availability and Dosages

Available Forms

Bark, fluid extract, powdered bark, tincture

Plant Parts Used: Dried bark

Dosages and Routes

Adult

All dosages listed are PO.

- Bark: 2-4 g qd (Blumenthal, 1998)
- Extract: 0.2-0.5 g qd (Blumenthal, 1998)
- Fluid extract: 2-4 g qd (Blumenthal, 1998)
- Infusion: 2 tsp powdered bark in 8 oz boiling water, let stand 15 min, take tid
- Tincture: 1-2 ml tid or 2 g qd (Blumenthal, 1998)
- Water extract: 0.2-0.5 g qd (Blumenthal, 1998)

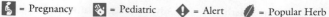
 = Pregnancy   = Pediatric   ◆ = Alert   = Popular Herb

C

Precautionary Information

Contraindications

Until more research is available, condurango should not be used during pregnancy and lactation, and it should not be given to children. Condurango should not be used by persons with hypersensitivity to this herb or any herb in the milkweed family, or by persons with hepatic disease or any seizure disorder.

Side Effects/Adverse Reactions

Central Nervous System: SEIZURES (overdose of bark)
Gastrointestinal: Nausea, vomiting, anorexia, HEPATOTOXICITY
Integumentary: Hypersensitivity reactions

Interactions with Condurango

Drug

Cardiac glycosides (digoxin): Absorption of digitoxin and digoxin may be reduced when used with condurango; avoid concurrent use (theoretical).

Iron products: Absorption of iron products may be reduced when used with condurango; avoid concurrent use (theoretical).

Medications metabolized by P-450 enzyme system (carbamazepine, bupropion, orphenadrine, cyclophosphamide, citalopram, azole antifungals, macrolide antibiotics, omeprazole): Use condurango cautiously with these drugs, especially in clients with hepatic disorders

Medications metabolized by CYP2A6 enzyme system (carbamazepine, paroxetine, ritonavir, sertraline): Use these medications cautiously with condurango.

Food	Herb	Lab Test
None known	None known	None known

🌍 Endangered Herb   Adverse effects: BOLD = life-threatening

Client Considerations

Assess

- Assess for hypersensitivity reactions. If present, discontinue use of condurango and administer antihistamine or other appropriate therapy.
- Assess for hepatotoxicity: increased AST, ALT, and bilirubin levels; jaundice, clay-colored stools, right upper-quadrant pain.
- Assess for adverse central nervous system reactions.
- Identify all medications taken by the client (see Interactions).

Administer

- Instruct the client to store condurango in a cool, dry place, away from heat and moisture.

Teach Client/Family

- Until more research is available, caution the client not to use condurango during pregnancy and lactation and not to give it to children.

Pharmacology

Pharmacokinetics

Pharmacokinetics and pharmacodynamics are unknown.

Primary Chemical Components of Condurango and Their Possible Actions		
Chemical Class	**Individual Component**	**Possible Action**
Tannin		Astringent
Glycoside	Condurango A, A0, A1, B0, C, C1, D0, E0, E2	Antitumor
Essential oil		
Resin		
Condurangin		
Caoutchouc		
Condruit		
Phytosterin		
Sitosterol		
Vanillin		
Coumarin		
Esculetin		

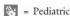

Primary Chemical Components of Condurango and Their Possible Action—cont'd		
Chemical Class	**Individual Component**	**Possible Action**
Flavonoid Acid	Caffeic acid; Cholorogenic acid	Bile stimulant
Strychnine-like alkaloid		

Actions

Antitumor Action

One study has evaluated the differentiation-inducing activity of condurango in the mouse myeloid leukemia cell line. Among the chemical components of the herb, the condurango glycosides were the most potent differentiation inducers of phagocytic cells after 24 hours of treatment with these compounds. This indicates the antitumor action of condurango (Umehara, 1994). Another study identified the antitumor activity of this herb against sarcomas (Hayashi, 1980).

Other Actions

The tannins in condurango possess astringent properties that contribute to its wound healing effects.

References

Blumenthal M, editor: *The complete German Commission E monographs: therapeutic guide to herbal medicines,* Austin, Tex, American Botanical Council; Boston, Integrative Medicine Communication, 1998.

Hayashi K et al: Antitumor active glycosides from condurango cortex, *Chem Pharm Bull* 28:1954-1958, 1980.

Umehara K et al: Studies on differentiation inducers IV: pregnane derivatives from condurango cortex. *Chem Pharm Bull (Tokyo)* 42(3): 611-616, 1994.

Coriander
(koe'ree-an-duhr)

Scientific names: *Coriandrum sativum, Coriandrum sativum* var. *vulgare, Coriandrum sativum* var. *microcarpum*

Other common names: Chinese parsley, cilantro, coriander

Class 1 (Fruit, Seed)

Origin: Coriander is found throughout the world.

Uses

Reported Uses
Coriander is used as an anthelmintic and appetite stimulant and as a treatment for arthritic conditions and dyspepsia. It is also used as a spice and flavoring in foods.

Product Availability and Dosages

Available Forms
Crude extract, tincture, whole herb

Plant Parts Used: Dried fruits

Dosages and Routes

Adult

Dosages vary widely. All dosages listed are PO.
- Decoction: 2 tsp crushed herb in 150 ml boiling water, let stand 15 min, strain, drink 8 oz ac
- Tincture: 10-20 drops after meals
- Whole herb: 3 g/day in divided doses (Blumenthal, 1998)

Precautionary Information

Contraindications
Until more research is available, coriander should not be used during pregnancy and lactation and should not be given to children. It should not be used by persons with hypersensitivity to this herb. Class 1 herb (fruit, seed).

Side Effects/Adverse Reactions
Gastrointestinal: Nausea, vomiting, anorexia, fatty liver tumors
Integumentary: Hypersensitivity reactions

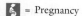 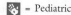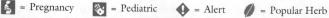

C

Interactions with Coriander

Drug
Oral antidiabetic agents: Coriander may increase the effects of oral antidiabetic agents; use together cautiously.

Food	Herb	Lab Test
None known	None known	None known

Client Considerations

Assess
- Assess for hypersensitivity reactions. If present, discontinue use of coriander and administer antihistamine or other appropriate therapy.
- Assess for the use of oral antidiabetic agents (see Interactions).

Administer
- Instruct the client to store coriander in a sealed container away from light and moisture.

Teach Client/Family

- Until more research is available, caution the client not to use coriander during pregnancy and lactation and not to give it to children.

Pharmacology

Pharmacokinetics
Pharmacokinetics and pharmacodynamics are unknown.

Primary Chemical Components of Coriander and Their Possible Actions

Chemical Class	Individual Component	Possible Action
Volatile oil	Coriandrol; D-linalol; Limonene; Alpha-pinenes; Cymene; Camphor; Camphene; Terpinene; Monoterpene; Phellandrene; Carvone; Geraniol; Borneol	
Sitosterol		
Triacontanol		
Flavonoid	Quercetin; Isoquercetin	Antiinflammatory
	Rutin	Antioxidant; astringent
	Glucuronide; Coriandrinol	
Tannin		
Fatty acid	Oleic acid; Petroselinic acid; Linolenic acid	
Coumarin	Scopoletin; Umbelliferone	

Actions

Antilipidemic Action

Three studies using laboratory rats fed a high-fat diet have evaluated the antilipidemic action of *Coriandrum sativum* (Chithra, 1997; Chithra, 1999; Chithra, 2000). In all three studies, the use of coriander seeds lowered the lipid level significantly, with levels of total cholesterol and triglycerides decreased. The levels of low-density lipoprotein (LDL) and very-low-density lipoprotein (VLDL) cholesterol decreased, while high-density lipoprotein (HDL) cholesterol levels increased.

Antidiabetic Action

In traditional herbal medicine, coriander has been used for many years to lower blood glucose. When streptozocin-diabetic mice were fed coriander in their diet and in their drinking

 = Pregnancy   = Pediatric   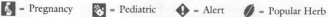 = Alert   = Popular Herb water, a significant reduction in blood glucose occurred. Sequential extraction revealed insulin-releasing activity (Gray, 1999). In an older study evaluating the antidiabetic action of several herbs, coriander was shown to decrease glucose levels in diabetic mice (Swanston-Flatt, 1990).

Other Actions

Fresh coriander seeds were found to exert abortifacient effects on female rats. An oral dose of 250-500 mg/kg produced an antiimplantation effect but failed to produce complete infertility (Al-Said, 1987). A mixed fraction of dill, cilantro, coriander, and eucalyptus essential oils showed additive, synergistic, or antagonistic effects depending on organism (Delaguis, 2002).

References

Al-Said MS et al: Post-coital antifertility activity of the seeds of *Coriandrum sativum* in rats, *J Ethnopharmacol* 21(2):165-173, 1987.

Blumenthal M, editor: *The complete German Commission E monographs: therapeutic guide to herbal medicines,* Austin, Tex, American Botanical Council; Boston, Integrative Medicine Communication, 1998.

Chithra V et al: Hypolipidemic effect of coriander seeds *(Coriandrum sativum):* mechanism of action, *Plant Foods Hum Nutr* 51(2):167-172, 1997.

Chithra V et al: *Coriandrum sativum* changes the levels of lipid peroxides and activity of antioxidant enzymes in experimental animals, *Indian J Biochem Biophys* 36(1):59-61, 1999.

Chithra V et al: *Coriandrum sativum:* effect on lipid metabolism in 1,2-dimethyl hydrazine induced colon cancer, *J Ethnopharmacol* 71(3): 457-463, 2000.

Delaguis PJ et al: Antimicrobial activity of individual and mixed fractions of dill, cilantro, coriander, and eucalyptus essential oils, *Int J Food Microbial* 74(1-2):101-109, 2002.

Gray AM et al: Insulin-releasing and insulin-like activity of the traditional anti-diabetic plant *Coriandrum sativum,* *Br J Nutr* 81(3):203-209, 1999.

Swanston-Flatt SK et al: Traditional plant treatments for diabetes: studies in normal and streptozotocin diabetic mice, *Diabetologia* 33(8):462-464, 1990.

Corkwood
(kawrk'wud)

Scientific name: *Duboisia myoporoides*
Other common name: Pituri

Origin: Corkwood is found in South America and Australia.

Uses

Reported Uses

Before commercial preparations of scopolamine were available, corkwood was used to prevent the nausea and vomiting associated with motion sickness. It has also been used to decrease spasms of the gastrointestinal system.

Product Availability and Dosages

Available Forms

Liquid, tablets

Plant Parts Used: Leaves, roots, stems

Dosages and Routes

Many different dosages are reported.

Precautionary Information

Contraindications

Until more research is available, corkwood should not be used during pregnancy and lactation, and it should not be given to children. It should not be used by persons with hypersensitivity to this herb or those with narrow-angle glaucoma, myasthenia gravis, or gastrointestinal/genitourinary obstruction. Persons with congestive heart failure, prostatic hypertrophy, hypertension, arrhythmia, or gastric ulcer should avoid the use of corkwood.

Side Effects/Adverse Reactions

Cardiovascular: Palpitations, tachycardia, postural hypotension
Central Nervous System: Confusion, anxiety, restlessness, irritability, headache, dizziness, flushing
Ears, Eyes, Nose, and Throat: Blurred vision

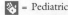

 = Pregnancy   = Pediatric   = Alert   = Popular Herb

C

Precautionary Information—cont'd
Side Effects/Adverse Reactions—cont'd
Gastrointestinal: Nausea, vomiting, anorexia, dry mouth, constipation, abdominal distress
Genitourinary: Hesitancy, retention
Integumentary: Hypersensitivity reactions

Interactions with Corkwood

Drug
An increased anticholinergic effect occurs when corkwood is used with alcohol, antihistimines, opioids, phenothiazines, and tricyclics.

Food	Herb	Lab Test
None known	None known	None known

Client Considerations

Assess

- Assess for hypersensitivity reactions. If present, discontinue use of corkwood and administer antihistamine or other appropriate therapy.
- Assess the client's mental status (mood, affect, anxiety, restlessness).
- Assess for urinary hesitancy or retention.
- Assess for medications used (see Interactions).

Administer

- Instruct the client to store corkwood products away from moisture and light.
- Advise the client to use hard candy, liquids, and chewing gum to alleviate dry mouth.

Teach Client/Family

- Until more research is available, caution the client not to use corkwood during pregnancy and lactation and not to give it to children.
- Advise the client to avoid driving and operating machinery if dizziness occurs.

Pharmacology
Pharmacokinetics
Pharmacokinetics and pharmacodynamics are unknown.

Primary Chemical Components of Corkwood and Their Possible Actions		
Chemical Class	Individual Component	Possible Action
Alkaloid	Scopolamine; Hyoscyamine Valtropine; Valeroidine	Anticholinergic

Actions
Anticholinergic Action
Two of the chemical components of corkwood, scopolamine and hyoscyamine, exert anticholinergic activity (Griffin, 1975). This action inhibits acetylcholine at receptor sites in the autonomic nervous system. The results are a decrease in secretions, an increase in blood pressure, blurred vision, and other visual disturbances.

References
Griffin WJ et al: Analysis of *Duboisia myoporoids* R. Br. and *Duboisia leichhardtii* F. Muell, *J Pharm Sci* 64(11):1821-1825, 1975.

Couchgrass
(kuch'gras)

Scientific names: *Agropyron repens, Elymus repens, Graminis rhizomo, Triticum repens* L.

Other common names: Cutch, dog grass, durfa grass, quack grass, quitch grass, Scotch quelch, triticum, twitch-grass, witch grass

Class 1

Origin: Couchgrass is found in Europe and is now grown in the United States.

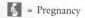 = Pregnancy  = Pediatric 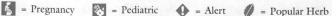 = Alert = Popular Herb

Uses
Reported Uses
Couchgrass is used in the treatment of cystitis, urethritis, and prostatitis; as an irrigant to treat urinary tract disorders with inflammation; for prevention of renal gravel; in the treatment of upper respiratory conditions; as a demulcent and an antimicrobial; and in the treatment of gout, rheumatism, and cough. The juice of the roots is used to treat cirrhosis of the liver, and some species are used to treat tumors and cancer. Couchgrass is not commonly used today.

Product Availability and Dosages
Available forms
Capsule, cut rhizome, fluid extract, tablet, tincture

Plant Parts Used: Rhizome

Dosages and Routes
Adult
No published dosage is available for irrigation. All dosages listed are PO.
- Decoction: place 2 tsp cut rhizome in 8 oz water, bring to a boil, simmer 10 min, use tid; a single dose consisting of approximately 3-10 g of the herb can also be used
- Fluid extract: a 1:1 dilution is recommended
- Tincture: use 2-4 ml tid (1:5 dilution recommended)

Precautionary Information
Contraindications
Do not use as an irrigant if edema caused by cardiac or renal conditions is present. Class 1 herb.

Side Effects/Adverse Reactions
None known

Interactions with Couchgrass

Drug	Food	Herb	Lab Test
None known	None known	None known	None known

Client Considerations

Assess

- Assess the client for cardiac and renal disorders. If edema is present, do not use couchgrass as an irrigant.

Administer

- Instruct the client to take couchgrass PO as a decoction or extract.
- Instruct the client to store the herb in a sealed container in a dry, dark environment.

Pharmacology

Pharmacokinetics

Mannitol, present in couchgrass, is poorly absorbed by oral route. Most other pharmacokinetics and pharmacodynamics are unknown.

Primary Chemical Components of Couchgrass and Their Possible Actions

Chemical Class	Individual Component	Possible Action
Polysaccharide	Triticin	
Mucilage		
Saponin		Cancer prevention
Sugar alcohol	Mannitol; Inositrol	Diuretic
Essential oil	Agropyrene	Antifungal
	Polyacetylene;	Antimicrobial
	Carvone	
Vanilloside		
Vanillin		
Phenolcarboxylic acid		
Silicic acid		
Silicate		
Lectin		
Vitamin	A; B complex	
Mineral	Iron	

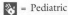 = Pregnancy   = Pediatric   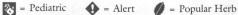 = Alert   = Popular Herb

Actions

No research is available on the actions of this herb. Existing studies focus on the composition of the chemical components of couchgrass.

Urolithiasis Action

Grasses (1995) reports that although the use of *Agropyron repens* does not improve urolithiasis of calcium oxalate stones, alterations in diet does affect the formation of calcium oxalate stones. This study compared three different diets: standard, high glucosidic, and high protein. An increase in citraturia occurred when *A. repens* was added to a high-protein diet, resulting in a reduction in stone formation.

Antimicrobial Action

Limited research is available on the antimicrobial action of couchgrass. The essential oil has been shown to possess antimicrobial effects (Bissett, 1994).

References

Bissett NG, editor: *Herbal drugs and phytopharmaceuticals,* Stuttgart, 1994, Medpharm.
Grasses F et al: Effect of *Herniaria hirsuta* and *Agropyron repens* on calcium oxalate urolithiasis risk in rats, *J Ethnopharmacol* 45:211-214, 1995.

Cowslip
(kow'slip)

Scientific name: *Primula veris*

Other common names: Artetyke, arthritica, buckles, crewel, drelip, fairy cup, herb Peter, key of heaven, key flower, may blob, mayflower, our lady's keys, paigle, palsywort, password, peagle, petty mulleins, plumrocks

Class 1 (Flower, Root)

Origin: Cowslip is found in the western region of the United States.

Uses

Reported Uses

Cowslip is used to treat insomnia, anxiety, and nervousness.

Endangered Herb   Adverse effects: **BOLD** = life-threatening

Product Availability and Dosages
Available Forms
Dried herb, fluid extract

Plant Parts Used: Flowers

Dosages and Routes
Adult
- PO fluid extract: 1-2 ml tid (1:1 dilution in alcohol 25%)
- PO infusion: 1-2 g dried herb, tid

Precautionary Information
Contraindications
Until more research is available, cowslip should not be used during pregnancy and lactation and should not be given to children. It should not be used by persons with hepatic disease, gastrointestinal conditions, or hypersensitivity to this herb. Class 1 herb (flower, root).

Side Effects/Adverse Reactions
Gastrointestinal: Nausea, vomiting, anorexia, diarrhea, gastritis, HEPATOTOXICITY
Integumentary: Hypersensitivity reactions, contact dermatitis

---

Interactions with Cowslip

Drug
Sedatives/hypnotics: Cowslip may increase the effect of antianxiety agents and sedatives/hypnotics; do not use concurrently.

Food	Herb	Lab Test
None known	None known	None known

Client Considerations
Assess
- Assess for hypersensitivity reactions including contact dermatitis. If present, discontinue use of cowslip and administer antihistamine or other appropriate therapy.
- Assess for hepatotoxicity (increased AST, ALT, bilirubin levels; jaundice; clay-colored stools; right upper-quadrant

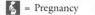 = Pregnancy    = Pediatric   = Alert   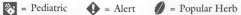 = Popular Herb

pain). If present, herb use should be discontinued and appropriate action taken.
- Assess for the use of antianxiety agents and sedative/hypnotics (see Interactions).

Administer
- Instruct the client to store cowslip products in a cool, dry place, away from heat and moisture.

Teach Client/Family
- Until more research is available, caution the client not to use cowslip during pregnancy and lactation and not to give it to children.
- Inform the client that scientific research is lacking to support any of the uses for or actions of cowslip.

Pharmacology

Pharmacokinetics
Pharmacokinetics and pharmacodynamics are unknown.

Primary Chemical Components of Cowslip and Their Possible Actions

Chemical Class	Individual Component	Possible Action
Flavonoid	Quercetin; Apigenin	Antiinflammatory; antispasmodic
	Kaempferol Luteolin; G1, 2, 3, 4, 5, 6, (Huck, 2000)	Antiinflammatory
Phenol	Primulaveroside; primveroside	
Saponin		Hypotensive; hypertensive
Tannin		Astringent
Volatile oil		
Carbohydrate		

Actions

Respiratory Action
One study conducted in Europe evaluated the effect of pharmacotherapeutic options and herbal remedies for bronchitis. The

herbal remedy *Primula veris* showed an effect equal to that of pharmacologic treatments (Ernst, 1997), as did several other combination herbal products with oil of eucalyptus, peppermint, anise, and ivy extract.

Other Actions

Other older studies have identified both hypotensive and hypertensive effects of saponins, chemical components in *Primula veris*. Two flavonoids, quercetin and apigenin, are responsible for the antiinflammatory and antispasmodic effects of cowslip. These effects are common in all herbs with these chemical components.

References

Ernst E et al: A controlled multi-centre study of herbal versus synthetic secrolytic drugs for acute bronchitis, *Phytomedicine* 4(4):287-293, 1997.

Huck CW et al: Isolation and characterization of methoxylated flavones in the flowers of *Primulaveris* by liquid chromatography and mass spectrometry, *J Chromatography A*, 870(1-2):453-462, 2000.

Cranberry
(kran′beh-ree)

Scientific names: *Vaccinium macrocarpon, Vaccinium oxycoccus, Vaccinium erythrocarpum*

Other common names: Bog cranberry, isokarpalo, marsh apple, mountain cranberry, pikkukarpalo

Origin: Cranberry is a small shrub found in the United States, from Tennessee to Alaska.

Uses

Reported Uses

Cranberry is used to prevent (but not to treat) urinary tract infections. It may be used to treat kidney stones.

Product Availability and Dosages

Available Forms

Capsules, fresh berries, juice

Plant Parts Used: Berries

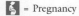 = Pregnancy   = Pediatric   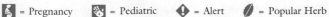 = Alert   = Popular Herb

Dosages and Routes
Adult
All dosages listed are PO.
- Capsules: 9-15 capsules/day (400-500 mg each) (McCaleb, 2000)
- Capsules (powdered concentrate): 2 capsules qd
- Juice: 1-2 cups qd (Murray, 1998)

Precautionary Information

Contraindications

Cranberry should not be used by persons with oliguria, anuria, or hypersensitivity to this herb.

Side Effects/Adverse Reactions

Gastrointestinal: Diarrhea (large doses)
Integumentary: Hypersensitivity reactions

Interactions with Cranberry

Drug	Food	Herb
None known	None known	None known
Lab Test		
Cranberry decreases urine pH.		

Client Considerations

Assess

- Assess for hypersensitivity reactions. If present, discontinue use of cranberry and administer antihistamine or other appropriate therapy.
- Assess the client's genitourinary status: urinary frequency, hesitancy, pain, or burning. If a urinary tract infection is present, refer the client for antibiotic therapy.

Administer

- Instruct the client to store cranberry products away from light and moisture.

🌱 Endangered Herb   Adverse effects: BOLD = life-threatening

Teach Client/Family

- Caution the client not to use cranberry in place of antibiotic therapy if urinary frequency, hesitancy, pain, or burning are present.
- Advise the client that cranberry is effective for preventing urinary tract infections but not for treating them.

Pharmacology

Pharmacokinetics

Pharmacokinetics and pharmacodynamics are unknown.

Primary Chemical Components of Cranberry and Their Possible Actions		
Chemical Class	**Individual Component**	**Possible Action**
Acid	Benzoic acid; Malic acid; Citric acid; Quinic acid	
Carbohydrate	Oligosaccharides Fructose	Antimicrobial
Anthocyanin		
Proanthocyanidins		
Flavonoids	Quercetin; Myricetin (Kandil, 2002)	
Glycosides	Epicatechin; Catechin (Kandil, 2002)	

Actions

Urinary Tract Action

Studies abound on the urinary tract action of cranberry. It is well known that cranberry juice is useful for the prevention of urinary tract infections (Jackson, 1997; Jepson, 2000). The increase in urine acidity causes a decrease in organism growth. However, cranberry juice is not effective for the treatment of urinary tract infections. Cranberry does decrease ionized calcium in urine by 50% and therefore may be used to treat recurrent kidney stones (Murray, 1998).

Antioxidant Action

A recent study has evaluated the antioxidant properties of blueberry and cranberry juice. Consumption of cranberry juice in-

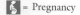 = Pregnancy   = Pediatric   = Alert    = Popular Herb

creased the ability of plasma to increase antioxidants. Blueberry juice did not exert this effect (Pedersen, 2000). However, this was a small study with only nine participants.

Oral Antiplaque Action

One study using a high-molecular-weight cranberry constituent found that the substance altered subgingival microbes and therefore would be able to control periodontal disease (Weiss, 1998).

References

Jackson B et al: Effect of cranberry juice on urinary pH in older adults, *Home Health Nurse* 15:198-202, 1997.

Jepson RG et al: Cranberries for preventing urinary tract infections, *Cochrane Database Syst Rev* 2:CD001321, 2000.

Kandil FE et al: Composition of chemopreventive proanthocyanidin-rich fraction from cranberry fruits responsible for the inhibition of 12-0-tetra decanoyl, *J Agric Food Chem* 50(5):1063-1069, 2002.

McCaleb R et al: *The encyclopedia of popular herbs: your complete guide to leading medicinal plants,* Roseville, Calif, 2000, Prima Health.

Murray M, Pizzorno J: *Encyclopedia of natural medicine,* 2 ed (revised), Roseville, Calif, 1998, Prima.

Pedersen CB et al: Effects of blueberry and cranberry juice consumption on the plasma antioxidant capacity of healthy female volunteers, *Eur J Clin Nutr* 54(5):405-408, 2000.

Weiss EI et al: Inhibiting interspecies coaggregation of plaque bacteria with a cranberry juice constituent, *J Am Dent Assoc* 129(12):1719-1723, 1998.

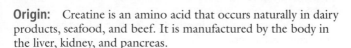

Creatine
(kree'uh-teen)

Origin: Creatine is an amino acid that occurs naturally in dairy products, seafood, and beef. It is manufactured by the body in the liver, kidney, and pancreas.

Uses

Reported Uses

Creatine is used to enhance athletic performance.

Product Availability and Dosages

Available Forms

Powder, tablets

Dosages and Routes

Different dosages are reported. Both dosages listed are PO.

Adult

- Normal dietary dose: 2 g/day
- To enhance athletic performance: 10-30 g/day

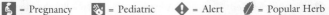

Precautionary Information

Contraindications

Until more research is available, creatine supplements should not be used during pregnancy and lactation, and they should not be given to children. Creatine supplementation is not recommended for persons with renal or cardiac disease.

Side Effects/Adverse Reactions

Gastrointestinal: Nausea, anorexia, bloating, weight gain, diarrhea

Systemic: Dehydration, cramping (high doses)

Interactions with Creatine

Drug

Caffeine: Increased caffeine intake may decrease the effects of creatine.

Glucose: Increased glucose intake may increase the storage of creatine in muscle tissue.

Food	Herb	Lab Test
None known	None known	None known

Client Considerations

Assess

- Assess for signs of abuse in athletes; creatine is used as a performance enhancer.
- Assess for caffeine and glucose use (see Interactions).

Administer

- Instruct the client to store creatine products in a sealed container in a cool, dry place, away from heat and moisture.

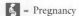 = Pregnancy    = Pediatric   = Alert   = Popular Herb

Teach Client/Family

- Until more research is available, caution the client not to use creatine supplements during pregnancy and lactation and not to give them to children.
- Advise the client not to use creatine to treat renal or cardiovascular disease. Research on the cardiovascular action of creatine is inconclusive.
- Inform the client that creatine has been used to increase endurance during intense exercise sessions lasting less than 1 hour.
- Caution the client that the effects of long-term creatine supplementation are unknown.

Pharmacology

Pharmacokinetics

Pharmacokinetics and pharmacodynamics are unknown.

Primary Chemical Components of Creatine and Their Possible Actions		
Chemical Class	**Individual Component**	**Possible Action**
Amino Acid	Arginine (precursors)	Enhancement of exercise endurance
	Glycine (precursors)	

Actions

Exercise Performance Enhancement

A group of athletes was evaluated for increased muscle strength after creatine supplementation. Measures used to determine muscle strength included knee extensor torque and ammonia and lactate levels. The study concluded that creatine supplementation increased muscle strength (Greenhaff, 1993).

Cardiovascular Action

A recent study focused on the effects of dietary creatine supplementation in patients with congestive heart failure. Muscle metabolism was measured using a cannula inserted into an antecubital vein. Maximum voluntary contraction was also measured. Researchers drew the participants' blood at rest and at 2 minutes after exercise to compare measurements of lactate and ammonia buildup. Results indicated increased muscle contractions. Researchers concluded that creatine supplementation increased skeletal muscle endurance and lessened abnormal skeletal muscle metabolic response to exercise (Andrews, 1998).

References

Andrews R et al: The effect of dietary creatine supplementation on skeletal muscle metabolism in congestive heart failure, *Eur Heart J* 19:617-622, 1998.

Greenhaff PL et al: Influence of oral creatine supplementation of muscle torque during repeated bouts of maximal voluntary exercise in man, *Clin Sci* 84:565-571, 1993.

Cucumber
(kyew-kuhm-bur)

Scientific name: *Cucumis sativus*
Other common names: Wild cucumber

Origin: Cucumber is a vegetable found in India.

Uses

Reported Uses

In traditional herbal medicine, cucumber is used to treat both hypertension and hypotension and as a diuretic. It is used topically to soothe irritated skin. The seeds may possess anthelmintic properties. Wild cucumber is not the same as cucumber available in grocery stores.

Product Availability and Dosages

Available Forms

Juice; seeds; shampoo, conditioner, and cosmetics with cucumber as a component

Plant Parts Used: Fruit, seeds

Dosages and Routes

Adult

- PO ground seeds: 1-2 oz prepared as a decoction steeped in water
- Topical: apply prn

 = Pregnancy    = Pediatric   = Alert   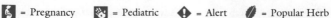 = Popular Herb

Precautionary Information

Contraindications

Until more research is available, cucumber should not be used during pregnancy and lactation and should not be given to children. Cucumber products should not be used by persons with hypersensitivity to this herb.

C

Side Effects/Adverse Reactions

Gastrointestinal: Heartburn, belching (fruits)

Interactions with Cucumber

Drug

Diuretics: Cucumber may increase the diuretic effect of other diuretics; avoid concurrent use.

Food	Herb	Lab Test
None known	None known	None known

Client Considerations

Assess

- Determine how much cucumber the client is using. The seeds should not be used in amounts greater than the recommended dosage.
- Assess for the use of diuretics (see Interactions).

Administer

- Instruct the client to store cucumber products in a cool, dry place, away from heat and moisture.

Teach Client/Family

- Until more research is available, caution the client not to use cucumber during pregnancy and lactation and not to give it to children.

Pharmacology

Pharmacokinetics

Pharmacokinetics and pharmacodynamics are unknown.

Primary Chemical Components of Cucumber and Their Possible Actions		
Chemical Class	**Individual Component**	**Possible Action**
Fatty acid Glycoside Resin	Cucurbitin	

Actions

Very little research has been done on wild cucumber. It has been used as a mild diuretic for many years (Duke, 1985). However, all of the available information on its uses comes from traditional herbal medicine and is not based on scientific research. Many studies have been done from a botanical rather than a medicinal perspective.

References

Duke J: *CRC handbook of medicinal herbs,* Boca Raton, Fla, 1985, CRC Press.

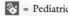 = Pregnancy   = Pediatric   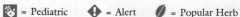 = Alert   = Popular Herb

Daffodil
(da'fuh-dil)

Scientific name: *Narcissus pseudonarcissus*

Other common names: Daffydown-dilly, fleur de coucou, Lent lily, narcissus, porillon

Origin: Daffodil is a flowering plant found in Europe and the United States.

Uses

Reported Uses

Daffodil is taken internally as an emetic and as a treatment for respiratory conditions such as congestion. It is used topically to relieve joint inflammation and pain and to treat burns and wounds.

Product Availability and Dosages

Available Forms

Extract, powder

Plant Parts Used: Bulb, flowers, leaves

Dosages and Routes

Different dosages are reported.

Adult

Emetic
• PO extract: 3 grains

Joint Pain, Inflammation, Wound Healing
• Topical: apply prn

Respiratory Conditions
• PO: 20 grains-2 drams

Precautionary Information

Contraindications

Daffodil should not be used during pregnancy and lactation and should not be given to children. Persons who are hypersensitive to daffodil should not use it. Daffodil bulbs and flowers should not be consumed. Serious and even fatal reactions can occur from flower and bulb consumption.

Continued

  Endangered Herb   Adverse effects: BOLD = life-threatening

> ### Precautionary Information—cont'd
>
> **Side Effects/Adverse Reactions**
> *Cardiovascular:* CARDIOVASCULAR COLLAPSE (bulbs)
> *Gastrointestinal:* Nausea, vomiting, anorexia
> *Integumentary:* Hypersensitivity reactions, contact dermatitis, daffodil itch
> *Respiratory:* RESPIRATORY COLLAPSE (bulbs)

Interactions with Daffodil			
Drug	Food	Herb	Lab Test
None known	None known	None known	None known

Client Considerations

Assess

- Assess for hypersensitivity reactions, contact dermatitis, and daffodil itch. If these are present, discontinue use of daffodil and administer antihistamine or other appropriate therapy.
- Assess for consumption of bulbs and flowers. Serious and even fatal reactions can occur.

Administer

- Instruct the client to avoid any use of daffodil products unless supervised by a qualified herbalist.

Teach Client/Family

- Until more research is available, caution the client not to use daffodil during pregnancy and lactation and not to give it to children.
- Strongly caution the client not to consume daffodil bulbs or flowers. Serious and even fatal reactions can occur.

Pharmacology

Pharmacokinetics

Pharmacokinetics and pharmacodynamics are unknown.

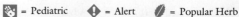

Primary Chemical Components of Daffodil and Their Possible Actions		
Chemical Class	**Individual Component**	**Possible Action**
Alkaloid	Narcissine	Emetic
	Lectin agglutinin (NPA)	Anti-HIV
	Masonin; Homolycorin; Hemanthamine; Galanthine; Galanthamine; Pluviine	
Acid	Chelidonic acid	
Polysaccharide	Sulphoevernan	Anti-HIV

Actions

Anti-HIV Action

Two studies have evaluated the anti-HIV action of daffodil (Weiler, 1990; Balzarini, 1991). The Weiler study determined that the polysaccharide component, sulphoevernan, binds to the virus rather than to the host cell. Similarly, the Balzarini study showed that a lectin component, NPA, also binds to the virus rather than to the host cell.

Anticancer Action

A recent study (Wang, 2000) focused on the effects of the lectins on differing carbohydrate-binding when daffodil is used to treat human hepatoma, human choriocarcinoma, mouse melanoma, and rat osteosarcoma. The lectins may be toxic to these cancers. The results showed *Narcissus pseudonarcissus* to be only mildly cytotoxic.

References

Balzarini J et al: Alpha-(1-3)- and alpha-(1-6)-D-mannose-specific plant lectins are markedly inhibitory to human immunodeficiency virus and cytomegalovirus infections in vitro, *Antimicrob Agents Chemother* 35(3):410-416, 1991.

Wang H et al: Effects of lectins with different carbohydrate-binding specificities on hepatoma, choriocarcinoma, melanoma and osteosarcoma cell lines, *Int J Biochem Cell Biol* 32(3):365-372, 2000.

Weiler BE et al: Sulphoevernan, a polyanionic polysaccharide, and the narcissus lectin potently inhibit human immunodeficiency virus infection by binding to viral protein, *J Gen Virol* 71(pt 1):1957-1963, 1990.

Daisy
(day'zee)

Scientific name: *Bellis perennis*

Other common names: Bairnwort, bruisewort, common daisy, day's eye, wild daisy

Origin: Daisy is a perennial found throughout the world.

Uses

Reported Uses

Daisy is used as a pain reliever and to treat diarrhea, cough, and gastrointestinal spasms. It is also used to relieve arthritis joint pain and inflammation and as a blood purifier and an antifungal.

Product Availability and Dosages

Available Forms

None available commercially

Plant Parts Used: Flowers, leaves

Dosages and Routes

Adult

- PO infusion: 1 tsp dried flowers steeped 20 min in 1 cup boiling water, drink 2-4 cups bid-qid
- PO tincture: 3-4 ml taken bid-tid
- Topical: apply a poultice of pressed leaves prn to affected area

Precautionary Information

Contraindications

Until more research is available, daisy should not be used during pregnancy and lactation and should not be given to children.

Side Effects/Adverse Reactions

None known

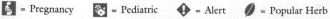

 = Pregnancy    = Pediatric   ◆ = Alert   ▮ = Popular Herb

Interactions with Daisy			
Drug	Food	Herb	Lab Test
None known	None known	None known	None known

D

Client Considerations

Assess
• Determine why the client is using daisy and suggest other alternatives.

Administer
• Instruct the client to store daisy in a cool, dry place, away from heat and moisture.

Teach Client/Family

• Until more research is available, caution the client not to use daisy during pregnancy and lactation and not to give it to children.

Pharmacology

Pharmacokinetics
Pharmacokinetics and pharmacodynamics are unknown.

Primary Chemical Components of Daisy and Their Possible Actions		
Chemical Class	Individual Component	Possible Action
Saponin	Polygalacteronic acid	
Tannin		Astringent
Organic acid		
Mucilage		
Essential oil		Antibacterial
Triterpenoid	Isohamnetin; Kaemferol	Antifungal
glycoside	(Gudej, 2001)	
Flavonol		
Glycosides		

Endangered Herb   Adverse effects: BOLD = life-threatening

Actions

Very little scientific research is available on daisy. Most of the research has focused on identifying its chemical components, which had not been studied previously.

Antimicrobial Action

One study revealed that the triterpenoid glycoside components of *Bellis perennis* L. are responsible for its antifungal activity. In this study these glycosides were effective against human pathogenic yeasts such as *Candida* and *Cryptococcus* spp. (Bader, 1990). Another study evaluated the essential oils of daisy for potential antimicrobial activity. Two of the oils exhibited activity against both gram-positive and gram-negative bacteria (Avato, 1997).

References

Avato P et al: Antimicrobial activity of polyacetylenes from *Bellis perennis* and their synthetic derivatives, *Planta Med* 63(6):503-507, 1997.

Bader G et al: The antifungal action of polygalacic acid glycosides, *Pharmazie* 45(8):618-620, 1990.

Gudej J et al: Flavonal glycosides from the flowers of *Bellis perennis*, *Fitoterpia*, 72(7):839-840, 2001.

Damiana
(dah-mee′ah-nah)

Scientific name: *Turnera diffusa*

Other common names: Herba de la pastora, Mexican damiana, old woman's broom, rosemary   Class 1 (Leaf)

Origin: Damiana is a shrub found in the United States and in Central and South America.

Uses

Reported Uses

Damiana is used as an aphrodisiac to increase sexual potency. It may irritate the urethra and increase sensitivity of the penis. Damiana may be used in combination with other herbs for sexual potency. This herb is also used as a diuretic and antidepressant, and it is thought to produce euphoric effects when smoked.

 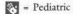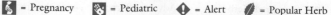

Investigational Uses

Damiana shows promise as an antidiabetic agent (Alarcon-Aguilar, 2002) and as a weight-loss agent (Anderson, 2001).

Product Availability and Dosages

Available Forms

Capsules, powder, tea, tincture

Plant Parts Used: Leaves

Dosages and Routes

Adult

All dosages listed are PO.
- Decoction: 18 g powder/500 ml water tid
- Tea: 1 cup tid (Murray, 1998)
- Tincture: 2.5 ml tid

Precautionary Information

Contraindications

Until more research is available, damiana should not be used during pregnancy and lactation and should not be given to children. It should not be used by persons with liver disease or hypersensitivity to this herb. Class 1 herb (leaf).

Side Effects/Adverse Reactions

Central Nervous System: Hallucinations, confusion
Gastrointestinal: Nausea, vomiting, anorexia, HEPATO-TOXICITY (high doses)
Genitourinary: Urethral irritation
Integumentary: Hypersensitivity reactions

Interactions with Damiana

Drug	Food	Herb	Lab Test
None known	None known	None known	None known

Client Considerations

Assess

- Assess for hypersensitivity reactions. If present, discontinue use of damiana and administer antihistamine or other appropriate therapy.
- Assess for hepatotoxicity: increasing ALT, AST, and bilirubin levels; clay-colored stools; right upper-quadrant pain. If hepatotoxicity occurs, use of herb should be discontinued and appropriate action taken.

Administer

- Instruct the client to store damiana products in a cool, dry place, away from heat and moisture.

Teach Client/Family

- Until more research is available, caution the client not to use damiana during pregnancy and lactation and not to give it to children.

Pharmacology

Pharmacokinetics

Pharmacokinetics and pharmacodynamics are unknown.

Primary Chemical Components of Damiana and Their Possible Actions		
Chemical Class	**Individual Component**	**Possible Action**
Volatile oil	Cineol Pinenes; Cymene	Choleretic; antibacterial
Thymol		
Sesquiterpene		
Glycoside	Cyanogenic; Arbutin	
Resin		
Tannin		Wound healing
Mucilage		
Gum		

Actions

Very little research is available for damiana. Two small studies have been done since 1998. One focused on the antihyperglycemic effects of damiana, testing 28 different plant species to de-

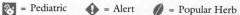

termine their antidiabetic effects. One herb that was found to be an effective antihyperglycemic was *Turnera diffusa* (Alarcon-Aguilar, 1998; Alarcon-Aguilar, 2002). Another study focused on the role of damiana in increasing the sexual behavior of male rats. This study seems to support the traditional use of *Turnera diffusa* as a sexual stimulant (Arletti, 1999).

D

References

Alarcon-Aguilar FJ et al: Study of the antihyperglycemic effect of plants used as antidiabetics, *J Ethnopharmacol* 61(2):101-110, 1998.

Alarcon-Aguilar FJ et al: Investigation on the hypoglycaemic effects of extracts of four Mexican medicinal plants in normal and alloxan-diabetic mice, *Phytother Res* 16(4):383-386, 2002.

Arletti R et al: Stimulating property of *Turnera diffusa* and *Pfaffia paniculata* extracts on the sexual behavior of male rats, *Psychopharmacology* 143(1):15-19, 1999.

Murray M, Pizzarno J: *The encyclopedia of natural medicine,* Roseville, Calif, 1998, Prima.

Dandelion
(dan'duh-ly-uhn)

Scientific names: *Taraxacum officinale, Taraxacum laevigatum*

Other common names: Blowball, cankerwort, lion's tooth, priest's crown, puffball, swine snout, white endive, wild endive

Class 1 (Leaf)

Origin: Dandelion is a weed found throughout the world. It is cultivated in parts of Europe.

Uses

Reported Uses

Dandelion has been used as a laxative, an antihypertensive, and a diuretic.

Investigational Uses

Dandelion is used experimentally as an antitumor agent and immunogenic and to treat chronic colitis. Dandelion has also been used to treat urolithiasis; however, other pharmacologic treatments are just as effective (Grases, 1994).

🌀 Endangered Herb　　　　Adverse effects: BOLD = life-threatening

Product Availability and Dosages
Available Forms
Capsule, fluid extract, fresh plant, juice, solid extract, tea, tincture

Plant Parts Used: Flowers, leaves, roots

Dosages and Routes
Adult
All dosages listed are PO.
- Decoction: 2-8 g dried root in 150 ml boiling water, let stand 15 min, tid
- Fluid extract: 4-10 ml (1:1 in alcohol 25%) tid (Blumenthal, 1998)
- Infusion: 4-10 g dried leaves in 8 oz water tid
- Infusion: 2-8 g dried root in 8 oz water tid
- Juice: 4-8 ml tid
- Tincture: 5-10 ml (1:5 in alcohol 45%) tid
- Whole herb: 4-10 g herb tid (Blumenthal, 1998)

Child
- PO root infusion: ¼-1 cup/day several times/wk (Romm, 2000)
- Topical root tincture: ¼-1 tsp bid (Romm, 2000)

Precautionary Information
Contraindications
Dandelion should not be used during pregnancy and lactation. It should not be used by persons with hypersensitivity to this product or other Asteraceae spp. (chamomile, yarrow root) and should be used cautiously by persons with diabetes mellitus or fluid and electrolyte imbalances.
Persons with irritable bowel syndrome, digestive diseases, bile duct obstruction, intestinal obstruction, or latex allergy should avoid the use of this herb. Class 1 herb (leaf).

Side Effects/Adverse Reactions
Gastrointestinal: Nausea, vomiting, anorexia, cholelithiasis, gallbladder inflammation
Integumentary: Hypersensitivity reactions, contact dermatitis

D

Interactions with Dandelion

Drug

Antihypertensives: Dandelion may increase the effects of antihypertensives; avoid concurrent use.

Diuretics: Dandelion may increase diuresis when used concurrently with diuretics, leading to fluid loss and electrolyte imbalances; avoid concurrent use.

Insulin: Dandelion may increase the effects of insulin; avoid concurrent use.

Lithium: Toxicity may occur as a result of sodium excretion if dandelion is used concurrently with lithium.

Oral antidiabetics: Dandelion may increase the effects of oral antidiabetics; avoid concurrent use.

Food	Herb	Lab Test
None known	None known	None known

Client Considerations

Assess

- Assess for hypersensitivity reactions and contact dermatitis. If either of these is present, discontinue use of dandelion and administer antihistamine or other appropriate therapy. Also, assess for hypersensitivity to other *Asteraceae* spp.
- Identify use of antihypertensives, diuretics, oral antidiabetics, insulin, and lithium. Use of dandelion should be avoided if client is taking these medications (see Interactions).
- Assess for fluid and electrolyte imbalances: check sodium chloride and potassium chloride levels.
- Assess blood pressure if the client is combining dandelion with antihypertensives.
- Assess blood glucose in the diabetic patient who is taking insulin or oral antidiabetics.

Administer

- Instruct the client to store dandelion products away from moisture and light.

Teach Client/Family

- Until more research is available, caution the client not to use dandelion during pregnancy and lactation.

- Caution clients with children taking diabetic medications not to use dandelion until approved by prescriber.
- Inform the client that dandelion may cause increased diuresis and that fluid and electrolyte imbalances may result.

Pharmacology

Pharmacokinetics

Pharmacokinetics and pharmacodynamics are unknown.

Primary Chemical Components of Dandelion and Their Possible Actions		
Chemical Class	**Individual Component**	**Possible Action**
Acid	Caffeic acid; Chlorogenic acid	Antitumor; analgesic
	Linoleic acid	Antiarteriosclerotic
	Oleic acid	Antiinflammatory; antitumor
	Palmitic acid	Antifibrinolytic
	Linolenic; Chicoric; Monocaffeyltartaric; Taraxacin; Taraxacum	
Coumarin	Cichoriin; Aesculin	
Flavonoid	Luteolin; Chrysoeriol	
Mineral		
Resin		
Taraxasterol		Antiinflammatory
Taraxerin		
Taraxerol		
Taraxalisin		
Terpenoid		
Vitamin	A; B; C; D	
Carotenoid		
Glycosides		
Sesquiterpene lactones	Dihydroconiferin; Syringin; Dihydrosyringin; 11beta; 13-Dihydrolactucin; Ixerin D; Ainslioside (Kisiel, 2000)	

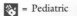

Actions

Antitumor/Immunogenic Action

One Chinese study evaluated immunomodulators used to restore suppressed immune functions in scald mice, including cell-mediated, humoral, and nonspecific immunity. The control group of scald mice all showed depressed immune function. *Taraxacum officinale* exhibited immunomodulating effects, with the effects directly related to the dose (Luo, 1993). A more recent study focused on nitric oxide production, which is an indicator of immune regulation and defense. *T. officinale* restored the ability of mouse peritoneal macrophages to inhibit nitric oxide production. The secretion of tumor necrosis factor-alpha (TNF-alpha) is responsible for this effect (Kim, 1998).

Anticolitic Action

One study documents the efficacy of *T. officinale* when used in combination with other herbs for the treatment of chronic colitis. Twenty-four patients with chronic nonspecific colitis were given an herbal combination of *T. officinale, Hypericum perforatum, Melissa officinalis, Calendula officinalis,* and *Foeniculum vulgare.* After 15 days of treatment, defecation occurred only once daily, and diarrhea was normalized in patients with diarrhea syndrome (Chakurski, 1981).

Other Actions

One of the traditional uses of *T. officinale* has been to treat urolithiasis. In one study the herb improved citraturia, calciuria, phosphaturia, urine pH, and diuresis. Its urolithiatic action is believed to result from its saponin components (Grases, 1994). However, other products that work equally well are available to treat urolithiasis.

References

Blumenthal M, editor: *The complete German Commission E monographs: therapeutic guide to herbal medicines,* Austin, Tex, American Botanical Council; Boston, Integrative Medicine Communication, 1998.

Chakurski I et al: Treatment of chronic colitis with a herbal combination of *Taraxacum officinale, Hipericum perforatum, Melissa officinaliss, Calendula officinalis* and *Foeniculum vulgare, Vutr Boles* 20(6):51-54, 1981.

Grases F et al: Urolithiasis and phytotherapy, *Int Urol Nephrol* 26(5):507-511, 1994.

Kim HM et al: *Taraxacum officinale* restores inhibition of nitric oxide production by cadmium in mouse peritoneal macrophages, *Immuno-pharmacol Immunotoxicol* 20(2):283-297, 1998.

Kisiel W et al: Futher sesquiterpenoids and phenolics from *Taraxacum officinale, Fitoterpia* 71(3):269-273, 2000.

Luo ZH: The use of Chinese traditional medicines to improve impaired immune functions in scald mice, *Chung Hua Cheng Hsing Shao Shang Wai Ko Tsa Chih* 9(1):56-58, 80, 1993 (in English).

Romm A: Better Nutrition's 2000 guide to children's supplements, *Better Nutrition* 62(10):38-43, 2000.

Devil's Claw
(dev'uhlz claw)

Scientific name: *Harpagophytum procumbens*

Other common names: Grapple plant, wood spider

Class 2d (Secondary Tuber)

Origin: Devil's claw grows wild in southwest Africa.

Uses

Reported Uses

Devil's claw is used to increase the appetite and to treat joint pain and inflammation, allergies, headache, heartburn, dysmenorrhea, gastrointestinal upset, malaria, gout, and nicotine poisoning.

Product Availability and Dosages

Available Forms

Capsules, dried powdered root, dry solid extract, tea, tincture

Plant Parts Used: Roots, tubers

Dosages and Routes

Adult

All dosages listed are PO.

Anorexia
• Infusion: 1.5 g herb tid (Blumenthal, 1998)

Gout
• Dried powdered root: 1-2 g tid (Murray, 1998)
• Tincture: 4-5 ml (1:5 dilution) tid (Murray, 1998)
• Dry solid extract: 400 mg tid (Murray, 1998)

Osteoarthritis
• Dried powdered root: 1-2 g tid (Murray, 1998)

 = Pregnancy    = Pediatric   = Alert   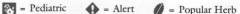 = Popular Herb

- Tincture: 4-5 ml (1:5 dilution) tid (Murray, 1998)
- Dry solid extract: 400 mg tid (Murray, 1998)

Other

- Infusion: ≤4.5 g herb (Blumenthal, 1998) in 300 ml boiling water, let stand 8 hr, strain and drink

D

Precautionary Information

Contraindications

Because it may stimulate the uterus and cause contractions, devil's claw should not be used during pregnancy. Until more research is available, this herb should not be used during lactation and should not be given to children. Persons with peptic or duodenal ulcer disease, cholecystitis, or hypersensitivity to this herb should avoid the use of devil's claw. Class 2d herb (secondary tuber).

Side Effects/Adverse Reactions

Gastrointestinal: Nausea, vomiting, anorexia
Integumentary: Hypersensitivity reactions

Interactions with Devil's Claw

Drug

Antiarrhythmics: Because two of the chemical components in devil's claw exert inotropic and chronotropic effects, use this herb cautiously with antiarrhythmics (theoretical).

Food	Herb	Lab Test
None known	None known	None known

Client Considerations

Assess

- Assess for hypersensitivity reactions. If present, discontinue use of devil's claw and administer antihistamine or other appropriate therapy.
- Assess cardiac status in any client with a cardiac condition: blood pressure, character of pulse. Identify what prescription drugs and herbal supplements the client is taking to treat this condition (see Interactions).

- Assess joint pain and inflammation in any client with an arthritic condition: pain location, duration, intensity, and alleviating and aggravating factors. Identify what prescription and herbal supplements the client is taking to treat this condition.

Administer

- Instruct the client to store devil's claw products in a cool, dry place, away from heat and moisture.

Teach Client/Family

- Because it may stimulate the uterus and cause contractions, caution the client not to use devil's claw during pregnancy. Until more research is available, caution the client to avoid the use of this herb during lactation and not to give it to children.

Pharmacology

Pharmacokinetics

Pharmacokinetics and pharmacodynamics are unknown.

Primary Chemical Components of Devil's Claw and Their Possible Actions		
Chemical Class	**Individual Component**	**Possible Action**
Triterpene Resin Flavonoid Monoterpenes	Kaempferol; Luteolin Harpagoside; Harpagide Procumbide	Negative chronotropic; positive inotropic
Stigmasterol Beta sitosterol Fatty acid		

Actions

Antiinflammatory Action

Several studies have evaluated the antiinflammatory properties of devil's claw in the treatment of joint conditions. The results are mixed. One Canadian study (Whitehouse, 1983) evaluated *Harpagophytum procumbens* for reduction of rat hind-foot edema. Devil's claw was completely ineffective, even at doses

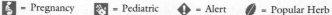

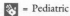 = Pregnancy    = Pediatric   ◆ = Alert   𝄢 = Popular Herb

greater than 100 times the recommended human dose. Another study produced similar results. No clinical significance was found when human subjects consumed devil's claw (Moussard, 1992). A more recent study (Baghdikian, 1997) reported conflicting results on harpagoside, one of the chemical components of the herb, which showed analgesic and antiinflammatory properties. *H. procumbens* was found to produce analgesic and antiinflammatory effects (Chantre, 2000; Gobel, 2001; Fiebich, 2001). The most recent study determined that the iridoid glycosides are responsible for the analgesic, antiinflammatory, and antiphlogistic effects of devil's claw (Wegener, 1999).

D

Cardiovascular Action

When rats and rabbits were studied to determine the cardiovascular effects of *H. procumbens,* a significant dose-dependent reduction occurred in arterial blood pressure, along with a reduction in heart rate at high doses. Harpagoside, one of the chemical components of the herb, exhibited less activity than did the extract of *H. procumbens.* The extract of *H. procumbens* produced a mild decrease in heart rate, with mild positive inotropic effects at low doses but a significant negative inotropic effect at higher doses. Harpagoside showed negative chronotropic and positive inotropic effects (Circosta, 1984). Another study demonstrated that devil's claw exerts a protective action in hyperkinetic ventricular arrhythmias in rats (Costa De Pasquale, 1985).

References

Baghdikian B et al: An analytical study, anti-inflammatory and analgesic effects of *Harpagophytum procumbens* and *Harpagophytum zeyheri, Planta Med* 63(2):171-176, 1997.

Blumenthal M, editor: *The complete German Commission E monographs: therapeutic guide to herbal medicines,* Austin, Tex, American Botanical Council; Boston, Integrative Medicine Communication, 1998.

Chantre P et al: Efficacy and tolerance of *Harpagophytum procumbens* versus diacerhein in treatment of osteoarthritis, *Phytomedicine* 7(3): 177-183, 2000.

Circosta C et al: A drug used in traditional medicine: *Harpagophytum procumbens* DC, II, cardiovascular activity, *J Ethnopharmacol* 11(3): 259-274, 1984.

Costa De Pasquale R et al: A drug used in traditional medicine: *Harpagophytum procumbens* DC, III, effects on hyperkinetic ventricular arrhythmias by reperfusion, *J Ethnopharmacol* 13(2):193-199, 1985.

Fiebich BL et al: Inhibition of TNF-alpha synthesis in LPS-stimulated primary human monocytes by *Harpagophytum* extract steittap 69, *Phytomedicine* 8(1):28-30, 2001.

Gobel H et al: Effects of *Harpagophytum procumbens* LI 174 (devil's claw) on sensory, motor and vascular muscle reagibility in the treatment of unspecific back pain, *Schmerz* 15(1):10-18, 2000.

Moussard C et al: A drug used in traditional medicine: *Harpagophytum procumbens*—no evidence for NSAID-like effect on whole blood eicosanoid production in humans, *Prostaglandins Leukot Essent Fatty Acids* 46(4):283-286, 1992.

Murray M, Pizzarno J: *The encyclopedia of natural medicine,* Roseville, Calif, 1998, Prima.

Wegener T: Therapy of degenerative diseases of the musculoskeletal system with South African devil's claw (*Harpagophytum procumbens* DC), *Wien Med Wochenschr* 149(8-10):254-257, 1999 (abstract).

Whitehouse LW et al: Devil's claw *(Harpagophytum procumbens):* no evidence for anti-inflammatory activity in the treatment of arthritic disease, *Can Med Assoc J* 129(3):249-251, 1983.

DHEA

Scientific name: Dehydroepiandrosterone

Origin: DHEA is naturally occurring in yam (see wild yam, p. 920).

Uses

Reported Uses

DHEA may be used to stimulate immunity and to treat atherosclerosis, hyperglycemia, and cancer. It is also used to prevent osteoporosis and to improve memory and cognitive functioning.

Investigational Uses

Research is underway to determine the efficacy of DHEA used by postmenopausal women in place of traditional hormone replacement therapy. DHEA may also reduce symptoms of depression, aging, asthma, rheumatoid arthritis, and lupus erythematosus.

Product Availability and Dosages

Available Forms

Capsules, cream, tablets

 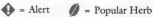

Dosages and Routes

Adult

All dosages listed are PO.

Rheumatoid Arthritis

• 50-200 mg/day (Murray, 1998)

Supplementation

• Men >50 yrs of age: 25-50 mg/day (Murray, 1998)
• Women >50 yrs of age: 15-25 mg/day (Murray, 1998)
• Men and women >70 yrs of age: 50-100 mg/day (Murray, 1998)

Precautionary Information

Contraindications

Until more research is available, DHEA should not be used during pregnancy and lactation and should not be given to children. Persons with estrogen-sensitive tumors (such as breast or uterine cancer), prostate cancer, or benign prostatic hypertrophy should not use this product.

Side Effects/Adverse Reactions

Cardiovascular: Irregular heart rhythm (high doses) (Sahelian, 1997)
Central Nervous System: Insomnia, restlessness, irritability, anxiety, increased mood, aggressiveness
Integumentary: Acne

Interactions with DHEA

Drug
Hormone replacement therapy: DHEA may interfere with estrogen and androgen therapy; avoid concurrent use (theoretical).

Food	Herb	Lab Test
None known	None known	None known

Client Considerations

Assess

• Assess for changes in mood and inability to sleep. Watch for increasing aggressiveness, irritability, and restlessness.

 Endangered Herb   Adverse effects: BOLD = life-threatening

- Determine whether the client is currently using hormone replacement therapy; if so, use of DHEA should be avoided (see Interactions).
- Assess for hormone-sensitive tumors; DHEA may stimulate the growth of these tumors.

Administer

- Instruct the client to store DHEA in a sealed container away from moisture and light.

Teach Client/Family

- Until more research is available, caution the client not to use DHEA during pregnancy and lactation and not to give it to children.
- Advise the client to lower the dosage of DHEA if acne develops.

Pharmacology

Pharmacokinetics

Pharmacokinetics and pharmacodynamics are unknown.

Actions

Hormonal Action

In the human body, DHEA is synthesized from a precursor steroid, pregnenolone, and then is converted into estrogens and testosterone in men and women (Baulieu, 1996). Reports confirm that levels of DHEA decline significantly after age 40. Some researchers suspect that this decline may be associated with insulin resistance, increased weight gain, and cardiovascular conditions (Sahelian, 1997). DHEA may provide an alternative to hormone replacement therapy in women (Takayanagi, 2002). However, supplementation should not be started before the client undergoes a thorough evaluation for hormone-sensitive tumors.

Cancer Stimulation/Cancer Inhibition

Conflicting studies have reported increased tumor flare in patients with prostate cancer. However, initiation of antihormone therapy caused the flare to retreat (Jones, 1997).

Cardiovascular Action

One study evaluated levels of DHEA in patients with congestive heart failure. The results showed that levels of DHEA are lower in patients with congestive heart failure, in proportion to the severity of the disease (Moriyama, 2000).

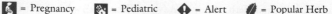

Immunoregulation Action

A new study (Cheng, 2000) has evaluated the effect of DHEA and DHEA sulfate on interleukin-10 (IL-10) in laboratory mice. The results indicated that DHEA and DHEA sulfate increase IL-10, and DHEA may also affect the functioning of B-lymphocytes.

Cognitive Function Action

In a recent study, DHEA levels were found to be significantly lower in patients with Alzheimer's disease and vascular dementia than in patients who did not have these diseases. Cortisol levels were found to be significantly higher. The usefulness of this information has not yet been determined (Bernardi, 2000).

References

Baulieu E et al: *J Endocrinol* 150:s221-s239, 1996.

Bernardi F et al: Allopregnanolone and dehydroepiandrosterone response to corticotropin-releasing factor in patients suffering from Alzheimer's disease and vascular dementia, *Eur J Endrocrinol* 142(5):466-471, 2000 (in-process citation).

Cheng GF et al: Regulation of murine interleukin-10 production by dehydroepiandrosterone, *J Interferon Cytokine Res* 20(5):471-478, 2000 (in-process citation).

Jones et al: Use of DHEA in a patient with advanced prostate cancer: a case report and review, *Urology* 50(5):784-788, 1997.

Moriyama Y et al: The plasma levels of dehydroepiandrosterone sulfate are decreased in patients with chronic heart failure in proportion to severity, *J Clin Endocrinol Metab* 85(5):1834-1840, 2000 (in-process citation).

Murray M, Pizzarno J: *The encyclopedia of natural medicine,* Roseville, Calif, 1998, Prima.

Sahelian R: New supplements and unknown, long-term consequences, *Am J Nat Med* 4(8):8-9, 1997.

Takayanagi R et al: DHEA as a possible source for estrogen formation in bone cells: correlation between bone mineral density and serum DHEA-sulfate concentration in postmenopausal women, *Mech Ageing Dev* 123(8):1107-1114, 2002.

Dill
(dil)

Scientific name: *Anethum graveolens*
Other common names: Dill seed, dillweed, garden dill, dilly

Class 1 (Fruit)

Origin: Dill is found throughout the world.

Uses
Reported Uses
In traditional herbal medicine dill is used to relieve flatulence and infant colic. It is also reported to exert antispasmodic effects.

Investigational Uses
Research is underway to confirm the uses of dill as an antihyperlipidemic and antihypercholesterolemic (Yazdanparest, 2001).

Product Availability and Dosages
Available Forms
Dried fruit, essential oil, water (concentrated and distilled)

Plant Parts Used: Flowers, fruit, seeds

Dosages and Routes
Adult
All dosages listed are PO.
- Dried fruit: 1-4 g tid
- Essential oil: 0.05-2 ml tid, or 0.1-0.3 g qd (Blumenthal, 1998)
- Seeds: 3 g qd (Blumenthal, 1998)
- Water, concentrated: 0.2 ml tid
- Water, distilled: 2-4 ml tid

Precautionary Information
Contraindications
As other than a food product, dill should not be used during pregnancy and lactation, and it should not be given to children except under the supervision of a qualified herbalist. Persons with a fluid or electrolyte imbalance and those with hypersensitivity to dill or other related spices should not use this herb. Class 1 herb (fruit).

🝒 = Pregnancy   **🐾** = Pediatric   **❶** = Alert   **∅** = Popular Herb

D

Precautionary Information—cont'd

Side Effects/Adverse Reactions

Endocrine: May alter sodium balance
Integumentary: Hypersensitivity reactions; photodermatitis
(fruit)

Interactions with Dill			
Drug	Food	Herb	Lab Test
None known	None known	None known	None known

Client Considerations

Assess

- Assess for hypersensitivity reactions and photodermatitis. If
these are present, discontinue use of dill and administer antihistamine or other appropriate therapy.
- Assess fluid and electrolytes in clients with known imbalances.

Administer

- Instruct the client to store dill products away from moisture
and light.

Teach Client/Family

- Until more research is available, caution the client not to use
dill during pregnancy and lactation. Caution the client not to
give dill to children unless under the supervision of a qualified herbalist.

Pharmacology

Pharmacokinetics

Pharmacokinetics and pharmacodynamics are unknown.

Primary Chemical Components of Dill and Their Possible Actions

Chemical Class	Individual Component	Possible Action
Furancoumarin		
Flavonoid	Quercetin; Kaempferol Glucuronide; Isohamnetin	Antiinflammatory
Volatile oil	Eugenol; Anethole Anethofuran; Carvone; Limonene (Zheng, 1992)	Antioxidant
Xanthone		
Triterpene		
Glucopyranosides	Hydroxypipentone; hydroxygeraniol	

Actions

Very little research is available for *Anethum graveolens*. Primary research has focused on determining the chemical components of this herb. Other information has come from anecdotal reports and traditional uses.

Antimicrobial Action

One study evaluated the volatile oil of dill for antimicrobial activity. The volatile oil taken from mature plants exerted the highest antimicrobial effect. Unlike many other herbs, the geographic area in which the plant was grown did not change its antimicrobial effect. Dill inhibited the growth of both yeast and lactic acid bacteria (Shcherbanovsky, 1975).

Other Actions

Rats were fed a diet high in cholesterol and fats. After feeding the rats a dill extract for 2 weeks, cholesterol was not reduced but triglycerides were reduced by 42% (Yazdanparast, 2001).

References

Blumenthal M, editor: *The complete German Commission E monographs: therapeutic guide to herbal medicines,* Austin, Tex, American Botanical Council; Boston, Integrative Medicine Communication, 1998.
Shcherbanovsky LR et al: Volatile oil of *Anethum graveolens* L. as an

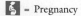 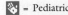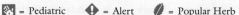

inhibitor of yeast and lactic acid bacteria, *Prikl Biokhim Mikrobiol* 11(3):476-477, 1975.

Yazdanparast R et al: Antihyperlipidaemic and antihypercholesterolemic effects of *Anethum graveolens* leaves after the removal of furocoumarins, *Cytobios* 105(410):185-191, 2001.

Zheng GQ et al: Anethofuran, carvone, and limonene: potential cancer chemopreventive agents from dill weed oil and caraway oil, *Planta Med* 58(4):338-341, 1992.

Dong Quai

Scientific name: *Angelica polymorpha* var. *sinensis*

Other common names: Chinese angelica, dang gui, dry-kuei, tanggwi, tang-kuei, toki, women's ginseng

Class 2b (Root)

Origin: Dong quai is a perennial found in Japan, China, and Korea.

Uses

Reported Uses

Dong quai has been used extensively in many to treat the symptoms of menopause. It is also used to treat menstrual irregularities such as dysmenorrhea, PMS, and menorrhagia. Other uses include treatment for headache, neuralgia, herpes infections, and malaria. In traditional Chinese medicine dong quai is used to treat vitiligo and anemia. Dong quai should not be confused with other *Angelica* spp.

Product Availability and Dosages

Available Forms

Capsules, fluid extract, raw roots (powdered), tablets, tea, tincture; available in many combination products; not available as a standardized extract

Plant Parts Used: Roots

Dosages and Routes

Adult

All dosages listed are PO.

Symptoms of Menopause and PMS

• Fluid extract: 1 ml (¼ tsp) tid (Murray, 1998)

- Powdered root: 1-2 g tid (Murray, 1998)
- Tea: 1-2 g tid (Murray, 1998)
- Tincture: 4 ml (1 tsp) (1:5 dilution) tid (Murray, 1998)

Other

- Capsules/tablets: 500 mg ≤ 6 times/day (Foster, 1998)
- Raw root: 1 g/day
- Tea: 1 cup bid-tid (Foster, 1998)
- Tincture: 5-20 drops (1:5 concentration) ≤ tid (Foster, 1998)

Precautionary Information

Contraindications

Until more research is available, dong quai should not be used during pregnancy and lactation and should not be given to children. In Chinese medicine, dong quai has been used during pregnancy, but its use must be monitored by a qualified herbalist. This herb should not be used by persons who are hypersensitive to it, or by those with bleeding disorders, excessive menstrual flow, or acute illness. Class 2b herb (root).

Side Effects/Adverse Reactions

Gastrointestinal: Nausea, vomiting, diarrhea, anorexia
Genitourinary: Increased menstrual flow
Integumentary: Hypersensitivity reactions, photosensitivity
Systemic: Fever, BLEEDING

Interactions with Dong Quai

Drug

Antiplatelets: Dong quai may increase the effects of antiplatelets.
Oral anticoagulants (anisindione, dicumarol, warfarin): Dong quai may increase the effects of oral anticoagulants.

Food

None known

Herb

Chamomile, dandelion, horse chestnut, red clover: Dong quai may potentiate anticoagulant activity.

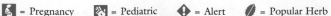

Interactions with Dong Quai—cont'd
Herb—cont'd
St. John's Wort: Dong quai may increase photosensitivity (theoretical).
Lab Test
None known

D

Client Considerations

Assess

- Assess for hypersensitivity reactions. If present, discontinue use of dong quai and administer antihistamine or other appropriate therapy.
- Determine whether the client is using oral anticoagulants; dong quai may increase bleeding tendencies (see Interactions).

Administer

- Instruct the client to store dong quai products in a sealed container away from moisture and heat.

Teach Client/Family

- Until more research is available, caution the client not to use dong quai during pregnancy and lactation and not to give it to children. Clients who wish to use dong quai during pregnancy should do so only under the direction of an experienced herbalist.
- Advise client that photosensitivity may occur. Sunscreen or protective clothing should be worn in sunlight.

Pharmacology

Pharmacokinetics

Pharmacokinetics and pharmacodynamics are unknown.

Primary Chemical Components of Dong Quai and Their Possible Actions

Chemical Class	Individual Component	Possible Action
Volatile oil	Safrole	Carcinogenic
	n-Butylphthalide; Ligustilide	Relaxes bronchial smooth muscles
	Carinene; Isosafrole; Carvacrol; Succinic acid; Nicotinic acid; Uracil	
Vitamin	B_{12}	
Coumarin	Osthole	Anticoagulant
	Psoralen; Bergapten; Imperatorin; Oxypeucedanin	
Ferulic acid		Anticoagulant; decreased uterine movement
Polysaccharide		Immunostimulation

Actions

Dong quai has been used since the sixth century as a blood and liver tonic. In Chinese medicine, it has been used to treat hormonal irregularities and anemia.

Hormonal Action

Research on the hormonal actions of dong quai shows conflicting results. One study showed no statistical difference between dong quai and a placebo in reducing menopausal symptoms (Hirata, 1997). During the 6-month study, participants took standardized capsules of 0.5 mg/kg of ferulic acid, one of the chemical components of dong quai, and were evaluated at 6, 12, and 24 weeks. Reported menopausal symptoms did not differ between the placebo group and the dong quai group. Researchers concluded that dong quai exerts no estrogenic effects and that it is not effective when used alone to treat menopausal symptoms. However, the herbal combination tokishakuyakusan, including peony, *Angelica*, alisma, and cnidium, increased progesterone secretion by means of its action in the corpora lutea (Usuki, 1991).

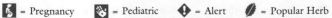

 = Pregnancy   = Pediatric   = Alert   = Popular Herb

Other Actions

A study evaluating the effects of *Angelica sinensis* root on melanocyte proliferation showed no stimulation of melanocyte division. Instead, cell cytotoxicity resulted at higher doses (Raman, 1996). Other actions include decreased intraocular pressure, decreased blood pressure (Yoshihiro, 1985), decreased premature ventricular contractions (Zhuang, 1991), inhibition of platelet aggregation (Li, 1989), increased tumor necrosis factor (TNF) (Haranaka, 1985), and decreased atherosclerosis. Antiinflammatory and mild analgesic properties have also been reported.

References

Foster S: *101 medicinal herbs,* Loveland, Colo, 1998, Interweave Press.

Haranaka K et al: Antitumor activities and tumor-necrosis factor producibility of traditional Chinese medicines and crude drugs, *Cancer Immunol Immunother* 20(1):1-5, 1985.

Hirata JD et al: Does dong quai have estrogenic effects in postmenopausal women? a double blind, placebo-controlled trial, *Fertility and Sterility* 68(6):981-986, 1997.

Li RZ et al: Studies of the active constituents of the Chinese drug "duhuo" *Angelica pubescents, Yao Hsueh Hsueh Pao* 24(7):546-551, 1989.

Murray M, Pizzarno J: *The encyclopedia of natural medicine,* 2 ed (revised), Roseville, Calif, 1998, Prima.

Raman A et al: Investigation of the effect of *Angelica sinensis* root extract on the proliferation of melanocytes in culture, *J Ethnopharmacol* 54(2-3):165-170, 1996.

Usuki S: Effects of herbal components of tokishakuyakusan on progesterone secretion by corpus luteum in vitro, *Am J Chin Med* 19(1):57-60, 1991.

Yoshihiro K: The physiological actions of tang kuei and cnidium, *Bull Oriental Healing Arts Institute of the USA* 10(7):269-278, 1985.

Zhuang XX: Protective effect of *Angelica* injection on arrhythmia during myocardial ischemia reperfusion in rat, *Chung Hsi I Chieh Ho Tsa Chih* 11(6):360-361, 326, 1991.

Echinacea

Scientific names: *Echinacea angustifolia, Echinacea pallida, Echinacea purpurea*

Other common names: American cone flower, black sampson, black susans, cock-up-hat, comb flower, coneflower, hedgehog, Indian head, Kansas snakeroot, Missouri snakeroot, purple coneflower, red sunflower, rudbeckia, sampson root, scurvy root, snakeroot

Class 1 (Root/Seed)

Origin: Echinacea is a perennial found in only three states: Missouri, Nebraska, and Kansas. It is cultivated in much of the world.

Uses

Reported Uses

Echinacea is used internally, primarily as an immune stimulant and for immune support, and as prophylaxis for colds, influenza, and other viral, fungal, and bacterial infections. It may be used topically to promote wound healing and to treat wounds, bruises, burns, scratches, and leg ulcers. Echinacea is more effective when taken at onset or first signs of an illness, not after illness is well-established.

Investigational Uses

Researchers are experimenting with the use of echinacea to stimulate the immune system of HIV/AIDS patients. It may also be used as a prophylaxis for colds or urinary tract infections.

Product Availability and Dosages

Available Forms

Capsules, fluid extract, juice, solid (dry powdered) extract, sublingual tablets, tablets, tea, tincture
NOTE: Some extracts may be standardized to 4% to 5% echinacoside; others are standardized to phenolics.

Plant Parts Used: Rhizome, roots; depending on developmental stage of growth: flowers, juice from the stem, leaves, whole plant

E

Dosages and Routes
Adult
- Parenteral: dose individualized to age of client and condition (NOTE: parenteral route not used in the United States; herb used parenterally in Germany)

The following dosages are PO.
- Capsules: 500 mg-1 g tid (McCaleb, 2000)
- Dried root: 0.5-1 g tid; can use as tea (Murray, 1998)
- Fluid extract: 1-2 ml tid (1:1 dilution) mixed in a little water (Bradley, 1992); 2-4 ml tid (Murray, 1998)
- Freeze dried plant: 325-650 mg tid (Murray, 1998)
- Pressed juice: 6-9 ml qd in divided doses (25:1 dilution in 22% alcohol) (McCaleb, 2000)
- Solid (dry powdered) extract: 150-300 mg tid (6.5:1 dilution or 3.5% echinacoside) (Murray, 1998)
- Tea: 2 tsp (4 g) powdered herb simmered 15 min in hot water.
- Tincture: 15-30 drops bid-qid or 30-60 drops bid (McCaleb, 2000); 2-4 ml tid (1:5 dilution) (Murray, 1998); other references suggest q1-2h when person is ill.

Child
Acute Infections
- PO root tincture: ½-1 tsp up to q2h (Romm, 2000)

Skin Infections
- Topical tincture: 1 tbsp root/¼ cup water, use as topical rinse (Romm, 2000)

To Prevent Colds and Infections
- PO root tincture: ½ tsp bid (Romm, 2000)

Precautionary Information
Contraindications
Until more research is available, echinacea should not be used during pregnancy (although one study showed no harmful effects during the first trimester [Gallo, 2001]) and lactation, and it should not be given to children younger than 2 years of age. It should not be used by persons who have autoimmune diseases such as lupus erythematosus, multiple sclerosis, HIV/AIDS, or collagen disease or by those with tuberculosis or hypersensitivity to *Bellis* sp. or composite family herbs. Immunosuppression may occur after extended therapy with this herb; do not use for longer than

Continued

Precautionary Information—cont'd

Contraindications—cont'd

8 weeks without a 3-week rest period. Class 1 herb (root/seed).

Side Effects/Adverse Reactions

Gastrointestinal: HEPATOTOXICITY (Chernecky, 2001)
Integumentary: Hypersensitivity reactions
Respiratory: ACUTE ASTHMA ATTACK (Mullins, 2002)
Systemic: ANAPHYLAXIS, ANGIOEDEMA (Mullins, 2002)

Interactions with Echinacea

Drug

Econazole vaginal cream: The action of this cream may be decreased by echinacea; avoid concurrent use.

Immunomodulators (azathioprine, basiliximab, cyclosporine, daclizumab, muromionab, mycophenolate, tacrolimus): Echinacea may decrease the effects of immunosuppressants and should not be used immediately before, during, or after transplant surgery.

Food

None known

Herb

None known

Lab Test

Echinacea may increase ALT, AST, lymphocyte counts *(Echinacea purpurea)*, serum immunoglobulin E (IgE), blood erythrocyte sedimentation rate (ESR).

Interference: High doses of herb interfere with sperm enzyme activity.

Client Considerations

Assess

- Assess for hypersensitivity reactions to this herb or members of the daisy family (genus *Bellis*) or composite family herbs. If hypersensitivity is present, discontinue use of this herb and administer antihistamine or other appropriate therapy.
- Assess for use of econazole vaginal cream (see Interactions).

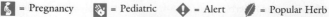

🍃 = Pregnancy   👶 = Pediatric   ❗ = Alert   🌿 = Popular Herb

Administer
- Instruct the client to store echinacea products in sealed container away from heat and moisture.
- Instruct the client not to use this herb for longer than 8 weeks without a 3-week rest period.

Teach Client/Family

- Until more research is available, caution the client not to use echinacea during pregnancy and lactation and not to give it to children younger than 2 years of age.
- Caution the client to be careful not to confuse this herb with other *Echinacea* spp. that have different uses.

Pharmacology

Pharmacokinetics

Very little is known about the pharmacokinetics in humans. Immunosuppression is thought to occur after extended therapy with echinacea.

Primary Chemical Components of Echinacea and Their Possible Actions

Chemical Class	Individual Component	Possible Action
Phenylpropenoid	Echinacoside glycosides	Antimicrobial
	Caffaric acid	Antioxidant
	Chicoric acid; Aynarine	
Alkylamide	Tartaric acid	Inhibits arachidonic metabolism
Alkaloid	Tussilagine; Isotussilagine; Tetraen acid; Isobutylamide	
Polysaccharide	Inulin	Antiinflammatory; antiviral; immune stimulation
	Heteroxylin; Arabinorhamnogalactans; Fructose	
Essential oil	Palmitic; Linolenic	
Flavonoid	Rutin	Antioxidant
Echinacin		Increases lymphocyte counts

 Endangered Herb   Adverse effects: BOLD = life-threatening

Actions

Echinacea has been studied extensively and found to be effective in both the prevention and treatment of acute colds and upper respiratory tract infections. Native Americans have used this herb to treat various illnesses. For the past several years echinacea has been among a group of herbs accepted by practitioners of mainstream medicine.

Immunostimulant Action

Echinacea stimulates the nonspecific immune response via phagocytosis, which plays a major role in the immune response. It also stimulates T-lymphocytes (Wagner, 1981). One study has demonstrated that echinacea significantly increases the phagocytosis of red blood cells (Vomel, 1984). A more recent study showed that 4 weeks of treatment with echinacea pressed juice enhanced interleukin-6 (IL-6) production in response to strenuous exercise. This study suggests that prophylactic treatment with echinacea counteracts the immunosuppressive effects of strenuous exercise (Berg, 1998).

Antiinfective Action

Echinacea has been shown to inhibit streptococcal growth and tissue hyaluronidase and to stabilize hyaluronic acid (Busing, 1955). Hyaluronidase is found in pathogenic organisms.

References

Berg A et al: Influence of Echinacin (EC31) treatment on the exercise-induced immune response in athletes, *J Clin Res* 1:367-380, 1998.

Bradley PR, editor: *British herbal compendium, vol 1,* London,1992, British Herbal Medicine Assoc, pp 81-83.

Busing KH: Hyaluronidase inhibition of some naturally occurring substances used in therapy, *Arzneimittelforschung* 5:320-322, 1955.

Chernecky CC, Berger BJ: Laboratory tests and diagnostic procedures, 2 ed, Philadelphia, Penn, 2001, Saunders.

Gallo M et al: Can herbal products be used safely during pregnancy? Focus on echinacea, *Can Fam Physician* 47:1727-1728, 2001.

McCaleb R et al: *The encyclopedia of popular herbs: your complete guide to the leading medicinal plants,* Roseville, Calif, 2000, Prima Health.

Mullins RJ et al: Adverse reactions associated with echinacea: the Australian experience, *Ann Allergy Asthma Immunol* 88(1):42-51, 2002.

Murray M, Pizzarno J: *The encyclopedia of natural medicine,* 2 ed (revised), Roseville, Calif, 1998, Prima.

Romm A: Better Nutrition's 2000 guide to children's supplements, *Better Nutrition* 62(10):38-43, 2000.

Vomel VT: Einflub eines unsezifischon immunstimulans auf die phagozytose vanerthrozyten, *Arzneim-Forsch/Drug Res* 34:691-695, 1984.

Wagner H et al: An immunostimulating active principal from *Echinacea purpurea, A. agnew, Phytother* 2(5):166-168, 171, 1981.

🐾 = Pregnancy   😾 = Pediatric   ❶ = Alert   🌿 = Popular Herb

E

Elderberry
(el'duhr-beh-ree)

Scientific names: *Sambucus nigra, Sambucus canadensis*

Other common names: Black elder, boretree, bountry, common elder, ellhorn, European elder, sweet elder   **Class 1 (Ripe Fruit, Flowers)**

Origin: Elderberry is a shrub found in the United States and Europe.

Uses
Reported Uses
Elderberry is used as a gargle in combination with sage, honey, and vinegar. It is also used as a treatment for colds, diaphoresis, toothache, headache, sinusitis, hay fever, wounds, skin disorders, hepatic conditions, and inflammation.

Investigational Uses
May be used orally for influenza.

Product Availability and Dosages
Available Forms
Oil, ointment, syrup, tea, tincture, wine

Plant Parts Used: Flowers, fruit

Dosages and Routes
Adult
• PO: use only cooked berries; bark and leaves are poisonous
• Topical: apply ointment to affected area prn
Child
All dosages listed are PO.
• Syrup: 1-2 tsp up to tid (Romm, 2000)
• Tea: ½-1 cup up to qid; serve hot (Romm, 2000)
• Tincture: ½-1 tsp up to qid (Romm, 2000)

Precautionary Information
Contraindications
Until more research is available, elderberry should not be used during pregnancy and lactation. It should not be used by persons with hypersensitivity to this plant or similar

Continued

 Endangered Herb   Adverse effects: BOLD = life-threatening

Precautionary Information—cont'd

Contraindications—cont'd

plants. Elderberry bark and leaves are toxic; use only the parts of the plant that are recommended. Class 1 herb (ripe fruit/flowers).

Side Effects/Adverse Reactions

Gastrointestinal: Nausea, vomiting, anorexia, diarrhea
Integumentary: Hypersensitivity reactions
Systemic: CYANIDE TOXICITY (bark, leaves, unripe berries)

Interactions with Elderberry

Drug
Iron salts: Elderberry may prevent absorption of iron salts, do not give concomitantly, space by at least 2 hours.

Food	Herb	Lab Test
None known	None known	None known

Client Considerations

Assess

- Assess for hypersensitivity reactions. If present, discontinue use of this herb and administer antihistamine or other appropriate therapy.
- ◆ Assess for consumption of bark and leaves, which are toxic.

Administer

- Instruct the client to store elderberry products in a cool, dry place, away from heat and moisture.

Teach Client/Family

- 🌿 Until more research is available, caution the client not to use elderberry during pregnancy or lactation.
- Caution the client to be careful not to confuse elderberry with other *Sambucus* spp., some of which are poisonous.
- Caution the client to use only the parts of elderberry recommended for use. Other parts are toxic.
- 🖐 Teach client that children should not play with the shafts of
- ◆ the plant; cyanide poisoning can occur.

🌿 = Pregnancy   🖐 = Pediatric   ◆ = Alert   🖋 = Popular Herb

Pharmacology
Pharmacokinetics
Pharmacokinetics and pharmacodynamics are unknown.

Primary Chemical Components of Elderberry and Their Possible Actions		
Chemical Class	**Individual Component**	**Possible Action**
Flavonoids	Rutin	Antioxidant
	Quercitrin	Antiinflammatory
	Hyperoside; Isoquercitrin; Astragalin; Nicotoflorin	
Glycoside	Sambunigrine	
Volatile oil	Palmitic acid	
Tannin		
Mucilage		
Anthocyanin		Antioxidant
Vitamin	C	
Caffeic acid	Chlorogenic	
Cyanogenins		
Lignans		

Actions
Initial research on elderberry has identified antioxidant, insulin-like, and diuretic actions for this herb. However, multiple studies to confirm these actions are not yet available.

Antioxidant Action
One study provides information on the antioxidant properties of elderberry, which result from the anthocyanins present in elderberry flavonoids. These anthocyanins are responsible for scavenging in the bloodstream and the colon. Other chemical components, aglycons and glycosides, also provide antioxidant protection (Pool-Zobel, 1999).

Insulin-Like Action
Because elderberry has been used as a traditional treatment for diabetes mellitus, the insulin-like action of this herb has been studied. In one study, the insulin-releasing and insulin-like

activity of *Sambucus nigra* produced a cumulative effect (Gray, 2000).

Diuretic Action

One study identified the diuretic activity of elderberry in rats. Rats treated with the herb experienced increased urine flow and sodium excretion (Beaux, 1999).

References

Beaux D et al: Effect of extracts of *Orthosiphon stamineus* Benth, *Hieracium pilosella* L., *Sambucus nigra* L., and *Arctostaphylos uva-ursi* (L.) Spreng. in rats, *Phytother Res* 13(3):222-225, 1999.

Gray AM et al: The traditional plant treatment, *Sambucus nigra* (elder), exhibits insulin-like and insulin-releasing actions in vitro, *J Nutr* 130(1):15-20, 2000.

Pool-Zobel BL et al: Anthocyanins are potent antioxidants in model systems but do not reduce endogenous oxidative DNA damage in human colon cells, *Eur J Nutr* 38(5):227-234, 1999.

Romm A: Better Nutrition's 2000 guide to children's supplements, *Better Nutrition* 62(10):38-43, 2000.

Elecampane
(eh-li-cam-payn′)

Scientific name: *Inula helenium*

Other common names: Aunee, elfdock, elfwort, horseheal, horse-elder, scabwort, velvet dock, wild sunflower

Class 2b (Rhizome, Root)

Origin: Elecampane is native to Asia and Europe. It has been naturalized to North America.

Uses

Reported Uses

Elecampane has been used as an antimicrobial, primarily against *Mycobacterium tuberculosis,* and as a relaxant for smooth muscles in the trachea and ileus. In traditional herbal medicine, elecampane has been used for its expectorant, antiseptic, and diuretic effects. It is also used to treat cough, whooping cough, the common cold, bronchitis, bronchiectasis, and asthma, and it may be used as an anthelmintic. Elecampane is a bitter that is used to stimulate digestion and the appetite.

Investigational Uses

Research is underway to confirm the blood glucose and blood pressure lowering uses of elecampane.

Product Availability and Dosages

Available Forms

Fluid extract, powder

Plant Parts Used: Rhizome (dried and fresh), roots

Dosages and Routes

Adult

All dosages listed are PO.

Expectorant
- Infusion: pour boiling water over 1 g ground herb (1 tsp = 4 g), let stand 15 min, strain, drink 1 cup tid

Other
- Dried root: 3 g tid
- Extract: 3 g dried root/10 ml water/20 ml alcohol tid
- Fresh root: 2 tbsp tid

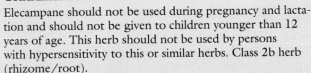

Precautionary Information

Contraindications

Elecampane should not be used during pregnancy and lactation and should not be given to children younger than 12 years of age. This herb should not be used by persons with hypersensitivity to this or similar herbs. Class 2b herb (rhizome/root).

Side Effects/Adverse Reactions

Central Nervous System: PARALYSIS (large doses)
Ears, Eyes, Nose, and Throat: Irritation of mucous membranes
Gastrointestinal: Nausea, vomiting, diarrhea, gastrointestinal spasms, anorexia (large amounts)
Integumentary: Hypersensitivity reactions, severe contact dermatitis

Interactions with Elecampane		
Drug		
Antidiabetics: May decrease blood glucose; avoid concurrent use (theoretical).		
Food	**Herb**	**Lab Test**
None known	None known	None known

Client Considerations

Assess

- Assess for hypersensitivity reactions, including contact dermatitis. If such reactions are present, discontinue use of elecampane and administer antihistamine or other appropriate therapy.
- Monitor for reactions indicating large dosages (nausea, vomiting, anorexia, paralysis).
- Assess for client use of antidiabetics; elecampane may increase the action of antidiabetics.

Administer

- Instruct the client to store elecampane products in a glass container away from moisture and heat. This herb should not be stored in plastic.
- In case of overdose, perform gastric lavage or administer activated charcoal. Overdose also may be treated with triflupromazine.

Teach Client/Family

- Until more research is available, caution the client not to use elecampane during pregnancy and lactation and not to give it to children younger than 12 years of age.

Pharmacology

Pharmacokinetics

Pharmacokinetics and pharmacodynamics are unknown.

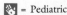 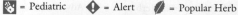

Primary Chemical Components of Elecampane and Their Possible Actions

Chemical Class	Individual Component	Possible Action
Volatile oil	Alantolactone	Antimycobacterial; expectorant
	Isoalantolactone; Dihydroisoalanto-lactone; Dihydroalantolactone	
Polyyne		
Lactone	Alantol; Alantic acid	
Polysaccharides	Inulin	

Actions

Very little controlled research is available for elecampane.

Antimycobacterial Action

The root extracts of elecampane have been studied for their antimycobacterial effects. Chromatographic fractions of the root showed significant activity against *Mycobacterium tuberculosis,* resulting from the volatile oils alantolactone and isoalantolactone (Cantrell, 1999).

Muscle Relaxant Action

One study using guinea pigs demonstrated that elecampane relaxes tracheal and ileal smooth muscles. Researchers studied the effects of volatile oils isolated from 22 different plant species and compared them with the effects of catecholamines and phosphodiesterase inhibitors. One of the most potent volatile oils studied was that from elecampane root extract (Reiter, 1985).

Anthelmintic Action

When rabbits infected with worms were given boiled extracts of *Inula helenium,* the result was necrosis, dilatation, and atrophy of the worms (Rhee, 1985). These results indicate that elecampane shows promise as an anthelmintic.

References

Cantrell CL et al: Antimycobacterial eudesmanolides from *Inula helenium* and *Rudbeckia subtomentosa, Planta Med* 65(4):351-355, 1999.

Reiter M et al: Relaxant effects of tracheal and ileal smooth muscles of the guinea pig, *Arzneimittelforschung* 35(1A):408-414, 1985.

Rhee JK et al: Structural investigation on the effects of the herbs on *Clonorchis sinensis* in rabbits, *Am J Chin Med* 13(1-4):119-125, 1985.

Ephedra
(i-feh′dah)

Scientific names: *Ephedra sinica, Ephedra nevadensis, Ephedra trifurca, Ephedra equisetina, Ephedra distachya*

Other common names: Brigham tea, cao ma huang, desert tea, epitonin, herba ephedrae, herbal ecstasy, joint fir, ma huang, mahuuanggen, Mexican tea, Mormon tea, muzei mu huang, natural ecstacy, popotillo, sea grape, squaw tea, teamster's tea, yellow astringent, yellow horse, zhong ma huang   **Class 2b/2c/2d (Whole Herb)**

Origin: Ephedra is an evergreen found throughout the world.

Uses

Reported Uses

Ephedra contains ephedrine, a central nervous system stimulant with amphetamine-like properties. It has been used in Chinese medicine to treat asthma, bronchitis, headache, pulmonary congestion, and joint pain and inflammation. More recently, it has been used for its stimulant effect and to promote weight loss.

Product Availability and Dosages

Available Forms

Capsules, extract, tablets, tea, tincture; available as a component of many combination products

Plant Parts Used: Leaves, seeds

Dosages and Routes

Adult

Dosages vary with the species of ephedra. Only *E. trifurca* and *E. nevadensis* are available as tea. Standardized products usually contain ephedrine and pseudoephedrine 6%. All dosages listed are PO.

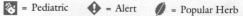

 = Pregnancy   = Pediatric   = Alert   = Popular Herb

- Capsules/tablets (crude herb): 500-1000 mg bid-tid (Foster, 1998)
- Extract: 12-25 mg total alkaloids, standardized to ephedrine, bid-tid (Foster, 1998)
- Tea: use 1.5-9 g herb in 1 pt boiling water, let stand 15 min, drink in divided doses
- Tincture: 15-30 drops bid-tid (Foster, 1998)

E

Precautionary Information

Contraindications

Ephedra should not be used during pregnancy and lactation, and it should not be given to children younger than 12 years of age. It should not be used by persons with hypersensitivity to sympathomimetics, narrow-angle glaucoma, seizure disorders, hyperthyroidism, diabetes mellitus, prostatic hypertrophy, arrhythmias, heart block, hypertension, psychosis, tachycardia, or angina pectoris. The FDA has considered restricting the use of ephedra because there have been many reports of adverse effects, including death. Class 2b/2c/2d herb (whole herb).

Side Effects/Adverse Reactions

NOTE: Side effects and adverse reactions are similar to those of ephedrine.

Cardiovascular: Palpitations, tachycardia, hypertension, chest pain, ARRHYTHMIAS, STROKE, MYOCARDIAL INFARCTION, CARDIAC ARREST

Central Nervous System: Anxiety, nervousness, insomnia, hallucinations, headache, dizziness, poor concentration, tremors, confusion, SEIZURES, psychosis (Tormey, 2001)

Gastrointestinal: Nausea, vomiting, anorexia, constipation or diarrhea, HEPATOTOXICITY

Genitourinary: Dysuria, urinary retention

Integumentary: Hypersensitivity reactions, EXFOLIATIVE DERMATITIS

Reproductive: Uterine contractions

Respiratory: Dyspnea

 Endangered Herb   Adverse effects: BOLD = life-threatening

Interactions with Ephedra

Drug

Anesthetics, halothane: Ephedra causes increased arrhythmias when used with halothane anesthetics; do not use concurrently.

Antidiabetics: Ephedra may cause an increase in blood glucose level; monitor carefully.

Beta-blockers: Ephedra causes increased hypertension when used with beta-blockers; avoid concurrent use.

Guanethidine: Ephedra may decrease the effect of guanethidine; monitor concurrent use carefully.

MAOIs: Hypertensive crisis occurs when ephedra is used with MAOIs; do not use concurrently.

Oxytocics: Ephedra causes severe hypertension when used with oxytocics; do not use concurrently.

Phenothiazines: Tachycardia may result if ephedra is used with phenothiazines; do not use concurrently.

Sympathomimetics, other: Ephedra increases the effect of sympathomimetics and also causes hypertension; do not use concurrently.

Tricyclics: Hypertensive crisis occurs when ephedra is used with tricyclics; do not use concurrently.

Urinary alkalizers: Ephedra increases the effect of urinary alkalizers; monitor concurrent use carefully.

Xanthines (caffeine, theophylline): Ephedra causes increased central nervous system stimulation; avoid concurrent use with xanthines.

Food

Caffeinated coffee, cola, "Red Bull," and tea may increase the stimulating effect of ephedra.

Herb

Concurrent use of ephedra with bitter orange, coffee, ginseng, green tea, guarana, Indian sida, kola nut, malvaceae, Siberian ginseng, soapwort, or yerba maté may increase hypertension and central nervous system stimulation; avoid concurrent use.

Lab Test

Ephedra may increase AST, ALT, total bilirubin, and urine bilirubin.

Client Considerations

Assess

- Assess for hypersensitivity reactions and exfoliative dermatitis. If these are present, discontinue use of ephedra and administer antihistamine or other appropriate therapy.
- Assess for increased cardiovascular side effects (hypertension, palpitations, arrhythmias, chest pain). If these are present, discontinue use of ephedra immediately.
- Assess for symptoms of increased central nervous system stimulation (poor concentration, insomnia, anxiety, nervousness, seizures, tremors, hallucinations). If these are present, discontinue use of ephedra.
 - Assess all medications and supplements the client is taking; many serious interactions can occur (see Interactions).

Administer

- Instruct the client not to take PO dosages exceeding 24 mg/day and not to take ephedra for longer than 1 week.
- Instruct the client to store ephedra products in a cool, dry place, away from heat and moisture.

Teach Client/Family

 - Because it can cause uterine contractions, caution the client not to use ephedra during pregnancy, Also, caution the client not to use this herb during lactation and not to give it to children younger than 12 years of age.
- Caution any client with hypersensitivity to sympathomimetics, narrow-angle glaucoma, seizure disorders, hyperthyroidism, diabetes mellitus, prostatic hypertrophy, arrhythmias, heart block, hypertension, psychosis, tachycardia, or angina pectoris not to use this herb.
- Caution the client that ephedra has been responsible for many deaths from seizure, stroke, myocardial infarction, and cardiac arrest.
- Advise the client to review all other medications and supplements taken for interactions; some interactions can be life threatening.

Pharmacology

Pharmacokinetics

Pharmacokinetics and pharmacodynamics for *ephedrine* are as follows: onset 15 to 60 minutes, duration 2 to 4 hours; metabolized in the liver, excreted unchanged in the urine and breast milk; crosses the blood-brain barrier and the placenta.

Primary Chemical Components of Ephedra and Their Possible Actions

Chemical Class	Individual Component	Possible Action
Alkaloid	Ephedrine	Central nervous system stimulant; bronchodilator; increased myocardial contractility
	Methylephedrine; Norephedrine; Ephedrine; Ephedroxane; Pseudoephedroxane	
Tannin		
Volatile oil		
Flavonoid		
Inulin		
Catechin		
Gallic acid		

Actions

Much research has been done on ephedrine, which is a prescription medication and a component of ephedra. Ephedrine acts primarily on beta-receptors in the heart and on alpha-receptors, causing vasoconstriction in blood vessels. It also exerts amphetamine-like effects, causing bronchodilation, decreased gastrointestinal motility, increased mydriasis, and central nervous system stimulation.

References

Foster S: *101 medicinal herbs,* Loveland, Colo, 1998, Interweave Press.

Skidmore-Roth L: *Mosby's nursing drug reference,* St Louis, 2001, Mosby.

Tormey WP et al: Acute psychosis due to the interaction of legal compounds—ephedra alkaloids in "vigueur fit" tablets, caffeine in "red bull" and alcohol, *Med Sci Law* 41(4):331-336, 2001.

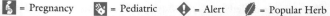

= Pregnancy   = Pediatric   = Alert   = Popular Herb

Eucalyptus
(yew-kuh-lip'tuhs)

Scientific name: *Eucalyptus globulus*

Other common names: Blue gum, fever tree, gum, red gum, stringy bark tree, Tasmanian blue gum   Class 2d (Leaf)

E

Origin: Eucalyptus is now cultivated throughout the world. It is native to Australia.

Uses

Reported Uses

Eucalyptus is used to treat nasal/pulmonary congestion and appears frequently as a component in combination products used for sinusitis and pharyngitis. It is also used as an antispasmodic to treat irritable bowel syndrome; as a treatment for gallstones, kidney stones, and cystitis; as a central nervous system stimulant; and as an aromatherapeutic agent. Eucalyptus can be used topically as an antiseptic for wounds.

Investigational Uses

Studies are underway to determine the efficacy of eucalyptus in the treatment of infections caused by bacteria or fungi, inflammation, and diabetes mellitus.

Product Availability and Dosages

Available Forms

Aqueous-alcoholic preparation, essential oil, fluid extract, lotion, semisolid preparation; eucalyptus is a component of various cosmetics and over-the-counter products used to treat sinusitis and pharyngitis

Plant Parts Used: Branch tips, leaves

Dosages and Routes

Adult

NOTE: Dilute internal dosages before use.
- PO eucalyptol: 0.05-0.2 ml
- PO eucalyptus oil: 0.05-2 ml or 0.3-0.6 g qd
- PO fluid extract: 3 g
- Topical aqueous-alcoholic preparation: 5%-10% prn
  (Blumenthal, 1998)

🌀 Endangered Herb   Adverse effects: BOLD = life-threatening

- Topical essential oil: several drops rubbed into skin prn (Blumenthal, 1998)
- Topical oil or semisolid preparations: 5%-20% prn (Blumenthal, 1998)

Precautionary Information

Contraindications

Until more research is available, eucalyptus should not be used during pregnancy and lactation and should not be given to children younger than 2 years of age. It should not be used near mucous membranes or on the face. Persons with hypersensitivity to eucalyptus and those with kidney, gastrointestinal, or severe hepatic disease should not use this herb. As little as 3.5 ml of eucalyptus oil taken internally can be fatal. Class 2d herb (leaf).

Side Effects/Adverse Reactions

Central Nervous System: Confusion, delirium, dizziness, SEIZURES
Gastrointestinal: Burning stomach, nausea, vomiting, anorexia
Integumentary: Hypersensitivity reactions

Interactions with Eucalyptus

Drug

Amphetamines: Eucalyptus may decrease the effectiveness of amphetamines; avoid concurrent use.
Barbiturates: Eucalyptus may decrease the effectiveness of barbiturates; avoid concurrent use.
Insulin: Eucalyptus may alter the effectiveness of insulin; do not use concurrently.
Oral antidiabetics: Eucalyptus may alter the effectiveness of oral antidiabetics; do not use concurrently.

Food	Herb	Lab Test
None known	None known	None known

 = Pregnancy    = Pediatric   = Alert   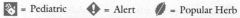 = Popular Herb

Client Considerations

Assess

- Assess for hypersensitivity reactions. If present, discontinue use of eucalyptus and administer antihistamine or other appropriate therapy.
- Assess for central nervous system reactions if the client is taking this herb internally.
- Assess for use of amphetamines, barbiturates, insulin, and oral antidiabetics (see Interactions).

Administer

- Instruct the client to store eucalyptus products in a cool, dry place, away from heat and moisture.
- Instruct the client to dilute all products used internally before use.

Teach Client/Family

- Until more research is available, caution the client not to use eucalyptus during pregnancy and lactation and not to give it to children younger than 2 years of age.
- Inform the client that eucalyptus may be used topically on children in combination with menthol and camphor.
- Alert the client that poisoning of children has occurred with only a few drops of eucalyptus.
- Caution clients with hypersensitivity to eucalyptus and those with kidney, gastrointestinal, or severe hepatic disease not to use this herb.

Pharmacology

Pharmacokinetics

Pharmacokinetics and pharmacodynamics are unknown.

Primary Chemical Components of Eucalyptus and Their Possible Actions		
Chemical Class	**Individual Component**	**Possible Action**
Volatile oil	Eucalyptol Cineole	Decongestant Decreased renal and biliary colic; antimicrobial
	Alpha-pinene; Aromadendrene; Globulol; Trans-pinocarveol; Limonene; Eucalyptus	
Flavonoid	Quercetin Rutin Hyperoside	Antiinflammatory Antioxidant
Tannin Fatty Acids Fatty Alcohol Aromatic compounds (Freire et al, 2002)		Wound healing

Actions

Antimicrobial Action

Cineole, a chemical component of eucalyptus, has been shown to exert significant antimicrobial effects. One study has shown that this substance is highly effective against both gram-positive and gram-negative bacteria, as well as some fungi (Saeed, 1995). Another study with similar findings investigated 21 different species of eucalyptus (Hajji, 1993). Of these, *Eucalyptus citriodora* was the most effective species, with the widest array of antimicrobial effects. Gundidza (1993) determined that the essential oil of *E. globulus maidenii* was active against the fungi *Candida albicans, Penicillium citrinum,* and *Aspergillus flavus,* as well as the bacteria *Klebsiella pneumoniae, Citrobacter freundii, Serratia marcescens, Clostridium sporogenes,* and *Bacillus subtilis* (Moleyar, 1992). Another study demonstrated that cineole acts against *Staphylococcus aureus, Pseudomonas aeruginosa, Enterococcus faecalis,* and *Bacillus subtilis* (Carson, 1995).

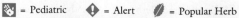 = Pregnancy   = Pediatric   = Alert   = Popular Herb

Decongestant Action

Because of its ability to improve respiratory function significantly, one of the most common uses of eucalyptus is as an inhalant. It eases breathing by opening the nasal passages and sinuses (Cohen, 1982). In one study, Vicks Vaporub, a combination of eucalyptus, camphor, and menthol, significantly reduced restlessness in children with upper-respiratory infections (Berger, 1978). It is postulated that the ingredients in Vicks Vaporub decrease the surface tension between water and air in the pulmonary system, increasing the surfactant of the lung.

Other Actions

Other studies have shown that cineole increases locomotor activity in laboratory animals (Kovar, 1987), acts as a spasmogenic in the duodenum of rats (Zarzuelo, 1987), and decreases drowsiness (Nakagawa, 1992).

References

Berger H et al: Effects of Vaporub on the restlessness of children with acute bronchitis, *J Intern Med Res* 6:491-493, 1978.

Blumenthal M, editor: *The complete German Commission E monographs: therapeutic guide to herbal medicines,* Austin, Tex, American Botanical Council; Boston, Integrative Medicine Communication, 1998.

Carson CF et al: Antimicrobial activity of the major components of the essential oil of *Melaleuca alternifolia, J Appl Biol* 78:264-269, 1995.

Cohen BM et al: Acute aromatics inhalation modifies the airways: effects of the common cold, *Respiration* 43:285-293, 1982.

Freire CSR et al: Identification of new hydroxy fatty acids and ferulic acid esters in the wood of *Eucalyptus globulus, Holzforschung,* 56(2):143-149, 2002.

Gundidza M et al: Antimicrobial activity of the essential oil from *Eucalyptus maidenii, Planta Med* 59:705-706, 1993.

Hajji F et al: Antimicrobial activity of twenty-one eucalyptus essential oils, *Fititerapia* 64(1):71-77, 1993.

Kovar K et al: Blood levels of 1, 8-cineole and locomotor activity of mice after inhalation and oral administration of rosemary oil, *Planta Med* 53(4):315-318, 1987.

Moleyar V et al: Antibacterial activity of essential oil components, *Int J Food Microbiol* 16:337-342, 1992.

Nakagawa M et al: Evaluation of drowsiness by EEGs-odours controlling drowsiness, *Fragrance J* 10:68-72, 1992.

Saeed MA et al: Antimicrobial studies of the constituents of Pakistani eucalyptus oils, *J Fac Pharm Gazi Univ* 12(2):129-140, 1995.

Zarzuelo A et al: Spasmolytic activity of *Thymus membranaceus* essential oil, *Phytotherapy Res* 1(3):114-116, 1987.

Endangered Herb   Adverse effects: BOLD = life-threatening

Evening Primrose Oil
(eev'ning prim'roes)

Scientific names: *Oenothera biennis, Primula elatior*

Other common names: Buckles, butter rose, cowslip, English cowslip, fairy caps, key flower, key of heaven, king's-cure-all, mayflower, our lady's key, palsywort, peagles, petty mulleins, plumrocks password

Origin: Evening primrose is found in North America.

Uses

Reported Uses

Evening primrose oil is used to treat cardiovascular disease, PMS, mastalgia, rheumatoid arthritis, multiple sclerosis, eczema, breast disorders, cough, bronchitis, irritable bowel syndrome, and other digestive disorders.

Product Availability and Dosages

Available Forms

Capsules

Plant Parts Used: Seeds

Dosage and Routes

Adult

Eczema
• PO capsules: 6 capsules/day (240 GLA)

Mastalgia
• PO capsules: 6 capsules/day (240 GLA)

Diabetic Neuropathy
• PO 8-12 capsules/day (320-480 mg GLA)

Premenstrual syndrome
• PO 6 capsules/day (240 GLA)

Child

Eczema
• PO capsules, ages 1-12: 160 mg-4 g qd (standardized to GLA 8%)

Precautionary Information

Contraindications

Until more research is available, evening primrose oil should not be used during pregnancy and lactation. This herb should not be used by persons with hypersensitivity to it or those with seizure disorders.

Side Effects/Adverse Reactions

Central Nervous System: Headache, TEMPORAL LOBE SEIZURES IN SCHIZOPHRENIA

Gastrointestinal: Nausea, vomiting, anorexia, diarrhea

Integumentary: Hypersensitivity reactions, rash

Miscellaneous: Inflammation, IMMUNOSUPPRESSION (with long-term use)

E

Interactions with Evening Primrose Oil

Drug

Phenothiazines: Phenothiazines (chlorpromazine) may cause seizures if used with evening primrose oil; do not use concurrently.

Food	Herb	Lab Test
None known	None known	None known

Client Considerations

Assess

- Assess for hypersensitivity reactions. If present, discontinue use of evening primrose oil and administer antihistamines or other appropriate therapy.
- Assess for phenothiazine use. Evening primrose oil should not be used with this medication.
- Assess for clients with seizure disorders, do not use evening primrose oil in clients with a seizure disorder.

Administer

- Instruct the client to store evening primrose oil in a sealed container away from heat and moisture.

Teach Client/Family

- Until more research is available, caution the client not to use evening primrose oil during pregnancy and lactation.

Pharmacology

Pharmacokinetics

Pharmacokinetics and pharmacodynamics are unknown.

Primary Chemical Components of Evening Primrose Oil and Their Possible Actions		
Chemical Class	**Individual Component**	**Possible Action**
Fatty acid	Linoleic acid	Decrease cholesterol
	Gamma linoleic acid (GLA)	Decrease hepatic injury
	Oleic acid; Stearic acid; Palmitic acid	
Flavonoid	Rutin; Gossypetin	
Triterpenoid Saponin	Protoprimuloside B	

Actions

Evening primrose oil has been used successfully to treat cardiovascular disease, breast disorders, PMS, mastalgia, rheumatoid arthritis, multiple sclerosis, atopic dermatitis, and other skin disorders. GLA has shown effectiveness in reversing neurologic damage caused by multiple sclerosis. It has been shown to decrease cardiovascular disease and obesity. Because the body does not manufacture the essential fatty acids in evening primrose oil, they must be obtained from the diet. A lack of GLA prevents the nerve cell membrane from functioning properly. GLA is needed for conduction of electrical impulses.

References

Duke J: *CRC handbook of medicinal herbs,* Boca Raton, Fla, 1985, CRC Press, pp 374-375.

Eyebright
(eye'brite)

Scientific name: *Euphrasia officinalis*

Other common names: Meadow eyebright, red eyebright

E

Origin: Eyebright is an annual that was originally found in Europe.

Uses

Reported Uses

Eyebright is used both internally and externally to relieve eye fatigue and to treat sty and eye infections such as conjunctivitis and blepharitis. It is also used to treat nasal catarrh in sinusitis, as well as hay fever.

Investigational Uses

It may be used for *Candida albicans* (Trovato, 2000) and to reduce blood glucose levels (Porchezhian, 2000).

Product Availability and Dosages

Available Forms

Internal: fresh herb, infusion, tablets, tincture; **topical:** infusion, fluid extract, fresh herb, lotion, poultice

Plant Parts Used: Flowering plant

Dosages and Routes

Adult

Ophthalmic

- Topical decoction: 5-10 drops (2%) in eye to cleanse, tid-qid
- Topical infusion: soak a towelette in infusion and apply over eye area prn

Other

- PO dried herb: 2-4 g tid as an infusion (Mills, 2000)
- PO fluid extract: 2-4 ml (1:2 dilution) tid (Mills, 2000)
- PO tea: cover 2-3 g finely cut herb with boiling water and let stand 10-15 min, strain, drink
- PO tincture: 2-6 ml (1:5 dilution) tid (Mills, 2000)

Precautionary Information

Contraindications

Eyebright should not be used by persons with hypersensitivity to this herb.

Side Effects/Adverse Reactions

Central Nervous System: Confusion, headache, weakness, fatigue

Ears, Eyes, Nose, and Throat: Nasal congestion, blurred vision, photophobia, lid swelling, sneezing

Integumentary: Hypersensitivity reactions

Interactions with Eyebright

Drug

Antidiabetics: May increase the effects of antidiabetics (theoretical) when *Euphrasia officinalis* is taken internally.

Iron salts: Eyebright may interfere with the absorption of iron salts; separate by at least 2 hours.

Food	Herb	Lab Test
None known	None known	None known

Client Considerations

Assess

- Assess for hypersensitivity reactions. If present, discontinue use of eyebright and administer antihistamine or other appropriate therapy.
- Assess the eye for swelling, lacrimation, redness, and exudate.

Administer

- Instruct the client to apply eyebright externally as a compress or drops.
- Instruct the client to store eyebright products in a cool, dry place, away from heat and moisture.

Teach Client/Family

- If an eye infection is present, instruct the client to wash hands frequently and not to share towels with others.
- Instruct client in the correct method for washing the eye with solution.

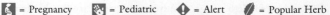

= Pregnancy   = Pediatric   = Alert   = Popular Herb

Pharmacology
Pharmacokinetics
Pharmacokinetics and pharmacodynamics are unknown.

Primary Chemical Components of Eyebright and Their Possible Actions		
Chemical Class	**Individual Component**	**Possible Action**
Tannin		Wound healing
Monoterpene	Aucubin	Antibacterial; hepatoprotective; antitumor
	Euphroside; Veronicoside; Catapol; Ixoroside; Verproside; Mussaenoside; Ladroside	
Alkaloid		
Sterol		
Phenolic acid		
Flavonoid		
Amino acid		

Actions
Very little research is available on eyebright. It has been used since the fourteenth century to treat eye conditions, although none of the available studies have confirmed any of its actions. One study has identified cytotoxic effects, however (Trovato, 1996). For that reason, eyebright is not recommended for any use. Aucubin, one of the chemical components of eyebright, has shown antibacterial (Rombouts, 1956), hepatoprotective (Chang, 1983), and antitumor activity (Isiguro, 1986). Two more recent studies (Trovato, 2000) have shown antimycotic activity in vitro on *Candida albicans* isolated from clinical samples from acute vaginitis. Another study (Porchezhian, 2000) showed decreased blood glucose levels when *Euphrasia officinale* was given to alloxan-diabetic rats. The diabetic rats' blood glucose levels were decreased, but normal rats showed a lack of hypoglycemic effects.

References

Chang IM et al: *Drug Chem Toxicol* 6(5):443-454, 1983.

Isiguro K et al: *Chem Pharm Bull* 34(6):2375-2379, 1986.

Mills S, Bone K: *Principles and practice of phytotherapy,* London, 2000, Churchill Livingstone.

Prochezhian E et al: Antihyperglycemic activity of *Euphrasia officinale* leaves, *Fitoterapia* 71(5):522-526, 2000.

Rombouts JE et al: *Experientia* 12(2):78-80, 1956.

Trovato A et al: In vitro anti-mycotic activity of some medicinal plants containing flavonoids, *Bull Chim Farm* 139(5):225-227, 2000.

Trovato A et al: In vitro cytotoxic effect of some medicinal plants containing flavonoids, *Bull Chim Farm* 135:263-266, 1996.

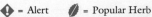

False Unicorn Root
(fawls yew'nuh-kawrn rewt)

Scientific name: *Chamaelirium luteum*

Other common names: Blazing star, devil's bit, drooping starwort, fairy-wand, fairywart, helonias dioica, helonias root, rattlesnake, starwort   **Class 2b (Rhizome)**

F

Origin: False unicorn root is a lily found in the eastern region of the United States. *Chamaelirium luteum* is a threatened species.

Uses
Reported Uses
False unicorn root has been used as a treatment for morning sickness and menstrual irregularities such as amenorrhea and dysmenorrhea, as a uterine and liver tonic, and as a diuretic, an emetic, and a genitourinary stimulant.

Product Availability and Dosages
Available Forms
Chopped root, dried root, tincture

Plant Parts Used: Roots

Dosages and Routes
Adult
- PO decoction: 1-2 tsp herb in 1 cup water, simmer 10-15 min, strain, drink tid
- PO tincture: 2-4 ml tid

Precautionary Information
Contraindications
Until more research is available, except under the direction of a qualified herbalist, false unicorn root should not be used during pregnancy and lactation. This herb should not be given to children. Persons with hypersensitivity to false unicorn root should not use it. Class 2b herb (rhizome).

Side Effects/Adverse Reactions
Integumentary: Hypersensitivity reactions

Interactions with False Unicorn Root			
Drug	Food	Herb	Lab Test
None known	None known	None known	None known

Client Considerations

Assess

- Assess for hypersensitivity reactions. If present, discontinue use of this herb and administer antihistamine or other appropriate therapy.

Administer

- Instruct the client to store products containing false unicorn root in a cool, dry place, away from heat and moisture.

Teach Client/Family

- Until more research is available, instruct the client not to use false unicorn root unless under the direction of a qualified herbalist. This herb should not be given to children.
- Inform the client that no research is available to confirm any of the uses of false unicorn root.

Pharmacology

Pharmacokinetics

Pharmacokinetics and pharmacodynamics are unknown.

Primary Chemical Components of False Unicorn Root and Their Possible Actions		
Chemical Class	Individual Component	Possible Action
Saponin	Chamaelirin; Helonin; Diosgenin	
Fatty acid	Oleic acid; Stearic acid; Linoleic acid	

 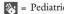

Actions

Very little research is available on false unicorn root. A few very old articles, ranging from the early 1900s to the mid-1940s, comprise most of the available information. The cited studies examined the gonadotropic effects of this herb on rats and its action on the uterus of the guinea pig and dog. These studies were unable to confirm any of the proposed actions of false unicorn root. One recent study (Brandt, 1996) proposes that the herb stimulates human chorionic gonadotropin.

References

Brandt D: A clinician's view, *HerbalGram* 36:75, 1996.

Fennel

(feh′nuhl)

Scientific name: *Foeniculum vulgare*

Other common names: Aneth fenouil, bitter fennel, carosella, fenchel, fenouil, fenouille, finocchio, Florence fennel, funcho, garden fennel, hinojo, large fennel, sweet fennel, wild fennel   **Class 1 (Fruit)**

Origin: Fennel is found in Asia and Europe and is cultivated in the United Kingdom and the United States.

Uses

Reported Uses

Fennel is used to increase the libido, aid digestion, treat indigestion, to treat menstrual irregularities, and to increase breast milk.

Investigational Uses

Investigation is underway to determine the usefulness of fennel for the treatment of infections. However, research supporting the use of this herb is limited.

Product Availability and Dosages

Available Forms

Internal: dried fruit, essential oil in water (bitter or sweet), fluid extract, tablets, tincture; **topical:** decoction, essential oil, extract

🌀 Endangered Herb   Adverse effects: ʙᴏʟᴅ = life-threatening

Plant Parts Used: Seeds

Dosages and Routes

Adult

All dosages listed are PO.

- Dried fruit infusion: 900-1800 mg/day (Mills, 2000)
- Essential oil: 5-20 drops/day (Mills, 2000)
- Fennel compound tincture: 5-7.5 g qd (Blumenthal, 1998)
- Fluid extract 3-6 ml/day (1:2 dilution) (Mills, 2000)
- Herb: 5-7 g herb qd (Blumenthal, 1998)
- Tincture: 7-14 ml/day (1:5 dilution) (Mills, 2000)

Precautionary Information

Contraindications

Until more research is available, fennel should not be used during pregnancy and lactation. The essential oil should not be given to infants or small children. Fennel should not be used by those with hypersensitivity to it, and it should not be used for extended periods. Class 1 herb (fruit).

Side Effects/Adverse Reactions

Central Nervous System: SEIZURES

Gastrointestinal: Nausea, vomiting, anorexia

Integumentary: Hypersensitivity reactions, contact dermatitis, photosensitivity

Systemic: PULMONARY EDEMA, POSSIBLE CANCERS

Interactions with Fennel

Drug

Ciprofloxacin: Fennel affects the absorption, distribution, and elimination of ciprofloxacin. If the two are used concurrently, their dosages should be separated by at least 2 hours (Zhu, 1999).

Food	Herb	Lab Test
None known	None known	None known

Client Considerations

Assess

- Assess for hypersensitivity reactions, contact dermatitis. If these are present, discontinue use of this herb and administer antihistamine or other appropriate therapy.
- Assess for use of ciprofloxacin (see Interactions).

Administer

- Instruct the client to store fennel in a sealed container away from moisture and heat.

Teach Client/Family

- Until more research is available, caution the client not to use fennel during pregnancy and lactation and not to give the essential oil to infants or small children.
- Warn the client of the life-threatening side effects of fennel.

Pharmacology

Pharmacokinetics

Pharmacokinetics and pharmacodynamics are unknown.

Primary Chemical Components of Fennel and Their Possible Actions		
Chemical Class	Individual Components	Possible Action
Volatile oil	Anethole	Phytoestrogen, TNF inhibitor (Chainy, 2000)
	Dianethole; Photoanethole; Fenchone; Estragole; Limonene; Camphene; Alpha-pinene	
Fixed oil	Oleic acid; Linoleic acid; Petroselinic acid	
Tocopherol		
Flavonoid	Kaempferol	Antiinflammatory
Vitamin		
Mineral		
Umbelliferone		
Terpinene		
Terpinolene		

🝙 Endangered Herb   Adverse effects: BOLD = life-threatening

Actions

Antimicrobial Action

Other organisms fennel has shown bacteriostatic action against include the following: *Aerobacter aerogenes, Bacillus subtilis, E. coli, Proteus vulgaris, Pseudomonas aeruginosa, Staphylococcus albius,* and *Staphylococcus aureus* (Kivanc, 1986). Among its proposed actions are an antimicrobial effect against *Listeria monocytogenes* and *Salmonella enteritidis,* an estrogenic effect in female rats (Malini, 1985).

Estrogenic Action

Anethole, one of the chemical components of fennel may influence milk secretion by competing with dopamine at receptor sites, thereby reducing the inhibition by dopamine of prolactin secretion (Albert-Puleo, 1980).

References

Albert-Puleo M: *J Ethnopharmacol* 2:337-344, 1980.

Blumenthal M, editor: *The complete German Commission E monographs: therapeutic guide to herbal medicines,* Austin, Tex, American Botanical Council; Boston, Integrative Medicine Communication, 1998.

Kivanc M et al: *Flavour Fragrance J* 1:175-179, 1986.

Malini T et al: The effects of *Foeniculum vulgare* mill seed extract on the genital organs of male and female rats, *Indian J Physiol Pharmacol* 29:21, 1985.

Mills S, Bone K: *Principles and practice of phytotherapy,* London, 2000, Churchill Livingstone.

Zhu M et al: Effect of oral administration of fennel *(Foeniculum vulgare)* on ciprofloxacin absorption and disposition in the rat, *J Pharm Pharmacol* 51:1391-1396, 1999.

Fenugreek
(fen'yuh-greek)

Scientific name: *Trigonella foenum-graecum*

Other common names: Bird's foot, Greek hayseed, trigonella

Class 2b (Seed)

Origin: Fenugreek is an annual found in Europe and Asia.

Uses

Reported Uses

Fenugreek is taken internally to treat gastrointestinal com-

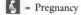 = Pregnancy    = Pediatric   = Alert   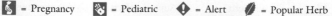 = Popular Herb

plaints, including constipation, dyspepsia, and gastritis; to promote lactation, for menstrual and menopausal discomfort. It is used topically to promote wound healing and to treat ulcers of the leg and cellulitis.

Investigational Uses

Studies are underway to determine the usefulness of fenugreek as an antioxidant and as a treatment for diabetes mellitus, gastric ulcers, hypercholesteremia, and infections such as tuberculosis.

Product Availability and Dosages

Available Forms

Capsules, crude herb, defatted fenugreek powder, fluid extract, powder (made from dried seeds)

Plant Parts Used: Seeds

Dosages and Routes

Adult

Diabetes Mellitus
• PO defatted fenugreek powder: 50 g/day (Murray, 1998)

Other
• PO: 1-6 g seeds tid
• PO: 6 g herb (Blumenthal, 1998)
• PO powdered seeds: 50 mg bid
• Topical: 50 g powdered herb dissolved in 250 ml water, qd (Blumenthal, 1998)

Precautionary Information

Contraindications

Because it can cause premature labor, fenugreek should not be used during pregnancy. Until more research is available, this herb should not be used during lactation and should not be given to children. Persons with hypersensitivity to fenugreek should not use it. Class 2b herb (seed).

Side Effects/Adverse Reactions

Integumentary: Hypersensitivity reactions
Systemic: Bruising, petechiae, BLEEDING

Interactions with Fenugreek

Drug

All medications: Because of the rapid rate at which this herb moves through the bowel and coats the gastrointestinal tract, fenugreek may cause reduced absorption of all medications used concurrently.

Anticoagulants (anisindione, dicumerol, heparin, warfarin): There is a possible increased risk of bleeding when fenugreek is used concurrently with anticoagulants.

Oral antidiabetics: Because fenugreek lowers blood glucose levels, increased hypoglycemia is possible when this herb is used concurrently with oral antidiabetics (theoretical).

Food	**Herb**
None known	None known

Lab Test

Fenugreek may decrease total cholesterol, blood glucose (decoctions, infusions), and LDL cholesterol.

Client Considerations

Assess

- Assess for hypersensitivity reactions. If present, discontinue use of this herb and administer antihistamine or other appropriate therapy.
- Assess for increased hypoglycemia in diabetic clients who are taking using antidiabetics (see Interactions).
- Assess for bleeding in clients who are using anticoagulants (see Interactions).

Administer

- Instruct the client to store fenugreek products in a sealed container away from heat and moisture.

Teach Client/Family

- Because it can cause premature labor, caution the client not to use fenugreek during pregnancy. Until more research is available, caution the client not to use this herb during lactation and not to give it to children.
- Instruct the client to report side effects and adverse reactions (bleeding, hypersensitivity, hypoglycemia) to the health care provider.

🐾 = Pregnancy 🖐 = Pediatric ◆ = Alert ∥ = Popular Herb

Pharmacology

Pharmacokinetics

Pharmacokinetics and pharmacodynamics are unknown.

Chemical Class	Individual Components	Possible Action
Saponin	Fenugreekine; Smilagenin; Diosgenin; Trigogenin; Gitogenin; Yamogenin; Neotigogenin; Neogitogenin	
Alkaloid	Gentianine; Carpaine; Choline; Trigonelline	
Amino acid	Lysine; Hydroxyisoleucine; Tryptophan; Histidine; Arginine	
Coumarin		
Vitamin		
Mineral		
Fiber		

Primary Chemical Components of Fenugreek and Their Possible Actions

F

Actions

Anticholesteremic Action

Fenugreek has been studied in diabetic rats to evaluate lipid peroxidation and antioxidant effects. Results revealed disruption of free radical metabolism in the diabetic animals (Ravikumar, 1999). Alpha-tocopherol levels increased significantly.

Analgesic Action

One study using laboratory rats evaluated tail-flick as a response to pain. When a large amount of fenugreek extract was given to the rats, tail-flicking behavior decreased, indicating a reduction in pain (Javen, 1997).

Antidiabetic Action

One study evaluated diabetic rats after they were fed fenugreek seed and its extracts (Ali, 1995). No effects were evident on fasting blood glucose levels with fenugreek alone, but when the rats received fenugreek simultaneously with glucose, a significant reduction in blood glucose occurred. Many other studies have confirmed the antidiabetic effects of fenugreek (Abdel-Barry, 1997; Abdel-Barry, 2000; Ghafghazi, 1977; Gupta, 1999; Gupta, 2001; Khosla, 1995; Ribes, 1986; Vats, 2002).

Other Actions

The effect of fenugreek seeds compared to omeprazole was evaluated on ethanol-induced gastric ulcers. The result was significant ulcer protective effects (Suja, 2002).

References

Abdel-Barry JA et al: Hypoglycaemic and antihyperglyceamic effects of *Trigonella foenum-graecum* leaf in normal and alloxan induced diabetic rats, *J Ethnopharmacol* 58(3):149-155, 1997.

Abdel-Barry JA et al: Hypoglycaemic effect of aqueous extract of the leaves of *Trigonella foenum-graecum* in healthy volunteers, *East Mediterr Health* 6(1):83-88, 2000.

Ali L et al: Characterization of the hypoglycemic effects of *Trigonella foenum graecum* seed, *Planta Med* 61(4):358-360, 1995.

Blumenthal M, editor: *The complete German Commission E monographs: therapeutic guide to herbal medicines,* Austin, Tex, American Botanical Council; Boston, Integrative Medicine Communication, 1998.

Ghafghazi T et al: Antagonism of cadmium and alloxan-induced hyperglycemia in rats by *Trigonella foenum graecum, Pahlavi Med* 8(1):14-25, 1977.

Gupta A et al: Modulation of some gluconeogenic enzyme activities in diabetic rat liver and kidney: effect of antidiabetic compounds, *Indian J Exp Biol* 37(2):196-199, 1999.

Gupta A et al: Effect of *Trigonella foenum-graecum* (fenugreek) seeds on glycaemic control and insulin resistance in type 2 diabetes mellitus: a double blind placebo controlled study, *J Assoc Physicians India* 49:1057-1061, 2001.

Khosla P et al: Effect of *Trigonella foenum graecum* (Fenugreek) on blood glucose in normal and diabetic rats, *Indian J Physiol Pharmacol* 39(2):173-174, 1995.

Javen M et al: Antinociceptive effects of *Trigonella foenum-graecum* leaves extract, *J Ethnopharmacol* 58(2):125-129, 1997.

Murray M, Pizzarno J: *The encyclopedia of natural medicine,* 2 ed (revised), Roseville, Calif, 1998, Prima.

Ravikumar P et al: Effect of fenugreek seeds on blood lipid peroxidation and antioxidants in diabetic rats, *Phytother Res* 13(3):197-201, 1999.

Ribes G et al: Antidiabetic effects of subfractions from fenugreek seeds in diabetic dogs, *Proc Soc Exp Biol Med* 182(2):159-166, 1986.

Suja P et al: Gastro protective effect of fenugreek seeds on experimental gastric ulcer in rats, 81(3):393-397, 2002.

⟨§⟩ = Pregnancy   **⟨🐾⟩** = Pediatric   **◆** = Alert   **⫮** = Popular Herb

Vats V et al: Evaluation of anti-hyperglycemic and hypoglycemic effect by *Trigonella foenum-graecum* Linn, *Ocimum sanctum* Linn, and *Pterocarpus marsupium* Linn in normal and alloxanized diabetic rats, *J Ethnopharmacol* 79(1):95-100, 2002.

F

Feverfew
(fee'vuhr-fyew)

Scientific name: *Chrysanthemum parthenium*

Other common names: Altamisa, bachelors' button, chamomile grande, featherfew, featherfoil, febrifuge plant, midsummer daisy, mutterkraut, nosebleed, Santa Maria, wild chamomile, wild quinine   **Class 2b (Whole Herb)**

Origin: Feverfew is a perennial found throughout the world.

Uses

Reported Uses
Feverfew is used traditionally to treat menstrual irregularities, threatened spontaneous abortion, arthritis, and fever.

Investigational Uses
Research is underway to determine whether feverfew is effective in the prevention and treatment of migraine headache.

Product Availability and Dosages

Available Forms
Capsules, crude herb (fresh), extract, tablets, tincture

Plant Parts Used: Leaves

Dosages and Routes
Adult
All dosages listed are PO.
Migraine Prophylaxis and Treatment
- Freeze dried extract: 25 mg qd
- Fresh leaves: 2 large or 4 small leaves/day chewed or mixed with food (McCaleb, 2000)
- Standardized extract: 275 mg/day (McCaleb, 2000) or 0.25-0.5 mg parthenolide (Murray, 1998); other sources report 50-100 mg of whole leaf extract
- Capsules/tablets: 300-400 mg tid-qid (Foster, 1998)

🌀 Endangered Herb   Adverse effects: **BOLD** = life-threatening

• Tincture: 15-30 drops per day (Foster, 1998) standardized to 0.2-0.7 mg parthenolide

Precautionary Information

Contraindications

Until more research is available, feverfew should not be used during pregnancy and lactation and should not be given to children. Feverfew should not be used by persons with hypersensitivity to it. Class 2b herb (whole herb).

Side Effects/Adverse Reactions

Ears, Eyes, Nose, and Throat: Mouth ulcers (chewed leaves)
Gastrointestinal: Nausea, vomiting, anorexia, abdominal pain
Integumentary: Hypersensitivity reactions
Musculoskeletal: Muscle stiffness, muscle and joint pain

Interactions with Feverfew

Drug

Anticoagulants (anisindione, dicumarol, heparin, warfarin): Feverfew may increase the anticoagulant properties of anticoagulants.
Antiplatelets: Feverfew may increase the action of antiplatelets; avoid concurrent use (theoretical).

Food
None known

Herb
None known

Lab Test

Feverfew may decrease platelet aggregation. It may increase prothrombin time (PT) and plasma partial prothrombin time (PTT) in clients taking warfarin concurrently.

Client Considerations

Assess

• Assess for hypersensitivity reactions. If present, discontinue use of this herb and administer antihistamine or other appropriate therapy.
• Assess for mouth ulcers and muscle and joint pain or stiffness.

 = Pregnancy   = Pediatric   = Alert   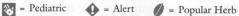 = Popular Herb

Administer
- Instruct the client to store feverfew products in a cool, dry place, away from heat and moisture.

Teach Client/Family

- Until more research is available, caution the client not to use feverfew during pregnancy and lactation and not to give it to children.

Pharmacology

Pharmacokinetics

Pharmacokinetics and pharmacodynamics are unknown.

Primary Chemical Components of Feverfew and Their Possible Actions		
Individual Class	**Individual Component**	**Possible Action**
Monoquiterpene		
Sesquiterpene		
Sesquiterpene lactone	Chrysanthemolide; Parthenolide Chrysanthemonin; Magnoliolide	Decreases serotonin Platelet inhibitor
Melatonin		Sleep regulation
Flavonoid	Apigenin; Luteolin; Chrysoeriol; Scutellarein; Santin	
Santamarin		
Tanaparthin		
Reynosin		

Actions

Antimigraine Action

Primary research has focused on the use of feverfew for the prevention and treatment of migraine headache. In a study of 57 patients with severe migraine headaches, use of feverfew significantly reduced pain intensity, vomiting, and noise sensitivity (Palevitch, 1997). Another study demonstrated that feverfew acts as a significant migraine preventive when taken for 4 months. The control group experienced severe migraine headaches, whereas the experimental group reported a 47% re-

F

duction in headaches. When the groups were switched after 4 months, migraine headache frequency increased in the control group but decreased in the experimental group (Murphy, 1988). One theory is that feverfew decreases platelet aggregation and inhibits production of prostaglandins and thromboxanes. One of the chemical components of this herb also prevents the release of serotonin from platelets. The release of serotonin from platelets is thought to stimulate migraine headache.

Antiinflammatory Action

Feverfew may decrease the release of polymorphonuclear leukocytes in joints that are arthritic and inflamed (Heptinstall, 1998). Another study has demonstrated that feverfew inhibits arachidonate metabolism in leukocytes that may increase inflammation (Williams, 1995).

References

Foster S: *101 medicinal plants,* Loveland, Colo, 1998, Interweave Press.

Heptinstall L et al: Feverfew: a review of its history, its biological and medicinal properties, and the status of commercial preparations of the herb. In Lawson L et al: *Phytomedicines of Europe: chemistry and biological activity,* Washington, DC, 1998, American Chemical Society, pp 158-175.

McCaleb R et al: *The encyclopedia of popular herbs: your complete guide to leading medicinal plants,* Roseville, Calif, 2000, Prima Health.

Murphy JJ et al: Randomised double-blind placebo controlled trial of feverfew in migraine prevention, *Lancet* pp 189-192, July 23, 1988.

Palevitch D et al: Feverfew as a prophylactic treatment for migraine: a double-blind placebo-controlled study, *Phytotherapy Res* 2:508-511, 1997.

Williams CA et al: *Phytochemistry* 38:267, 1995.

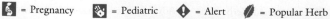

F

Figwort
(fig'wuhrt)

Scientific names: *Scrophularia nodosa, Scrophularia ningpoensis*

Other common names: Carpenter's square, common figwort, kernelwort, knotty rooted figwort, rose-noble, scrofula plant, square stalk, stinking christopher, throatwort

Class 2d (*S. ningpoensis* Whole Herb/Root)

Origin: Figwort is found in China.

Uses

Reported Uses

Figwort is most often used topically to treat skin disorders such as acne, eczema, contact dermatitis, urticaria, psoriasis, and pruritus. Figwort is used internally to decrease gastrointestinal symptoms, stimulate cardiac function, and reduce inflammation.

Product Availability and Dosages

Available Forms

Fluid extract, soak, tincture

Plant Parts Used: Dried flowers, dried leaves

Dosages and Routes

Adult
- PO fluid extract: 2-8 ml (1:2) qd-bid
- PO infusion: 2-8 g herb qd
- PO tincture: 2-4 ml (1:5 dilution) qd-bid
- Topical: use as a soak or apply by compress prn

Precautionary Information

Contraindications

Until more research is available, figwort should not be used during pregnancy and lactation, and it should not be given to children. Figwort should not be used by persons with hypersensitivity to this herb or those who have serious cardiac disease. Class 2d herb (*S. ningpoensis* whole herb/root).

Continued

 Endangered Herb　　　Adverse effects: **BOLD** = life-threatening

> ## Precautionary Information—cont'd
> **Side Effects/Adverse Reactions**
> *Cardiovascular:* Decreased heart rate, HEART BLOCK, ASYSTOLE
> *Gastrointestinal:* Nausea, vomiting, anorexia, diarrhea
> *Integumentary:* Hypersensitivity reactions

> ### Interactions with Figwort
>
> **Drug**
> *Antiarrhythmics:* The action of figwort may increase the effects of antiarrhythmics; do not use concurrently.
> *Beta-blockers:* The action of figwort may increase the effects of beta-blockers; do not use concurrently.
> *Cardiac glycosides:* The action of figwort may be increased by cardiac glycosides; do not use concurrently.
>
> | Food | Herb |
> |------|------|
> | None known | None known |
>
> **Lab Test**
> Figwort may decrease blood glucose.

Client Considerations

Assess

- Assess for hypersensitivity reactions. If present, discontinue use of figwort and administer antihistamine or other appropriate therapy.
- Assess cardiac status, including blood pressure and pulse (character). Watch for decreasing pulse. Patients with cardiac disorders should not take figwort.
- Assess for other cardiovascular drugs the client may be using. Figwort should not be used concurrently with antiarrhythmics, cardiac glycosides, or beta-blockers (see Interactions).

Administer

- Instruct the client to store figwort products in a cool, dry place, away from heat and moisture.

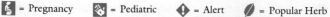
 = Pregnancy   = Pediatric   = Alert   = Popular Herb

Teach Client/Family

- Until more research is available, caution the client not to use figwort during pregnancy and lactation and not to give it to children.
- Warn the client of the life-threatening side effects of figwort.
- Advise the client that research is lacking and therefore any use or action of figwort is speculative.

Pharmacology

Pharmacokinetics

Pharmacokinetics and pharmacodynamics are unknown.

Primary Chemical Components of Figwort and Their Possible Actions		
Chemical Class	**Individual Component**	**Possible Action**
Amino acid	Isoleucine; Leucine; Alanine; Lysine; Tyrosine; Phenylalanine; Threonine; Valine	
Flavonoid	Aucubin; Catalpol Diosmetin; Harpagide; Harpagoside; Isoharpagoside; Procumbid; Iridoids	Laxative
Phenolic acid	Ferulic acid Vanillic acid; Caffeic acid; Cinnamic acid	Antiinflammatory
Glycosides	Ningposides A, B, C (Li, 2000), Sibirioside A, Cistanoside D, Angoroside C acteoside, Decaffeoy lactoside, Cistanoside F	
Saponin Asparagine		

Actions

Very little research is available on figwort. This herb is classified as an iridoid glycoside and is related to the foxglove plant, from which digitalis is derived. Therefore some of the actions of figwort are similar to those of digitalis-like drugs. However, no primary research supports the possible cardiac actions of this herb.

Miscellaneous Actions

Figwort has been tested for its insulin-binding reaction (Liu, 1991), its antiprotozoacidal activity (Martin, 1998), its antiinflammatory activity (Fernandez, 1998), and its possible antitoxic effects in chemotherapy (Liu, 1993). The 1991 Liu study determined that figwort did not alter insulin binding in any way. Martin, et al., evaluated 60 plant species and found that figwort was active against *Trichomonas vaginalis* and *Leishmania infantum* (Martin, 1998).The Fernandez study found that figwort used topically exerts stronger antiinflammatory action than does figwort used orally. The action of this herb used topically is influenced by migration of neutrophils into the infected area. The 1993 Liu study found that figwort prevents toxicity in chemotherapy (Liu, 1993). When chemotherapeutic agents were combined with several Chinese herbs, the group treated with the herbs suffered fewer toxic reactions at a statistically significant level. Stevenson (2002) identified the wound healing activity of glycosides in *Scrophularia nodosa*.

References

Fernandez MA et al: Anti-inflammatory activity in rats and mice of phenolic acids isolated from *Scropularia frutescens, J Pharm Pharmacol* 50:1183-1186, 1998.

Li YM et al: Phenylpropanoid glycosides from *Scrophularia ningpoensis, Phytochemistry* 54(8):923-925, 2000.

Liu GL et al: Effect of water extract of 4 Chinese herbal drugs on the binding of insulin with human erythrocyte insulin receptor, *Zhong Xi Yi Jie He Za Zhi* 11(10):581-582, 606-607, 1991.

Liu JQ et al: 32 cases of postoperative osteogenic sarcoma treated by chemotherapy combined with Chinese medicinal herbs, *Zhongguo Zhong Xi Yi Jie He Za Zhi* 13(3):132, 150-152, 1993.

Martin T et al: Screening for protozoacidal activity of Spanish plants, *Pharm Biol* 36(1):56-62, 1998.

Stevenson PC et al: Wound healing activity of acylated iridoid glycosides from *Scrophularia nodosa, Phytother Res* 16(1):33-35, 2002.

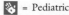

= Pregnancy = Pediatric = Alert = Popular Herb

Flax
(flaks)

Scientific name: *Linum usitatissimum*

Other common names: Flaxseed, linseed, lint bells, linen flax, linum

Class 2d (Seed)

Origin: Flax is a flowering annual found in the United States, Canada, and Europe.

Uses

Reported Uses

Flax generally is used internally as a laxative and an anticholesteremic. Topically it is used as an inflammatory.

Investigational Uses

Researchers are experimenting with the use of flax to treat inflammatory conditions such as colitis, irritable bowel syndrome, diverticulitis, osteoarthritis, psoriasis, and eczema. It may also be effective in the treatment of allergies and autoimmune disorders such as multiple sclerosis, cancer, lupus erythematosus, and rheumatoid arthritis, as well as learning disorders such as attention deficit disorder with or without hyperactivity and dyslexia. It is also used experimentally to treat hypertension and agoraphobia.

Product Availability and Dosages

Available Forms

Capsules, oil, powder, softgel capsules

Plant Parts Used: Seeds

Dosages and Routes

Flax may be standardized to 58% alpha-linolenic acid.

Adult

Agoraphobia
- PO: 2-6 tbsp/day (Rudin, 1981)

Diabetes Mellitus
- PO: 1 tbsp/day (Murray, 1998)

Eczema
- PO: 1 tbsp/day (Murray, 1998)

General Use
- PO oil: 1-2 tbsp qd in divided doses.

 Endangered Herb   Adverse effects: BOLD = life-threatening

- PO seeds: 2 ½ tsp ground seeds bid-tid (McCaleb, 2000); whole flaxseed can be ground at home using a small food processor to break the hard portion of the outside of the seed; ground flax should be mixed in 6-8 oz water and eaten within 15 min

Hypertension
- PO: 1 tbsp/day (Murray, 1998)

Inflammation
- Topical: 30-40 g flax flour (Blumenthal, 1998), moistened to form a paste, prn

Multiple Sclerosis
- PO: 1 tbsp/day (Murray, 1998)

Rheumatoid Arthritis
- PO: 1 tbsp/day (Murray, 1998)

Precautionary Information

Contraindications

Until more research is available, flax should not be used during pregnancy and lactation, and it should not be given to children. This herb should not be used by persons with bowel obstruction or dehydration or by persons with hypersensitivity to it. Flax poultice should not be used on open wounds. Only mature seeds should be used; immature seeds are toxic. Class 2d herb (seed).

Side Effects/Adverse Reactions

Gastrointestinal: Nausea, vomiting, anorexia, diarrhea, flatulence
Integumentary: Hypersensitivity reactions
Overdose: WEAKNESS, INCOORDINATION, DYSPNEA, TACHYPNEA, PARALYSIS, SEIZURES, DEATH

Interactions with Flax

Drug

All oral medications: Absorption of medications may be decreased if taken concurrently with flax.
Laxatives: Flax may increase the action of laxatives, resulting in diarrhea.

Food	Herb	Lab Test
None known	None known	None known

= Pregnancy   = Pediatric   = Alert   = Popular Herb

Client Considerations

Assess
- Assess for hypersensitivity reactions. If present, discontinue use of this herb and administer antihistamine or other appropriate therapy.

- Assess for overdose reactions.
- Assess for use of medications, including laxatives (see Interactions).

Administer
- Instruct the client to refrigerate flax products to prevent fatty acid breakdown.

Teach Client/Family
- Until more research is available, caution the client not to use flax during pregnancy and lactation and not to give it to children.
- Inform the client that flax may decrease the absorption of all other medications.
- Warn the client to use only mature seeds; the immature seeds are toxic.
- Inform the client of the symptoms of overdose (see Side Effects).

Pharmacology

Pharmacokinetics

Pharmacokinetics and pharmacodynamics are unknown.

Primary Chemical Components of Flax and Their Possible Actions		
Chemical Class	**Individual Component**	**Possible Action**
Fatty acid	Linolenic acid	Decreases cholesterol
	Linoleic acid; Oleic acid	
Mucilage	Galactose; Xylose; Arabinose; Rhamnose	
Protein		
Flavonoid	Equol	Antitumor
Lignan	Secoisolariciresinol diglucoside (Degenhardt, 2002)	Anticancer

Actions

Adequate levels of zinc and acidophilus are needed to metabolize flax.

Anticancer Action

One study showed a significantly reduced incidence of breast cancer when women consumed high levels of phytoestrogens such as the lignans found in flax products (Ingram, 1997). This study compared 144 women with breast cancer with 144 women without breast cancer. The women were matched demographically. Investigators determined that the largest reduction in breast cancer was associated with a high intake of equol, one of the flavone components, and enterolactone, a substance formed by the breakdown of flax.

Anticholesteremic Action

In a 6-week double-blind crossover study, 38 postmenopausal women with elevated cholesterol were given whole flaxseed and sunflower seed. In the experimental group, cholesterol dropped by nearly 15% (Arjmandi, 1999). Other studies have confirmed that the addition of flax to the diet reduces risk factors for coronary artery disease, thrombotic disorders, and cerebrovascular accident.

References

Arjmandi BH et al: Whole flaxseed consumption lowers serum LDL-cholesterol and lipoprotein concentrations in postmenopausal women, *Nutr Res* 18(7):1203-1214, 1999.

Blumenthal M, editor: *The complete German Commission E monographs: therapeutic guide to herbal medicines,* Austin, Tex, American Botanical Council; Boston, Integrative Medicine Communication, 1998.

Degenhardt A et al: Isolation of the lignan secoisolariciresinol diglucoside from flaxseed (*Linum usitatissimum* L.) by high speed counter-current chromatography, *J Chromatogr A* 943(2):299-302, 2002.

Ingram D et al: Case-control study of phytoestrogens and breast cancer, *Lancet* 350:990-994, 1997.

McCaleb R et al: *The encyclopedia of popular herbs: your complete guide to leading medicinal plants,* Roseville, Calif, 2000, Prima Health.

Murray M, Pizzarno J: *The encyclopedia of natural medicine,* 2 ed (revised), Roseville, Calif, 1998, Prima.

Rudin DO: The major psychoses and neuroses as omega-3 essential fatty acid deficiency syndrome: substrate pellagra, *Biol Psychiatry* 16(9):837-850, 1981.

Fo-ti
(foe′tee)

Scientific name: *Polygonum multiflorum*

Other common names: Chinese cornbind, Chinese knotweed, flowery knotweed, ho shou wu

Origin: Fo-ti is a climbing perennial found in China.

Uses

Reported Uses

In traditional Chinese medicine, fo-ti is used as a general tonic. It is also used to slow the aging process and to treat insomnia, autoimmune disorders, and diabetes mellitus. It may also be used to treat diverticular disease and hemorrhoids. A laxative action is present in the chemical components of fo-ti.

Investigational Uses

Research is underway to confirm the myocardial protective use of *Polygonum multiflorum,* as well as the cognitive enhancing use.

Product Availability and Dosages

Available Forms

Sliced root; available in combination in many herbal tonics

Plant Parts Used: Roots

Dosages and Routes

No published dosages are available.

Precautionary Information

Contraindications

Until more research is available, fo-ti should not be used during pregnancy and lactation and should not be given to children. It should not be used by persons with diarrhea or those with hypersensitivity to this herb.

Side Effects/Adverse Reactions

Gastrointestinal: Nausea, vomiting, anorexia, diarrhea, laxative dependence (long-term use)

Integumentary: Hypersensitivity reactions

 Endangered Herb   Adverse effects: BOLD = life-threatening

Interactions with Fo-ti			
Drug	**Food**	**Herb**	**Lab Test**
None known	None known	None known	None known

Client Considerations

Assess

- Assess for hypersensitivity reactions. If present, discontinue use of this herb and administer antihistamine or other appropriate therapy.

Administer

- Instruct the client to take fo-ti PO.
- Inform the client that dark roots are the most potent. Roots with white streaks are of a lesser quality.
- Instruct the client to store fo-ti in a cool, dry place, away from heat and moisture.

Teach Client/Family

- Until more research is available, caution the client not to use fo-ti during pregnancy and lactation and not to give it to children.
- Advise the client that long-term use of this herb may lead to laxative dependence.

Pharmacology

Pharmacokinetics

Pharmacokinetics and pharmacodynamics are unknown.

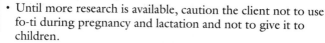

Primary Chemical Components of Fo-Ti and Their Possible Actions		
Chemical Class	**Individual Component**	**Possible Action**
Anthraquinone	Emodin Rhein	Laxative
Chrysophanol Chrysophanic acid		

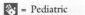 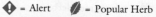

Actions

Information on fo-ti is lacking. Most of the available information comes from Chinese literature published in the early- to mid-1990s. A few studies are available documenting the cholesterol-lowering action of this herb in animals (Hong, 1994; Chevallier, 1996), and the root has been shown to lower triglyceride accumulations in animal livers (Liu, 1992). A newer study (Yim, 2000) has shown a myocardial protective action against ischemia-reperfusion injury when *Polygonum multiflorum* extract is used. Hsieh (2000) showed no cognitive enhancing properties of *Polygonum multiflorum* when studied with other Chinese herbs.

References

Chevallier A: *Encyclopedia of medicinal plants,* New York, 1996, DK, p 121.

Hong Y et al: *Am J Chin Med* 22(1):63-70, 1994.

Hsieh MT et al: The ameliorating effects of the cognitive-enhancing Chinese herbs on scopolamine-induced amnesia in rats, *Phytother Res* 14(5):375-377, 2000.

Liu C et al: *Chung Kuo Chung Yao Tsa Chih* 17(10):595-596, 1992.

Yim TK et al: Myocardial protection against ischaemia-reperfusion injury by a *Polygonum multiflorum* extract supplemented "Dang-Gui decoction for enriching blood," a compound formulation, ex vivo, *Phytother* 14(3):195-199, 2002.

Fumitory
(fyew′muh-toe-ry)

Scientific name: *Fumaria officinalis*

Other common names: Earth smoke, hedge fumitory, wax dolls

Origin: Fumitory is an annual bush or shrub found in Africa, Europe, the United States, Canada, Asia, and Australia.

Uses

Reported Uses

Fumitory is taken internally as a laxative, a diuretic, and a treatment for biliary illness. Topically, it may be used to treat various skin disorders such as eczema, psoriasis, and scabies.

🜲 Endangered Herb   Adverse effects: ʙᴏʟᴅ = life-threatening

Investigational Uses

Researchers are experimenting with the usefulness of fumitory in the treatment of arrhythmias.

Product Availability and Dosages

Available Forms

Dried herb, extract, tincture

Plant Parts Used: Flowering parts, leaves

Dosages and Routes

Adult

- PO dried herb: 6 g/day (Blumenthal, 1998)
- PO fluid extract: 2-4 ml (1:1 dilution) in 25% alcohol, tid
- PO tea: 2-4 g tid
- PO tincture: 1-4 ml (1:5 dilution) in 45% alcohol, tid
- Topical: apply dried herb prn

Precautionary Information

Contraindications

Until more research is available, fumitory should not be used during pregnancy and lactation, and it should not be given to children. This herb should not be used by persons with seizure disorders or increased intraocular pressure, and it should not be used by those with hypersensitivity to it.

Side Effects/Adverse Reactions

Cardiovascular: Decreased blood pressure, decreased pulse
Central Nervous System: **Seizures** (overdose)
Ears, Eyes, Nose, and Throat: Increased intraocular pressure
Gastrointestinal: Nausea, vomiting, anorexia
Integumentary: Hypersensitivity reactions

 = Pregnancy   = Pediatric    = Alert   = Popular Herb

Interactions with Fumitory		
Drug		
Antiarrhythmics: The actions of fumitory may increase the effects of antiarrhythmics; do not use concurrently.		
Beta-blockers: The actions of fumitory may increase the effects of beta-blockers; do not use concurrently.		
Cardiac glycosides: The actions of fumitory may increase the effects of cardiac glycosides; do not use concurrently.		
Food	Herb	Lab Test
None known	None known	None known

F

Client Considerations

Assess

- Assess for hypersensitivity reactions. If present, discontinue use of fumitory and administer antihistamine or other appropriate therapy.
- Assess the client's cardiac status, including blood pressure and pulse (character). Watch for decreasing pulse.
- Assess for other cardiovascular drugs the client may be taking. Fumitory should not be taken concurrently with antiarrhythmics, cardiac glycosides, or beta-blockers (see Interactions).

Administer

- Instruct the client to store fumitory products in a cool, dry place, away from heat and moisture.

Teach Client/Family

- Until more research is available, caution the client not to use fumitory during pregnancy and lactation and not to give it to children.

Pharmacology

Pharmacokinetics

Pharmacokinetics and pharmacodynamics are unknown.

Primary Chemical Components of Fumitory and Their Possible Actions		
Chemical Class	**Individual Component**	**Possible Action**
Alkaloid	Fumarine	Negative chronotropic; Antihistaminic
	Cryptopine	Negative chronotropic
	Aurotensine; Coridaline; Sinactine; Stylopine, Cryptocavine; Sanguinarine; Bulbocapnine	
Fumaric acid	Fumaricine; Fumritine; Fumariline	
Flavonoid	Quercetin; Isoquercetin	Antiinflammatory
Mucilage		
Resin		
Fumaric acid		Bile stimulant/ antispasmodic
Caffeic acid		Bile stimulant/ antispasmodic

Actions

A review of the literature reveals very few studies supporting the use of fumitory as a treatment for skin disorders, a diuretic, or a laxative. In Germany, fumitory is approved for treatment of colicky pain in the gallbladder or biliary system. Only two studies have evaluated the possible use of fumitory in the treatment of cardiac disorders. The first study, using dogs, evaluated the efficacy of its alkaloid components in treating temporary disorders of coronary blood flow. The injected alkaloids significantly reduced ischemic shifts (Gorbunov, 1980). The second study evaluated a number of different plant species grown in Bulgaria. Results showed that fumitory exerted a healing effect on ischemic heart disease, atherosclerosis, and hypertension (Petkov, 1979). A more recent study (Rao, 1998) showed *Fumaria indica,* a different *Fumaria* sp. from that used for the preparations that are typically available, to be hepatoprotective.

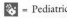 = Pregnancy 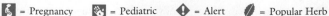 = Pediatric = Alert 𝄾 = Popular Herb

References

Blumenthal M, editor: *The complete German Commission E monographs: therapeutic guide to herbal medicines,* Austin, Tex, American Botanical Council; Boston, Integrative Medicine Communication, 1998.

Gorbunov NP et al: Pharmacological correction of myocardial ischemia and arrhythmias in reversible coronary blood flow disorders and experimental myocardial infarct in dogs, *Kardiologiia* 20(5):84-87, 1980.

Petkov V: Plants and hypotensive, antiatheromatous and coronarodilatating action, *Am J Chin Med* 7(3):197-236, 1979.

Rao KS et al: Antihepatotoxic activity of monomethyl fumarate isolated from *Fumaria indica, J Ethnopharmacol* 60:207-213, 1998.

F

Galanthamine
Scientific name: *Galanthus nivalis*

Origin: Galanthamine is a bulb plant found throughout the world.

Uses
Reported Uses
Galanthamine is used widely in other countries to treat Alzheimer's disease, myasthenia gravis, and paralysis caused by polio.

Product Availability and Dosages
Available Forms
Ampules, tablets

Plant Parts Used: Bulb

Dosages and Routes
Adult
- PO ampules or tablets: 5 mg tid; dosage may be increased gradually to 40 mg qd

Precautionary Information
Contraindications
Until more research is available, galanthamine should not be used during pregnancy and lactation and should not be given to children. This herb should not be used by persons with exposure to organophosphate fertilizers or those with hypersensitivity to it.

Side Effects/Adverse Reactions
Central Nervous System: Dizziness, anxiety, agitation, restlessness, insomnia
Gastrointestinal: Nausea, vomiting, anorexia, abdominal cramping and pain, diarrhea
Integumentary: Hypersensitivity reactions

Interactions with Galanthamine		
Drug		
MAOIs: Do not use galanthamine concurrently with MAOIs; hypertensive crisis may occur.		
Food	**Herb**	**Lab Test**
None known	None known	None known

Client Considerations

Assess

- Assess for hypersensitivity reactions. If present, discontinue use of this herb and administer antihistamine or other appropriate therapy.
- Assess for the use of MAOIs and organophosphate fertilizers, neither of which should be used concurrently with galanthamine (see Interactions).

Administer

- Instruct the client to store galanthamine products in a cool, dry place, away from heat and moisture.

Teach Client/Family

- Until more research is available, caution the client not to use galanthamine during pregnancy and lactation and not to give it to children.
- Inform the client that conventional treatments may be more effective than galanthamine.

Pharmacology

Pharmacokinetics

Pharmacokinetics and pharmacodynamics are unknown. However, the components of galanthamine are known to cross the blood-brain barrier.

Primary Chemical Components of Galanthamine and Their Possible Actions		
Chemical Class	**Individual Component**	**Possible Action**
Alkaloid		Acetylcholinesterase inhibitor

 Endangered Herb   Adverse effects: BOLD = life-threatening

Actions

Acetylcholinesterase Inhibition

Research has identified galanthamine as an acetylcholinesterase inhibitor, which can reverse the effects of nondepolarizing muscle relaxants (Schuh, 1976). The use of galanthamine has produced both positive and negative effects in clients with Alzheimer's disease. In two studies (Bores, 1996; Iliev, 2000; Kewitz, 1994), a course of galanthamine produced an improvement in cognitive functioning in humans and animals. However, another study showed no such improvement (Dal-Bianco, 1991).

Antiinfective Action

In a recent study of rats infected with salmonella, the rats were fed *Galanthus nivalis* agglutininfor 3 days preinfection and 6 days postinfection. *G. nivalis* significantly reduced salmonella numbers in the small bowel and large intestine of the infected rats (Naughton, 2000). In another study, in vitro, *G. nivalis* inhibited the growth of *Chlamydia trachomatis* by binding a glycoprotein present in the infecting organism (Amin, 1995). A strong immune response resulted when the glycoproteins of HIV-1, HIV-2, and SIV were purified with *G.nivalis* (Gilljam, 1993).

References

Amin K et al: Binding of *Galanthus nivalis* lectin to *Chlamydia trachomatis* and inhibition of in vitro infection, *APMIS* 103(10):714-720, 1995.

Bores GM et al: Pharmacological evaluation of novel Alzheimer's disease therapeutics: acetylcholinesterase inhibitors related to galanthamine, *J Pharmacol Exp Ther* 277:728-738, 1996.

Dal-Bianco P et al: Galanthamine treatment in Alzheimer's disease, *J Neural Transm Suppl* 33:59-63, 1991.

Gilljam G: Envelope glycoproteins of HIV-1, HIV-2, and SIV purified with *Galanthus nivalis, AIDS Res Hum Retroviruses* 9(5):431-438, 1993.

Iliev AI et al: A post-ischaemic single administration of galanthamine, a cholinesterase inhibitor, improves learning ability in rats, *J Pharm Pharmacol* 52(9):1151-1156, 2000.

Kewitz H et al: Galanthamine, a selective nontoxic acetylcholinesterase inhibitor is significantly superior over placebo in the treatment of SDAT, *Neuropsychopharmacology* 10(suppl 2):130, 1994.

Naughton PJ et al: Modulation of salmonella infection by the lectins of *Canavalia ensiformis* (Con A) and *Galanthus nivalis* (GNA) in a rat model in vivo, *J Appl Microbiol* 88(4):720-727, 2000 (in-process citation).

$\boxed{\text{S}}$ = Pregnancy   ✥ = Pediatric   ◆ = Alert   ✿ = Popular Herb

Schuh FT: On the molecular mechanism of action of galanthamine, an antagonist of nondepolarizing muscle relaxants: *Anaesthesist* 25(9): 444-448, 1976.

Garcinia
(gar-sin-ee′uh)

Scientific names: *Garcinia cambogia, G. indica, G. hanburyi*

Other common names: Camboge, gorikapuli, gutta cambodia, HCA, hydroxycitric acid, malabar tamarind, tom rong

G

Origin: *Garcinia cambogia* comes from the Indian brindall berry.

Uses
Reported Uses
Traditionally, garcinia is used for constipation because it possesses a strong laxative effect.

Investigational Uses
New studies are underway using garcinia for weight loss.

Product Availability and Dosages
Available Forms
Tablets, capsules, powder, and as a component in snack bars and breakfast bars. Garcinia may be standardized to a fixed HCA amount.

Plant Parts Used: Ground drug from resin

Dosage and Routes
Adult
• PO: 250-1000 mg tid

Precautionary Information
Contraindications
Garcinia should not be used in hypersensitivity, pregnancy, or lactation; for children; or in hepatic or renal disease.

Side Effects/Adverse Reactions
Gastrointestinal: Severe diarrhea, abdominal pain, nausea, vomiting
Systemic: **DEATH** (>4 g of herb)

 Endangered Herb   Adverse effects: BOLD = life-threatening

Interactions with Garcinia			
Drug	Food	Herb	Lab Test
None known	None known	None known	None known

Client Considerations
Assess
- Assess the reason client is using garcinia.
- Monitor weight while taking this product.

Administer
- Keep garcinia in a dry area, away from direct sunlight.

Teach Client/Family

- Teach the client that garcinia should not be used in pregnancy, in lactation, or for children until more research is completed with these populations.
- Advise the patient that the herb should be used under the supervision of a qualified herbalist, because overdose can cause death.

Pharmacology
Pharmacokinetics
Pharmacokinetics and pharmacodynamics are unknown.

Primary Chemical Components of Garcinia and Their Possible Actions		
Chemical Class	Individual Component	Possible Action
Resins Xanthones	Benzophenones Gambogin; Morelin dimethyl acetal; Isomoreolin B; Moreolic acid; Gambogenic acid; Gambogenin; Isogambogenin; Desoxygambogenin; Gambogenin dimethyl acetal; Isomorellin; Morellic acid; Desoxymorellin	Cytotoxic (Asano, 1996)
Mucilages		

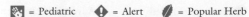

= Pregnancy   = Pediatric   = Alert   = Popular Herb

Actions

There is little research for garcinia's use in weight loss. One small study (Heymsfield, 1998) identified its use to reduce fatty acid synthesis and food intake and thus reduction in weight. In another study (Mahendran, 2002), rats with indomethacin-induced gastric ulcers showed improvement when fed *G. cambogia*.

References

Asano J et al: Cytotoxic xanthones from *Garcinia hanburyi*, *Phytochemistry* 41(3):818-820, 1996.

Heymsfield SB et al: *Garcinia cambogia* as a potential antiobesity agent: a randomized controlled trial, *JAMA* 280:1596-1600, 1998.

Mehendran P et al: The antiulcer activity of *Garcinia cambogia* extract against indomethacin-induced gastric ulcer in rats. *Phytother Res* 16(1):80-83, 2002.

G

Garlic
(gahr'lik)

Scientific name: *Allium sativum*

Other common names: Ail, allium, camphor of the poor, da-suan, knoblaunch, la-suan, nectar of the gods, poor-man's treacle, rustic treacle, stinking rose

Class 2c (Bulb)

Origin: Garlic is a perennial bulb found throughout the world.

Uses

Reported Uses

Garlic is used as an antilipidemic, antimicrobial, antiasthmatic, and antiinflammatory. It is a possible antihypertensive and is used to treat some types of heavy metal poisoning.

Investigational Uses

Studies are underway to determine the role of garlic as an anticancer agent, antioxidant, antiplatelet, and antidiabetic.

Product Availability and Dosages

Available Forms

Bulbs, capsules, extract , fresh garlic, oil, powder, syrup, tablets, tea

Plant Parts Used: Bulb (root)

Dosages and Routes

Garlic may be standardized to its allicin (active ingredient) content.

Adult

All dosages listed are PO.

Chronic Candidiasis
- Fresh garlic: 4 g qd (Murray, 1998)

General Use
- Extract, aged: 4 ml qd (McCaleb, 2000)
- Fresh garlic: 4 g qd (Blumenthal, 1998; McCaleb, 2000)
- Oil, perles: 10 mg qd (McCaleb, 2000)

Hypercholesteremia/Hypertension
- 40,000 µg qd (allicin) (Murray, 1998)
- Capsules/powder/tablets: 600-900 mg qd to decrease lipids (McCaleb, 2000)

Child

All dosages listed are PO.

General Use
- Fresh garlic: ½-3 cloves qd (Romm, 2000)
- Syrup: 1-2 tsp/day (Romm, 2000)
- Tea: 1 cup qd; may give up to 4 cups qd to treat colds (Romm, 2000)

Precautionary Information

Contraindications

Because garlic may stimulate labor and cause colic in infants, it should not be used medicinally during pregnancy or lactation. Dietary amounts are acceptable. Because garlic may reduce iodine uptake, it should not be used by persons with hypothyroidism. Because garlic may cause clotting time to be increased, it should not be used by persons who recently have had or are about to have surgery. Garlic should not be used by persons with stomach inflammation, gastritis, or hypersensitivity to this herb. Class 2c herb (bulb).

🜂 = Pregnancy   ✋ = Pediatric   ◆ = Alert   ∅ = Popular Herb

Precautionary Information—cont'd

Side Effects/Adverse Reactions

Central Nervous System: Dizziness, headache, irritability
Gastrointestinal: Nausea, vomiting, anorexia
Genitourinary: Hypothyroidism
Integumentary: Hypersensitivity reactions, contact dermatitis
Systemic: Diaphoresis, garlic odor, irritation of the oral cavity, decreased red blood cells

G

Interactions with Garlic

Drug

Anticoagulants (anisindione, dicumerol, heparin, warfarin): Garlic may increase bleeding when used with anticoagulants; do not use concurrently.
Insulin: Because of the hypoglycemic effects of garlic, insulin dosages may need to be adjusted.
Oral antidiabetics (acetohexamide, chlorpropamide, glipizide, metformin, tolazamide, tolbutamide, troglitazone): Because of the hypoglycemic effects of garlic, oral antidiabetic dosages may need to be adjusted.

Food

None known

Herb

Acidophilus: Acidophilus may decrease the absorption of garlic. If taken concurrently, separate the dosages by 3 hours.

Lab Test

Garlic may decrease LDL cholesterol (aged extract taken continuously), platelet aggregation (aged extract of garlic taken over extended period of time), triglycerides (aged extract of garlic taken over extended period of time), blood lipid profile. Garlic may increase prothrombin time and serum immunoglobulin E (IgE).

🍀 Endangered Herb   Adverse effects: BOLD = life-threatening

Client Considerations

Assess

- Because garlic is a common allergen, assess for hypersensitivity reactions and contact dermatitis. If such reactions are present, discontinue use of garlic and administer antihistamine or other appropriate therapy.
- Assess lipid levels if the client is using garlic to decrease lipids.
- Monitor CBC and coagulation studies if the client is using garlic at high doses or with anticoagulants. Identify anticoagulants the client is using, including salicylates (see Interactions).
- Determine whether the client is diabetic and is using insulin or oral antidiabetics; dosages may need to be adjusted (see Interactions).

Administer

- Instruct the client to avoid the daily use of medicinal garlic, unless under the supervision of a qualified herbalist. Blood clotting may be affected.
- Instruct the client to store garlic products in a sealed container away from heat and moisture.

Teach Client/Family

- Because garlic may stimulate labor and cause colic in infants, caution the client not to use this herb during pregnancy or lactation. However, some studies have indicated that garlic may be helpful in treating children with hypercholesterolemia (McCindle, 1998).
- Advise the client to inform all health care providers of garlic use.
- Caution the client to discontinue use of garlic before undergoing any invasive procedure in which bleeding may occur.

Pharmacology

Pharmacokinetics

Pharmacokinetics and pharmacodynamics are unknown.

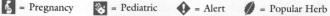

Primary Chemical Components of Garlic and Their Possible Actions

Chemical Class	Individual Component	Possible Action
Volatile oil	Alliin	Decreased platelet aggregation
	Allicin	
Alliinase		
Ajoene		Antiplatelet effect
Terpene	Citral; Geraniol; Linalool	
Diallyl sulfide		
Vitamin	A; B; C; E	
Mineral	Selenium	Antioxidant
	Germanium; Zinc; Magnesium	
Amino acid		
Glycoside		

G

Actions

The main actions attributed to garlic are antimicrobial, antilipidemic, antitriglyceride, antiplatelet, antioxidant, and cancer preventative.

Antimicrobial Action

A study using aqueous extracts of garlic in vitro showed that garlic inhibits both gram-positive and gram-negative organisms (Elmma, 1983; Sovova, 2002). Other studies have demonstrated the antimicrobial action of garlic against *Mycobacterium tuberculosis* (Hughes, 1991) and *Staphylococcus aureus* (Gonzalez-Fandos, 1994). Between 1983 and 1996, various studies identified the antifungal, antiviral, and antiparasitic actions of garlic.

Cardiovascular Action

Garlic has been shown to exert cholesterol-lowering, triglyceride-lowering, and antiplatelet actions.

Cholesterol-Lowering and Triglyceride-Lowering Actions
In one study, the cholesterol-lowering action of garlic was equal to that of bezafibrate, a prescription drug available in Germany (Holzgartner, 1992). However, results of other studies have been mixed. One study showed no difference in cholesterol levels between the experimental and the control group (Neil,

1996). However, a more recent study showed an 11% reduction in the cholesterol levels of male subjects after 12 weeks of garlic treatment (Adler, 1997). The chemical component believed to be responsible for the anticholesterol action is allicin, which is believed to reduce cholesterol production by preventing gastric lipase fat digestion and fecal excretion of sterols and bile acids (Gebhardt, 1993).

Antiplatelet Action

The antiplatelet effect of garlic has been demonstrated, with ajoene apparently functioning as the chemical component responsible (Apitz-Castro, 1994). Several investigations have demonstrated the ability of garlic to reduce platelet aggregation and cyclooxygenase (Bordia, 1996; Ali, 1995; Apitz-Castro, 1994). Among the documented results are improved circulation, decreased atherosclerosis, and improved intermittent claudication.

Cancer Prevention

A large amount of evidence is available to support the beneficial effects of garlic in the prevention of cancer and the slowing of its progression. One study showed a decrease in the development of gastric cancer when garlic was added to the diet (Buiatti, 1989). Another study has shown that the addition of vegetables in the *Allium* family (onions, leeks, garlic) to the diet prevents gastric cancer (Dorant, 1996). The protective effects may be due to the antioxidant properties of these vegetables and their ability to inhibit cancer cell proliferation.

Other Actions

Garlic has been shown to inhibit free radicals, which may be responsible for cancer proliferation, and to decrease lipid peroxidation (Rietz, 1995). Other actions have been proposed, such as the hypoglycemic effects of garlic and its role as a protectant against lead, cadmium, and radiation poisoning, but to date little research supports these claims.

References

Adler AJ et al: Effect of garlic and fish-oil supplementation on serum lipid and lipoprotein concentrations in hypercholesterolemic men, *Am J Clin Nutr* 65(2):445-450, 1997.

Ali M: Mechanism by which garlic inhibits cyclooxygenase activity: effect of raw versus boiled garlic extract on the synthesis of prostanoids, *Prostaglandins Leukot Essent Fatty Acids* 53(6):397-400, 1995.

Apitz-Castro R et al: Evidence for direct coupling of primary agonist receptor interaction to the exposure of functional IIb-IIIa complexes in

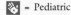

human blood platelet result from studies with the antiplatelet compound ajoene, *Biochim Biophys Acta* 1094:269-280, 1994.

Bordia A et al: Effect of garlic on platelet aggregation in humans: a study in healthy subjects and patients with coronary artery disease, *Prostaglandins Leukot Essent Fatty Acids* 55(3):201-205, 1996.

Blumenthal M, editor: *The complete German Commission E monographs: therapeutic guide to herbal medicines,* Austin, Tex, American Botanical Council; Boston, Integrative Medicine Communication, 1998.

Buiatti E et al: A case controlled study of gastric cancer and diet in Italy, *Int J Cancer* 44:611-616, 1989.

Dorant E et al: Consumption of onions and a reduced risk of stomach carcinoma, *Gastroenterology* 110(1):12-20, 1996.

Elmma E et al: The antimicrobial activity of garlic and onion extracts, *Pharmazie* 38:747-748, 1983.

Gebhardt R: Multiple inhibitory effects of garlic extracts on cholesterol biosynthesis in hepatocytes, *Lipids* 28(7):613-619, 1993.

Gonzalez-Fandos E et al: Staphylococcal growth and enterotoxins (A-D) and thermonuclease synthesis in the presence of dehydrated garlic, *J Appl Bacteriol* 77(5):549-552, 1994.

Holzgartner H et al: Comparison of the efficacy and tolerance of a garlic preparation versus bezafibrate, *Arzneimittelforschung* 42:1473-1477, 1992.

Hughes B et al: Antimicrobial effects of *Allium sativum, Allium ampeloprasum* and *Allium cepa,* garlic compounds and commercial garlic supplement products, *Phytother Res* 5:154-158, 1991.

McCaleb R et al: *The encyclopedia of popular herbs: your complete guide to leading medicinal plants,* Roseville, Calif, 2000, Prima Health.

McCindle BW, Conner WT: Garlic extract therapy in children with hypercholesterolemia, *Arch Pediatr Adolesc Med* 152(11):1089-1094, 1998.

Murray M, Pizzarno J: *The encyclopedia of natural medicine,* 2 ed (revised), Roseville, Calif, 1998, Prima.

Neil HA et al: Garlic powder in the treatment of moderate hyperlipidaemia: a controlled trial and meta-analysis, *J R Coll Physicians Lond* 30(4):329-334, 1996.

Rietz B et al: The radical scavenging ability of garlic examined in various models, *Boll Chim Farm* 134(2):69-76, 1995.

Romm A: Better Nutrition's 2000 guide to children's supplements, *Better Nutrition* 62(10):38-43, 2000.

Sovovo M et al: Pharmaceutical importance of *Allium sativus* L. II. antibacterial effects, *Ceska Slov Farm* 51(1):11-61, 2002.

Gentian
(jehn'shuhn)

Scientific names: *Gentiana lutea* L., *Gentiana acaulis* L.

Other common names: Bitter root, bitterwort, feltwort, gall weed, pale gentian, stemless gentian, yellow gentian

Class 2d (Root)

Origin: Gentian is a flowering perennial found in Europe and Asia.

Uses

Reported Uses

Gentian has been used to stimulate the appetite and to treat digestive disorders such as colitis, irritable bowel syndrome, colic, gallstones, biliary pain, peptic ulcer, and heartburn. It is also used as a component in alcoholic beverages (bitters).

Product Availability and Dosages

Available Forms

Fluid extract, infusion, root, tea, tincture

Plant Parts Used: Rhizome, roots

Dosages and Routes

Adult

All dosages listed are PO.
- Fluid extract: 2-4 g qd (Blumenthal, 1998)
- Infusion: no dosage consensus
- Root: 2-4 g qd (Blumenthal, 1998)
- Tea: Place ½ tsp in 4 oz water, boil and strain, take tid ac
- Tincture: 1-3 g qd (Blumenthal, 1998); 2 ml tid (1:5 dilution) (Mills, 2000)

Precautionary Information

Contraindications

Until more research is available, gentian should not be used during pregnancy, and it should not be given to children. Gentian should not be used by persons with hypersensitivity to this herb, those with stomach irritability or inflammation, or those with stomach or duodenal ulcers. Class 2d herb (root).

🐾 = Pregnancy   🐾 = Pediatric   ❶ = Alert   🌿 = Popular Herb

Precautionary Information—cont'd
Side Effects/Adverse Reactions
Central Nervous System: Headache
Gastrointestinal: Nausea, vomiting, anorexia
Integumentary: Hypersensitivity reactions

Interactions with Gentian

Drug
Iron salts: Gentian may interfere with absorption of iron salts;
separate by at least 2 hours.

Food	Herb	Lab Test
None known	None known	None known

G

Client Considerations
Assess
- Assess for hypersensitivity reactions. If present, discontinue use of this herb and administer antihistamine or other appropriate therapy.

Administer
- Instruct the client to store gentian products in a cool, dry place, away from heat and moisture.

Teach Client/Family

- Until more research is available, caution the client not to use gentian during pregnancy and not to give it to children.

Pharmacology
Pharmacokinetics
Pharmacokinetics and pharmacodynamics are unknown.

Primary Chemical Components of Gentian and Their Possible Actions		
Chemical Class	**Individual Component**	**Possible Action**
Gentiopicrin Gentiamarin Gentiin Gentisin Gentianose Gentisic acid		Increased salivation, digestive juice secretions

Actions

Very little primary research is available for gentian. It is typically used to stimulate the appetite and is usually mixed in alcoholic products. However, no studies support this use.

References

Blumenthal M, editor: *The complete German Commission E monographs: therapeutic guide to herbal medicines,* Austin, Tex, American Botanical Council; Boston, Integrative Medicine Communication, 1998.

Duke J: *CRC handbook of medicinal herbs,* Boca Raton, Fla, 1985, CRC Press.

Mills S, Bone K: *Principles and practice of phytotherapy,* London, 2000 Churchill Livingstone.

 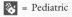 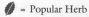

= Pregnancy   = Pediatric   = Alert   = Popular Herb

Ginger

(jin-juhr)

Scientific name: *Zingiber officinale*
Other common names: Black ginger, race ginger, zingiber

Class 1 (Fresh Root)
Class 2b/2d (Dried Root)

Origin: Ginger is found in the tropics of Asia and is now culti-vated in the tropics of South America, China, India, Africa, the Caribbean, and parts of the United States.

Uses

Reported Uses

Ginger is used as an antioxidant; to prevent and relieve motion and morning sickness; to relieve sore throat, nausea, and vomiting; and to treat migraine headaches.

Investigational Uses

Preliminary research is available that documents the efficacy of ginger in decreasing the pain and inflammation associated with arthritis and other joint disorders. Some evidence indicates that it may also reduce platelet aggregation.

Product Availability and Dosages

Available Forms

Capsules, dried root, extract, fresh root, powder, tablets, tea, tincture

Plant Parts Used: Rhizome

Dosages and Routes

Ginger may be standardized to its volatile oil (4%) or essential oil (8%).

Adult

All dosages listed are PO.

General Use

- Dried ginger capsules: 1 g/day (McCaleb, 2000)
- Dried root equivalent: 500 mg bid-qid (Mills, 2000)
- Fluid extract: 0.7-2 ml/day (1:2 dilution) (Mills, 2000)
- Fresh root equivalent: 500-1000 mg tid (Mills, 2000)
- Tablets: 500 mg bid-qid (Mills, 2000)
- Tincture: 1.7-5 ml/day (1:5 dilution) (Mills, 2000)

Migraine
- Dried ginger: 500 mg qid
- Extract:100-200 mg, standardized to 20% ginerol and shogol
- Fresh ginger: 10 g/day (¼-in slice) (Murray, 1998)

Motion and Morning Sickness Prevention
- Extract:100-200 mg, standardized to 20% ginerol and shogol
- Powder: 1-2 g ½-1 hr before traveling or upon arising
- Tea, dried root: 1½ tsp ground dried root in 1 cup water, boil 5-10 min, drink prn
- Tea, fresh root: 1 tsp fresh root in 1 cup water, infuse 5 min, drink prn

Rheumatoid Arthritis
- Extract: 100-200 mg, standardized to 20% ginerol and shogol (Murray, 1998)
- Fresh ginger: 8-10 g/day (Murray, 1998)

Sore Throat
- Fresh root tea: 1 tsp fresh root in 1 cup water, infuse 5 min, gargle prn (Murray, 1998)

Child

All dosages listed are PO.

General Use
- Ginger root tea: ¼-1 cup prn (Romm, 2000)
- Tincture: 5-25 drops in water prn (Romm, 2000)

Precautionary Information

Contraindications

Because it is an abortifacient in large amounts, until more research is available, ginger should not be used during pregnancy and lactation. It should not be used by persons with hypersensitivity to it. Unless directed by a physician, ginger should not be used by persons with cholelithiasis. Class 1 herb (fresh root); class 2b/2d herb (dried root).

Side Effects/Adverse Reactions

Gastrointestinal: Nausea, vomiting, anorexia
Integumentary: Hypersensitivity reactions

Interactions with Ginger

Drug

All oral medications: Ginger may increase absorption of all medications taken orally.

Anticoagulants (ardeparin, anisindione, aspirin, dicumerol, dalteparin, heparin, warfarin): Ginger may increase the risk of bleeding when used concurrently with anticoagulants (theoretical).

Antiplatelets (abciximab): Ginger may increase the risk of bleeding when used concurrently with antiplatelets (theoretical).

Food	Herb
None known	None known

Lab Test

Ginger may increase plasma partial prothrombin time (PTT) in clients taking warfarin concurrently and may increase prothrombin time (PT).

Client Considerations

Assess

- Assess for hypersensitivity reactions. If present, discontinue use of this herb and administer antihistamine or other appropriate therapy.
- Assess all medications used (see Interactions).

Administer

- Instruct the client to store ginger products in a cool, dry place, away from heat and moisture.

Teach Client/Family

- Until more research is available, caution the client not to use ginger during pregnancy and lactation.

Pharmacology

Pharmacokinetics

Information on the pharmacokinetics and pharmacodynamics of ginger is limited. Its metabolites are known to be eliminated via urinary excretion within 24 hours, and it is 90% bound to plasma proteins (Monge, 1976).

Primary Chemical Components of Ginger and Their Possible Actions

Chemical Class	Individual Component	Possible Action
Pungent	Gingerol	Antioxidant; antiulcer
	Zingerone	Antioxidant
	Shogaol	
Volatile oil	Bisabolene; Zingiberene; Zingiberol	
Proteolytic enzyme		
Gingesulphonic acid		Antiulcer
Sesquiterpene		Antiviral

Actions

Antiemetic and Antinausea Actions

Several studies have documented the antiemetic and antinausea actions of ginger. When dried ginger powder was evaluated against dimenhydrinate and a placebo, ginger was found to reduce nausea and vomiting more effectively than dimenhydrinate (Mowrey, 1982). This effect is postulated to result from action on the digestive tract instead of the central nervous system. Ginger lacks any anticholinergic effects. Since these studies were completed, several other studies have also confirmed the antiemetic and antinausea effects of ginger (Fischer-Rasmussen, 1990; Bone, 1990; Liu, 1990).

Antiinflammatory Action

In one study, the ability of ginger to decrease induced paw edema in laboratory animals was equal to that of aspirin. Its ability to inhibit arachidonic acid metabolism is believed to be responsible. Ginger has been used in traditional medicine to treat rheumatic disorders (Srivastava, 1989).

Other Actions

Other actions for ginger include improved digestive function; antiulcer, antiplatelet, antipyretic, antiinfective, antioxidant, and antidiabetic action; and positive inotropic action.

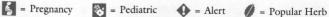

Improved Digestive Functioning

Improved digestive functioning may occur as a result of increased amylase and salivary production (Yamahara, 1985). Ginger has been shown to increase the absorption of other drugs and to prevent degradation during the first hepatic pass (Chang, 1987).

Antiulcer Action

The antiulcer effects of ginger may be due to two of its chemical components, gingerol and gingesulphonic acid. Improvements in ulcer patients occurred with the use of ginger decocted in water. However, relapse was common, and complete cure did not occur (Chang, 1987).

Antiplatelet Action

The antiplatelet action of ginger may be a result of the inhibition of thromboxane formation. Increases occurred in ADP, collagen, arachidonic acid, and epinephrine when ginger was used (Srivastava, 1984).

Antipyretic Action

The antipyretic effect of ginger is due to its prostaglandin inhibition. Ginger is as effective as aspirin in reducing fever (Mascolo, 1989).

Antiinfective Action

Ginger exerts antiinfective action against both gram-positive and gram-negative bacteria. Its antiinfective action was very weak when tested; however, one class of chemical components, the sesquiterpenes, did exert significant action against antirhinoviral infections (Denyer, 1994).

Antioxidant Action

The antioxidant effects of ginger may be the result of the actions of gingerol and zingerone, two of its chemical components. These components inhibit lipoxygenase and eliminate the radicals superoxide and hydroxyl (Cao, 1993). Another study (Ahmed, 2000) identified a significant lowered lipid peroxidation by maintaining activities of the antioxidant enzymes, again strengthening the supportive evidence for use of ginger as an antioxidant.

Antidiabetic Action

Ginger may be useful in the treatment of hyperglycemia. Rabbits treated with ginger exhibited a hypoglycemic effect (Mascolo, 1989).

Positive Inotropic Action

In one study, the cardiovascular actions of ginger included a positive inotropic effect. When subjects were asked to chew fresh ginger, their blood pressure increased. This action resulted from the pressor response, but it was short term (Chang, 1987).

References

Ahmed RS et al: Influence of dietary ginger on antioxidant defence system in rat: comparison with ascorbic acid, *Indian J Exp Biol* 38(6):604-606, 2000.

Bone ME et al: Ginger root—a new antiemetic: the effect of ginger root on postoperative nausea and vomiting after major gynaecological surgery, *Anaesthesia* 45(8):669-671, 1990.

Cao ZF et al: Scavenging effects of ginger on superoxide anion and hydroxyl radical, *Chung Kuo Chung Yao Tsa Chih* 18(12):750-751, 1993.

Chang HM et al: *Pharmacology and applications of Chinese materia medica*, Singapore, 1987, Scientific.

Denyer CL et al: Isolation of antirhinoviral sesquiterpenes from ginger (*Zingiber officinale*), *J Nat Prod* 57(5):658-662, 1994.

Fischer-Rasmussen W et al: Ginger treatment of *Hyperemesis gravidarum*, *Eur J Obstet Gynecol Reprod Biol* 38:19-24, 1990.

Liu WHD: Ginger root: a new antiemetic, *Anaesthesia* 45(12):1085, 1990.

Mascolo N et al: Ethnopharmacologic investigation of ginger, *J Ethnopharmacol* 27:129-140, 1989.

McCaleb R et al: *The encyclopedia of popular herbs: your complete guide to leading medicinal plants*, Roseville, Calif, 2000, Prima Health.

Mills S, Bone K: *Principles and practice of phytotherapy*, London, 2000, Churchill Livingstone.

Monge P et al: The metabolism of zingerone, a pungent principle of ginger, *Xenobiotic* 6(7):411-423, 1976.

Mowrey DB et al: Motion sickness, ginger and psychophysics, *Lancet* 1(8273):655-657, 1982.

Murray M, Pizzarno J: *The encyclopedia of natural medicine*, 2 ed (revised), Roseville, Calif, 1998, Prima.

Romm A: Better Nutrition's 2000 guide to children's supplements, *Better Nutrition* 62(10):38-43, 2000.

Srivastava KC: Effects of aqueous extracts of onion, garlic and ginger on platelet aggregation and metabolism of arachidonic acid in the blood vascular system: in vitro study, *Prostagland Leukot Med* 13(2):227-235, 1984.

Srivastava KC et al: Ginger (*Zingiber officinale*) and rheumatic disorders, *Med Hypotheses* 29:25-28, 1989.

Yamahara J et al: Cholagogic effect of ginger and its active constituents, *J Ethnopharmacol* 13(2):217-225, 1985.

Ginkgo
(ging'koe)

Scientific name: *Gingko biloba*

Other common names: Maidenhair tree, rokan, sophium, tanakan, tebofortan, tebonin   Class 1 (Leaf)

Origin: Ginkgo is a tree native to China and Japan. It is now also found in the United States and Europe.

Uses
Reported Uses
Gingko is used to decrease disturbances of cerebral functioning and peripheral vascular insufficiency in persons with Alzheimer's disease or other types of age-related dementia. It is also used as an antioxidant, to improve peripheral artery disease, and to enhance circulation throughout the body. Other reported uses include the treatment of depressive mood disorders, sexual dysfunction, asthma, glaucoma, menopausal symptoms, multiple sclerosis, headaches, tinnitus, dizziness, arthritis, altitude sickness, and intermittent claudication.

Product Availability and Dosages
Available Forms
Capsules, fluid extract, tablets, tincture

Plant Parts Used: Leaves

Dosages and Routes
Ginkgo may be standardized to 24% ginkgo flavonglycosides and 6% terpene trilactones.
Adult
All dosages listed are PO.
Alzheimer's Disease
- Capsules/extract/tablets: 80 mg tid standardized to 24% flavonglycosides (Murray, 1998)
Asthma
- Extract 80 mg tid (Murray, 1998)
Cerebral Vascular Insufficiency
- Extract: 80 mg tid standardized to 24% flavonglycosides (Murray, 1998)
General Use
- Standardized extract: 40 mg tid

🍃 Endangered Herb   Adverse effects: **BOLD** = life-threatening

Glaucoma
- Extract 40-80 mg tid standardized to 24% flavonglycosides (Murray, 1998)

Impotence From Arterial Insufficiency
- Extract: 80 mg tid standardized to 24% flavonglycosides (Murray, 1998)

Menopause
- Extract: 40 mg tid standardized to 24% flavonglycosides (Murray, 1998)

Multiple Sclerosis
- Extract: 40-80 mg tid standardized to 24% flavonglycosides (Murray, 1998)

Precautionary Information

Contraindications

Until more research is available, ginkgo should not be used during pregnancy or lactation, and it should not be given to children. It should not be used by persons with coagulation or platelet disorders, hemophilia, or hypersensitivity to this herb. Class 1 herb (leaf).

Side Effects/Adverse Reactions

Central Nervous System: Transient headache, anxiety, restlessness
Gastrointestinal: Nausea, vomiting, anorexia, diarrhea
Integumentary: Hypersensitivity reactions, rash

Interactions with Ginkgo

Drug

Anticonvulsants (carbamazepine, gabapentin, phenobarbital, phenytoin): Ginkgo components may decrease the anticonvulsant effect; avoid concurrent use.
Anticoagulants (anisindione, dalteparin, dicumerol, heparin, salicylates, warfarin): Because of the increased risk of bleeding, ginkgo should not be taken concurrently with anticoagulants.
MAOIs: MAOI action may be increased if taken with ginkgo; do not use concurrently (theoretical).

Interactions with Ginkgo—cont'd

Drug—cont'd

Platelet inhibitor (abciximab): Because of the increased risk of bleeding, ginkgo should not be taken concurrently with platelet inhibitors.

Food	Herb
None known	None known

Lab Test

Ginkgo may increase prothrombin time (PT) and blood salicylate, and may decrease platelet activity; Ginkgo may cause increased bleeding (partial thromboplastin time, ASA tolerance test).

G

Client Considerations

Assess

- Assess for hypersensitivity reactions. If present, discontinue use of this herb and administer antihistamine or other appropriate therapy.
- Assess for use of anticoagulants, platelets inhibitors, or MAOIs (see Interactions).

Administer

- Inform the client that ginkgo takes 1 to 6 months before it becomes effective.

Teach Client/Family

- Until more research is available, caution the client not to use ginkgo during pregnancy and lactation and not to give it to children.
- Caution the client not to use ginkgo with anticoagulants, platelet inhibitors, trazadone, or MAOIs.

Pharmacology

Pharmacokinetics

Excretion < 30% of metabolites. Bioavailability is unaffected by food.

Primary Chemical Components of Ginkgo and Their Possible Actions

Chemical Class	Individual Component	Possible Action
Flavonoid	Kaempferol; Quercetin Isorhamnetin; Myricetin	Antiinflammatory
Diterpene	Ginkgolides	Platelet inhibitor; neuroprotective effects
Sesquiterpene Triterpene Ginkgetin	Bilobalide Sterols; Benzoic; Ginkgolic	Antiinflammatory; antiarthritic

Actions

Much research is available documenting the uses and actions of *Ginkgo biloba* L. Ginkgo has been used in China since ancient times. Initial research began in Europe in the 1960s.

Cognitive Enhancement Action

The cognitive enhancement action of ginkgo is a result of the flavonoids present in the extract. The pharmacologic actions involve increased release of neurotransmitters, including catecholamines, and inhibition of monoamine oxidase (MAO). Approximately 50 controlled studies between 1975 and 1997 have demonstrated the positive effects of gingko in the treatment of cerebral insufficiency. All studies incorporated various dosages and varying lengths of treatment, and all results were positive (Hadjiivanova, 2002; Schulz, 1997).

Vasoprotective and Tissue-Protective Actions

The vasoprotective and tissue-protective actions of ginkgo result from several factors: its ability to relax blood vessels, to protect against capillary permeability, to inhibit platelet aggregation, and to decrease ischemia and edema. More recent studies have confirmed this effect in rabbits (Monboisse, 1993).

Other Actions

Gingko has been studied for its antioxidant effects, its relief of altitude sickness, its antiarthritic and analgesic effects, and its relief of ischemia in intermittent claudication.

 = Pregnancy   = Pediatric   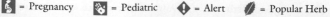 = Alert   = Popular Herb

Antioxidant Action

Gingko has been studied for its antioxidant effects. It has been found to eliminate free radicals and is able to inhibit polymorphonuclear neutrophils (Monboisse, 1993).

Altitude Sickness Relief

Gingko can also relieve altitude sickness. One study involving two groups of mountain climbers focused on the effects of gingko when traveling to high altitudes. One group took 160 mg of gingko daily while climbing while the other received a placebo. Both groups ascended to 14,700 feet and made other ascents from that point. None of the gingko group reported full-blown altitude sickness, whereas 82% of the placebo group did (Feng, 1989). Another study (Gertsch, 2002) was designed to identify the time needed to prevent acute mountain sickness (AMS). One day of pretreatment with ginkgo 60 mg tid significantly reduced the severity of AMS.

Antiarthritic and Analgesic Actions

Ginkgetin, a chemical component of gingko, has been studied for its antiarthritic and analgesic effects. Ginkgetin given in dosages of 10-20 mg/kg/day reduced arthritic inflammation in laboratory animals by 86% at the highest dose given (Kim, 1999).

References

Feng SH et al: Effects of shengmaiyin and danshen-chuanxiong decoction on preventing cardiopulmonary changes in adults caused by a high-altitude environment, *Zhong Xi Yi Jie He Za Zhi* 9(11):643, 650-652, 1989.

Gertsch JH et al: *Ginkgo biloba* for the prevention of severe acute mountain sickness (AMS) starting one day before rapid ascent, *High Alt Med Biol* 3(1):29-37, 2002.

Hadjiivanova CH et al: Effect of *Ginkgo biloba* extract on beta-adrenergic receptors in different rat brain regions, *Phytother* 16(5):488-490, 2002.

Kim HK et al: Inhibition of rat adjuvant-induced arthritis by ginkgetin, a biflavone from *Ginkgo biloba* leaves, *Planta Med* 65:465-467, 1999.

Monboisse JC et al: Advances in *Gingko biloba* extract research 2:123-128, 1993.

Murray M, Pizzarno J: *The encyclopedia of natural medicine,* 2 ed (revised), Roseville, Calif, 1998, Prima.

Schulz V et al: Clinical trials with phyto-psychopharmacological agents, *Phytomedicine* 4(4):379-387, 1997.

Ginseng
(jin'sing)

Scientific names: *Panax quinquefolius, Panax ginseng*

Other common names: American ginseng, Asiatic ginseng, Chinese ginseng, five-fingers, Japanese ginseng, jintsam, Korean ginseng, ninjin, Oriental ginseng, schinsent, seng and sang, tartar root, Western ginseng

Class 2d (Root)

Origin: Ginseng is now found throughout the world. *Panax quinquefolius* is native to North America; *Panax ginseng* is native to the Far East.

Uses

Reported Uses

Ginseng has been used for a variety of purposes for about 5000 years. It has been used to increase physical endurance and lessen fatigue, to improve the ability to cope with stress, and to improve concentration. It also may improve overall well being. Many herbalists consider it a tonic.

Investigational Uses

Initial research is exploring the use of ginseng to improve cognitive functioning and to treat diabetes mellitus, hyperlipidemia, seizure disorders, cancer, male infertility, male erectile dysfunction, to enhance immunity, emphysema, for tuberculosis children, and rheumatoid arthritis.

Product Availability and Dosages

Available Forms

Capsules, dried root used for decoction, extract, powder, standardized extract, tea, tincture; may be found in creams and lotions used to treat wrinkles

Plant Parts Used: Roots

Dosages and Routes

Standardized extracts contain 5% ginsenosides (an aglycone chemical component believed to act as a stimulant).
Adult
All dosages listed are PO.

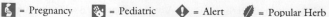
🍃 = Pregnancy   🔅 = Pediatric   ◆ = Alert   🍂 = Popular Herb

General Use
- Capsules: 200-500 mg extract qd (Blumenthal, 1998)
- Infusion: pour boiling water over 3 g herb, let stand 10 min, strain; may be taken tid for 3-4 wk
- Powdered root: 1-4 g qd
- Standardized extract: 200-500 mg qd (Blumenthal, 1998)
- Tincture: 1-2 ml extract qd (1:1 dilution) (Blumenthal, 1998)

Male Infertility
- Crude herb (root, high quality): 1.5-2 g tid (Murray, 1998)
- Extract: 100-200 mg tid standardized to 5% ginsenosides (Murray, 1998)

Rheumatoid Arthritis
- Crude herb: 4.5-6 g/day in divided doses
- Extract: 500 mg qd-tid

G

Precautionary Information

Contraindications

Until more research is available, ginseng should not be used during pregnancy and lactation and it should not be given to children. Ginseng should not be used by persons with hypertension, cardiac disorders, or hypersensitivity to it. Class 2d herb (root).

Side Effects/Adverse Reactions

Cardiovascular: Hypertension, chest pain, palpitations
Central Nervous System: Anxiety, insomnia, restlessness (high doses), headache
Gastrointestinal: Nausea, vomiting, anorexia, diarrhea (high doses)
Ginseng Abuse Syndrome: EDEMA, INSOMNIA, HYPERTONIA
Integumentary: Hypersensitivity reactions, rash
Cardiovascular: Decreased diastolic blood pressure, increase QTc interval.

Interactions with Ginseng

Drug

Anticoagulants (anisindione, dicumarol, heparin, warfarin): Ginseng may decrease the action of anticoagulants.
Anticonvulsants: Ginseng may provide an additive anticonvulsant action (theoretical).

Continued

Interactions with Ginseng—cont'd

Drug—cont'd

Immunosuppressants (azathioprine, basiliximab, cyclosporine, daclizumab, muromonab, mycophenolate, tacrolimus): Ginseng may diminish the effect of immunosuppressants; do not use immediately before, during, or after transplant surgery.

Insulin: Because ginseng is known to decrease blood glucose levels, it may increase the hypoglycemic effect of insulin; avoid concurrent use.

MAOIs (isocarboxazid, phenelzine, tranylcypromine): Concurrent use of MAOIs with ginseng may result in manic-like syndrome.

Oral antidiabetics (acetohexamide, chlorpropamide, glipizide, metformin, tolazamide, tolbutamide, troglitazone): Because ginseng is known to decrease blood glucose levels, it may increase the hypoglycemic effect of antidiabetics; avoid concurrent use.

Stimulants: Use of stimulants (e.g., xanthines) concurrently with ginseng is not recommended; overstimulation may occur.

Food

Overstimulation may occur when ginseng is used with caffeinated coffee, cola, and tea; avoid concurrent use.

Herb

Ephedra: Concurrent use of ephedra and ginseng may increase hypertension and central nervous system stimulation; avoid concurrent use.

Lab Test

Ginseng may decrease blood glucose (decoctions, infusions). It may increase plasma partial thromboplastin time (PTT) and have an additive effect on serum and 24-hour urine estrogens. Ginseng may falsely increase serum digoxin.

Client Considerations

Assess

- Assess for hypersensitivity reactions and rash. If these are present, discontinue use of this herb and administer antihistamine or other appropriate therapy.

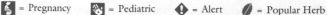

 = Pregnancy   = Pediatric   ◆ = Alert   ∅ = Popular Herb

- Assess for ginseng abuse syndrome: insomnia, edema, and hypertonia.
- Assess for the use of stimulants, anticoagulants, MAOIs, and antidiabetics (see Interactions).

Administer

- Instruct the client to store ginseng products in a cool, dry place, away from heat and moisture.
- Instruct the client to avoid the continuous use of ginseng. The recommendation is to use this herb for no more than 3 continuous months, taking a break between courses (Mills, 2000).

G

Teach Client/Family

- Until more research is available, caution the client not to use this herb during pregnancy and lactation and not to give it to children.
- Advise the client to use other stimulants and antidiabetics carefully if taking concurrently with ginseng (see Interactions).
- Warn the client of the life-threatening side effects of ginseng abuse syndrome.
- Instruct the client that *Siberian ginseng* and *Panax ginseng* are not the same.

Pharmacology
Pharmacokinetics

Pharmacokinetics and pharmacodynamics are unknown.

Primary Chemical Components of Ginseng and Their Possible Actions

Chemical Class	Individual Component	Possible Action
Agylcone	Ginsenosides	Stimulant inhibits platelet activating factor, anticancer
Triterpene saponin		
Sesquiterpene		
Polyacetylenes	Falcarinol; Falcarintriol	
Polysaccharide	Panaxans A-U	Antidiabetic
Adenosine		Antidiabetic
Essential Oil		
Peptides		

🌀 Endangered Herb   Adverse effects: BOLD = life-threatening

Actions

Most of the available research on ginseng comes from Asia, where this herb has been studied extensively. Investigators have completed research on the ability of ginseng to decrease fatigue, increase physical performance, and improve mental functioning. Studies have also been done on its anticancer and antidiabetic effects.

Decreased Fatigue, Increased Physical Performance, and Improved Mental Function

Decreased Fatigue

One study used a questionnaire to identify participants with fatigue. The subjects were treated with either ginseng or a placebo. Results showed significant improvement in fatigue with the use of ginseng as compared with the use of a placebo (Le Gal, 1996).

Increased Physical Performance

Studies using both human subjects and laboratory animals indicate that ginseng increases physical performance. In one study, male athletes took 200 mg of standardized ginseng daily. Their performance increased significantly, as demonstrated by measurements including increased oxygen utilization and improved reaction time (Forgo, 1985).

Improved Mental Function

In both animal and human studies, ginseng has been shown to improve mental functioning. One study revealed improved learning and memory in rats (Saito, 1977).

Anticonvulsant Action

Generalized tonic-clonic convulsions were induced in rats by chemical means, then *Panax ginseng* was given to one group every day: 100 mg/kg ½ hour before administration of convulsive chemical (Gupta, 2001). There was significant protection in the group treated with *Panax ginseng*. *Panax ginseng* may show promise as an anticonvulsant.

Anticancer Action

A significant reduction in cancer risk occurred when a large group of human subjects was divided into control and experimental groups, matched for multiple risk factors, and given ginseng. Those taking ginseng had a lower cancer risk than those in the control group (Yun, 1990). Another study indicates that long-term administration of ginseng inhibits tumor growth (Yun, 1983).

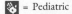 = Pregnancy   = Pediatric   = Alert   = Popular Herb

Antidiabetic Action

Ginseng has been used for centuries to treat diabetes mellitus. Its antidiabetic action results from the chemical components from adenosine, known as panaxans, and others (Ng, 1985).

References

Blumenthal M, editor: *The complete German Commission E monographs: therapeutic guide to herbal medicines,* Austin, Tex, American Botanical Council; Boston, Integrative Medicine Communication, 1998.

Forgo I et al: The duration of effect of the standardized ginseng extract G115 in healthy competitive athletes, *Notobene Medici* 15(9):636-640, 1985.

Gupta YK et al: Antiepileptic activity of *Panax ginseng* against pentylene-tetrazole induced kindling in rats, *Indian J Physiol Pharmacol* 45(4): 502-506, 2001.

Le Gal M et al: Pharmation capsules in the treatment of functional fatigue: a double-blind study versus placebo evaluated by a new methodology, *Phytotherapy Res* 10:49-53, 1996.

Mills S, Bone K: *Principles and practice of phytotherapy,* London, 2000, Churchill Livingstone.

Murray M, Pizzarno J: *The encyclopedia of natural medicine,* 2 ed (revised), Roseville, Calif, 1998, Prima.

Ng TB et al: Hypoglycemic constituents of *Panax ginseng, Gen Pharmacol* 6:549-552, 1985.

Saito H et al: Effects of *Panax ginseng* root on conditional avoidance response in rats, *Japan J Pharm* 27:509-516, 1977.

Yun TK et al: Anticarcinogenic effect of long-term oral administration of newborn mice exposed to various chemical carcinogens, *Cancer Detect Prev* 6:515-525, 1983.

Yun TK et al: A case-control study of ginseng intake and cancer, *Int J Epidemiol* 19(4):871-876, 1990.

Glucomannan
(glew-koe-man′uhn)

Scientific name: *Amorphophallus konjac*

Other common names: Konjac, konjac mannan

Origin: Glucomannan is purified from konjac flour by chemical processing.

Uses

Reported Uses

Glucomannan is useful as a bulk laxative.

 Endangered Herb   Adverse effects: BOLD = life-threatening

Investigational Uses

Researchers are studying glucomannan for its lipid-lowering action and it antidiabetic effects. It has also shown some efficacy in promoting weight loss.

Product Availability and Dosages

Available Forms

Capsules, powder, tablets

Plant Parts Used: Tubers

Dosages and Routes

Adult

Diabetes Mellitus

- PO capsules/tablets: up to 7.2 g qd; treatment of longer than 3 mo may be required

Lipid Lowering

- PO capsules/tablets: no consensus on dosage

Weight Loss

- PO capsules/tablets: 1.5 g bid for 2 months or longer

Precautionary Information

Contraindications

Until more research is available, glucomannan should not be used during pregnancy and lactation and should not be given to children. Persons with hypersensitivity to glucomannan should not use it.

Side Effects/Adverse Reactions

Endocrine: Hypoglycemia

Gastrointestinal: Nausea, vomiting, anorexia, diarrhea, flatulence, cramping, dyspepsia, GASTROINTESTINAL OBSTRUCTION OR PERFORATION

Integumentary: Hypersensitivity reactions

Interactions with Glucomannan

Drug

All medications: Glucomannan may decrease the absorption of medications if taken concurrently; separate dosages by at least 2 hours.

Antilipidemics: Glucomannan may increase the action of antilipidemics.

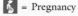 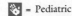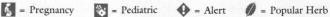

Interactions with Glucomannan—cont'd		
Drug—cont'd		
Insulin: Glucomannan may increase the hypoglycemic effect of insulin.		
Oral antidiabetics: Glucomannan may increase the hypoglycemic effect of oral antidiabetics.		
Food	Herb	Lab Test
None known	None known	None known

G

Client Considerations

Assess

- Assess for hypersensitivity reactions. If present, discontinue use of glucomannan and administer antihistamine or other appropriate therapy.
- Assess for use of medications. Concurrent glucomannan use may decrease their absorption or increase their effects (see Interactions).

Administer

- Instruct the client to store glucomannan products in a cool, dry place, away from heat and moisture.

Teach Client/Family

- Until more research is available, caution the client not to use glucomannan during pregnancy and lactation and not to give it to children.
- Caution the client that gastrointestinal obstruction and perforation have occurred in conjunction with use of this product.

Pharmacology

Pharmacokinetics

Pharmacokinetics and pharmacodynamics are unknown.

Primary Chemical Components of Glucomannan and Their Possible Actions		
Chemical Class	**Individual Component**	**Possible Action**
Polysaccharide	Mannose	Laxative; hypoglycemic; anticholesteremic
	Glucose	

Actions

Because some of the chemical components are the same (mannose and a similar polysaccharide, galactose), glucomannan has many of the same properties as guar gum. For this reason, the actions of guar gum and glucomannan may be expected to be the same. Glucomannan has been used as an antidiabetic, an anticholesteremic, an aid to weight reduction, and a laxative.

Antidiabetic Action

Glucomannan has been shown to delay absorption of glucose from the intestine (Jenkins, 1978). In one study in which diabetic clients received glucomannan for 3 months, fasting blood glucose levels decreased by approximately one third, and dosages of antidiabetics were able to be reduced (Doi, 1979).

Anticholesteremic Action

In one study using laboratory rats, cholesterol levels were reduced when glucomannan was added to the rats' diet (Kiriyama, 1969). When overweight individuals with high cholesterol levels were given 100 ml of a 1% glucomannan solution for 11 weeks, cholesterol levels decreased by a mean of 18%. In another study, men's cholesterol levels decreased by approximately 10% (Arvill, 1995).

Weight Reduction

Results have been mixed when glucomannan is used for weight reduction. One study showed a decrease in weight of 2.2 kg at the end of 2 months when 1.5 g of glucomannan was added to the diet twice a day (Reffo, 1990).

Laxative Action

Because the addition of water to the polysaccharides glucose and mannose causes them to swell, these substances are used as

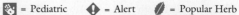

bulk laxatives. Viscosity of the intestinal contents is increased and gastric emptying is slowed. This may be of benefit for chronic constipation in neurologically impaired children (Staiano, 2000).

References

Arvill A et al: *J Clin Nutr* 61(3):585, 1995.
Doi K et al: *Lancet* 1:987, 1979.
Jenkins DJ et al: *Br Med J* 1(6124):1392, 1978.
Kiriyama S et al: *J Nutr* 97(3):382, 1969.
Reffo GC et al: *Curr Ther Res* 47:753, 1990.
Staiano A et al: Effect of the dietary fiber glucomannan on chronic constipation in neurologically impaired children, *J Pediatr* 136(1):41-45, 2000.

G

Glucosamine
(glew-koe'suh-meen)

Scientific name: 2-amino-2-deoxyglucose

Other common names: Chitosamine, GS

Origin: Glucosamine is found in mucopolysaccharides, chitin, and mucoproteins. Glucosamine is a naturally occurring substance; glucosamine sulfate is manufactured synthetically.

Uses

Reported Uses

Glucosamine typically is used in conjunction with chondroitin to treat joint conditions such as those associated with arthritis.

Investigational Uses

Investigators are working to determine whether glucosamine may be effective in the treatment of diabetes mellitus.

Product Availability and Dosages

Available Forms

Capsules, tablets

Dosages and Routes

Adult

General Use

• PO capsules/tablets: 1500 mg glucosamine and 1200 mg chondroitin for average-weight individuals; lower doses for

🌿 Endangered Herb   Adverse effects: BOLD = life-threatening

underweight individuals; higher doses for overweight individuals

Osteoarthritis

- PO capsules/tablets: 1500 mg/day (Murray, 1998)

Precautionary Information

Contraindications

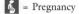

Until more research is available, glucosamine should not be used during pregnancy and lactation and, because its effects on them are unknown, it should not be given to children. Glucosamine should not be used by persons with hypersensitivity to it.

Side Effects/Adverse Reactions

Central Nervous System: Drowsiness, headache

Gastrointestinal: Nausea, vomiting, anorexia, constipation or diarrhea, heartburn, epigastric pain and cramps, indigestion

Integumentary: Hypersensitivity reactions, rash (rare)

Interactions with Glucosamine

Drug

Antidiabetics: Glucosamine may increase the effects of antidiabetics (theoretical).

Food	Herb	Lab Test
None known	None known	None known

Client Considerations

Assess

- Assess for hypersensitivity reactions, rash (rare). If these are present, discontinue use of glucosamine and administer antihistamine or other appropriate therapy.
- Assess for joint pain, stiffness, and aggravating or ameliorating factors.
- Monitor blood glucose in diabetic patients (see Interactions).

Administer

- Instruct the client to take glucosamine PO with food to reduce gastric upset.

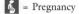 = Pregnancy   = Pediatric   = Alert   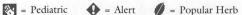 = Popular Herb

- Instruct the client to store glucosamine products in a cool, dry place, away from heat and moisture.

Teach Client/Family

- Until more research is available, caution the client not to use glucosamine during pregnancy and lactation and not to give it to children.
- Inform the diabetic client that glucosamine may lower blood glucose levels.

Pharmacology

Pharmacokinetics

Pharmacokinetics and pharmacodynamics are unknown.

Chemical Properties

Glucosamine sulfate is a synthetically manufactured product or is derived from chitin (marine exoskeletons). Glucosamine is required for synthesis of certain proteins needed for tendons, ligaments, and cartilage.

Actions

Antiarthritic Action

The primary action of glucosamine is to protect against and prevent osteoarthritis. Several studies have focused on the results of glucosamine use as compared with that of nonsteroidal antiinflammatories and placebos. In one study more than 200 people were given either 500 mg of glucosamine or a placebo 3 times daily for 4 weeks. The experimental group showed significant improvement in movement and pain control (Noack, 1994). Another study comparing the benefits of glucosamine versus ibuprofen showed the two treatments to be equally effective after the second week of treatment. Study participants were then given 500 mg of glucosamine or 400 mg of ibuprofen 3 times daily for 4 weeks. The glucosamine group reported fewer side effects (Muller-Fassbender, 1994). A further study compared the effects of glucosamine and piroxicam. Subjects were given glucosamine, piroxicam, both, or a placebo for 3 months. The glucosamine group reported significant improvement as measured by the Lequesne index (Rovati, 1994). These results were achieved with fewer dropouts and fewer side effects. Studies are being added yearly that support the use of glucosamine in arthritic conditions (Rubin, 2001; *Altern Med Rev*, 1999).

References

Glucosamine sulfate, *Altern Med Rev* 4(3):193-195, 1999.

Muller-Fassbender H et al: Glucosamine sulfate compared to ibuprofen in osteoarthritis of the knee, *Osteoarthritis Cartilage* 2:61-69, 1994.

Murray M, Pizzarno J: *The encyclopedia of natural medicine,* 2 ed (revised), Roseville, Calif, 1998, Prima.

Noack W et al: Glucosamine sulfate in osteoarthritis of the knee, *Osteoarthritis Cartilage* 2:51-59, 1994.

Rovati LC et al: A large, randomized placebo controlled, double-blind study of glucosamine sulfate vs. piroxicam and vs. their association, on the kineses of the symptomatic effect in knee osteoarthritis, *Osteoarthritis Cartilage* 2:56, 1994.

Rubin BR et al: Oral polymeric *N*-acetyl-D-glucosamine and osteoarthritis, *J Am Osteopath Assoc* 101(6):339-344, 2001.

Goat's Rue
(goets rew)

Scientific name: *Galega officinalis*

Other common names: French honeysuckle, French lilac, Italian fitch

Origin: Goat's rue is a perennial found in parts of Europe and Iran.

Uses
Reported Uses

Goat's rue has been reported to function as both a diuretic and an antidiabetic. It is used to increase milk production in dairy cows.

Product Availability and Dosages
Available Forms

Dried leaves

Plant Parts Used: Dried leaves, flowers, stalks

Dosages and Routes
Adult

- PO infusion: pour 8 oz boiling water over 1 tsp dried leaves, let stand 15 min, strain, drink bid

---

🛡 = Pregnancy   👣 = Pediatric   ❗ = Alert   ✒ = Popular Herb

Precautionary Information
Contraindications
Until more research is available, goat's rue should not be used during pregnancy and lactation and should not be given to children. Goat's rue should not be used by persons with hypersensitivity to it.

Side Effects/Adverse Reactions
Central Nervous System: Headache, restlessness, weakness
Gastrointestinal: Nausea

G

Interactions with Goat's Rue		
Drug		
Antidiabetics: Goat's rue may increase the effects of antidiabetics (theoretical).		
Food	Herb	Lab Test
None known	None known	None known

Client Considerations
Assess
- Assess for hypersensitivity reactions. If these are present, discontinue use of glucosamine and administer antihistamine or other appropriate therapy.
- Monitor blood glucose in diabetic patients (see Interactions).

Administer
- Instruct the client to take this herb PO only after steeping for 15 minutes in boiling water and straining.

Teach Client/Family
- Until more research is available, caution the client not to use goat's rue during pregnancy and lactation and not to give it to children.

Pharmacology
Pharmacokinetics
Pharmacokinetics and pharmacodynamics are unknown.

 Endangered Herb   Adverse effects: BOLD = life-threatening

Primary Chemical Components of Goat's Rue and Their Possible Actions		
Chemical Class	**Individual Components**	**Possible Action**
Tannin		Wound healing
Alkaloid	Galegine	Possible toxicity
	Paragalegine; Peganine	

Actions

Very little primary research is available for goat's rue, and no scientific studies confirm any of its reported actions. However, it has been used in Europe for many years to treat hyperglycemia. Toxicity may result from two of its chemical components, galegine and paragalegine. In one study (Palit, 1999) *Galega officinalis* has shown a novel weight-reducing action that is independent of reduction of food intake in mice. Another study (Atanasov, 2000) identified the inhibiting and disaggregating effect of *Galega officinalis* on platelet aggregation.

References

Atanasov AT et al: Inhibiting and disaggregating effect of gel-filtered *Galega officinalis* L. herbal extract on platelet aggregation, *J Ethnopharmacol*, 69(3):235-240, 2000.

Palit P et al: Novel weight-reducing activity of *Galega officinalis* in mice, *J Pharm Pharmacol* 51(11):1313-1319, 1999.

Goldenrod
(goeld-uhn-rahd)

Scientific name: *Solidago virgaurea*

Other common names: Aaron's rod, blue mountain tea, denrod, European gosweet goldenrod, woundwort

Class 2d (Whole Herb)

Origin: Goldenrod is a flowering plant found in Europe and the United States.

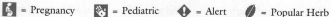

🔥 = Pregnancy 🐾 = Pediatric ❗ = Alert 🌿 = Popular Herb

Uses

Reported Uses

Goldenrod may be used as a diuretic, an antispasmodic, an analgesic, and an antiinflammatory. In many countries, goldenrod is used to prevent urolithiasis and to help eliminate calculi that have already been formed. Goldenrod also may be used to induce abortion. It has been given to children to treat otitis media and for its anticatarrh effect (Mills, 2000).

Product Availability and Dosages

Available Forms

Alcoholic extract, aqueous extract, dried herb

Plant Parts Used: Flowers, leaves

Dosages and Routes

Adult

All dosages listed are PO.

- Decoction: 2 tsp chopped dried herb in 8 oz water, boil 15 min, let stand 2 min, strain, take 1 tbsp tid-qid
- Dried herb: 6-12 g qd (Blumenthal, 1998)
- Infusion of flowers and leaves: 2 tsp herb in 8 oz water, infuse 10-15 min, strain, drink all, take tid

Precautionary Information

Contraindications

Because it is an abortifacient, goldenrod should not be used during pregnancy. Until more research is available, it should not be used during lactation and should not be given to children. Without medical advice, goldenrod should not be used by persons with congestive heart failure or renal disease. This herb should not be used by persons with hypersensitivity to it or other Asteraene family herbs. Class 2d herb (whole herb).

Side Effects/Adverse Reactions

Gastrointestinal: Nausea, vomiting, anorexia
Integumentary: Hypersensitivity reactions, rash
Respiratory: Asthma, difficult respirations
Toxicity: GASTROINTESTINAL HEMORRHAGE, ENLARGED SPLEEN, EDEMA OF ABDOMEN, EMACIATION, TACHYPNEA, SEVERE VOMITING, DEATH

 Endangered Herb   Adverse effects: BOLD = life-threatening

Interactions with Goldenrod

Drug
Lithium: Goldenrod taken with lithium may result in dehydration and lithium toxicity; avoid concurrent use.

Food	Herb	Lab Test
None known	None known	None known

Client Considerations

Assess

- Assess for hypersensitivity reactions, including asthma, rash, and difficult respirations. If such reactions are present, discontinue use of goldenrod and administer antihistamine or other appropriate therapy.
- Assess for symptoms of toxicity: gastrointestinal hemorrhage, enlarged spleen, severe emesis, and tachypnea.

Administer

- Instruct the client to take goldenrod PO after preparing a decoction.
- Instruct the client to store goldenrod in a cool, dry place, away from heat and moisture.

Teach Client/Family

- Because it is an abortifacient, caution the client not to use goldenrod during pregnancy. Until more research is available, caution the client not to use this herb during lactation and not to give it to children.
- Warn the client of the life-threatening side effects of goldenrod.

Pharmacology

Pharmacokinetics

Pharmacokinetics and pharmacodynamics are unknown.

Primary Chemical Components of Goldenrod and Their Possible Actions

Chemical Class	Individual Component	Possible Action
Phenolic glucoside	Lelocarposide; Isoschaftoside	
Titerpene	Bisdesmoside	
Flavonoid	Rutin	Diuretic; antioxidant, increased urine volume; increased sodium excretion
	Hyperoside; Isoquercitrin	
Caffeoylguinic acids		
Saponin		Diuretic
Carotenoid		
Tannin		Wound healing; astringent
Nitrate		
Volatile oil	Gamma-cadinene	
Polysaccharide		

G

Actions

The primary actions of goldrenrod are diuretic, antispasmodic, and antiinflammatory. However, little or no primary research is available to confirm most of its proposed actions and uses. One small study has evaluated the ability of goldenrod and several other herbs to reduce paw edema induced in laboratory rats. Goldenrod was found to reduce paw edema significantly (Ghazaly, 1992). Another study identified the analgesic effects of several herbs, including goldenrod. The analgesic effect is due to selective action to a single receptor (Sampson, 2000).

References

Blumenthal M, editor: *The complete German Commission E monographs: therapeutic guide to herbal medicines,* Austin, Tex, American Botanical Council; Boston, Integrative Medicine Communication, 1998.

Ghazaly M et al: Study of the anti-inflammatory activity of *Populus tremula, Solidago virgaurea, Fraxinus excelsior, Arzneimittelforschung* 42:333-336, 1992.

Mills S, Bone K: *Principles and practice of phytotherapy,* London, 2000, Churchill Livingstone.

Sampson JH et al: Ethnomedicinally selected plants as sources of potential analgesic compounds: indication of in vitro biological activity in receptor binding assays. *Phytother Res* 14(1):24-29, 2000.

Goldenseal
(goeld'uhn-seel)

Scientific name: *Hydrastis canadensis*

Other common names: Eye balm, eye root, goldsiegel, ground raspberry, Indian dye, Indian turmeric, jaundice root, orange root, turmeric root, yellow paint, yellow puccoon, yellow root, wild curcuma

Class 2b (Rhizome, Root)

Origin: Goldenseal is a perennial originally found in the Ohio River Valley and now cultivated.

Uses

Reported Uses

Goldenseal is used to treat various conditions. Its most common uses include the treatment of gastritis, gastrointestinal ulceration, peptic ulcer disease, mouth ulcer, bladder infection, sore throat, and postpartum hemorrhage. It may also be used to treat skin disorders such as pruritus, boils, hemorrhoids, anal fissures, and eczema, as well as cancer and tuberculosis. Goldenseal may also be used to promote wound healing and reduce inflammation.

Investigational Uses

Studies are underway to determine the efficacy of goldenseal in the treatment of cholera, *Giardia*, shigella, *Enterobacteriaceae*, and salmonella.

Product Availability and Dosages

Available Forms

Capsules, dried herb, fluid extract, powder, tablets, tea, tincture

Plant Parts Used: Air-dried rhizome

Dosages and Routes

Adult

Dosages should be standardized to berberine content. All dosages listed are PO unless noted.

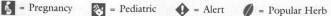

= Pregnancy   = Pediatric   = Alert   = Popular Herb

Bladder Infection
- Dried root/tea: 1-2 g tid (Murray, 1998)
- Tincture: 4-6 ml (1-1½ tsp) tid (1:5 dilution) (Murray, 1998)
- Fluid extract: 0.5-2.0 ml (¼-½ tsp) tid (Murray, 1998)
- Freeze-dried root: 500-1000 mg tid (Murray, 1998)
- Powdered solid extract: 250-500 mg tid (8% alkaloids) (Murray, 1998)

Boils
- Topical poultice: 1 tbsp root powder mixed with water or egg white to make a paste, apply to area, cover with adsorbent material, use bid (Murray, 1998)

General Use
- Infusion/tea: 2-4 g dried rhizome, drink in divided doses tid
- Fluid extract: 250 mg (1:1 dilution) tid
- Powder: 250-500 mg tid
- Tincture: 6-12 ml (1:5 dilution) tid
- Capsules: 500-600 mg qid
- Powdered root: ½-1 g divided into 3 daily doses (McCaleb, 2000)
- Tincture: 2-4 ml (1:10 dilution) (McCaleb, 2000)

Sore Throat
- Dried root/tea: 2-4 g tid (Murray, 1998)
- Tincture: 6-12 ml (1½-3 tsp) (1:5 dilution) tid (Murray, 1998)
- Fluid extract: 2-4 ml (½-1 tsp) (1:1 dilution) tid (Murray, 1998)
- Powdered solid extract: 250-500 mg (8%-12% alkaloids) tid (Murray, 1998)

Precautionary Information
Contraindications

Because it is a uterine stimulant, goldenseal should not be used during pregnancy. Until more research is available, it should not be used during lactation and should not be given to children. This herb should not be used by persons who have cardiovascular conditions such as heart block, arrhythmias, or hypertension, or by those who are hypersensitive to it. Goldenseal should not be used locally by persons with purulent ear discharge or by those with a ruptured eardrum. Class 2b herb (rhizome, root).

Continued

 Endangered Herb   Adverse effects: BOLD = life-threatening

Precautionary Information—cont'd

Side Effects/Adverse Reactions

Cardiovascular: BRADYCARDIA, ASYSTOLE, HEART BLOCK
Central Nervous System: Hallucinations, delirium (prolonged use); CENTRAL NERVOUS SYSTEM DEPRESSION, SEIZURES; PARALYSIS (increased doses), PARESTHESIA
Gastrointestinal: Nausea, vomiting, anorexia, diarrhea, or constipation, abdominal cramping, mouth ulcers
Integumentary: Hypersensitivity reactions, rash, contact dermatitis; phototoxicity (topical)
Respiratory: DYSPNEA (prolonged use)
Toxicity: RESTLESSNESS, NERVOUSNESS, IRRITABILITY, CENTRAL NERVOUS SYSTEM DEPRESSION, SEIZURES, CARDIOVASCULAR COLLAPSE, COMA, DEATH

Interactions with Goldenseal

Drug

Alcohol: Goldenseal may increase the effects of alcohol; do not use concurrently.
Antiarrhythmics: Goldenseal may increase the effects of antiarrhythmics; do not use concurrently.
Anticoagulants: Goldenseal may decrease the effects of anticoagulants; do not use concurrently.
Antihypertensives: Goldenseal may increase the effects of antihypertensives; do not use concurrently.
Azole antifungals: Goldenseal may slow the metabolism of azole antifungals; avoid concurrent use.
Benzodiazepines: Goldenseal may slow the metabolism of benzodiazepines; avoid concurrent use.
Beta-blockers: Goldenseal may increase the effects of beta-blockers; do not use concurrently.
Calcium channel blockers: Goldenseal may slow the metabolism of calcium channel blockers; avoid concurrent use.
Cardiac glycosides: Goldenseal may decrease the effects of cardiac glycosides; do not use concurrently.
Central nervous system depressants: Goldenseal may increase the effects of central nervous system depressants; do not use concurrently.

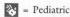 = Pregnancy   = Pediatric   = Alert   = Popular Herb

> ## Interactions with Goldenseal—cont'd
>
> **Drug—cont'd**
>
> ***Statins:*** Goldenseal may slow the metabolism of statins; avoid concurrent use.
>
> ***Vitamin B:*** Goldenseal may decrease the absorption of vitamin B; do not use concurrently.
>
> | Food | Herb |
> |------|------|
> | None known | None known |
>
> **Lab Test**
>
> Goldenseal may increase blood osmolality and serum or urine plasma sodium.

G

Client Considerations

Assess

- Assess for hypersensitivity reactions, including rash and contact dermatitis. If these are present, discontinue use of this herb and administer antihistamine or other appropriate therapy.
- Assess the client's use of central nervous system depressants, beta-blockers, antihypertensives, antiarrhythmics, anticoagulants, cardiac glycosides, and antihypertensives. None of these drugs should be used concurrently with goldenseal (see Interactions).
- Assess for symptoms of toxicity (see Side Effects).

Administer

- Instruct the client to take goldenseal PO as an extract or as a dried rhizome.
- Instruct the client to store goldenseal products in a cool, dry place, away from heat and moisture.
- Advise the client to avoid the sun or wear protective clothing when using goldenseal topically (Inbaraj, 2001).

Teach Client/Family

- Until more research is available, caution the client not to use goldenseal during pregnancy and lactation and not to give it to children.
- Warn the client of the many life-threatening side effects of goldenseal.

 Endangered Herb   Adverse effects: BOLD = life-threatening

- Advise the client not to perform hazardous activities such as driving or operating heavy machinery until physical response to the herb can be evaluated.

Pharmacology

Pharmacokinetics

Pharmacokinetics and pharmacodynamics are unknown.

Primary Chemical Components of Goldenseal and Their Possible Actions		
Chemical Class	**Individual Components**	**Possible Action**
Alkaloid	Berberine	Immunostimulant, antibacterial, antisecretory, anticholinergic
	Hydrastine Berberastine Canadine Candaline	Antibacterial
	Beta-Hydrastine	Astringent, antibacterial
Resin **Phytosterin** **Chlorogenic acid**		

Actions

Goldenseal is used for its antiinfective, immunostimulant, antipyretic, and anticancer actions. Native Americans have used it for many years. Because it has been overused, this herb is now becoming endangered in the wild. Efforts are currently underway to cultivate goldenseal.

Antiinfective Action

One of the chemical components of goldenseal, berberine, has been shown to be effective against a number of bacteria, fungi, and protozoa. It is effective against *Staphylococcus* sp., *Streptococcus* sp., *Eshericia coli, Chlamydia* sp., *Salmonella typhi, Corynebacterium diphtheria, Diplococcus pneumoniae, Pseudomonas* sp., *Shigella dysenteriae, Entamoeba histolytica, Trichomonas vaginalis, Neisseria gonorrhoeae, Treponema pallidum, Giardia lamblia, Leishmania donovani,* and *Candida albicans.*

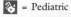 = Pregnancy   = Pediatric   = Alert   = Popular Herb

Many other organisms have been shown to be sensitive to goldenseal in vitro (Amin, 1969; Johnson, 1952).

Immunostimulant Action

Berberine increases the blood supply to the spleen, with possible immune stimulant effects (Sabir, 1971). Berberine has also been found to increase the action of macrophages.

Anticancer Action

Berberine has been shown to destroy brain tumor cells in rats at rates more double those of nitrosurea (Rong-Xun, 1990). An additive effect also accrues from combining berberine with nitrosurea.

References

Amin AH et al: Berberine sulfate: antimicrobial activity, bioassay and mode of action, *Can J Microbiol* 15:1067-1076, 1969.

Inbaraj JJ et al: Photochemistry and photocytotoxicity of alkaloids from Goldenseal l. Berberine, *Chem Res Toxicol* 14(1):1529-1534, 2001.

Johnson CC et al: Toxicity of alkaloids to certain bacteria, *Acta Pharmacol Toxicol* 8:71-78, 1952.

McCaleb R et al: *The encyclopedia of popular herbs: your complete guide to leading medicinal plants,* Roseville, Calif, 2000, Prima Health.

Murray M, Pizzarno J: *The encyclopedia of natural medicine,* 2 ed (revised), Roseville, Calif, 1998, Prima.

Rong-Xun Z et al: Laboratory studies of berberine used alone and in combination with 1,3-bis(2-chloroethyl)-1-nitrosurea to treat malignant brain tumors, *Chin Med J* 103:658-665, 1990.

Sabir M et al: Study of some pharmacologic actions of berberine, *Indian J Physiol Pharmacol* 15:111-132, 1971.

Gossypol
(gah'suh-pawl)

Scientific name: *Gossypium hirsutum*

Other common names: American upland cotton, common cotton, cotton, upland cotton, wild cotton

Origin: Gossypol is found in cotton and is made synthetically.

Uses

Reported Uses

Gossypol is used as a male contraceptive, as a vaginal spermicide female contraceptive, to induce labor and delivery, and to treat dysmenorrhea. Gossypol is used for uterine fibroids, endometriosis, and dysfunctional uterine bleeding.

Product Availability and Dosages

Available Forms

Extract

Plant Parts Used: Roots, seeds, stems

Dosages and Routes

Adult

Male Contraceptive

- PO extract: 20 mg qd for 2-3 mo until sperm count drops to < 4 million sperm/ml, then 75-100 mg every 2 wk for maintenance

Precautionary Information

Contraindications

Because it can induce labor, gossypol should not be used during pregnancy except under the direction of a qualified herbalist. Until more research is available, this herb should not be used during lactation and should not be given to children. Persons with hypersensitivity to gossypol or those with hepatic or renal damage should not use it. Males may have a lowered sperm count for >90 days.

Side Effects/Adverse Reactions

Cardiovascular: HEART FAILURE, CIRCULATORY COLLAPSE
Gastrointestinal: Nausea, vomiting, anorexia, diarrhea
Integumentary: Hypersensitivity reactions
Musculoskeletal: Muscle fatigue, weakness, PARALYSIS
Genitourinary: Male sterility (prolonged use)

Interactions with Gossypol

Drug

Antifungals: Use of gossypol with antifungals may cause nephrotoxicity; do not use concurrently.
Diuretics (bumetanide, ethacrynic acid, furosemide, hydrochlorothiazide, torsemide, triamterene): Use of gossypol with diuretics may cause severe hypokalemia; do not use concurrently.

 = Pregnancy   = Pediatric   = Alert   = Popular Herb

Interactions with Gossypol—cont'd

Drug—cont'd

NSAIDs (diclofenac, etodolac, fenoprofen, fluroprofen, indomethacin, ketoprofen, ketorolac, meclofenamate, nabumetone, naproxen, oxaprozin, piroxicam, sulindac, tolmetin): Gossypol used with NSAIDs may result in gastrointestinal distress and gastrointestinal tissue damage.

Salicylates (aspirin): Gossypol used with salicylates may result in tissue damage.

Food	Herb	Lab Test
None known	None known	None known

G

Client Considerations

Assess

- Assess for hypersensitivity reactions. If present, discontinue use of gossypol and administer antihistamine or other appropriate therapy.
- Assess for use of antifungals or diuretics, which should not be used concurrently with gossypol (see Interactions). Monitor potassium levels, which may be decreased with gossypol use.
- Assess for cardiovascular reactions, including arrhythmias.

Administer

- Instruct the client to take extract PO.
- Instruct the client to store gossypol products in a cool, dry place, away from heat and moisture.

Teach Client/Family

- Because it can induce labor, caution the client not to use gossypol during pregnancy unless under the direction of a qualified herbalist. Until more research is available, caution the client not to use this herb during lactation and not to give it to children.
- Warn the client of the life-threatening cardiovascular side effects of gossypol.

Pharmacology

Pharmacokinetics

Pharmacokinetics and pharmacodynamics are unknown.

 Endangered Herb   Adverse effects: BOLD = life-threatening

Primary Chemical Components of Gossypol and Their Possible Actions		
Chemical Class	**Individual Component**	**Possible Action**
Enantiomers		

Actions

Male Contraception

The primary action of gossypol is contraceptive. Extensive testing began in China about 30 years ago. Studies have demonstrated the contraceptive effectiveness of this herb in both male and female laboratory animals. As a male contraceptive, gossypol decreases sperm production by inhibiting lactate dehydrogenase X, which is needed for sperm production. Sperm recovered from rats and hamsters treated with gossypol were found to be immotile, with heads or tails not attached (Chang, 1980). No changes in libido or hormone levels occurred. The recommended dose for males is 20 mg per day until the sperm count is reduced to less than 4 million per ml (after about 90 days), then 75 to 100 mg given two times per month as a maintenance dose to keep the sperm count low. One study found gossypol to be more than 99% effective when used at the proposed levels (Wu, 1989). Sperm production usually returns to normal 90 days after termination of therapy. However, some men continue to experience lowered sperm production beyond 90 days.

Female Contraception

In female rats, gossypol has been shown to inhibit implantation and also possibly to affect luteinizing hormone (LH) levels (Lin, 1985).

References

Chang MC: *Contraception* 21:461, 1980.
Lin YC et al: *Life Sci* 37:39, 1985.
Wu: *Drugs* 38:333, 1989.

Gotu Kola
(goe-tew'koe-lah)

Scientific name: *Centella asiatica*

Other common names: Centella, hydrocotyle, Indian pennywort, Indian water navelwort, talepetrako, teca, water pennywort

Origin: Gotu kola is a creeping plant found in the swamps of Africa, Sri Lanka, and Madagascar.

Uses

Reported Uses

Gotu kola is taken internally as a stimulant; to increase fertility; and to treat hypertension, cancer, hepatic disorders, leprosy, and varicose veins. It also may be taken internally to treat chronic interstitial cystitis, cellulite, and periodontal disease. Gotu kola may be used externally to promote wound healing and to treat skin disorders such as psoriasis, eczema, and keloids.

Investigational Uses

New studies are underway for use of Gotu kola as preventing gastric ulcers.

Product Availability and Dosages

Available Forms

Capsules, cream, dried herb, extract

Plant Parts Used: Dried leaves

Dosages and Routes

All dosages listed are PO. No topical dosages are available.
Adult
Cellulite
• Extract: 30 mg triterpenes tid (Murray, 1998)
General Use
• Capsule: 450 mg qd
• Dried leaf: 0.3-0.6 g tid
Periodontal Disease
• Extract: 30 mg triterpenes bid (Murray, 1998)
Varicose Veins
• Extract: 30-60 mg triterpenes qd (Murray, 1998)

🍀 Endangered Herb   Adverse effects: BOLD = life-threatening

Precautionary Information

Contraindications

Until more research is available, gotu kola should not be used during pregnancy and lactation and should not be given to children. It should not be used by persons with hypersensitivity to this herb or to members of the celery family.

Side Effects/Adverse Reactions

Central Nervous System: Sedation
Integumentary: Hypersensitivity reactions such as burning (topical use), contact dermatitis, rash, pruritus
Systemic: Increased blood glucose, increased cholesterol levels

Interactions with Gotu Kola

Drug
Antidiabetics: Gotu kola may decrease the effectiveness of antidiabetics; do not use concurrently.
Antilipidemics: Gotu kola may decrease the effectiveness of antilipidemics; avoid concurrent use.

Food	Herb	Lab Test
None known	None known	None known

Client Considerations

Assess

- Assess for hypersensitivity reactions: burning (topical), contact dermatitis, rash, and pruritus. If these are present, discontinue use of this herb and administer antihistamine or other appropriate therapy.
- Assess for medications used (see Interactions).

Administer

- Instruct the client to store gotu kola products in a cool, dry place, away from heat and moisture.

Teach Client/Family

- Until more research is available, caution the client not to use gotu kola during pregnancy and lactation and not to give it to children.

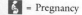 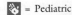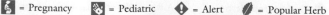

- Explain to the client that gotu kola is not the same as other cola spp.

Pharmacology

Pharmacokinetics

Pharmacokinetics and pharmacodynamics are unknown.

Primary Chemical Components of Gotu Kola and Their Possible Actions		
Chemical Class	**Individual Component**	**Possible Action**
Glycoside	Madecassoside; Madecasoside Asiaticoside Brahmoside; Brahminoside Centelloside	Antiinflammatory Wound healing Sedative
Madecassol Acid	Madecassic acod; Centellic acid; Centoic acid; Asiatic acid; Asiaticentoic acid	
Tannin		Wound healing
Phytosterol		
Flavonoid	Kaempferol; Quercetin	Antiinflammatory

Actions

Wound Healing Action

Gotu kola is used primarily as a topical preparation to promote wound healing. In one study using laboratory rats, gotu kola penetrated tissues in high concentrations and produced a faster rate of healing with topical administration than with oral. Increased collagen was found in the cell layer in the form of fibronectin (Tenni, 1988). One of the chemical components of gotu kola, the glycoside madecassoside, decreases inflammation while another glycoside, asiaticoside, may be responsible for wound healing.

Antiinfertility Action

In a preliminary study, gotu kola was shown to decrease infertility in female mice. The mechanism of action is unknown (Dutta, 1968).

Other Actions

Other possible uses of gotu kola that have not been investigated to any great degree include its antihypertensive, anticancer, peridontal disease, cellulite, and connective tissue regulation actions. One study has confirmed the gastroprotective effects of *Centella asiatica*. Rats were induced with gastric lesions by ethanol; the oral administration of *Centella* extract significantly inhibited gastric lesions (Cheng, 2000).

References

Cheng CL et al: Effects of *Centella asiatica* on ethanol-induced gastric mucosal lesions in rats, *Life Sci* 67(21):2647-2653, 2000.

Dutta T et al: *Indian J Exp Biol* 6(30):181, 1968.

Murray M, Pizzarno J: *The encyclopedia of natural medicine,* 2 ed (revised), Roseville, Calif, 1998, Prima.

Tenni R et al: *Ital J Biochem* 37(2):69, 1988.

Grapeseed
(grayp'seed)

Scientific name: *Vitis vinifera*

Other common name: Muskat

Origin: Grapeseed is found throughout the world.

Uses

Reported Uses

Grapeseed may be used as an antioxidant and an anticancer treatment; to treat varicose veins and circulatory problems; and to treat vision problems such as cataracts and improve vision by lessening eye strain.

Investigational Uses

Researchers are experimenting with the use of grapeseed to treat diabetes mellitus and inflammatory, degenerative, diverticular, and heart diseases.

Product Availability and Dosages

Available Forms

Capsules, tablets

Plant Parts Used: Seeds

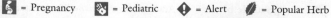

Dosages and Routes

Dosages are standardized to 85%-95% procyanidins.

Adult

Supplementation
- PO capsules/tablets: 50-100 qd (McCaleb, 2000)

Therapeutic Use
- PO capsules/tablets: 150-300 mg qd for 21 days, then 50-80 mg qd maintenance (McCaleb, 2000)

G

Precautionary Information

Contraindications

Until more research is available, grapeseed should not be used pregnancy and lactation and should not be given to children.

Side Effects/Adverse Reactions

Central Nervous System: Dizziness
Gastrointestinal: Nausea, anorexia, HEPATOTOXICITY (theoretical)
Integumentary: Rash

Interactions with Grapeseed

Drug	Food	Herb	Lab Test
None known	None known	None known	None known

Client Considerations

Assess

- If the client is using grapeseed to improve cardiovascular disorders, assess cardiovascular status: edema in legs, improvement in atherosclerosis, and improvement in varicose veins. Monitor blood pressure and pulse.
- Identify other cardiovascular medications taken by the client.
- Assess for hepatotoxicity.

Administer

- Instruct the client to take grapeseed PO only once per day.
- Instruct the client to store grapeseed products in a cool, dry place, away from heat and moisture.

Teach Client/Family

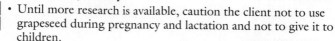

- Until more research is available, caution the client not to use grapeseed during pregnancy and lactation and not to give it to children.

Pharmacology

Pharmacokinetics

Pharmacokinetics and pharmacodynamics are unknown.

Primary Chemical Components of Grapeseed and Their Possible Actions		
Chemical Class	**Individual Component**	**Possible Action**
Flavonoid	Kaempferol; Quercetin	Antiinflammatory, antioxidant
Tannin **Tocopherol** **Fatty acid**	Proanthocyanidins	

Actions

Vision Improvement

Grapeseed has produced beneficial effects in people with vision problems. One study focused on participants with computer-related visual stress. People who worked at a video display terminal (VDT) for at least 6 hours a day were assigned to one of three groups, receiving either grapeseed, bilberry, or a placebo. After 2 months, the grapeseed group reported much less visual stress, with improvements even greater than those seen in the bilberry group (Fusi, 1990). An earlier study had shown grapeseed to be significantly more effective than a placebo in improving night vision. This earlier study included 98 people who experienced prolonged nighttime visual glare or visual stress caused by VDTs (Corbe, 1988).

Other Actions

Grapeseed has shown protective effects against carbon tetra-chloride hepatic poisoning in mice (Oshima, 1995), as well as photoprotective properties of melanins (Novikov, 2001).

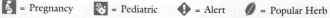

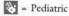 = Pregnancy   = Pediatric   = Alert   = Popular Herb

References

Corbe CH et al: Chromatic sense and chorioretinal circulation: a study of the effects of OPC (Endotelon), *J Fr Ophtamol* 1(5):453-460, 1988.

Fusi L et al: Effects of procyanidolic oligomers from *Vitis vinifera* in subjects working at video-display units, *Ann Ottalmologia Clin Oculista* 116:575, 1990.

McCaleb R et al: *The encyclopedia of popular herbs: your complete guide to leading medicinal plants,* Roseville, Calif, 2000, Prima Health.

Novikov DA et al: Photoprotective properties of melanins from grape and black tea, *Radiats Biol Radioecol* 41(6):664-670, 2001.

Oshima Y et al: *Experientia* 51(1):63, 1995.

G

Green Tea
(green tee)

Scientific name: *Camellia sinensis*
Other common name: Matsu-cha

Origin: Green tea is a shrub found in Asia.

Uses

Reported Uses

Green tea is used as a general antioxidant, anticancer agent, diuretic, antibacterial, antilipidemic, and antiatherosclerotic.

Investigational Uses

Research is underway to confirm its use in treating HIV, increasing muscle health, reducing total cholesterol, and for vascular protection.

Product Availability and Dosages

Available Forms

Capsules, extract, tea

Plant Parts Used: Dried leaves

Dosages and Routes

Green tea is standardized to 60% polyphenols.

Adult
- PO extract: 250-400 mg/day of standardized to 90% polyphenols (McCaleb, 2000)
- PO tea: 1 tsp tea leaves in 8 oz hot water, drink 2-5 cups/day (McCaleb, 2000)

Endangered Herb   Adverse effects: BOLD = life-threatening

Precautionary Information

Contraindications

Green tea should not be used by persons with hypersensitivity to this product or by those with kidney inflammation, gastrointestinal ulcers, insomnia, cardiovascular disease, or increased intraocular pressure. This herb contains caffeine, although decaffeinated tea is available.

Side Effects/Adverse Reactions

Cardiovascular: Increased blood pressure, palpitations, irregular heartbeat (high doses)
Central Nervous System: Anxiety, nervousness, insomnia (high doses)
Gastrointestinal: Nausea, heartburn, increased stomach acid (high doses)
Integumentary: Hypersensitivity reactions

Interactions with Green Tea

Drug

Antacids: Antacids may decrease the therapeutic effects of green tea (theoretical).
Bronchodilators: Large amounts of green tea increase the action of some bronchodilators.
MAOIs (isocarboxazid, phenelzine, tranylcypromine): Green tea used in large amounts taken with MAOIs can lead to hypertensive crisis, do not use together.
Xanthines (theophylline): Large amounts of green tea increase the action of xanthines.

Food

Dairy products: Dairy products may decrease the therapeutic effects of green tea.

Herb

Ephedra: Concurrent use of ephedra and caffeinated green tea may increase hypertension and central nervous system stimulation; avoid concurrent use with caffeinated green tea products.

Lab Test

None known

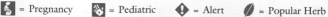

Client Considerations

Assess

- Assess for hypersensitivity reactions. If present, discontinue use of this herb and administer antihistamine or other appropriate therapy.
- Assess for other conditions that are contraindications to green tea use, including cardiovascular and renal disease and increased intraocular pressure.
- Assess for use of antacids, dairy products, and ephedra (see Interactions).

Administer

- Instruct the client to store green tea in a cool, dry place, protected from heat and moisture.

Teach Client/Family

- Because this herb contains caffeine, caution the client with renal or cardiovascular disease or increased intraocular pressure not to use caffeinated green tea products.

Pharmacology

Pharmacokinetics

Pharmacokinetics and pharmacodynamics are unknown.

G

Primary Chemical Components of Green Tea and Their Possible Actions		
Chemical Class	**Individual Component**	**Possible Action**
Tannin		Wound healing; antiinflammatory
Flavonoid	Epigallocatechin gallate	Antioxidant; anti-HIV (Fassina, 2002)
	Catechin	Chemoprotective
	Epicatechin; Epicatechin gallate; Proanthocyanidins	
Xanthines	Caffeine; Theobromine; Theophylline	Central nervous system stimulant
Lignin		
Organic acid		
Protein		
Vitamin	C	Lipolytic

Actions

Green tea and black tea come from the same plant, *Camellia sinensis*. Black tea is produced by allowing the leaves to oxidize, while green tea is cut and steamed. The major actions of green tea result from its antioxidant, anticancer, and antilipidemic properties.

Antioxidant and Anticancer Actions

Green tea exerts protective effects against gastrointestinal cancers of the stomach, intestine, colon, rectum, and pancreas. One study showed a significant reduction in these cancers when green tea was used (Ji, 1997). Green tea also has been shown to decrease the incidence of breast cancer in vitro by inhibiting the interaction with estrogen receptors (Komori, 1993). In one study laboratory-induced lung cancer in rats was shown to be decreased in those that received a 2% solution of green tea. The cancer rates for the green tea group were 16%, as compared with 46% in the group that drank only water (Luo, 1995). In many studies, black tea has been shown to increase cancer risk in the endometrium and gallbladder. The chemical component epigallocatechin gallate from green tea was able to strongly inhibit the replication of two strains of HIV when tested on blood lymphocytes (Fassina, 2002).

Antilipidemic Action

In one study, green tea produced a significant increase in HDL and a decrease in LDL lipoproteins. These reactions occurred in direct proportion to the amount of green tea consumed (Imai, 1995).

Other Actions

Green tea was able to improve muscle health by reducing or delaying necrosis in mice by an antioxidant mechanism (Buetler, 2002). Another new action being studied is the consumption of green tea to reduce lipids and lipoproteins (Tokunaga, 2002).

References

Buetler TM et al: Green tea extract decreases muscle necrosis in mice and protects against reactive oxygen species, *Am J Clin Nutr* 75(4):749-753, 2002.

Fassina G et al: Polyphenolic antioxidant epigallocatechin-3-gallate from green tea as a candidate anti-HIV agent, *AIDs* 16(6):939-941, 2002.

Imai K et al: Cross sectional study of effects of drinking green tea on cardiovascular and liver disease, *Br Med J* 310:693-696, 1995.

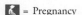 = Pregnancy    = Pediatric   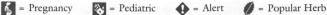 = Alert   = Popular Herb

Ji HT et al: Green tea consumption and the risk of pancreatic and colon cancer, *Int J Cancer* 7:255-258, 1997.

Komori A et al: Anticarcinogenic activity of green tea polyphenols, *Jpn J Clin Oncol* 23:186-190, 1993.

Luo SQ et al: Inhibitory effect of green tea extract on the carcinogenesis induced with asbestos plus benzo(a)pyrene in rat, *Biomed Environ Sci* 8(1):54-58, 1995.

McCaleb R et al: *The encyclopedia of popular herbs: your complete guide to leading medicinal plants,* Roseville, Calif, 2000, Prima Health.

Tokunaga S et al: Green tea consumption and serum lipids and lipoproteins in a population of healthy workers in Japan. *Ann Epidemiol* 12(3):157-165, 2002.

G

Ground Ivy

Scientific name: *Glechoma hederacea*

Other common names: Alehoof, cat's foot, creeping Charlie, haymaids, hedgemaids

Origin: Ground ivy is a flowering plant found in the United Kingdom.

Uses
Reported Uses
Many herbalists recommend ground ivy to treat sinusitis, allergic conditions, bronchitis, and various conditions of the ears, nose, and throat. It may also be used to treat disorders of the gastrointestinal system such as diarrhea.

Product Availability and Dosages
Available Forms
Fluid extract, infusion, tincture

Plant Parts Used: Flowers, leaves

Dosages and Routes
Adult
• PO fluid extract: 14-28 grains tid
Child
• Ages 6 years and older: to prevent toxicity use very low dose, only under the supervision of an herbalist

---

🌀 Endangered Herb   Adverse effects: BOLD = life-threatening

Precautionary Information

Contraindications

Until more research is available, ground ivy should not be used during pregnancy and lactation and should not be given to children younger than 6 years of age. It should not be used by persons with hypersensitivity to it.

Side Effects/Adverse Reactions

Gastrointestinal: Nausea, vomiting, anorexia
Integumentary: Hypersensitivity reactions
Toxicity: DIAPHORESIS, BRONCHIAL CONGESTION AND EDEMA, CYANOSIS, PUPIL DILATATION

Interactions with Ground Ivy

Drug
Iron salts: Ground ivy may decrease the absorption of iron salts; avoid concurrent use.

Food	Herb	Lab Test
None known	None known	None known

Client Considerations

Assess

- For hypersensitivity reactions. If present, discontinue use of this herb and administer antihistamine or other appropriate therapy.
- Assess for toxicity (see Side Effects).

Administer

- Instruct the client to store ground ivy in a cool, dry place, away from heat or moisture.

Teach Client/Family

- Until more research is available, caution the client not to use ground ivy during pregnancy and lactation and not to give it to children younger than 6 years of age. With older children, ground ivy should be used only in very small amounts under the supervision of an herbalist.
- Advise the client that toxicity has occurred in animals.

 = Pregnancy   = Pediatric   = Alert   = Popular Herb

Pharmacology
Pharmacokinetics
Pharmacokinetics and pharmacodynamics are unknown.

Primary Chemical Components of Ground Ivy and Their Possible Actions		
Chemical Class	Individual Component	Possible Action
Flavonoid		
Volatile oil		
Tannin		Wound healing
Saponin		
Resin		
Sesquiterpene		
Bitter	Glechomine	

Actions
Very little information is available on ground ivy other than anecdotal evidence. Although this herb is reported to clear sinusitis, rhinitis, and upper respiratory congestion, it is not recommended for any use because no scientific studies are available.

References
Duke J: *CRC handbook of medicinal herbs,* Boca Raton, Fla, 1985, CRC Press.

Guar Gum
(gwahr guhm)

Scientific name: *Cyamopsis tetragonolobus*

Other common names: Guar flour, gucran, Indian cluster bean, jaguar gum   Class 2d (Seed)

Origin: Guar gum is an annual found in India, the United States, and the tropics of Asia.

🌍 Endangered Herb   Adverse effects: **BOLD** = life-threatening

Uses
Reported Uses
Guar gum has been used to treat hyperlipidemia, diabetes mellitus, and obesity.

Product Availability and Dosages
Available Forms
Flour

Plant Parts Used: Endosperm

Dosages and Routes
Adult
No published dosages are available.

Precautionary Information
Contraindications
Until more research is available, guar gum should not be used during pregnancy and lactation and should not be given to children. It should not be used by persons with hypersensitivity to this product. Persons with bowel obstruction or dehydration should not use guar gum; these conditions will worsen. Class 2d herb (seed).

Side Effects/Adverse Reactions
Gastrointestinal: Flatulence, nausea, vomiting, anorexia, GASTROINTESTINAL OBSTRUCTION
Integumentary: Hypersensitivity reactions

Interactions with Guar Gum

Drug
All oral medications: Guar gum may decrease the absorption and action of all oral medications.
Insulin: Guar gum may delay glucose absorption when used with insulin; insulin dose may need to be decreased.

Food	Herb
None known	None known

Lab Test
Guar gum may decrease blood cholesterol and blood glucose levels.

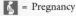 = Pregnancy  = Pediatric 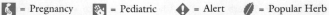 = Alert   = Popular Herb

Client Considerations

Assess

- Assess for hypersensitivity reactions. If are present, discontinue use of guar gum and administer antihistamine or other appropriate therapy.

Administer

- Instruct the client to store guar gum products in a cool, dry place, away from heat and moisture.
- Assess for medications used (see Interactions).

Teach Client/Family

- Until more research is available, caution the client not to use this herb during pregnancy and lactation and not to give it to children.
- Caution the client not to use guar gum with bowel obstruction or dehydration. These conditions will worsen.
- Take with adequate fluids to prevent bowel obstruction, dehydration.

Pharmacology

Pharmacokinetics

Pharmacokinetics and pharmacodynamics are unknown. Guar gum is not absorbed.

Primary Chemical Components of Guar Gum and Their Possible Actions		
Chemical Class	**Individual Component**	**Possible Action**
Polysaccharide	Galactomannan	Antidiabetic; antihyperlipidemic

Actions

The primary actions of guar gum are bulk laxative, antihyperlipidemic, and antidiabetic.

Antihyperlipidemic Action

Guar gum has been shown to decrease cholesterol and LDL levels with little or no effect on triglyceride HDL levels. Its cholesterol-lowering effect may be due to increased bile excretion of cholesterol. This action mirrors that of bile sequestering drugs. Guar gum used in combination with other antihyperlipidemics lowers cholesterol to a much greater extent than either used alone (Uusitupa, 1992).

Antidiabetic Action

The antidiabetic action of guar gum may result from the increased transit of gastrointestinal tract contents through the gastrointestinal system or from adsorbing glucose in the gut. Studies have shown guar gum to decrease blood glucose (Landin, 1992).

Weight Reduction

One study (Pittler, 2001) showed that guar gum is not useful for weight loss primarily due to the adverse reactions of abdominal pain, flatulence, diarrhea, and cramps.

References

Landin K et al: *Am J Clin Nutr* 56:1061, 1992.
Pittler MH et al: Guar gum for body weight reduction: meta-analysis of randomized trials, *Am J Med* 110(9):724-730, 2001.
Uusitupa MI et al: *Arterioscler Thromb Vasc Biol* 12:806, 1992.

Guarana
(gwah'rah-nuh)

Scientific names: *Paullinia cupana, Paullinia sorbilis*

Other common names: Brazilian cocoa, guarana gum, guarana paste, zoom   **Class 2d (*Paullinia cupana* Seed)**

Origin: Guarana is a paste made from seeds of a shrub found in the Amazon and Brazil.

Uses

Reported Uses

Guarana traditionally has been used as a stimulant and typically is used in combination with other products to promote weight loss.

Product Availability and Dosages

Available Forms

Capsules, elixir, extract, tablets, tea; component in various supplements, drinks, flavorings, weight-loss products, and gum

 = Pregnancy    = Pediatric   = Alert   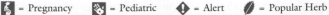 = Popular Herb

Plant Parts Used: Seeds

Dosages and Routes

Dosages vary widely depending on the form used.

Adult

• PO: do not exceed 3 g/day

Precautionary Information

Contraindications

Because of its caffeine content, until more research is available, guarana should not be used during pregnancy (caffeine crosses placenta) and lactation (caffeine enters breast milk) and should not be given to children. Guarana should not be used by persons with cardiovascular diseases such as hypertension, arrhythmias, or heart block, or by persons with duodenal ulcers, diabetes, renal disease, or hypersensitivity to this product. Class 2d herb (*P. cupana* seed).

Side Effects/Adverse Reactions

Cardiovascular: Hypertension, palpitations, TACHYCARDIA, ARRHYTHMIAS

Central Nervous System: Headache, anxiety, nervousness, restlessness, insomnia, tremors, SEIZURES

Gastrointestinal: Nausea, vomiting, anorexia; diarrhea

Integumentary: Hypersensitivity reactions

Interactions with Guarana

Drug

Adenosine: Guarana may decrease the adenosine response.

Antihypertensives: Guarana may decrease the effects of antihypertensives (theoretical).

Beta-blockers: Guarana may increase the effects of beta-blockers such as metoprolol (theoretical).

Bronchodilators: Guarana may increase the action of bronchodilators due to caffeine content.

MAOIs (isocarboxazid, phenelzine, tranylcypromine): Guarana in large amounts taken with MAOIs can result in hypertensive crisis; do not use together.

Continued

Interactions with Guarana—cont'd

Drug—cont'd

Xanthines: Xanthines such as theophylline and caffeine may increase pulse rate, blood pressure, and arrhythmias when used with guarana; avoid concurrent use.

Food

None known

Herb

Ephedra: Concurrent use of ephedra and guarana may increase hypertension and central nervous system stimulation; avoid concurrent use.

Lab Test

None known

Client Considerations

Assess

- Assess for hypersensitivity reactions. If present, discontinue use of this herb and administer antihistamine or other appropriate therapy.
- Assess for use of medications and ephedra (see Interactions).

Administer

- Instruct the client to store guarana products in a cool, dry place, away from heat and moisture.

Teach Client/Family

- Because of the caffeine content, until more research is available, caution the client not to use this herb during pregnancy and lactation and not to give it to children.
- Warn the client of the life-threatening side effects of guarana.

Pharmacology

Pharmacokinetics

Caffeine crosses the placenta and enters breast milk. Other pharmacokinetics and pharmacodynamics are unknown.

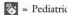

Primary Chemical Components of Guarana and Their Possible Actions

Chemical Class	Individual Component	Possible Action
Tannin	Catechutannic acid	Wound healing
	Tannic acid; Catechol; Catechin	Antioxidant
Saponin	Timbonine	Skin softener
Xanthine	Caffeine	Central nervous system stimulator

G

Actions

Very few studies corroborate any of the uses or actions of guarana in humans.

Antioxidant Action

One study examined the antioxidant effects of guarana (Mattei, 1998). The herb was found to possess antioxidant components.

Stimulant/Weight Loss Action

Guarana has been used for centuries in Brazil for its stimulant properties, which result from its high caffeine content. Weight loss occurs when ephedra is combined with caffeine products. Because guarana has a significant caffeine content, weight loss may be expected when it is combined with ephedra. However, central nervous system stimulation may be increased significantly when the two are combined. Delayed gastric emptying and promotion of fullness may be responsible for the weight reduction effect of guarana (Andersen, 2001).

References

Andersen T et al: Weight loss and delayed gastric emptying following a South American herbal preparation in overweight patients, *J Hum Nutr Diet* 14(3):243-250, 2001.

Mattei R et al: Guarana *(Paullinia cupana):* toxic behavioral effects in laboratory animals and antioxidants activity in vitro, *J Ethnopharmacol* 60(2):111-116, 1998.

🍀 Endangered Herb   Adverse effects: BOLD = life-threatening

Guggul
(gew'guhl)

Scientific name: *Commiphora mukul*

Other common names:
Mukul myrrh tree, myrrh   Class 2b (Prepared Gum Resin)

Origin: Guggul is found in India.

Uses

Reported Uses

Guggul is used to decrease high cholesterol and to treat arthritic conditions. It is used in Ayurvedic medicine to treat obesity and increase fat metabolism. Guggul is believed to increase thyroid function, but no studies confirm this. Guggul may be used to treat gum infections (gingivitis, pyorrhea, mouth ulcers).

Product Availability and Dosages

Available Forms

Alcoholic extract, crude gum, gugulipid, guggulsterone, petroleum ether extract

Plant Parts Used: Resin

Dosages and Routes

Adult

All dosages listed are PO.
- Alcoholic extract: 4.5 g qd
- Crude gum guggul: 10 g qd
- Gugulipid: 500 mg, standardized to 5% guggulsterones
- Guggulsterone: 25 mg tid
- Petroleum ether extract: 1.5 g qd

Precautionary Information

Contraindications

Because it can cause uterine contractions, guggul should not be used during pregnancy. Until more research is available, this herb should not be used during lactation and should not be given to children. Persons with hypersensitivity to guggul should not use it. Class 2b herb (prepared gum resin).

※ = Pregnancy   **※** = Pediatric   **◆** = Alert   **∥** = Popular Herb

Precautionary Information—cont'd

Side Effects/Adverse Reactions
Gastrointestinal: Nausea, vomiting, anorexia, diarrhea
Genitourinary: Kidney irritation (large doses)
Integumentary: Hypersensitivity reactions, rash

Interactions with Guggul			
Drug	Food	Herb	Lab Test
None known	None known	None known	None known

Client Considerations

Assess
- Assess for hypersensitivity reactions. If present, discontinue use of guggul and administer antihistamine or other appropriate therapy.

Administer
- Instruct the client to take guggul PO.
- Instruct the client to store guggul products in a cool, dry place, away from heat and moisture.

Teach Client/Family
- Because it can cause uterine contractions, caution the client not to use guggul during pregnancy. Until more research is available, caution the client not to use this herb during lactation and not to give it to children.

Pharmacology

Pharmacokinetics
Pharmacokinetics and pharmacodynamics are unknown.

Primary Chemical Components of Guggul and Their Possible Actions		
Chemical Class	**Individual Components**	**Possible Action**
Guggulsterones	E; Z	Lipid lowering; bile acid antagonist
Aromatic acid Nonaromatic acid Steroidal compound		

Actions

Anticholesterol Action

Guggulsterones have been shown to decrease cholesterol synthesis in the hepatic system and promote the breakdown and excretion of cholesterol (Satyavati, 1991; Wu, 2002; Urizar, 2002). Three studies have investigated the use of guggul for the reduction of cholesterol and triglyceride levels, and all showed a significant reduction of both (Nityanand, 1989; Verma, 1988; Agarwal, 1986). Two of the studies used guggulipid, and the third used gum guggul.

Antiobesity Action

More studies are needed to confirm the efficacy of guggul in reducing obesity and stimulating thyroid function. To date, no studies have confirmed these potential actions.

References

Agarwal RC et al: Clinical trial of guggulipid: a new hypolipidemic agent of plant origin in primary hyperlipidemic agent of plant origin in primary hyperlipidemia, *Indian J Med Res* 84:626-634, 1986.

Nityanand S et al: Clinical trials with guggulipid: a new hypolipidemic agent, *J Assoc Physicians India* 37(5):323-328, 1989.

Satyavati G: Guggulipid: a promising hypolipidaemic agent from gum guggul *(Commiphora wightii)*. In Wagner H et al, editors: *Economic and medicinal plant research,* vol 5, San Diego, 1991, Academic Press.

Urizar NL et al: A natural product that lowers cholesterol as an antagonist ligand for FXR, *Science* 296(5573):1703-1706, 2002.

Verma SK et al: Effect of *Commiphora mukul* (gum guggulu) in patients of hyperlipidemia with special reference to HDL-cholesterol, *Indian J Med Res* 87:356-360, 1988.

Wu J et al: The hypolipidemic natural product guggulsterone acts as an antagonist of the bile acid receptor, *Mol Endocrinol* 16(7):1590-1597, 2002.

🔥 = Pregnancy   🐾 = Pediatric   ◆ = Alert   🌿 = Popular Herb

Gum Arabic
(guhm eh'ruh-bik)

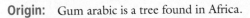

Scientific name: *Acacia senegal*

Other common names: Egyptian thorn, senega

Origin: Gum arabic is a tree found in Africa.

Uses

G

Reported Uses

Gum arabic is used to lower cholesterol and to improve renal status in persons with chronic renal failure. Gum arabic chewing gum has been used to improve gingival health and to reduce oral plaque formation. Other reported traditional uses include treatment of diarrhea, sore throat, inflammation, and cough.

Product Availability and Dosages

Available Forms

Gum, powder, syrup

Plant Parts Used: Gum from tree

Dosages and Routes

Adult

To Lower Cholesterol

• PO powder: 10-50 g qd

To Promote Dental Health

• PO gum: may be chewed qd; no specific dosages are reported

Precautionary Information

Contraindications

Until more research is available, gum arabic should not be used during pregnancy and lactation and should not be given to children. It should not be used by persons with hypersensitivity to gum arabic or those with contact dermatitis.

Side Effects/Adverse Reactions

Gastrointestinal: Diarrhea, bloating, flatulence; HEPATOTOXICITY (intravenous use)

Continued

 Endangered Herb   Adverse effects: BOLD = life-threatening

> **Precautionary Information—cont'd**
> **Side Effects/Adverse Reactions—cont'd**
> *Genitourinary:* NEPHROTOXICITY (INCREASED BLOOD UREA NITROGEN [BUN] AND CREATININE LEVELS) (intravenous use)
> *Integumentary:* Hypersensitivity reactions, contact dermatitis, other skin lesions

Interactions with Gum Arabic			
Drug	Food	Herb	Lab Test
None known	None known	None known	None known

Client Considerations
Assess
- Assess for hypersensitivity reactions, contact dermatitis, and other skin lesions. If these are present, discontinue use of gum arabic and administer antihistamine or other appropriate therapy.

- Assess for hepatotoxicity (increased ALT, AST, and bilirubin levels) and nephrotoxicity (increased BUN and creatinine levels) if herb was used intravenously.

Administer
- Instruct the client to store gum arabic in a cool, dry place, away from heat and moisture.

Teach Client/Family

- Until more research is available, caution the client not to use gum arabic during pregnancy and lactation and not to give it to children.
- Warn the client of the life-threatening side effects of gum arabic.
- Warn the client not to use this herb parenterally.

Pharmacology
Pharmacokinetics
Pharmacokinetics and pharmacodynamics are unknown.

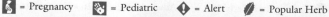

Chemical Class	Individual Component	Possible Action
Primary Chemical Components of Gum Arabic and Their Possible Actions		
Tannin		Wound healing; astringent
Mineral	Calcium; Potassium; Magnesium	
Glycoside		Antimicrobial
Polysaccharide		
Oxidase		
Peroxidase		Antimicrobial
Pectinase		Antimicrobial

G

Actions

Dental Health Promotion

In traditional herbal medicine, gum arabic is often used to promote dental health. Because several of its chemical components inhibit the growth of microbes, there may be reason for its use to reduce dental plaque and decrease periodontal disease. Although few studies are available to support the anecdotal reports for this use, one study has demonstrated that gum arabic decreases the number of microbes present in periodontal areas of the mouth (Clark, 1993).

Antilipidemic Action

Other studies have evaluated the possible antilipidemic action of gum arabic. Results have been poor, and at present gum arabic appears to exert no antilipidemic effects.

Renal Action

One study evaluated the excretion of fecal nitrogen content in patients with chronic renal failure (Bliss, 1996). Fecal nitrogen content and serum urea nitrogen was decreased significantly with the use of gum arabic.

Other Actions

Gum arabic has been used in topical preparations for its demulcent and soothing qualities.

🍀 Endangered Herb   Adverse effects: BOLD = life-threatening

References

Bliss DZ et al: Supplementation with gum Arabic fiber increases fecal nitrogen excretion and lowers serum urea nitrogen concentration in chronic renal failure patients consuming a low-protein diet, *Am J Clin Nutr* 63:392-398, 1996.

Clark DT et al: The effects of *Acacia arabica* gum on the in vitro growth and protease activities of periodontopathic bacteria, *J Clin Periodontol* 20:238-243, 1993.

Gymnema

Scientific name: *Gymnema sylvestre*

Other common names: Gurmar, meshashringi, merasingi

Origin: Gymnema is found in India and Africa.

Uses

Reported Uses

Gymnema has been used traditionally in Ayurvedic medicine to treat diabetes mellitus, to treat malaria, and as a laxative.

Investigational Uses

Studies are underway for the use of gymnema to lower lipids.

Product Availability and Dosages

Available Forms

Extract

Plant Parts Used: Leaves

Dosages and Routes

Adult

Diabetes Mellitus

• PO extract: 200 mg bid (Murray, 1998).

Precautionary Information

Contraindications

Until more research is available, gymnema should not be used during pregnancy and lactation and should not be given to children. Persons with hypersensitivity to this herb should not use it.

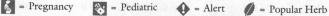

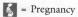 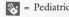

Precautionary Information—cont'd

Side Effects/Adverse Reactions

Gastrointestinal: Nausea, vomiting, anorexia, inhibition of bitter/sweet taste

Integumentary: Hypersensitivity reactions

Interactions with Gymnema

G

Drug

Insulin: Gymnema may increase the action of insulin (theoretical).

Oral antidiabetics (acetohexamide, chlorpropamide, glipizide, glyburide, metformin, tolazamide, tolbutamide, troglitazone): Gymnema may increase the action of oral antidiabetics (theoretical).

Food	Herb
None known	None known

Lab Test

Gymnema may cause decreased blood glucose (decoctions, infusions), decreased LDL cholesterol, and total cholesterol.

Client Considerations

Assess

- Assess for hypersensitivity reactions. If present, discontinue use of gymnema and administer antihistamine or other appropriate therapy.
- Assess for use of insulin and oral antidiabetics (see Interactions).

Administer

- Instruct the client to store gymnema in a cool, dry place, away from heat and moisture.

Teach Client/Family

- Until more research is available, caution the client not to use this herb during pregnancy and lactation and not to give it to children.

Pharmacology

Pharmacokinetics

Pharmacokinetics and pharmacodynamics are unknown.

Primary Chemical Components of Gymnema and Their Possible Actions		
Chemical Class	**Individual Component**	**Possible Action**
Gymnemic acid Triterpene glycosides	Longispinogenin	Antidiabetic

Actions

Antidiabetic Action

Several studies have investigated the antidiabetic action of gymnema. In one study, rats were fed gymnema at doses of 100 mg/kg for 30 days. Blood glucose levels dropped significantly by the second week (Gupta, 1962). Another study evaluated gymnema against the antidiabetic drug tolbutamide. The reduction in blood glucose from gymnema was equivalent to that of tolbutamide (Gupta, 1964). The antidiabetic action of this herb may be due to its ability to stimulate functioning beta cells in the pancreas to release insulin.

Lipid-Lowering Action

A few studies have shown the lipid-lowering effect of *Gymnema* (Shigematsu, 2001; Shigematsu, 2001).

References

Gupta SS et al: *Indian J Med Res* 50:1, 1962.
Gupta SS et al: *Indian J Med Res* 52:200, 1964.
Murray M, Pizzarno J: *The encyclopedia of natural medicine,* 2 ed (revised), Roseville, Calif, 1998, Prima.
Shigematsu N et al: Effect of administration with the extract of *Gymnema sylvestre* R. Br. leaves on lipid metabolism in rats; *Biol Pharm Bull* 24(6):713-717, 2001.
Shigematsu N et al: Effect of long-term administration with *Gymnema sylvestre* R. Br. on plasma and liver lipid in rats, *Biol Pharm Bull* 24(6):643-649, 2001.

 = Pregnancy   = Pediatric    = Alert   = Popular Herb

Hawthorn
(haw'thawrn)

Scientific name: *Crataegus* spp.

Other common names: Li 132, may, maybush, quickset, thorn-apple tree, whitethorn

Class 1 (Flowers, Fruit, Leaves)

Origin: Hawthorn is a bush or tree found throughout the United States, Canada, Europe, and Asia.

H

Uses
Reported Uses
Hawthorn is one of the most commonly used herbs. It is used to treat cardiovascular disorders such as hypertension, arrhythmias, arteriosclerosis, congestive heart failure, Buerger's disease, and stable angina pectoris.

Product Availability and Dosages
Available Forms
Capsules of berries, extended release capsules, fluid extract, leaves, solid extract, tea, tincture, topical cream

Plant Parts Used: Flowers, fruit, leaves

Dosages and Routes
Adult
All dosages listed are PO.
Angina
- Berries of flowers, dried: 3-5 g tid or as a tea (Murray, 1998)
- Fluid extract: 1-2 ml (¼-½ tsp) tid (1:1 dilution) (Murray, 1998)
- Solid extract: 100-250 mg tid (10% procyanidin or 1.8% vitexin-4'-rhamnoside) (Murray, 1998)
- Tincture: 4-6 ml (1-1½ tsp) tid (1:5 dilution) (Murray, 1998)

Coronary Artery Disease
- Solid extract: 100-250 mg tid (10% procyanidin content or 1.8% vitexin-4'-rhamnoside) (Murray, 1998)

General Use
- Solid extract: 120-240 mg tid of a standardized product (18.75% procyanidines or 2.2% flavonoids)
- Tea: 1-2 tsp berries, steep in 8 oz water for 15 min, strain, drink tid

🌍 Endangered Herb   Adverse effects: **BOLD** = life-threatening

- Tincture: 5 ml tid (1:5 dilution)

Moderate Hypertension
- Solid extract 100-250 mg tid (10% procyanidin content or 1.8% vitexin-4′-rhamnoside) (Murray, 1998)

 Child

General Use
- PO tea: 1 cup several times/wk (Romm, 2000)
- PO tincture: ¼-1 tsp up to tid (Romm, 2000)
- Topical cream: apply prn (Romm, 2000)

Precautionary Information

Contraindications

Until more research is available, hawthorn should not be used during pregnancy and lactation. It should not be used by persons with hypersensitivity to this herb or *Rosaceae* spp. Class 1 herb (flowers, fruit, leaves).

Side Effects/Adverse Reactions

Cardiovascular: Hypotension, arrhythmias
Central Nervous System: Fatigue, sedation
Gastrointestinal: Nausea, vomiting, anorexia
Integumentary: Hypersensitivity reactions

Interactions with Hawthorn

Drug

Antihypertensives (beta-blockers): Hawthorn may increase hypotension when used with antihypertensives; avoid concurrent use.
Cardiac glycosides: Hawthorn may increase the effects of cardiac glycosides; monitor concurrent use carefully.
Central nervous system depressants: Hawthorn may increase the sedative effects of central nervous system depressants such as alcohol, barbiturates, and psychotropics; avoid concurrent use.
Iron salts: Hawthorn tea may decrease the absorption of iron salts; separate by at least 2 hr.

Food

None known

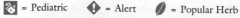

= Pregnancy   = Pediatric   = Alert   = Popular Herb

Interactions with Hawthorn—cont'd

Herb

Adonis: Hawthorn increases the action of *Adonis vernalis* when taken concurrently.

Lily of the valley: Hawthorn increases the action of *Convallaria majalis* when taken concurrently.

Squill: Hawthorn increases the action of *Scillae bulbus* when taken concurrently.

Lab Test

Hawthorn may cause false increase of serum digoxin.

H

Client Considerations

Assess

- Assess for hypersensitivity reactions. If present, discontinue use of hawthorn and administer antihistamine or other appropriate therapy.
- Assess cardiovascular status if the client is taking hawthorn to treat congestive heart failure.
- Assess for other cardiovascular drugs the client may be taking, including beta-blockers, cardiac glycosides, central nervous system depressants, and antihypertensives; assess for use of the herbs adonis and lily of the valley (see Interactions).

Administer

- Instruct the client to take hawthorn PO as an extract, tincture, or tea.
- Instruct the client to store hawthorn products in a cool, dry place, away from heat and moisture.

Teach Client/Family

- Until more research is available, caution the client not to use hawthorn during pregnancy and lactation.
- Caution the client to check with the prescriber before giving hawthorn to a child who is taking cardiovascular medications (Romm, 2000).
- Advise the client not to use this herb if allergic to *Rosaceae* spp.

Endangered Herb   Adverse effects: BOLD = life-threatening

Pharmacology

Pharmacokinetics

Pharmacokinetics and pharmacodynamics are unknown.

Primary Chemical Components of Hawthorn and Their Possible Actions

Chemical Class	Individual Components	Possible Action
Flavonoid	Quercetin Rutin Hyperoside; Vitexin; Vitexin-rhamnoside	Antiinflammatory Antioxidant
Proanthocyanidin	Procyanidin C-1	Angiotensin-converting enzyme (ACE) inhibitor; chronotropic Antiviral (Shahatt, 2002)
Catechin Epicatechin Eudesmanolide		

Actions

Cardiovascular Action

Hawthorn exerts both antihypertensive and antihyperlipidemic effects (Wegrowski, 1984). It increases blood supply to the heart, increases the force of contractions (Petkov, 1981), and indirectly inhibits angiotensin-converting enzyme (ACE) (Uchida, 1987). The proanthocyanidins, among the chemical components of hawthorn, have been shown to inhibit ACE in a manner similar to that of the drug captopril. Hawthorn also stabilizes collagen, reduces atherosclerosis, and decreases cholesterol (Wegrowski, 1984). The collagen-stabilizing action of hawthorn helps to keep the artery strong and free of plaque development. Hawthorn can be used with cardiac glycosides in the treatment of congestive heart failure. In one study, participants received 600 mg of standardized hawthorn extract or a placebo daily. The treatment group experienced increased

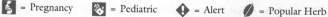
= Pregnancy   = Pediatric   = Alert   = Popular Herb

cardiac working capacity and reduced blood pressure (Schmidt, 1994; Schmidt, 2000).

References

Murray M, Pizzarno J: *The encyclopedia of natural medicine,* 2 ed (revised), Roseville, Calif, 1998, Prima.

Petkov E et al: Inhibitory effect of some flavonoids and flavonoid mixtures on cyclic AMP phosdiesterase activity of rat heart, *Planta Med* 43:183-186, 1981.

Romm A: *Better Nutrition's* 2000 guide to children's supplements, *Better Nutr* 62:10, 2000.

Schmidt U et al: Effects of an herbal crataegus-camphor combination on the symptoms of cardiovascular diseases, *Arzneimittelforschung* 50(7): 613-619, 2000.

Schmidt U et al: Efficacy of the hawthorn *(Crataegus)* preparation LI 132 in 78 patients with chronic congestive heart failure defined as NYHA functional class II, *Phytomedicine* 1:17-24, 1994.

Shahatt AA et al: Antiviral and antioxidant activity of flavonoids and proanthocyanidins from *Crataegus sinaicu*, *Planta Med* 68(6):539-541, 2002.

Uchida S et al: Inhibitory effects of condensed tannins on angiotensin converting enzyme, *Jpn J Pharmacol* 43:242-245, 1987.

Wegrowski J et al: The effect of procyanidolic oligomers on the composition of normal and hypercholesterolemic rabbit aortas, *Biochem Pharmacol* 33:3491-3497, 1984.

H

Hops
(hahps)

Scientific name: *Humulus lupulus*   Class 2d (Strobiles)

Origin: The hop plant is a perennial that is cultivated throughout the world.

Uses

Reported Uses

Hops traditionally have been used as an analgesic, antidepressant, and anthelmintic and as a sedative/hypnotic to treat insomnia. They are also used to treat menopausal symptoms and to wean patients off conventional sedative prescriptions.

Product Availability and Dosages
Available Forms
Cut herb, dry extract, extract, powdered dry herb, tea

Plant Parts Used: Whole hops

Dosages and Routes
Adult
All dosages listed are PO.
- Infusion: pour 8 oz boiling water over 0.4 g (1 tsp) ground hops cone, let stand 15 min
- Extract: 2-4 mg
- Cut herb 0.5 g as a single dose (Blumenthal, 1998)

Precautionary Information
Contraindications
Hops should not be used by persons who are hypersensitive to this product; persons who have breast, uterine, or cervical cancers; or those who suffer from a depressive condition. Hops are for short-term or intermittent use only. Class 2d herb (strobiles).

Side Effects/Adverse Reactions
Central Nervous System: Sedation, dizziness, decreased reaction time
Gastrointestinal: Nausea, vomiting, anorexia
Integumentary: Hypersensitivity reactions, including dermatitis and ANAPHYLAXIS

Interactions with Hops

Drug
Antidepressants: Hops may cause increased central nervous system effects when taken concurrently with antidepressants.
Antipsychotics: Hops may cause increased central nervous system effects when taken concurrently with antipsychotics.
Antihistamines: Hops may cause increased central nervous system effects when taken concurrently with antihistamines.
Alcohol: Hops may cause increased central nervous system effects when taken in conjunction with alcohol.

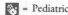 = Pregnancy   = Pediatric   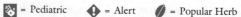 = Alert   = Popular Herb

Interactions with Hops—cont'd

Drug—cont'd

Central nervous system depressants: Hops may cause increased central nervous system effects when taken concurrently with CNS depressants.

Cytochrome P-450 (carbamazepine, bupropion, orphenadrine, cyclophosphamide, citalopram, azole antifungals, macrolide antibiotics, omeprazole, warfarin, theophylline): Hops may decrease the levels of these drugs.

Estrogens: Hops may cause increased hormonal levels when taken in conjunction with estrogen (theoretical).

Iron salts: Hops tea may decrease the absorption of iron salts; separate by at least 2 hr.

Food	Herb	Lab Test
None known	None known	None known

H

Client Considerations

Assess

- Assess for hypersensitivity reactions and dermatitis. If these are present, discontinue use of hops and administer antihistamine or other appropriate therapy.
- Assess for anaphylaxis.
- Assess for central nervous system reactions: sedation, dizziness, and decreased reaction time.
- Assess for medications used (see Interactions).

Administer

- Instruct the client to store hops in a cool, dry place, away from heat and moisture.

Teach Client/Family

- Advise the client not to perform hazardous tasks such as driving or operating heavy machinery if sedation, dizziness, or decreased reaction time occurs.

Pharmacology

Pharmacokinetics

Pharmacokinetics and pharmacodynamics are unknown.

Primary Chemical Components of Hops and Their Possible Actions		
Chemical Class	**Individual Component**	**Possible Action**
Acylphloro-glucinol		
Volatile oil	Humulene; Linalool; Lupulone Myrcene	Antineoplastic; antimicrobial
Hormone	Estradiol	Estrogenic
Colupulone		Antiinfective
Flavonoid	Xanthohumol; Prenylnaringenin; Isoxanthohumol	Cytochrome P450 inhibitor (Henderson, 2000)
Avermectin		Antiinfective
Phenolic acid	Ferulic acid; Caffeic acid	
Tannin		

Actions

Hops have been used by the food and liquor industries as a flavoring for food and beer. Three medicinal uses for hops are described here, although little reliable research exists for any uses or actions.

Estrogenic Action

Hops are believed to possess estrogen-like activity due to the phytoestrogen components of the hop plant and its ability to exert direct estrogenic effects (Zava, 1998). One older study demonstrated estrogenic activity in an acid fraction of the plant (Zenisek, 1960). However, many of the other available studies contain conflicting information regarding the estrogenic action. At this point it is uncertain whether the hop plant does exert estrogen-like activity.

Sedative/Hypnotic Action

The sedative/hypnotic effects of hops may be due to the volatile oils present in the plant (Tyler, 1987). The same volatile oils may also be responsible for the antispasticity effect.

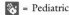 = Pregnancy   = Pediatric   ◆ = Alert   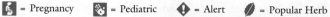 = Popular Herb

Antimicrobial Action

One small study shows that the antimicrobial effects of hops result from the bitter acid components (volatile oils) lupulone, humulene, and linalool (Leung, 1980).

References

Blumenthal M, editor: *The complete German Commission E monographs: therapeutic guide to herbal medicines,* Austin, Tex, American Botanical Council; Boston, Integrative Medicine Communication, 1998.

Henderson MC et al: In vitro inhibition of human P450 enzymes by prenylated flavonoids from hops, *Humulus lupulus, Xenobiotica* 30(3): 235-251, 2000.

Leung AY: *Encyclopedia of common natural ingredients used in food, drugs, and cosmetics,* New York, 1980, John Wiley & Sons.

Tyler VE: *The new honest herbal,* Philadelphia, 1987, GF Stickley.

Zava DT et al: Estrogen and progestin bioactivity of foods, herbs and spices, *Proc Soc Exp Biol Med* 217:369-378, 1998.

Zenisek et al: Contribution to the identification of the estrogen activity of hops, *Am Perfumer Arom* 75:61, 1960.

Horehound
(hoer′hound)

Scientific name: *Marrubium vulgare*

Other common names: Common horehound, hoarhound, houndsbane, marvel, white horehound

Class 2b (Whole Herb)

Origin: Horehound is a perennial found in Asia, Europe, the United States, and Canada.

Uses

Reported Uses

In traditional herbal medicine, horehound has been used internally to increase diuresis; to treat upper respiratory congestion, whooping cough, anorexia, asthma, bronchitis, tuberculosis, and diarrhea; to aid digestion; and as an anthelmintic and a laxative. Its topical form has been used to promote wound healing.

Investigational Uses

Researchers are beginning to investigate the potential role of horehound in the treatment of hyperglycemia.

🌿 Endangered Herb   Adverse effects: BOLD = life-threatening

Product Availability and Dosages
Available Forms
Capsules, cough lozenges, extract, powder, pressed juice, syrup, tea

Plant Parts Used: Dried leaves, flowering tops, fresh leaves

Dosages and Routes
Adult
All dosages listed are PO.
- Extract: 10-40 drops in a small amount of water, tid
- Infusion: pour 8 oz boiling water over herb, let stand 10 min, strain; take 1-2 g up to tid
- Lozenges: use prn
- Powder: 1-2 g tid; 4.5 g qd (Blumenthal, 1998)
- Pressed juice: 2-6 tbsp qd (Blumenthal, 1998)

Precautionary Information
Contraindications
Because horehound is an abortifacient, it should not be used during pregnancy. Until more research is available, this herb should not be used during lactation and should not be given to children. Horehound should not be used by persons who are hypersensitive to it or who have arrhythmias. Class 2b herb (whole herb).

Side Effects/Adverse Reactions
Cardiovascular: Arrhythmias
Endocrine: Decreased blood glucose
Gastrointestinal: Nausea, vomiting, anorexia, diarrhea
Integumentary: Hypersensitivity reactions

Interactions with Horehound

Drug
Antiarrhythmics: Antiarrhythmics may produce an increased serotonin effect when used with horehound; avoid concurrent use (theoretical).
Antidiabetics: Horehound may enhance hypoglycemia when used with antidiabetics; avoid concurrent use (theoretical).

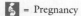 = Pregnancy    = Pediatric   = Alert   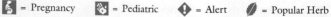 = Popular Herb

Interactions with Horehound—cont'd

Drug—cont'd

Emetics: Emetics such as granisetron and ondansetron may produce an increased serotonin effect when used with horehound; avoid concurrent use.

Ergots: Ergots may produce an increased serotonin effect when used with horehound; avoid concurrent use (theoretical).

Iron salts: Horehound tea may decrease the aborption of iron salts; separate by 2 hr.

Sumatriptan: Sumatriptan may produce an increased serotonin effect when used with horehound; avoid concurrent use.

Food	Herb	Lab Test
None known	None known	None known

H

Client Considerations

Assess

- Assess for hypersensitivity reactions. If present, discontinue use of horehound and administer antihistamine or other appropriate therapy.
- Assess blood glucose levels in diabetic clients. Identify other antidiabetic agents the client is taking.
- Assess cardiac status: blood pressure, pulse, and ECG changes in clients with cardiac disorders.
- Assess for medications used (see Interactions).

Administer

- Horehound products should be kept away from heat and moisture.
- Use horehound for short-term use (<2 wk).

Teach Client/Family

- Because it is an abortifacient, caution the client not to use horehound during pregnancy. Until more research is available, caution the client not to use this herb during lactation and not to give it to children.
- Advise the diabetic client that horehound may increased hypoglycemia and to use caution when taking horehound with antidiabetic medications.

 Endangered Herb   Adverse effects: BOLD = life-threatening

- Because of its many drug interactions, advise the client to consult a qualified herbalist before using horehound in any form other than lozenges.

Pharmacology

Pharmacokinetics

Pharmacokinetics and pharmacodynamics are unknown.

Primary Chemical Components of Horehound and Their Possible Actions		
Chemical Class	**Individual Component**	**Possible Action**
Volatile oil	Camphene; Cymene; Fenchene	
Diterpene bitter	Marrubiin	Bile secretion, expectorant
	Premarrubiin	
Tannin		Wound healing
Flavonoid	Chrysoeriol; Luteolin; Apigenin; Vicenin II	
Phenylethanoid glycoside	Marruboside	
	Acteside 2; Forsythoside; Arenarioside; Ballotetroside	

Actions

Horehound has been used primarily in Mexico, Europe, and Asia. Currently, horehound's use as an ingredient in throat lozenges is common in the United States. Although its most common use is as an expectorant, no studies are available to support this action, and few studies support any uses or actions of this herb. However, one study using laboratory rabbits found that horehound acted as a hypoglycemic (Roman, 1992). Another proposed action is an inhibitory effect on serotonin (Cahen, 1970). Evidence also suggests that one of the chemical components, marrubiin, may affect bile secretion (Krejci, 1959). One study (El Bardai, 2001) showed the hypotensive activity of horehound in hypertensive rats.

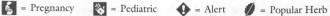

References

Blumenthal M, editor: *The complete German Commission E monographs: therapeutic guide to herbal medicines,* Austin, Tex, American Botanical Council; Boston, Integrative Medicine Communication, 1998.

Cahen R: Pharmacological spectrum of *Marrubium vulgare, C R Seances Soc Biol Fil* 164:1467, 1970.

El Bardai S et al: Pharmacological evidence of hypotensive activity of *Marrubium vulgare* and *Foeniculum vulgare* in spontaneously hypertensive rat, *Clin Exp Hypertens* 23(4):329-343, 2001.

Krejci I et al: *Planta Med* 7:1, 1959.

Roman RR et al: Hypoglycemic effect of plants used in Mexico as antidiabetics, *Arch Med Res* 23(1):59, 1992.

H

Horse Chestnut

(hoers chehs'nuht)

Scientific names: *Aesculus hippocastanum, Aesculus california, Aesculus glabra*

Other common names: Aescin, buckeye, California buckeye, chestnut, escine, Ohio buckeye

Origin: Horse chestnut is a tree or shrub found worldwide.

Uses

Reported Uses

Traditional uses of horse chestnut include treatment of fever, phlebitis, hemorrhoids, prostate enlargement, edema, inflammation, and diarrhea. It is commonly used in Germany to treat varicose veins.

Investigational Uses

Researchers are investigating the use of horse chestnut for treatment of venous insufficiency and varicose veins.

Product Availability and Dosages

Available Forms

Standardized extract, tincture

Plant Parts Used: Seeds, young bark

Dosages and Routes

Adult

• PO standardized extract: 100-150 mg qd in two divided doses
• PO tincture: 1-2 ml in ½ cup water, bid-qid (Smith, 1999)

🌀 Endangered Herb   Adverse effects: BOLD = life-threatening

Precautionary Information

Contraindications

Until more research is available, horse chestnut should not be used during pregnancy and lactation and it should not be given to children.

Side Effects/Adverse Reactions

Gastrointestinal: Nausea, vomiting, anorexia, **hepatotoxicity**

Genitourinary: NEPHROPATHY, NEPHROTOXICITY

Integumentary: Pruritus, hypersensitivity, rash, urticaria

Musculoskeletal: Spasms

Systemic: Bruising, SEVERE BLEEDING, SHOCK; SEEDS ARE TOXIC

Interactions with Horse Chestnut

Drug

Anticoagulants (anisindione, dicumarol, heparin, warfarin): Because of the presence of hydroxycoumarin, a chemical component of the herb that possesses anticoagulant activity, concurrent use of horse chestnut and anticoagulants increases the risk of severe bleeding. Do not use concurrently.

Antidiabetics: May increase the hypoglycemic effects of diabetic medications.

Aspirin and other salicylates: Because of the presence of hydroxycoumarin, a chemical component of the herb that possesses anticoagulant activity, concurrent use of horse chestnut and aspirin or other salicylates increases the risk of severe bleeding. Do not use concurrently.

Iron salts: Horse chestnut tea may decrease the absorption of iron salts; separate by 2 hr.

Food	Herb	Lab Test
None known	None known	None known

Client Considerations

Assess

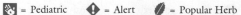

• Assess for symptoms of hepatotoxicity (increasing AST, ALT, and bilirubin levels; clay-colored stools; jaundice; right

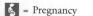 = Pregnancy    = Pediatric   = Alert   = Popular Herb

upper-quadrant pain). If any of these symptoms is present, discontinue use of this herb.
- Assess for bleeding and bruising. If these are present, discontinue use of this herb.
- Assess for allergic reactions such as rash or itching. If these occur, discontinue use of this herb.
- Assess kidney function if high dosage is suspected. Obtain blood urea nitrogen (BUN) and creatinine levels. Monitor for nephrotoxicity.
- Assess for medications used (see Interactions).
- Assess for toxicity (see Side Effects).

Administer
- Instruct the client to store horse chestnut in a cool, dry place, away from heat and moisture.

Teach Client/Family
- Until more research is available, caution the client not to use horse chestnut during pregnancy and lactation and not to give it to children.
- Warn the client of the life-threatening side effects of horse chestnut; not to use older bark, it is poisonous.

Pharmacology
Pharmacokinetics
Pharmacokinetics and pharmacodynamics are unknown.

Primary Chemical Components of Horse Chestnut and Their Possible Actions

Chemical Class	Individual Component	Possible Action
Steroid	Stigmasterol; Alpha-spinasterol; Beta-sitosterol	Antiinflammatory
Triterpene glycoside	Aescin	Decreased permeability of venous capillaries
Flavonoid	Quercetin; Kaempferol Astragalin; Iso-quercetin; Rutin	Antiinflammatory
Coumarin	Aesculetin; Fraxin; Scopolin	
Allantoin		
Choline		

Continued

Primary Chemical Components of Horse Chestnut and Their Possible Actions—cont'd		
Chemical Class	**Individual Component**	**Possible Action**
Phytosterol Amino acid Citric acid Tannin		Wound healing; antiinflammatory
Seeds Also Contain Oleic acid		

Actions

Antiinflammatory Action

Several studies have focused on the antiinflammatory action of horse chestnut. The chemical component aescin, a saponin present in horse chestnut, is responsible for its antiinflammatory properties (Matsuda, 1997). In another study of 30 patients with Widmer stage I or II CVI (central venous insufficiency), horse chestnut decreased the activity of lysosomal enzymes associated with venous insufficiency. The study participants received treatment with either tablets containing the substance (aescin) or a placebo. Those who received tablets containing aescin experienced significant improvement in ankle edema and venous filling rate. Subjective symptoms showed very little improvement (Shah, 1997).

References

Matsuda H et al: Effects of escins Ia, Ib, IIa, and IIb horse chestnut, the seeds of *Aesculus hippocastanum* L., on acute inflammation in animals, *Biol Pharm Bull* 20(10):1092-1095, 1997.

Shah D et al: Aescula force in chronic venous insufficiency, *Schweiz Zschr Ganzheitsmedizin* 9(2):86-91, 1997.

Smith E: *Therapeutic herb manual*, Williams, Ore, 1999, Author.

Horseradish
(hawrs'ra-dish)

Scientific name: *Armoracia rusticana*

Other common names: Great mountain root, pepperrot, great raifort, red cole

Class 2d (Rhizome, Root)

Origin: Horseradish is a perennial native to Europe but now found throughout the world.

Uses
Reported Uses
Horseradish is used to decrease joint inflammation; to reduce edema; and as an anthelmintic, diuretic, and antibacterial. It may also be used to treat sinusitis and whooping cough. Horseradish is a pungent, warming herb.

Product Availability and Dosages
Available Forms
Fresh root, paste, powder

Plant Parts Used: Roots

Dosages and Routes
Adult
- PO fresh root: 2-4 g ac
- Topical: 2% mustard oil maximum, applied prn

Precautionary Information
Contraindications
Because it is an abortifacient, horseradish should not be used during pregnancy. Until more research is available, this herb should not be used during lactation and should not be given to children younger than 4 years of age. Persons with hypothyroidism, hyperthyroidism, renal disease, gastrointestinal ulcers, or hypersensitivity to this herb should avoid its use. Horseradish is toxic if used internally in large quantities. Class 2d herb (rhizome/root).

Continued

 Endangered Herb   Adverse effects: **BOLD** = life-threatening

Precautionary Information—cont'd

Side Effects/Adverse Reactions

Ear, Eye, Nose, and Throat: Mucous membrane irritation
Gastrointestinal: Nausea, vomiting, anorexia, diarrhea
Integumentary: Hypersensitivity reactions

Interactions with Horseradish

Drug	Food	Herb	Lab Test
None known	None known	None known	None known

Client Considerations

Assess

- Assess for hypersensitivity reactions. If present, discontinue use of horseradish and administer antihistamine or other appropriate therapy.

Administer

- Instruct the client to store horseradish products in a cool, dry place, away from heat and moisture. Fresh roots should be kept buried.

Teach Client/Family

- Because it is an abortifacient, caution the client not to use horseradish during pregnancy. Until more research is available, caution the client not to use this herb during lactation and not to give it to children younger than 4 years of age.
- Because the horseradish plant is toxic if used internally in large quantities, advise the client to use horseradish internally only as a food flavoring.

Pharmacology

Pharmacokinetics

Pharmacokinetics and pharmacodynamics are unknown.

Primary Chemical Components of Horseradish and Their Possible Actions		
Chemical Class	**Individual Component**	**Possible Action**
Coumarin	Scopoletin; Aesculetin; Caffeic acid; Hydroxycinnamic acid	
Vitamin	C	
Peroxidase enzyme		
Resin		
Flavonoid	Quercetin; Kaempferol	Antiinflammatory
Asparagine		
Glucosinolate	Mustard oil	

H

Actions

Very little research is available on the actions of horseradish. Because the plant is poisonous, it should be used only as a flavoring in food unless under the supervision of a qualified herbalist. One study did show a hypotensive reaction in cats given horseradish IV (Sjaastad, 1984).

References

Duke J: *CRC handbook of medicinal herbs,* Boca Raton, Fla, 1985, CRC Press.

Sjaastad OV et al: Hypotensive effects in cats caused by horseradish peroxidase mediated metabolites of arachidonic acid, *J Histochem Cytochem* 32:1328-1330, 1984.

Horsetail
(hawrs'tayl)

Scientific name: *Equisetum arvense*

Other common names: Bottle brush, corn horsetail, dutch rushes, horse willow, horsetail grass, paddock pipes, pewterwort, scouring rush, shave grass, toadpipe

Class 2d (Whole Herb)

Origin: Horsetail is a perennial pteridophyte found throughout Europe and in parts of Asia.

Uses
Reported Uses
Horsetail is used internally to increase the strength of bones, teeth, nails, and hair. It also has been used internally as an antiinfective, diuretic, and anticancer treatment, as well as to decrease gout, prevent urinary stones, treat menorrhagia, and increase strength. It is used externally to promote wound healing.

Product Availability and Dosages
Available Forms
Crude herb, fluid extract; component in combination products

Plant Parts Used: Dried green aerial stems

Dosages and Routes
Adult
- PO fluid extract: initially, 20-40 drops tid-qid; maintenance 20-40 drops bid-tid (1:1 dilution in 25% alcohol)
- PO infusion: place 1.5 g herb in 8 oz water; take 2-4 g/day
- PO tea: pour 8 oz boiling water over 2-3 g herb, boil 5 min, let stand 15 min, strain
- Topical: 10 g herb/L water, used as a compress or bath prn

Precautionary Information
Contraindications
Until more research is available, horsetail should not be used during pregnancy and lactation and should not be given to children. This herb should not be used by persons with hypersensitivity to it or those with edema, cardiac disease, renal disease, or nicotine sensitivity. Horsetail contains nicotine

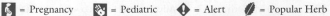

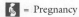 = Pregnancy    = Pediatric   = Alert   = Popular Herb

Precautionary Information—cont'd

Contraindications—cont'd

and should not be used for prolonged periods. The active chemicals in this herb are absorbed through the skin and can cause death. Class 2d herb (whole herb).

Side Effects/Adverse Reactions

Gastrointestinal: Nausea, vomiting, anorexia
Integumentary: Hypersensitivity reactions
Nicotine toxicity: WEAKNESS, DIZZINESS, FEVER, LOSS OF WEIGHT, FEELING OF COLD IN EXTREMITIES (VERY LARGE QUANTITIES)
Systemic: Thiamine deficiency

H

Interactions with Horsetail

Drug

Cardiac glycosides (digoxin): Horsetail may increase the toxicity of cardiac glycosides and increase hypokalemia.
Cerebral stimulants: Horsetail may cause increased central nervous system effects when used with cerebral stimulants; avoid concurrent use.
Diuretics: Horsetail may increase the effect of diuretics; avoid concurrent use (theoretical).
Lithium: Horsetail taken with lithium may cause dehydration and lithium toxicity.
Xanthines: Horsetail may cause increased central nervous system stimulation when used with xanthines such as caffeine and theophylline; avoid concurrent use.

Food

Horsetail may cause increased central nervous system stimulation when used with caffeinated coffee, tea, or cola; avoid concurrent use.

Herb

Adonis: Horsetail increases the action of *Adonis vernalis* when taken concurrently.
Lily of the valley: Horsetail increases the action of *Convalleria majalis* when taken concurrently.

Continued

Interactions with Horsetail—cont'd
Herb—cont'd **Squill:** Horsetail increases the action of *Scillae* bulbs when taken concurrently. **Tobacco:** Horsetail may cause increased central nervous system stimulation when used with tobacco; avoid concurrent use. Lab Test None known

Client Considerations

Assess

- Assess for hypersensitivity reactions. If present, discontinue use of horsetail and administer antihistamine or other appropriate therapy.
- Assess for the use of medications, caffeinated foods, and tobacco. Xanthines, cerebral stimulants, nicotine, coffee, tea, cola, and tobacco will cause increased central nervous system stimulation when used in conjunction with horsetail (see Interactions).
 - Assess for nicotine toxicity: weakness, dizziness, fever, weight loss, and feeling of cold in extremities. Horsetail would have to be taken in large quantities to cause a toxic reaction.

Administer

- Instruct the client to store horsetail products in sealed container away from heat and moisture.

Teach Client/Family

 - Until more research is available, caution the client not to use horsetail during pregnancy and lactation and not to give it to children.
- Caution the client not to confuse medicinal horsetail with other *Equisetum* spp.
- Warn the client about possible nicotine toxicity and the many drug, food, and herb interactions of horse chestnut.
- Warn the client to keep horsetail away from children. The active chemicals in this herb are absorbed through the skin and can cause death.

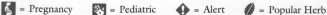
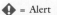

Pharmacology

Pharmacokinetics

Pharmacokinetics and pharmacodynamics are unknown.

Primary Chemical Components of Horsetail and Their Possible Actions		
Chemical Class	**Individual Component**	**Possible Action**
Flavonoid	Isoquercitrin; Equisetrin; Galuteolin	
Sterol	Cholesterol; Campesterol; Isofucosterol; Beta-sitosterol	
Alkaloid	Nicotine	Central nervous system stimulant
	Palustrinine; Palustrine	
Thiaminase		Thiamine deficiency

Actions

No data are available to confirm any uses or actions of horsetail. This herb exerts mild diuretic activity but is not recommended to treat any condition. Horsetail may increase sodium and water excretion. Anecdotal reports characterize it as an astringent used to stop bleeding, decrease inflammation, and promote wound healing. However, no evidence supports any of these claims.

References

Duke J: *CRC handbook of medicinal herbs,* Boca Raton, Fla, 1985, CRC Press.

Hyssop
(hi'suhp)

Scientific name(s): *Hyssopus officinalis*

Class 2b (Whole Herb)

Origin: Hyssop is a perennial found in the Mediterranean, the United States, and Canada.

Uses

Reported Uses

Hyssop has been used as a fragrance in soaps, perfumes, and cosmetics, as well as a flavoring in food. It has been used as an antiasthmatic and expectorant, as well as to treat sore throat (used as a gargle).

Investigational Uses

Initial evidence indicates that hyssop may be useful as an antiviral to treat HIV infections. Hyssop has also been used to treat herpes infections.

Product Availability and Dosages

Available Forms

Essential oil, fluid extract, tea, tincture

Plant Parts Used: Essential oil from leaves and flower tips

Dosages and Routes

Adult
- PO tea: cover 1 tsp herb with 8 oz boiling water, let stand 15 min, may take tid
- PO tincture: 2-4 ml tid

Precautionary Information

Contraindications

Because hyssop is an abortifacient, it should not be used during pregnancy. Until more research is available, this herb should not be used during lactation and should not be given to children younger than 2 years of age. Persons with hypersensitivity to hyssop should not use it. Class 2b herb (whole herb).

Precautionary Information—cont'd

Side Effects/Adverse Reactions

Central Nervous System: SEIZURES
Gastrointestinal: Nausea, vomiting, anorexia, diarrhea
Integumentary: Hypersensitivity reactions

Interactions with Hyssop			
Drug	Food	Herb	Lab Test
None known	None known	None known	None known

H

Client Considerations

Assess

- Assess for hypersensitivity reactions. If present, discontinue use of hyssop and administer antihistamine or other appropriate therapy.
- Determine the reason the client is using hyssop and suggest more effective alternatives.

Administer

- Children, geriatric clients, and clients who are emaciated should use only low doses of hyssop.

Teach Client/Family

- Because hyssop is an abortifacient, caution the client not to use it during pregnancy. Until more research is available, caution the client not to use this herb during lactation and not to give it to children younger than 2 years of age.
- Advise the client to use hyssop only under the direction of a qualified herbalist if using the herb for an extended period.
- Warn the client not to confuse *Hyssopus officinalis* with other plants commonly called "hyssop." These other plants are not members of the *Hyssopus* genus or its family, Labiatae.

Pharmacology

Pharmacokinetics

Pharmacokinetics and pharmacodynamics are unknown.

Primary Chemical Components of Hyssop and Their Possible Actions

Chemical Class	Individual Component	Possible Action
Terpenoid	Marrubiin; Ursolic acid; Oleanolic acid	Cardioactive; stimulates bronchial secretions
Volatile oil	Linalool; Camphor; Pinochamphone; Thujone; Alpha-pinene; Beta-pinene; Limonene; Camphene; Alphaterpinene; Bornylacetate; Isopinocamphone	Muscle relaxant (Lu, 2002)
Flavonoid	Hesperidiin Diosmetin	
Tannin		Wound healing; antiviral
Resin		
Acid	Caffeic acid	Antiviral
Polysaccharide	MAR-10	Anti-HIV

Actions

Hyssop is a member of the mint family. Little research is available to confirm any of its uses or actions.

Antiretroviral/Antiviral Action

Initial research indicates that hyssop may be useful in the treatment of HIV-1 infections (Gollapudi, 1995) and possibly herpes infections. One polysaccharide isolated from hyssop was shown to inhibit HIV replication. Another study showed that the tannins and caffeic acid found in hyssop exerted antiviral activity (Kreis, 1990).

Other Actions

Anecdotal reports suggest the use of hyssop as a stimulant, expectorant, sedative, and antispasmodic.

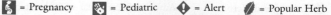

= Pregnancy　　 = Pediatric　　◆ = Alert　　 = Popular Herb

References

Gollapudi S et al: Isolation of a previously unidentified polysaccharide (Mar-10) from *Hyssopus officinalis* that exhibits strong activity against human immunodeficiency virus type 1, *Biochem Biophys Res Commun* 210(1):145, 1995.

Kreis W et al: Inhibition of HIV replication by *Hyssopus officinalis* extracts, *Antiviral Res* 14(6):323, 1990.

Lu M et al: Muscle relaxing activity of *Hyssopus officinalis* essential oil on isolated intestinal preparations, *Planta Med* 68(3):213-216, 2002.

H

Iceland Moss
(ise'luhnd maws)

Scientific name: *Cetraria islandica*

Other common names: Consumption moss, eryngo-leaved liverwort, Iceland lichen

Class 1 (Decoction, Infusion)
Class 2d (Alcoholic Extract, Powder, Thallus)

Origin: Iceland moss is a lichen found in Iceland and other parts of the Northern hemisphere.

Uses

Reported Uses

Iceland moss has been used to treat the common cold, cough, bronchitis, inflammation, and anorexia.

Investigational Uses

Initial research documents the use of Iceland moss to treat bacterial and HIV-1 infections.

Product Availability and Dosages

Available Forms

Capsules, creams, crude herb, lozenges, tincture

Plant Parts Used: All parts of the lichen

Dosages and Routes

Adult

Cough and Cold
- PO lozenges: take one lozenge prn

Other
- PO decoction: mix 1 tsp shredded moss in 8 oz water, boil 3 min, strain, take bid
- PO tincture: 1-2 ml bid-tid

Precautionary Information

Contraindications

Until more research is available, Iceland moss should not be used during pregnancy and lactation and should not be given to children. This herb should not be used by persons with gastric or duodenal ulcers or by those with hypersen-

Precautionary Information—cont'd

Contraindications—cont'd

sitivity to it. Class 1 herb (decoction, infusion); class 2d herb (alcoholic extract, powder, thallus).

Side Effects/Adverse Reactions

Gastrointestinal: Nausea, vomiting, gastritis, anorexia, HEPATOTOXICITY

Integumentary: Hypersensitivity reactions

Interactions with Iceland Moss			
Drug	Food	Herb	Lab Test
None known	None known	None known	None known

Client Considerations

Assess

- Assess for hypersensitivity reactions. If present, discontinue use of Iceland moss and administer antihistamine or other appropriate therapy.
- Determine the reason the client is using Iceland moss.
- Assess for signs of hepatotoxicity: jaundice, clay-colored stools, and right upper-quadrant pain. Monitor liver function studies: AST, ALT, and bilirubin.

Administer

- Instruct the client to store Iceland moss in a cool, dry place, away from heat and moisture.

Teach Client/Family

- Until more research is available, caution the client not to use Iceland moss during pregnancy and lactation and not to give it to children.
- Advise the client that very little research is available that documents any actions or uses of Iceland moss.

Pharmacology

Pharmacokinetics

Pharmacokinetics and pharmacodynamics are unknown.

Primary Chemical Components of Iceland Moss and Their Possible Actions		
Chemical Class	**Individual Component**	**Possible Action**
Polysaccharide Lichenic acid	Lichenin; Isolichenin Protolichesterinic acid Fumarprotocetraric acid; Lichesterinic acid	Antimicrobial

Actions

Antioxidant, Antimicrobial, Antiretroviral, and Anticancer Actions

Iceland moss has demonstrated significant antimicrobial effects against *Streptococcus pyogenes, Staphylococcus aureus, Mycobacterium tuberculosis,* and *Helicobacter pylori* (Ingolfsdottir, 1985, 1997). The chemical component responsible is protolichesterinic acid. Iceland moss has also been shown to exert significant activity against HIV-1 infection and certain cancers (Ingolfsdottir, 1994). *Cetraria islandica* showed significant antioxidant effect depending on concentration of sample. The conclusion was that *C. islandia* is a potential source of natural antioxidant (Gulcin, 2002).

References

Gulcin I et al: Determination of antioxidant activity of lichen *Cetraria islandica, J Ethnopharmacol* 79(3):325-329, 2002.

Ingolfsdottir K et al: In vitro evaluation of the antimicrobial activity of lichen metabolites as potential preservatives, *Antimicrob Agents Chemother* 28:289-292, 1985.

Ingolfsdottir K et al: Immunologically active polysaccharide from *Cetraria islandica, Planta Med* 60:527-531, 1994.

Ingolfsdottir K et al: In vitro susceptibility of *Helicobacter pylori* to protolichesterinic acid from the lichen *Cetraria islandica, Antimicrob Agents Chemother* 41(1):215-217, 1997.

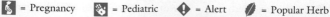

Indigo
(in'di-goe)

Scientific name: *Indigofera* spp.
Other common names: Qingdai

Origin: Indigo is a perennial shrub found in several regions of the world.

Uses

Reported Uses
Indigo has been used in traditional Chinese medicine to purify the liver and to treat inflammation, pain, and fever. Other uses include treatment of diabetes and mumps.

Investigational Uses
Indigo may be used to treat bacterial fungal infections.

Product Availability and Dosages

Available Forms
Powder, tablets

Plant Parts Used: Branches, leaves

Dosages and Routes
No dosage consensus exists.

Precautionary Information

Contraindications
Because birth defects have occurred in babies born to animals given *Indigofera spicata,* indigo should not be used during pregnancy. Until more research is available, this herb should not be used during lactation and should not be given to children. Persons who are hypersensitive to indigo should not use it.

Side Effects/Adverse Reactions
Ear, Eye, Nose, and Throat: Redness of the eye
Gastrointestinal: Nausea, vomiting, anorexia
Integumentary: Hypersensitivity reactions, dermatitis

Interactions with Indigo			
Drug	Food	Herb	Lab Test
None known	None known	None known	None known

Client Considerations

Assess

- Assess for hypersensitivity reactions and dermatitis. If these are present, discontinue use of indigo and administer antihistamine or other appropriate therapy.

Administer

- Instruct the client to store indigo in a cool, dry place, away from heat and moisture.

Teach Client/Family

- Because birth defects have occurred in babies born to animals given *Indigofera spicata,* caution the client not to use indigo during pregnancy. Until more research is available, caution the client not to use this herb during lactation and not to give it to children.
- Advise the client to avoid getting indigo in the eye.
- Advise the client to learn to distinguish false, wild, and bastard indigo *(Baptisia tinctoria)* from *Indigofera* spp. used for medicinal purposes.

Pharmacology

Pharmacokinetics

Pharmacokinetics and pharmacodynamics are unknown.

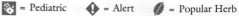

 = Pregnancy   = Pediatric   = Alert   = Popular Herb

Primary Chemical Components of Indigo and Their Possible Actions		
Chemical Class	**Individual Component**	**Possible Action**
Glucoside	Indican	Dye
Xanthene	Tetrahydroxanthene	
Indigofera spicata *Also Contains*		
Indospicine		Teratogenic; hepatotoxic
Indigtone		Hepatoprotective (Singh, 2001)

I

Actions

One species of indigo *(Indigofera spicata)* contains substances that are hepatotoxic and teratogenic. Other indigo species do not cause these toxicities. *Indigofera tinctoria* has been shown to prevent hepatotoxicity in the case of carbon tetrachloride poisoning (Anand, 1981). Some species have shown promise in the inhibition of certain cancers. However, insufficient research supports this action at this time.

References

Anand KK et al: Histological evidence of protection of *Indigofera tinctoria* Linn against carbon tetrachloride induced hepatotoxicity—an experimental study, *Indian J Exp Biol* 19:298, 1981.

Singh B et al: Hepatoprotective activity of indigtone: a bioactive fraction from *Indigofera* tincture Linn., *Phytother Res* 15(4):294-297, 2001.

Irish Moss
(ire′ish maws)

Scientific name: *Chondrus crispus*

Other common names: Carrageen, carageenan, chondrus

Origin: Irish moss is a seaweed found in Europe and on the coasts of Canada.

🌀 Endangered Herb   Adverse effects: BOLD = life-threatening

Uses

Reported Uses

Irish moss is used to treat diarrhea, gastritis, and bronchitis.

Investigational Uses

Research is underway to determine the effectiveness of Irish moss as an antiinflammatory and as a vehicle for delivery of gastrointestinal drugs.

Product Availability and Dosages

Available Forms

Component of: cream, lotion, ointment, toothpaste; granules in combination with other herbs

Plant Parts Used: Whole moss

Dosages and Routes

No published dosages are available.

Precautionary Information

Contraindications

Until more research is available, Irish moss should not be used during pregnancy and lactation and should not be given to children. This herb should not be used by persons with active gastrointestinal bleeding or a history of peptic ulcers, or by those with hypersensitivity to it.

Side Effects/Adverse Reactions

Cardiovascular: Decreased blood pressure
Gastrointestinal: Nausea, vomiting, anorexia, diarrhea, abdominal pain, GASTROINTESTINAL BLEEDING
Genitourinary: Renal changes (theoretical)
Integumentary: Hypersensitivity reactions

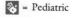 = Pregnancy   = Pediatric   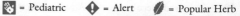 = Alert   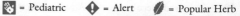 = Popular Herb

Interactions with Irish Moss

Drug

Anticoagulants (heparin, warfarin): Irish moss may increase the effects of anticoagulants; avoid concurrent use.

Salicylates (aspirin): Irish moss may pose an increased risk of bleeding when used with salicylates; avoid concurrent use.

Antihypertensives: Irish moss may increase the effects of antihypertensive; avoid concurrent use.

Food	Herb	Lab Test
None known	None known	None known

Client Considerations

Assess

- Assess for hypersensitivity reactions. If present, discontinue use of Irish moss and administer antihistamine or other appropriate therapy.
- Assess for suspected gastrointestinal bleeding: black tarry stools, guaiac stools.
- Assess for use of antihypertensives, anticoagulants, and salicylates (see Interactions).
- Determine the reason the client is using Irish moss.

Administer

- Instruct the client to store Irish moss in a cool, dry place, away from heat and moisture.

Teach Client/Family

- Until more research is available, caution the client not to use Irish moss during pregnancy and lactation and not to give it to children.

Pharmacology

Pharmacokinetics

Pharmacokinetics and pharmacodynamics are unknown.

Primary Chemical Components of Irish Moss and Their Possible Actions		
Chemical Class	**Individual Component**	**Possible Action**
Carrageenan		Antiinflammatory
Iodine		
Bromine		
Mineral	Iron; Magnesium; Calcium; Sodium	
Vitamin	A; B	

Actions

Traditionally, Irish moss has been used to treat cough, bronchitis, and diarrhea. However, no research supports these traditional uses, and little research is available on this herb in general. One recent study of laboratory animals did show an antiinflammatory action when carrageenan, one of the chemical components, was injected into inflamed paws. Other proposed actions that have not been studied include potential use as an anticholesteremic, anticoagulant, and antihypertensive. The food and drug industries use Irish moss as a binder, emulsifier, and stabilizer.

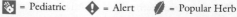

Jaborandi Tree
(zhah-boer-ahn'dee)

Scientific names: *Pilocarpus jaborandi, Pilocarpus microphyllus, Pilocarpus pinnatifolius*

Other common names: Arruda brava, arruda do mato, Indian hemp, jamguarandi, juarandi, pernambuco jaborandi

Class 2b (Leaf)

Origin: Jaborandi tree is found in Brazil.

Uses

Reported Uses

The primary use of jaborandi tree is to reduce the intraocular pressure caused by glaucoma and to treat xerostomia. It is also used to treat diabetes and nephritis and has been used topically to treat skin disorders such as psoriasis and eczema.

Product Availability and Dosages

Available Forms

Essential oil, extract, powder, tincture
NOTE: For information about pilocarpine (eye drops), refer to the pharmacologic literature.

Plant Parts Used: Leaves

Dosages and Routes

Adult
Ophthalmic
• Topical drops: 1-2 gtt tid
Other
• PO extract: 20-30 drops
• PO powdered leaves: 10-60 grains
• PO tincture: 1 dram

Precautionary Information

Contraindications

Until more research is available, jaborandi tree should not be used during pregnancy and lactation and should not be given to children. This herb should not be used by persons with uncontrolled asthma, angle-closure glaucoma, or

Continued

 Endangered Herb   Adverse effects: BOLD = life-threatening

Precautionary Information—cont'd

Contraindications—cont'd

iritis, or by persons with hypersensitivity to it. Persons with chronic obstructive pulmonary disease (COPD), bronchitis, cardiac disease, biliary tract disease, cholelithiasis, retinal disease, psychiatric disorders, neurologic disorders, or cognitive disorders should avoid the use of jaborandi tree. Class 2b herb (leaf).

Side Effects/Adverse Reactions

Cardiovascular: Hypertension, tachycardia, edema
Central Nervous System: Tremors, dizziness, headache, weakness
Ear, Eye, Nose, and Throat: Rhinitis, amblyopia, epistaxis; blurred vision, stinging, eye pain (ophthalmic use)
Gastrointestinal: Nausea, vomiting, anorexia, dysphagia
Genitourinary: Urinary frequency
Integumentary: Hypersensitivity reactions, flushing, sweating

Interactions with Jaborandi Tree

Drug

Anticholinergic: The effects of jaborandi tree are decreased when used internally with anticholinergics.
Beta-blockers: Adverse cardiovascular reactions are increased when jaborandi tree is used internally with beta-blockers; do not use concurrently.
Bethanechol: Increased cholinergic effects occur when jaborandi tree is used internally with bethanechol.
Cholinergics, ophthalmic: Increased cholinergic effects occur when jaborandi tree is used internally with ophthalmic cholinergics.
NSAIDs, topical: The action of jaborandi tree (ophthalmic route) is decreased when it is used with topical NSAIDs; do not use concurrently.

Food	Herb	Lab Test
None known	None known	None known

Client Considerations

Assess

- Assess for hypersensitivity reactions. If these are present, discontinue use of jaborandi tree and administer antihistamine or other appropriate therapy.
- Assess for dizziness, headache, weakness, blurred vision, hypertension, and tremors. If these are present, the herb dose may need to be reduced.
- Assess for medication use (see Interactions).

Administer

- Instruct the client to use the lowest PO dose possible.
- Store in dry, cool environment.
- Use by ophthalmic route tid.

Teach Client/Family

- Until more research is available, caution the client not to use jaborandi tree during pregnancy and lactation and not to give it to children.
- Advise the client that visual changes such as blurred vision may occur. The client should avoid driving or operating machinery until the particular effects are known.
- Advise the client that when jaborandi tree is used via the ophthalmic route, the eyes initially may sting and headache, brow ache, and decreased night vision may occur.

Pharmacology

Pharmacokinetics

Jaborandi tree is absorbed well when taken internally. It is excreted via urine, metabolized as an unchanged drug.

Primary Chemical Components of Jaborandi Tree and Their Possible Actions		
Chemical Class	**Individual Component**	**Possible Action**
Alkaloid	Pilocarpine	Direct-acting miotic; cholinergic
	Isopilocarpine; Pilocarpidine	
Jaborine **Pilosine**		

Continued

 Endangered Herb   Adverse effects: BOLD = life-threatening

Primary Chemical Components of Jaborandi Tree and Their Possible Actions—cont'd		
Chemical Class	**Individual Component**	**Possible Action**
Tannic acid Jaboric acid Pilocarpic acid Volatile oil		

Actions

The chemical component pilocarpine is responsible for the pharmacologic action of jaborandi tree. Most of the information available on this herb is derived from the mainstream pharmacologic literature on pilocarpine. Jaborandi may be administered either orally or ophthalmically. When taken orally, it acts on the cholinergic receptors, stimulating the exocrine glands and producing muscarinic effects. Gastric and bronchial secretions increase, as does motility of the urinary tract and gallbladder.

Ophthalmic Action

When used as an ophthalmic, jaborandi tree is a direct-acting miotic. This herb duplicates the muscarinic effects of acetylcholine. The result is pupillary constriction, increased aqueous humor outflow, and decreased intraocular pressure.

References

Duke J: *CRC handbook of medicinal herbs,* Boca Raton, Fla, 1985, CRC Press.
Skidmore-Roth L: *Mosby's nursing drug reference,* St Louis, 2001, Mosby.

Jamaican Dogwood
(jah-may'kuhn dawg'wood)

Scientific name: *Piscidia erythrina*

Other common names: Fish poison tree, fishfuddle, West Indian dogwood

Origin: Jamaican dogwood is now found in the West Indies, the northern portion of South America, and the southern portion of the United States.

🐾 = Pregnancy   👣 = Pediatric   ◆ = Alert   ✎ = Popular Herb

Uses

Reported Uses

Jamaican dogwood has been used to treat insomnia, menstrual disorders such as dysmenorrhea, asthma, migraine, dental pain, nerve pain, and the pain of labor. Most of its uses are intended to produce mild to moderate analgesia. Because of its toxicity, this herb is rarely used to treat any condition.

Product Availability and Dosages

Available Forms

Bark strips, dried bark, dried roots, fluid extract, tincture

Plant Parts Used: Bark, roots

Dosages and Routes

Adult

All dosages listed are PO.

- Dried bark/dried roots: 2-4 g qd divided tid
- Fluid extract: 5-20 drops, increasing to a maximum of 1-2 drams qd
- Tea: 1 tsp in 8 oz water, simmer 10-15 min
- Tincture: 2-3 ml bid-tid (taken hs if used to treat insomnia)

Precautionary Information

Contraindications

Until more research is available, Jamaican dogwood should not be used during pregnancy and lactation and should not be given to children. This herb should not be used by elderly persons, those with cardiovascular disease such as arrhythmias or hypotension, or those with hypersensitivity to it. Jamaican dogwood should not be used intravenously. This is a toxic herb that is not recommended for use.

Side Effects/Adverse Reactions

Central Nervous System: Dizziness, sedation
Gastrointestinal: Nausea, vomiting, anorexia
Integumentary: Hypersensitivity reactions
Toxicity: SWEATING, TREMORS

Interactions with Jamaican Dogwood

Drug

Alcohol: Jamaican dogwood may increase the effects of alcohol; avoid concurrent use.

Antihistamines: Antihistamines may produce an increased effect when used with Jamaican dogwood; avoid concurrent use.

Antihypertensives: Jamaican dogwood may increase the effects of antihypertensives; avoid concurrent use (theoretical).

Barbiturates: Jamaican dogwood may increase the effects of barbiturates; avoid concurrent use.

Opioids: Jamaican dogwood may increase the effects of opioids; avoid concurrent use.

Food	Herb	Lab Test
None known	None known	None known

Client Considerations

Assess

- Assess for hypersensitivity reactions. If present, discontinue use of Jamaican dogwood and administer antihistamine or other appropriate therapy.
- Assess for cardiovascular disease such as hypotension, bradycardia, and arrhythmias.
- Assess for use of alcohol, antihistamines, antihypertensives, barbiturates, and opioids (see Interactions).
- Assess for toxicity symptoms (sweating, tremors).

Administer

- Inform the client that Jamaican dogwood may be taken PO in the form of dried products (bark, root, or bark strips), extract, tincture, or tea.
- Instruct the client to store Jamaican dogwood products in a cool, dry place, away from heat and moisture.

Teach Client/Family

- Until more research is available, caution the client not to use Jamaican dogwood during pregnancy and lactation and not to give it to children.
- Because Jamaican dogwood causes drowsiness and sedation, advise the client not to perform hazardous activities such as

---

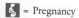 = Pregnancy   = Pediatric   = Alert   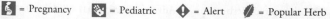 = Popular Herb

driving or operating heavy machinery until physical response to the herb can be evaluated.
- Warn the client that this herb cannot be recommended for any use or action because of its toxicity.

Pharmacology

Pharmacokinetics

Pharmacokinetics and pharmacodynamics are unknown.

Primary Chemical Components of Jamaican Dogwood and Their Possible Actions		
Chemical Class	**Individual Component**	**Possible Action**
Isoflavone		Spasmolytic
Rotenoid	Millettone; Isomillettone; Sumatrol; Dehydromillettone; Rotenone	
Tannin		Wound healing
Soflavone	Piscidone; Listetin; Erythbigenin; Piscerythrone; Ichthynone	
Tataric acid	Piscidic fukiic; Methlfukiic	

Actions

Very little information is available on Jamaican dogwood, and no primary research is available for any of its uses or actions. It is believed to exert an antispasmodic action, but research does not confirm this. Because of its toxicity, this herb is no longer in use to any significant extent. Its use should be discouraged and safer alternatives recommended.

Jambul
(jam-bewl′)

Scientific name: *Syzygium cuminii*

Other common names: Black plum, jamba, jambolana, jambolo, jambool, jambu, jambula, jambulon plum, java plum

Origin: Jambul is a tree found in India and Sri Lanka.

Uses

Reported Uses

Jambul has been used in traditional herbal medicine to treat diarrhea and diabetes mellitus.

Investigational Uses

Initial research indicates that jambul decreases inflammation.

Product Availability and Dosages

Available Forms

Decoction, tea

Plant Parts Used: Fruit, leaves, seeds

Dosages and Routes

No dosage consensus exists.

Precautionary Information

Contraindications

Until more research is available, jambul should not be used during pregnancy and lactation and should not be given to children. This herb should not be used by persons with hypersensitivity to it.

Side Effects/Adverse Reactions

Gastrointestinal: Nausea, anorexia
Integumentary: Hypersensitivity reactions

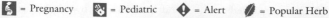

= Pregnancy   = Pediatric   = Alert   = Popular Herb

Interactions with Jambul

Drug
Antidiabetics: Jambul may increase the effects of antidiabetics; avoid concurrent use (theoretical).

Food	Herb	Lab Test
None known	None known	None known

Client Considerations
Assess
- Assess for hypersensitivity reactions. If present, discontinue use of jambul and administer antihistamine or other appropriate therapy.
- Monitor blood glucose in diabetic clients; identify antidiabetics used (see Interactions).

Administer
- Instruct the client to store jambul products in a cool, dry place, away from heat and moisture.

Teach Client/Family
- Until more research is available, caution the client not to use jambul during pregnancy and lactation and not to give it to children.

Pharmacology
Pharmacokinetics
Pharmacokinetics and pharmacodynamics are unknown.

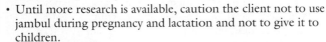

Primary Chemical Components of Jambul and Their Possible Actions

Chemical Class	Individual Component	Possible Action
Fatty acid	Oleic acid; Myristic acid; Linoleic acid; Palmitic acid	
Flavonoid	Quercetin	Antiinflammatory
Tannin	Corilagin; Ellagic; Galloyglucose	
Essential Oils		Antibacterial (Shafi, 2002)

 Endangered Herb   Adverse effects: BOLD = life-threatening

Actions

Hypoglycemic Action

Jambul has been used in Brazil for its hypoglycemic action. However, in one study using laboratory animals with streptozocin-induced diabetes, no difference was found in blood glucose levels when the animals were given jambul tea for 14 to 95 days as a water substitute (Teixera, 1997).

References

Shafi P et al: Antibacterial activity of *Syzygium cumini* and *Syzygium travancoricum* leaf essential oils, Fitoterapia 73(5):414, 2002.

Teixera CC et al: The effect of *Syzygium cumini* L. skeels on post-prandial blood glucose levels in non-diabetic rats and rats with streptozotocin-induced diabetes mellitus, *J Ethnopharmacol* 56(3):209-213, 1997.

DO NOT INGEST

Jimsonweed
(jim'suhn-weed)

Scientific name: *Datura stramonium*

Other common names: Angel's trumpet, angel tulip, apple-of-Peru, devil weed, devil's apple, devil's trumpet, Estramonio, green dragon, gypsyweed, inferno, Jamestown weed, loco seeds, locoweed, mad apple, moon weed, stramoine, stechapfel, stinkweed, thorn apple, tolguacha, trumpet lily, zombie's cucumber

---

Origin: Jimsonweed is a weed found in most temperate and subtropical parts of the world.

Uses

Reported Uses

Although jimsonweed is highly toxic, it has been used to treat asthma, Parkinsonism, and irritable bowel syndrome, as well as to reduce gastrointestinal secretions. It also has been used as a hallucinogen.

Product Availability and Dosages

Available Forms

Cigarettes, crude herb, rectal suppositories

Plant Parts Used: Flowering tops, leaves, roots

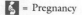 = Pregnancy    = Pediatric   = Alert   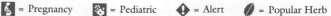 = Popular Herb

Dosages and Routes

Adult

• PO: 75 mg (Clause, 1961)

No dosage consensus exists.

Precautionary Information

Contraindications

Until more research is available, jimsonweed should not be used during pregnancy and lactation and should not be given to children. It should not be used by persons with hypersensitivity to this plant or belladonna alkaloids. Jimsonweed should not be used by persons with angle-closure glaucoma, obstruction of the gastrointestinal or urinary system, central nervous system disorders such as myasthenia gravis, thyrotoxicosis, ulcerative colitis, prostatic hypertrophy, tachycardia, tachyarrhythmia, asthma, acute hemorrhage, hepatic disease, or myocardial ischemia. Persons with spastic paralysis, gastric ulcers, hyperthyroidism, chronic obstructive pulmonary disease, hypertension, congestive heart failure, and renal disease should avoid its use. The jimsonweed plant is toxic, especially the seeds.

Side Effects/Adverse Reactions

Central Nervous System: Headache, dizziness, confusion, anxiety, flushing, drowsiness, insomnia, weakness, involuntary movements, decreased sweating, increased body temperature; COMA, SEIZURES, DEATH (plant ingestion)

Cardiovascular: Hypotension, paradoxical bradycardia, angina, premature ventricular contractions (PVCs), hypertension, tachycardia, ectopic ventricular beats

Ear, Eye, Nose, and Throat: Blurred vision, photophobia, eye pain, pupil dilatation, nasal congestion

Gastrointestinal: Nausea, vomiting, anorexia, dry mouth, abdominal pain, constipation, abdominal distention, altered taste

Genitourinary: Retention, hesitancy, impotence, dysuria

Integumentary: Hypersensitivity reactions, rash, urticaria, contact dermatitis, dry skin, flushing

J

Interactions with Jimsonweed

Drug

Amantadine: Increased anticholinergic effects result when jimsonweed is used with amantadine.

Antacids: Antacids decrease the action of jimsonweed.

Anticholinergics: Increased anticholinergic effects result when jimsonweed is used with anticholinergics.

MAOIs: Increased anticholinergic effects result when jimsonweed is used with MAOIs.

Phenothiazines: Jimsonweed decreases the action of phenothiazines.

Tricyclic antidepressants: Increased anticholinergic effects result when jimsonweed is used with tricyclics.

Food

None known

Herb

The action of jimsonweed is increased in cases of chronic use or abuse of aloe, buckthorn, cascara sagrada, chinese rhubarb, or senna.

Lab Test

None known

Client Considerations

Assess

- Assess for hypersensitivity reactions, such as rash, urticaria, and contact dermatitis. If these are present, discontinue use of jimsonweed and administer antihistamine or other appropriate therapy.
- Assess respiratory status, including rate, rhythm, wheezing, dyspnea, and engorged neck veins. If any of these symptoms is present, jimsonweed use should be discontinued immediately.
- Assess for increased intraocular pressure, including blurred vision, nausea, vomiting, and increased tearing. If any of these symptoms is present, jimsonweed use should be discontinued immediately.
- Assess cardiac status, including rate, rhythm, character, and blood pressure.
- Assess for medications and herbs used (see Interactions).

 = Pregnancy   = Pediatric   ◆ = Alert   ✿ = Popular Herb

Administer

- Instruct the client to increase bulk and water in the diet if constipation occurs.
- Instruct the client to use hard candy or gum and rinse the mouth frequently if dryness of the mouth occurs.

Teach Client/Family

- Until more research is available, caution the client not to use jimsonweed during pregnancy and lactation and not to give it to children.
- Warn the client that the jimsonweed plant is toxic, especially the seeds.
- Caution the client to report blurred vision, chest pain, and allergic reactions immediately.
- Because heat stroke may occur, caution the client not to perform strenuous activities in high temperatures while using jimsonweed.
- Advise the client to avoid consumption of jimsonweed because its alkaloid chemical components are similar to those of the deadly nightshade plant. Very little research exists on jimsonweed.
- Caution the client to use jimsonweed only under the supervision of a qualified herbalist. This herb is considered unsafe.

Pharmacology

Pharmacokinetics

The atropine component is well absorbed, metabolized by the liver, and excreted by the kidneys. It crosses the placenta and is excreted in breast milk.

Primary Chemical Components of Jimsonweed and Their Possible Actions		
Chemical Class	**Individual Component**	**Possible Action**
Seeds and Leaves Contain		
Alkaloid	Atropine; Scopolamine; Hyoscyamine; Hyoscine	Anticholinergic
Seeds Also Contain		
Fatty acid	Palmitic acid; Stearic acid; Oleic acid; Linoleic acid; Lignoceric acid	
All Plant Parts Contain		
Tannin Coumarin		Wound healing

Actions

Most of the information available on jimsonweed comes from mainstream pharmacologic literature regarding its component alkaloids. Its chemical components exert anticholinergic properties and block acetylcholine at parasympathetic neuroeffector sites. The blocking of vagal stimulation in the heart increases both cardiac output and heart rate and dries secretions. The chemical components responsible for these actions are atropine, hyoscine, scopolamine, and hyoscyamine. This herb is very poisonous to animals and humans, if it is not used correctly.

References

Clause EP: *Pharmacognosy,* ed 4, Philadelphia, 1961, Lea & Febnger.
Duke J: *CRC handbook of medicinal herbs,* Boca Raton, Fla, 1985, CRC Press.
Skidmore-Roth L: *Mosby's nursing drug reference,* St Louis, 2001, Mosby.

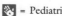 = Pregnancy = Pediatric 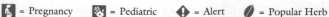 = Alert = Popular Herb

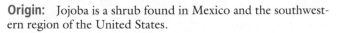

DO NOT INGEST

Jojoba
(hoe-hoe'bah)

Scientific name: *Simmondsia chinesis, Simmondsia californica*

Other common names: Deernut, goatnut, pignut

Origin: Jojoba is a shrub found in Mexico and the southwestern region of the United States.

Uses
Reported Uses
Jojoba has been used primarily to treat skin disorders including chapped, dry skin; scaling; eczema; psoriasis; and seborrhea. It is a component of many common skin products. Anecdotal information promotes the use of jojoba to treat hair loss and acne and to decrease the appearance of wrinkles.

Product Availability and Dosages
Available Forms
Beads; butter; crude wax; component of Chapstick, cream, dandruff shampoo, lipstick, lotion, soap

Plant Parts Used: Oil from seeds

Dosages and Routes
No dosage information is available.

> **Precautionary Information**
> **Contraindications**
> No known contraindications.
>
> **Side Effects/Adverse Reactions**
> *Integumentary:* Hypersensitivity reactions, contact dermatitis

Interactions with Jojoba			
Drug	**Food**	**Herb**	**Lab Test**
None known	None known	None known	None known

 Endangered Herb   Adverse effects: BOLD = life-threatening

Client Considerations

Assess

- Assess for hypersensitivity reactions and contact dermatitis. If these are present, discontinue use of jojoba and administer antihistamine or other appropriate therapy.

Administer

- Instruct the client to use jojoba topically only. If jojoba is ingested, toxicity will occur.

Teach Client/Family

- Caution the client not to consume any part of the jojoba plant. Toxicity will occur.

Pharmacology

Pharmacokinetics

Pharmacokinetics and pharmacodynamics are unknown.

Primary Chemical Components of Jojoba and Their Possible Actions		
Chemical Class	**Individual Component**	**Possible Action**
Fatty acid	Alpha-tocopherol	Emollient
Alcohol		
Simmondsin		
Vitamin	B; E	
Mineral	Chromium; Zinc; Copper	

Actions

Jojoba has been used for many years as a component in cosmetics, suntan lotions, shampoos, and hair conditioners. Primary research is lacking, and only two studies are available that relate to the medicinal uses of jojoba. One study evaluated rabbits given a 2% jojoba dietary supplement. After supplementation, cholesterol levels decreased by 40%. However, the mechanism of action was not studied (Clarke, 1981). Another study evaluated the antioxidant effects of jojoba, which are believed to result from its alpha-tocopherol content (Mallet, 1994). Most of the uses of jojoba are based on years of anecdotal information.

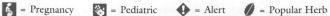

References

Clarke JA et al: Effects of ingestion of jojoba oil on blood cholesterol and lipoprotein patterns in New Zealand white rabbits, *Biochem Biophys Res Commun* 102(4):1409, 1981.

Mallet JE et al: Antioxidant activity of plant leaves in relation to their alpha-tocopherol content, *Food Chem Toxicol* 49(1):61, 1994.

Juniper
(jew'nuh-puhr)

Scientific names: *Juniperus communis, Juniperus oxycedrus* L.

Other common names: A'ra'r a'di, ardic, baccal juniper, common juniper, dwarf, gemener, genievre, ground juniper, hackmatack, harvest, horse savin, juniper mistletoe, yoshu-nezu, zimbro   **Class 2b (*Juniperus oxycedrus* L. Fruit, Berry)**

Origin: Juniper is an evergreen found in the United States, Canada, Europe, and Asia.

Uses

Reported Uses

Traditionally, juniper has been used as a diuretic (for both adults and children) and an antiflatulent, as well as to treat urinary tract infections, diabetes mellitus, inflammation, and gastrointestinal disorders.

Product Availability and Dosages

Available Forms

Berry juice, capsules, essential oil, liquid, tablets

Plant Parts Used: Dried fruit

Dosages and Routes

Adult

All dosages listed are PO.

Diabetes Mellitus

• Capsules/tablets: 250-500 mg qd

Gastrointestinal Disorders

• 0.05-0.1 ml essential oil

🌀 Endangered Herb   Adverse effects: BOLD = life-threatening

Inflammation
• 0.2-0.3 mg/ml
Urinary Tract Infection
• 20 mg/ml
Child
Urinary Tract Infection
• PO berry juice: dilute in water

Precautionary Information
Contraindications
Because it is an abortifacient, juniper should not be used
during pregnancy. Until more research is available, this herb
should not be used during lactation and should not be given
to children younger than 2 years of age. Juniper should not
be used by persons with hypersensitivity to it. Persons with
diabetes mellitus and gastrointestinal disorders should use
this herb with caution. Persons with urinary tract infections
or inflammation should use this herb only under the supervision of a qualified herbalist. Class 2b herb (*Juniperus oxycedrus* L. fruit, berry).

Side Effects/Adverse Reactions
Gastrointestinal: Nausea, vomiting, anorexia, diarrhea
Genitourinary: Increased diuresis
Integumentary: Hypersensitivity reactions, skin irritation,
burning, redness (topical)

Interactions with Juniper

Drug
Lithium: Juniper taken with lithium may result in dehydration
and lithium toxicity.

Food	Herb	Lab Test
None known	None known	None known

 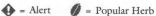

Client Considerations

Assess

- Assess for hypersensitivity reactions, skin irritation, burning and redness. If these are present, discontinue use of juniper and administer antihistamine or other appropriate therapy.
- Assess for lithium use; juniper should not be used with lithium.

Administer

- Instruct the client to give juniper to children 2 years of age or older PO diluted in water. It should not be given to children younger than 2 years of age.
- Instruct the client not to use juniper for longer than 4 weeks. Renal damage may occur.

Teach Client/Family

- Because it is an abortifacient, caution the client not to use juniper during pregnancy. Until more research is available, caution the client not to use this herb during lactation and not to give it to children younger than 2 years of age.

Pharmacology

Pharmacokinetics

Pharmacokinetics and pharmacodynamics are unknown.

Primary Chemical Components of Juniper and Their Possible Actions		
Chemical Class	**Individual Component**	**Possible Action**
Cresole Guaiacol Volatile oil	Piene; Sabinene; Mycrene; Limonene; Germacrene D; Gamma-Muurolene (Salido, 2002)	
Sesquiterpene	Cadinene	
Terpinen		Diuretic
Juniperin		
Resin		
Acid	Malic acid; Formic acid	
Protein		

Actions

Juniper has been used for its hypoglycemic, antiinflammatory, and antimicrobial actions. However, few studies support these uses.

Hypoglycemic Action

In one study, juniper was given to both diabetic and nondiabetic laboratory animals. The dried berries were shown to reduce hyperglycemia in rats with streptozocin-induced diabetes (Sanchez de Medina, 1994; Swanston-Flatt, 1990).

Antiinflammatory Action

Juniper has been shown to inhibit prostaglandin synthesis and decrease platelet activating factor. It has been used in Sweden as an antiinflammatory (Tunon, 1995).

References

Salido S et al: Chemical studies of essential oils of *Juniperus oxycedrus* ssp. *badia, J Ethnopharmacol* 81(1):129-134, 2002.

Sanchez de Medina F et al: Hypoglycemic activity of juniper berries, *Planta Med* 60(3):197-200, 1994.

Swanston-Flatt S et al: Traditional plant treatments for diabetes: studies in normal and streptozotocin diabetic mice, *Diabetologia* 33(8):462-464, 1990.

Tunon NH et al: Evaluation of anti-inflammatory activity of some Swedish medicinal plants: inhibition of prostaglandin biosynthesis and PAF-induced exocytosis, *J Ethnopharmacol* 48(2):61-76, 1995.

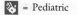 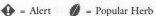

Kaolin
(kay'uh-luhn)

Scientific names: Kaolin, hydrated aluminum silicate

Origin: Kaolin is a naturally occurring clay that is treated for impurities.

Uses
Reported Uses
Kaolin is often combined with pectin and used as an antidiarrheal.

Product Availability and Dosages
Available Forms
Liquid

Dosages and Routes
No dosage consensus exists.

Precautionary Information
Contraindications
Until more research is available, kaolin should not be used during pregnancy and lactation and should not be given to children younger than 6 years of age. It should not be used by persons with hypersensitivity to this product.

Side Effects/Adverse Reactions
Gastrointestinal: Nausea, anorexia; constipation (chronic use)

Interactions with Kaolin

Drug
All medications: Kaolin decreases the absorption of all drugs; separate dosages by at least 2 hours.

Food
None known

Continued

 Endangered Herb   Adverse effects: BOLD = life-threatening

> **Interactions with Kaolin—cont'd**
>
> Herb
> ***All herbs:*** Kaolin decreases the absorption of all herbs; separate dosages by at least 2 hours.
>
> Lab Test
> None known

Client Considerations

Assess

- Assess the client's bowel pattern before administration of kaolin. Monitor for rebound constipation.
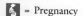 - Assess for dehydration in children.
- Assess for medications and herbs used. Separate dosages by at least 2 hours for proper absorption (see Interactions).

Administer

- Instruct the client not to use kaolin for more than 48 hours. If diarrhea is not relieved, a health care provider should be consulted.

Teach Client/Family

- Until more research is available, caution the client not to use kaolin during pregnancy and lactation and not to give it to children younger than 6 years of age.

Pharmacology

Pharmacokinetics

Pharmacokinetics and pharmacodynamics are unknown.

Actions

Most of the information available on kaolin comes from the mainstream pharmacologic literature. Kaolin decreases both gastric motility and stool water content. It has adsorbent and demulcent properties.

References

Duke J: *CRC handbook of medicinal herbs,* Boca Raton, Fla, 1985, CRC Press.
Skidmore-Roth L: *Mosby's nursing drug reference,* St Louis, 2003, Mosby.

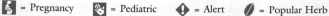

 = Pregnancy    = Pediatric   = Alert   ✱ = Popular Herb

Karaya Gum
(kuh-ry'uh guhm)

Scientific names: *Sterculia urens, Sterculia* spp.

Other common names: Indian tragacanth, kadaya, kadira, katila, kullo, mucara, sterculia gum

Origin: Karaya gum is a tree found in India and Pakistan.

Uses

Reported Uses

Karaya gum is used primarily as a bulk laxative. It is also used as an adhesive for colostomy appliances and dentures, and lozenges made from karaya gum are used to relieve sore throat. In addition, karaya gum is used as an emulsifier in foods.

Product Availability and Dosages

Available Forms

Powder

Plant Parts Used: Dried sap

Dosages and Routes

No specified dosages are available. Products that include karaya gum identify the amount included.

Precautionary Information

Contraindications

Until more research is available, karaya gum should not be use during pregnancy and lactation and should not be given to children.

Side Effects/Adverse Reactions

Gastrointestinal: Nausea, vomiting, anorexia, abdominal pain, diarrhea, GASTROINTESTINAL OBSTRUCTION

 Endangered Herb   Adverse effects: BOLD = life-threatening

Interactions with Karaya Gum

Drug
All medications: Karaya gum causes decreased absorption of all drugs; separate dosages by at least 2 hours.

Food
None known

Herb
All herbs: Karaya gum causes decreased absorption of all herbs; separate dosages by at least 2 hours.

Lab Test
None known

Client Considerations

Assess
- Determine the reason the client is using karaya gum. If karaya gum is used as a bulk laxative, assess the amount of bulk and water in the diet and the client's exercise habits.
- Assess for medications and herbs used. Separate dosages by at least 2 hours for proper absorption (see Interactions).

Administer
- Instruct the client to store karaya gum products in a cool, dry place, away from heat and moisture.

Teach Client/Family

- Until more research is available, caution the client not to use karaya gum during pregnancy and lactation and not to give it to children.

Pharmacology

Pharmacokinetics
Karaya gum is not absorbed and not digested.

Primary Chemical Component of Karaya Gum and Its Possible Actions

Chemical Class	Individual Component	Possible Action
Polysaccharide		

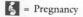 = Pregnancy    = Pediatric   = Alert   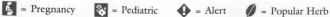 = Popular Herb

Actions

Karaya gum has been used primarily as a bulk laxative. It swells in the bowel and decreases the transit time of intestine contents. Karaya gum has also been used as a protectant and adhesive for dentures and other appliances such as colostomy devices. Initial evidence indicates that karaya may decrease lipids and may also decrease blood glucose levels in diabetics. However, no studies confirm these actions at this time.

Kava
(kah'vah)

Scientific name: *Piper methysticum*

Other common names: Ava, awa, kava-kava, kawa, kew, sakau, tonga, yagona **Class 2b/2c/2d (Rhizome, Root)**

K

Origin: Kava is a shrub found on the South Sea Islands.

Uses

Reported Uses

Kava is used as an anxiolytic, antiepileptic, antidepressant, and antipsychotic. It is also used as a muscle relaxant and to promote wound healing.

Product Availability and Dosages

Available Forms

Capsules, beverage, extract, tablets, tincture

Plant Parts Used: Dried rhizome, dried roots

Dosages and Routes

Adult

All dosages listed are PO.

Anxiolytic
- Extract, standardized: 45-70 mg kava lactones tid (Murray, 1998)

Depression
- Extract, standardized: 45-70 mg kava lactones tid (Murray, 1998)

General Use
- Extract, standardized: 70 mg kava lactones tid (Foster, 1998)

- Capsules/tablets: 400-500 mg up to 6 times/day (Foster, 1998)
- Tincture: 15-30 drops (dilution 1:2) taken tid in water (Foster, 1998)

Sedative

- Extract, standardized: 190-200 mg kava lactones 60 min hs

Precautionary Information

Contraindications

Until more research is available, kava should not be used during pregnancy and lactation and should not be given to children younger than 12 years of age. This herb should not be used by persons with major depressive disorder or Parkinson's disease, or by those with hypersensitivity to it. Class 2b/2c/2d herb (rhizome, root).

Side Effects/Adverse Reactions

Most side effects and adverse reactions occur when high doses are taken for a long period.

Central Nervous System: Increased reflexes

Ear, Eye, Nose, and Throat: Blurred vision, red eyes

Gastrointestinal: Nausea, vomiting, anorexia, weight loss, LIVER DAMAGE

Genitourinary: Hematuria

Hematologic: Decreased platelets, lymphocytes, bilirubin, protein, and albumin; increased red blood cell volume

Integumentary: Hypersensitivity reactions; skin yellowing and scaling (high doses)

Respiratory: Shortness of breath, PULMONARY HYPERTENSION

Interactions with Kava

Drug

Antiparkinsonians (carbidopa, levodopa): Antiparkinsonian drugs may increase symptoms of parkinsonism when used with kava; do not use concurrently.

Antipsychotics (chlorpromazine, fluphenazine, loxapine, mesoridazine, molindone, perphenazine, prochlorperazine, promazine, thioridazine, thiothixene, trifluoperazine, triflupromazine): Antipsychotics taken with kava may result in neuroleptic movement disorders.

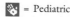 = Pregnancy   = Pediatric   = Alert   = Popular Herb

Interactions with Kava—cont'd

Drug—cont'd

Barbiturates (amobarbital, aprobarbital, butabarbital, phenobarbital, secobarbital): Barbiturates taken with kava may result in increased sedation.

Benzodiazepines: Increased sedation and coma (theoretical) may result when kava is used with benzodiazepines, including alprazolam; do not use concurrently.

Central nervous system depressants: Central nervous system depressants such as alcohol, benzodiazepines, and barbiturates may cause increased sedation when used with kava; avoid concurrent use.

Food

Increased absorption of kava occurs when it is taken with food.

Herb	Lab Test
None known	None known

K

Client Considerations

Assess

- Assess for hypersensitivity reactions. If present, discontinue use of kava and administer antihistamine or other appropriate therapy.
- Assess for use of other central nervous system depressants, including alcohol, barbiturates, benzodiazepines, antianxiety medications, and sedatives/hypnotics (see Interactions).

Administer

- Instruct the client to store kava products in a cool, dry place, away from heat and moisture.
- Instruct the client not to use kava for longer than 3 months unless under the direction of an herbalist. This herb may be habit forming.
- Inform the client that kava absorption is increased when kava is taken with food.

Teach Client/Family

- Until more research is available, caution the client not to use kava during pregnancy and lactation and not to give it to children younger than 12 years of age.

🌀 Endangered Herb   Adverse effects: BOLD = life-threatening

- Inform the client that excessive doses may result in daytime drowsiness. Advise the client not to operate heavy machinery or engage in hazardous activities if drowsiness occurs.
- Caution the client not to use kava with other central nervous system depressants (see Interactions).

Pharmacology

Pharmacokinetics

Most pharmacokinetics and pharmacodynamics are unknown. Kava lactones are more readily absorbed orally when taken as an extract of the root than as kava lactones alone. Kava may cross the placenta and enter breast milk.

Primary Chemical Components of Kava and Their Possible Actions		
Chemical Class	**Individual Components**	**Possible Action**

Kava lactone	Kavain
	Marindinine;
	  Methysticin;
	  Dehydromethysticin;
	  Yangonin;
	  Desmethoxyyangonin
		Sedative; anxiolytic

Chalcone
Kavain
Dihydrokavain
Pipermethystine
Bornyl esters
	Cinnamic acid;
	  Pinostrobin;
	  Flavokawain B;
	  Dimethoxyflavanone
		Cox-1, 2 inhibition (Wu, 2002)

Actions

Kava acts as a sedative, an analgesic, and an anxiolytic. It has been used for ceremonial purposes in Micronesia and Polynesia for thousands of years in the place of alcoholic beverages, which have not always been available.

Sedative Action

The sedative action of kava is unlike any other. It appears to act directly on the limbic system. Kava lactones may actually

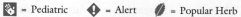

= Pregnancy   = Pediatric   = Alert   = Popular Herb

modify receptor areas rather than bind to receptor binding sites (Holm, 1991).

Anxiolytic Action

There appears to be no lack of effectiveness, even at large doses over time. Several studies confirm the ability of kava to decrease anxiety. One study used 84 volunteers with anxiety conditions who received kavain, a kava lactone, in doses of 400 mg/day. In the experimental group, the result was an increase in memory and reaction time (Scholing, 1977). A more recent study showed a significant reduction of anxiety symptoms with the use of kava (Pittler, 2000). One group of volunteers was given 100 mg of kava extract three times daily, while the other received a placebo. After 4 weeks, when the subjects were evaluated using the Hamilton Anxiety Scale, the kava group reported a significant decrease in anxiety symptoms (Kinzler, 1991).

Analgesic Action

The analgesic effect of kava appears to be unrelated to that of other pain relievers. Kava does not bind to opiate receptors and does not block pain impulses in the central nervous system. Its mechanism of action is unknown at present.

References

Foster S: *101 medicinal herbs*, Loveland, Colo, 1998, Interweave Press.

Holm E et al: Studies on the profile of the neurophysiological effects of D, L-kavain: cerebral sites of action and sleep-wakefulness-rhythm in animals, *Arzneimittelforschung* 41:673-683, 1991.

Kinzler E et al: Clinical efficacy of a kava extract in patients with anxiety syndrome: double-blind placebo controlled study over 4 weeks, *Arzneimittelforschung* 41:584-588, 1991.

Murray M, Pizzarno J: *The encyclopedia of natural medicine*, 2 ed (revised), Roseville, Calif, 1998, Prima.

Pittler MH et al: Efficacy of kava extract for treating anxiety: systematic review and meta-analysis, *J Clin Psychopharmacol* 20(1):84-89, 2000.

Scholing WE et al: On the effect of d, I-kavain: experience with neuronika, *Med Klin* 72:1301-1306, 1977.

Wu D et al: Novel compounds from *Piper methysticum* roots and their effect on cyclooxygenase enzyme, *J Agric Food Chem* 50(4):701-705, 2002.

K

Kelp
(kehlp)

Scientific names: *Laminaria digitata, Laminaria japonica, Laminaria saccharina, Marcrocystis pyrifera*

Other common names: Brown algae, horsetail, sea girdles, seaweed, sugar wrack, tangleweed

Origin: Kelp is an algae found in the northern Atlantic and Pacific oceans.

Uses

Reported Uses

Kelp has been used as an antiobesity and anticancer treatment and as an antihypertensive, antioxidant, abortifacient, and anticoagulant. It may be used for its high iodine content to treat goiter.

Product Availability and Dosages

Available Forms

Capsules, extract, powder, tablets

Plant Parts Used: Fronds

Dosages and Routes

Adult

- PO Capsules/tablets: 500-650 mg qd
- *Laminaria* tent: Insert to facilitate surgical abortion

Precautionary Information

Contraindications

Because of its abortifacient properties, kelp should not be used during pregnancy. Until more research is available, kelp should not be used during lactation and should not be given to children. Kelp should not be used by persons with hypersensitivity to *Laminaria* spp. or those with hyperthyroidism.

Side Effects/Adverse Reactions

Cardiovascular: Decreased blood pressure
Gastrointestinal: Nausea, vomiting, anorexia

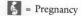 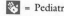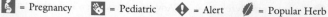

Precautionary Information—cont'd

Side Effects/Adverse Reactions—cont'd

Hematologic: ABNORMAL ERYTHROPOIESIS, THROMBOCYTOPENIA

Integumentary: Hypersensitivity reactions, acne-like eruptions

Reproductive: Uterine contractions, ABORTION

Systemic: BLEEDING

Interactions with Kelp

Drug

Anticoagulants (heparin, warfarin): Use of kelp with anticoagulants may pose an increased risk of bleeding; avoid concurrent use.

Antihypertensives: Antihypertensives may increase the hypotensive effects of kelp; avoid concurrent use.

Food	Herb	Lab Test
None known	None known	None known

K

Client Considerations

Assess

- Assess for hypersensitivity reactions. If present, discontinue use of kelp and administer antihistamine or other appropriate therapy.
- Assess for use of antihypertensives and anticoagulants (see Interactions). Monitor blood pressure.
- Assess blood work, including complete blood count and platelets; watch for bruising, black tarry stools, or frank blood.

Administer

- Instruct the client to store kelp products in a cool, dry place, away from heat and moisture.

Teach Client/Family

- Because of its abortifacient properties, caution the client not to use kelp during pregnancy. Until more research is available, caution the client not to use kelp during lactation and not to give it to children.
- Advise the client not to use kelp tents to increase dilatation

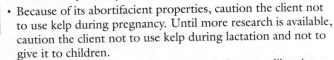

🍀 Endangered Herb   Adverse effects: BOLD = life-threatening

during labor. Use of kelp tents may cause contamination leading to infection and toxic shock syndrome.

Pharmacology

Pharmacokinetics

Pharmacokinetics and pharmacodynamics are unknown.

Primary Chemical Components of Kelp and Their Possible Actions		
Chemical Class	**Individual Components**	**Possible Action**
Fucoidan **Glucan** **Polysaccharide**	Laminarin Algin	Cervical dilatation
Vitamin **Iodine** **Mineral**		

Actions

Cervical Dilatation

Laminaria has been used intravenously with prostaglandin E2 to terminate second trimester pregnancies with fetal abnormalities. In one study, 106 pregnant women underwent insertion of a laminaria tent, followed by administration of prostaglandin E2 (Sulprostone IV) the following morning to induce uterine contractions. This is considered a satisfactory way to terminate second-trimester pregnancies (Chung, 1999). Another study found the use of laminaria to be a satisfactory means of dilating the cervix for various procedures (Mayr, 1998). There is growing concern that contamination may occur in some alga species and that kelp therefore should not be used for cervical tents.

References

Chung YP et al: *Laminaria* and sulprostone in second-trimester pregnancy termination for fetal abnormalities, *Int J Gynaecol Obstet* 65(1): 47-52, 1999.

Mayr NA et al: The use of laminarias for osmotic dilation of the cervix in gynecological brachytherapy applications, *Int J Radiat Oncol Biol Phys* 42(5):1049-1053, 1998.

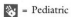 = Pregnancy   = Pediatric   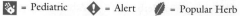 = Alert   = Popular Herb

Kelpware
(kelp'wehr)

Scientific name: *Fucus vesiculosus*

Other common names: Black-tang, bladder fucus, bladder-wrack, blasen-tang, quercus marina, sea wrack, sea-oak, seetang

Origin: Kelpware is a seaweed found in the Atlantic and Pacific oceans.

Uses
Reported Uses
In traditional herbal medicine, kelpware has been used to treat obesity and menorrhagia, to increase iodine levels in goiter, and to reduce inflammation of the renal system.

Investigational Uses
In preliminary research kelpware has shown promise as an anticoagulant, antioxidant, and antimicrobial.

Product Availability and Dosages
Available Forms
Fluid extract, gel tabs, soft extract, tablets, whole plant (dried)

Plant Parts Used: Whole plant

Dosages and Routes
Adult
All dosages listed are PO.
- Bruised plant: put 16 g herb in 500 ml water, take 2 oz tid-qid
- Fluid extract: 4-8 ml ac
- Gel tabs/tablets: 3 tabs qd, then gradually increase to 24 qd
- Soft extract: 200-600 mg qd

Precautionary Information
Contraindications
Until more research is available, kelpware should not be used during pregnancy and lactation and should not be given to children. Kelpware should not be used by persons with cardiac disorders such as recent myocardial infarction,

Continued

Precautionary Information—cont'd

Contraindications—cont'd

congestive heart failure, or severe angina pectoris. It also should not be used by the elderly or persons who have cancer, thyroid disorders (except goiter), renal or hepatic disease, diabetes mellitus, or hypersensitivity to it.

Side Effects/Adverse Reactions

Endocrine: Hyperglycemia

Gastrointestinal: Nausea, vomiting, anorexia, increased hunger

Genitourinary: Increased urinary output, NEPHROTOXICITY

Integumentary: Hypersensitivity reactions

Interactions with Kelpware

Drug

Anticoagulants (heparin, warfarin): Use of kelpware with anticoagulants may pose an increased risk of bleeding; avoid concurrent use.

Thyroid hormones: Kelpware may decrease the effects of thyroid hormones; avoid concurrent use.

Food	Herb	Lab Test
None known	None known	None known

Client Considerations

Assess

- Assess for hypersensitivity reactions. If these are present, discontinue use of kelpware and administer antihistamine or other appropriate therapy.
- Assess for anticoagulant and thyroid hormone therapy (see Interactions).
- ◆ Assess blood work, including CBC and platelets. Watch for bruising, black tarry stools, and frank blood.
- ◆ Assess for symptoms of nephrotoxicity (increased BUN and creatinine levels), which may result from heavy metal contaminants in kelpware.

🝚 = Pregnancy   🝚 = Pediatric   ◆ = Alert   ⫽ = Popular Herb

Administer
- Instruct the client to store kelpware products in a cool, dry place, away from heat and moisture.

Teach Client/Family
- Until more research is available, caution the client not to use kelpware during pregnancy and lactation and not to give it to children.

Pharmacology

Pharmacokinetics

Pharmacokinetics and pharmacodynamics are unknown.

Primary Chemical Components of Kelpware and Their Possible Actions		
Chemical Class	**Individual Component**	**Possible Action**
Polysaccharide	Algin; Fucoidan	
Vitamin		
Iodine		
Mineral	Bromine; Cadmium; Lead	

Actions

Anticoagulant Action

Kelpware has been shown to exert significant anticoagulant action. One study showed that activated partial thromboplastin time was prolonged in vitro (Durig, 1997).

Antimicrobial, Antioxidant Action

Kelpware has shown antimicrobial activity against *Escherichia coli, Neisseria meningitidis, Candida guilliermondii,* and *Candida krusei* (Craido, 1984). One study identified the antioxidant properties of kelpware (Ruperez, 2002).

References

Craido MT et al: Toxicity of an algal mucopolysaccharide for *Escherichia coli* and *Neisseria meningitidis* strains, *Rev Esp Fisiol* 40:227-230, 1984.
Durig J et al: Anticoagulant fucoidan fractions from *Fucus vesiculosus* induced platelet activation in vitro, *Thromb Res* 85(6):479-491, 1997.
Ruperez P et al: Potential antioxidant capacity of sulfated polysaccharides from the edible marine brown seaweed *Fucas vesiculosus, J Agric Food Chem* 50(4):840-845, 2002.

 Endangered Herb   Adverse effects: BOLD = life-threatening

Khat
(kaht)

Scientific name: *Catha edulis*

Other common names: Cat, chat, gad, kaht, kat, miraa, tschut

Origin: Khat is a tree found in Africa and on the Arabian Peninsula.

Uses

Reported Uses

Khat has been used in traditional herbal medicine to treat fatigue, obesity, depression, and peptic ulcer.

Product Availability and Dosages

Available Forms

Raw leaves

Plant Parts Used: Raw leaves

Dosages and Routes

Adult

- PO raw leaves: 100-200 g chewed, followed by fluids

Precautionary Information

Contraindications

Until more research is available, khat should not be used during pregnancy and lactation and should not be given to children. Persons with hypersensitivity to khat should not use it, and those with renal, cardiac, or hepatic disease should avoid its use.

Side Effects/Adverse Reactions

Cardiovascular: Increased heart rate, arrhythmias, increased blood pressure, PULMONARY EDEMA, CIRCULATORY COLLAPSE, DEATH

Central Nervous System: Restlessness, insomnia, headache, psychosis, hallucinations, decreased reaction time, hyperthermia, sweating

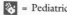 = Pregnancy   = Pediatric   ◆ = Alert   / = Popular Herb

Precautionary Information—cont'd

Side Effects/Adverse Reactions—cont'd

Gastrointestinal: Nausea, vomiting, anorexia, constipation, abdominal pain, stomatitis, HEPATOTOXICITY, abdominal spasms

Genitourinary: Decreased sperm count, decreased libido

Integumentary: Hypersensitivity reactions

Systemic: CEREBRAL HEMORRHAGE

Interactions with Khat

Drug

Khat may increase the action of amphetamines, antihistamines, antihypertensives, antiarrhythmics, beta-blockers, calcium channel blockers, cardiac glycosides, decongestants, and MAOIs.

Food	Herb	Lab Test
None known	None known	None known

Client Considerations

Assess

- Assess for hypersensitivity reactions. If these are present, discontinue use of khat and administer antihistamine or other appropriate therapy.
- Assess for use of other medications, including antihypertensives, cardiac glycosides, beta-blockers, antiarrhythmics, calcium channel blockers, amphetamines, antihistamines, and decongestants (see Interactions).
- Monitor liver function studies periodically (AST, ALT, and bilirubin levels); if elevated, discontinue use of khat.

Administer

- Instruct the client to store khat products in a cool, dry place, away from heat and moisture.

Teach Client/Family

- Until more research is available, caution the client not to use khat during pregnancy and lactation and not to give it to children.
- Warn the client of the life-threatening side effects of khat.

Endangered Herb   Adverse effects: BOLD = life-threatening

Pharmacology

Pharmacokinetics

Pharmacokinetics and pharmacodynamics are unknown.

Primary Chemical Components of Khat and Their Possible Actions		
Chemical Class	Individual Component	Possible Action
Alkaloid	Cathine	Increased adrenocortical function
	Cathinone	Amphetamine-like; increased adrenocortical function
	Eduline; Ephidrine; Cathinine; Cathidine	
Tannin		
Phenylpentenylamine		
Phenylpropyl		

Actions

Analgesic Action

In a comparative study of khat, amphetamines, and ibuprofen performed to identify pain-reducing qualities, all three were found to reduce pain (Connor, 2000).

Stimulant Action

Khat has been evaluated for its amphetamine-like action, which results from one of its alkaloid chemical components, cathinone (Ahmed, 1993; Kalix, 1996). Khat has been shown to be teratogenic and embryotoxic in rats (Islam, 1994).

Antiinflammatory Action

One study used the flavonoid fraction of khat to evaluate its antiinflammatory action in rats with carrageenan-induced paw edema and paw granuloma. Administration of khat produced a significant antiinflammatory action, comparable to that of oxyphenbutazone (Al-Meshal, 1986).

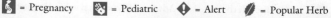 = Pregnancy　　 = Pediatric　　 = Alert　　 = Popular Herb

References

Ahmed MB et al: Biochemical effects of *Catha edulis,* cathine and cathinone on adrenocortical functions, *J Ethnopharmacol* 39(3):213-216, 1993.

Al-Meshal IA et al: Anti-inflammatory activity of the flavonoid fraction of khat (*Catha edulis* Forsk), *Agents Actions* 17(3-4):379-380, 1986.

Connor J et al: Comparison of analgesic effects of khat (*Catha edulis* Forsk) extract, D-amphetamine and ibuprofen in mice, *J Pharm Pharmacol* 52(1):107-110, 2000.

Islam MW et al: Evaluation of teratogenic potential of khat (*Catha edulis* Forsk) in rats, *Drug Chem Toxicol* 17(1):51-68, 1994.

Kalix P: *Catha edulis,* a plant that has amphetamine-like effects, *Pharm World Sci* 18(2):69-73, 1996.

Khella
(keh'luh)

Scientific name: *Ammi visnaga*

Other common names: Ammi, bishop's weed, khellin, visnagin

Origin: Khella is found in Egypt and Pakistan.

Uses

Reported Uses

Traditionally, khella has been used in combination with other herbs to treat angina pectoris. It has also been used to relieve abdominal cramping, dysmenorrhea, and biliary colic.

Investigational Uses

Researchers are working to determine whether khella is useful for the reduction of cholesterol levels, the prevention of bronchial asthma, and the treatment of atherosclerosis and severe allergic reactions.

Product Availability and Dosages

Available Forms

Capsules, dried powdered root extract, tablets, tea

Plant Parts Used: Fruit, roots, seeds

Dosages and Routes
Adult
Angina
- PO dried powdered root extract: 100 mg tid (12% khellin) (Murray, 1998)

Precautionary Information
Contraindications
Because it is a uterine stimulant, khella should not be used during pregnancy. Until more research is available, this herb should not be used during lactation and it should not be given to children. Persons with hypersensitivity to khella should not use it, and persons with liver disease, severe cardiac disorders, bleeding disorders, or hypotension should avoid its use. It is now considered a disapproved herb, since there are many potential risks.

Side Effects/Adverse Reactions
Central Nervous System: Insomnia, dizziness, headache
Gastrointestinal: Nausea, vomiting, anorexia, constipation, elevated liver function studies
Integumentary: Hypersensitivity reactions, phototoxicity; skin cancer (topical use)

Interactions with Khella

Drug
Anticoagulants (heparin, warfarin): Khella increases the risk of bleeding when used with anticoagulants such as heparin, warfarin, and aspirin; avoid concurrent use.
Antihypertensives: Increased hypotension is possible when khella is used with antihypertensives; avoid concurrent use.
Calcium channel blockers: Increased hypotension is possible when khella is used with calcium channel blockers; avoid concurrent use.
Diuretics: Increased hypotension is possible when khella is used with diuretics; avoid concurrent use.

Food	Herb	Lab Test
None known	None known	None known

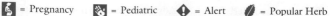

 = Pregnancy   = Pediatric   = Alert   = Popular Herb

Client Considerations

Assess

- Assess for hypersensitivity reactions. If present, discontinue use of khella and administer antihistamine or other appropriate therapy.
- Monitor liver function studies, including AST, ALT, and bilirubin, at least every 6 weeks.
- Assess for use of anticoagulants, salicylates, antihypertensives, calcium channel blockers, and diuretics (see Interactions).

Administer

- Instruct the client to store khella products in a cool, dry place, away from heat and moisture.

Teach Client/Family

- Until more research is available, caution the client not to use khella during pregnancy and lactation and not to give it to children.
- Because dizziness can occur, advise the client not to perform hazardous activities such as driving or operating heavy machinery until physical response to the herb can be evaluated.

Pharmacology

Pharmacokinetics

Pharmacokinetics and pharmacodynamics are unknown.

Primary Chemical Components of Khella and Their Possible Actions		
Chemical Class	Individual Component	Possible Action
Visnagin		
Khellin		Anticholesterol
Furanochromone		
Flavonoid	Quercetin; Kaempferol Isorhamnetin	Antiinflammatory
Essential Oil	Camphor; Terpineol; Terpinen; Linalool	
Psoralen	Methoxypsoralen	
Protein		

Actions

Among the possible actions of khella are antidiabetic effects, calcium channel blocking effects, and alteration of high-density lipoproteins (HDLs). Because as of this writing only one study is available to confirm each action, no conclusions can be drawn from research. However, khella may dilate coronary vessels and bronchioles.

Antidiabetic Actions

An extensive survey was taken of 130 participants who had agreed to provide information about plant-based hypoglycemic treatments used in Israel. *Ammi visnaga* L. was among the plants listed (Yaniv, 1987).

Calcium Channel Blocking Action

In a study that screened medicinal plants for their calcium-antagonistic action, one of the furanochromones present in khella, visnagin, was shown to inhibit potassium spasms. This inhibitory action results in a vasodilator response, suggesting that khella exerts a calcium-antagonistic effect (Rauwald, 1994).

Alteration of High-Density Lipoproteins

In a study focusing on the HDL-increasing effect of khella, participants with normal weight and normal lipid levels were given khellin, one of the furochromones present in *Ammi visnaga*. The participants received 50 mg four times daily for 4 weeks, and their lipid levels measured each week. Total cholesterol and triglyceride levels remained unchanged, although HDL levels increased and low-density lipoprotein (LDL)/HDL ratios decreased (Harvengt, 1983).

References

Harvengt C et al: HDL-cholesterol increase in normolipaemic subjects on khellin: a pilot study, *Int J Clin Pharmacol Res* 3(5):363-366, 1983.

Murray M, Pizzarno J: *The encyclopedia of natural medicine*, 2 ed (revised), Roseville, Calif, 1998, Prima.

Rauwald HW et al: The involvement of a Ca2$^+$ channel blocking mode of action in the pharmacology of *Ammi visnaga* fruits, *Planta Med* 60(2):101-105, 1994.

Yaniv Z et al: Plants used for the treatment of diabetes in Israel, *J Ethnopharmacol* 19(2):145-151, 1987.

Kudzu
(kuhd′zew)

Scientific name: *Pueraria lobata*

Other common names: Japanese arrowroot,
kudzu vine, ge gen   Class 1 (Root)

Origin: Kudzu is a vine found in China and Japan.

Uses
Reported Uses
Traditionally, kudzu has been used for suppression of alcoholism and as a treatment for arrhythmias, muscular aches and pains, and measles.

Product Availability and Dosages
Available Forms
No commercially prepared forms are available.

Plant Parts Used: Root

Dosages and Routes
Adult
• PO decoction: cut root into 0.4-0.7 cm slices, place in water 12-15 times the weight of the root; decoct 30 min (Yang, 1989)

Precautionary Information
Contraindications
Until more research is available, kudzu should not be used during pregnancy and lactation and should not be given to children. This herb should not be use by persons with hypersensitivity to it and should be used cautiously by persons who have heart disease. Class 1 herb (root).

Side Effects/Adverse Reactions
Gastrointestinal: Nausea, vomiting, anorexia
Integumentary: Hypersensitivity reactions

 Endangered Herb   Adverse effects: ʙᴏʟᴅ = life-threatening

Interactions with Kudzu
Drug
Kudzu may enhance the effects of cardiac medications such as antiarrhythmics and cardiac glycosides; do not use concurrently.

Food	Herb	Lab Test
None known	None known	None known

Client Considerations

Assess

- Assess for hypersensitivity reactions. If these are present, discontinue use of kudzu and administer antihistamine or other appropriate therapy.
- Assess cardiac status, including rate, rhythm, and character. Identify cardiac conditions and cardiac medications used (see Interactions).

Administer

- Instruct the client to store kudzu products in a cool, dry place, away from heat and moisture.

Teach Client/Family

- Until more research is available, caution the client not to use kudzu during pregnancy and lactation and not to give it to children.

Pharmacology

Pharmacokinetics

Pharmacokinetics and pharmacodynamics are unknown.

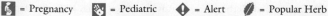

Primary Chemical Components of Kudzu and Their Possible Actions		
Chemical Class	**Individual Component**	**Possible Action**
Glycoside	Kudzusaponins A1, A2, Ar, SA4, SB1 (Arao, 1997)	
Sterol		
Isoflavone	Daidzin; Daidzein; Puerarin; Rutin; Furylfuramide;	Alcoholism suppression; antioxidant; antimutagenic (Miyazawa, 2001)

Actions

Suppression of Alcoholism

Kudzu has been used in traditional herbal medicine to suppress alcoholism. Research shows the presence of reversible inhibitors of an enzyme needed to metabolize alcohol in humans (Keung, 1993a). One study showed that kudzu decreased alcoholism in hamsters. Researchers identified the hamsters' baseline water and ethanol intake and then administered kudzu. The volume of ethanol intake decreased by approximately 50%. After the kudzu was stopped, alcohol intake returned to pretreatment levels (Keung, 1993b). Daidzin and daidzein, two of the chemical components of kudzu, were identified as being responsible for the suppression of alcoholism (Keung, 1998).

Cardiovascular Action

Kudzu has been shown to increase cerebral blood flow and decrease myocardial oxygen consumption in patients with diagnosed arteriosclerosis. Kudzu has been used successfully to treat cardiovascular disorders such as hypertension, angina, and cardiac ischemia (Qicheng, 1980).

Other Actions

Some of the other proposed actions of kudzu include antipyretic and contraceptive effects. This herb may also be useful for the reduction of muscle pain. More research is needed to determine the validity of these claims.

K

References

Arao T et al: Oleanene-type triterpene glycosides from puerariae radix, IV: six new saponins from *Pueraria lobata, Chem Pharm Bull (Tokyo)* 45(2):362-366, 1997.

Keung W: Biochemical studies of a new class of alcohol dehydrogenase inhibitors from radix puerariae, *Alcohol Clin Exp Res* 17:1254, 1993a.

Keung W et al: Daidzin and daidzein suppress free-choice ethanol intake by Syrian Golden hamsters, *Proc Natl Acad Sci USA* 90:10008-10012, 1993b.

Keung W et al: Kudzu root: an ancient Chinese source of modern antidipsotropic agents, *Phytochemistry* 47(4):499-506, 1998.

Miyazawa M et al: Antimutagenic activity of isoflavone from *Pueraria lobata, J Agric Food Chem* 49(1):336-341, 2001.

Qicheng F: Some current study and research approaches relating to the use of plants in the traditional Chinese medicine, *J Ethnopharmacol* 2(1):57-63, 1980.

Yang YH et al: Study on decocting conditions for *Pueraria lobata* Ohui in qiweibaizhu bage, *Chung Kuo Chung Yao Tsa Chih* 14(4):221-223, 254, 1989.

 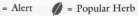

= Pregnancy   = Pediatric   ◆ = Alert   ✍ = Popular Herb

Lady's Mantle
(lay'deez man'tuhl)

Scientific names: *Alchemilla mollis, Alchemilla vulgaris*

Other common names: Bear's foot, dewcup, leontopodium, lady's mantle, lion's foot, nine hooks, stellaria

Class 1 (Whole Herb)

Origin: Lady's mantle is a flowering plant found in Europe, the United States, and Canada.

Uses

Reported Uses

Traditional uses of lady's mantle include control of bleeding (when used topically), treatment of menorrhagia, and relief of menstrual cramps, menopausal symptoms, and diarrhea. It is also used as an astringent.

Product Availability and Dosages

Available Forms

Extract, tea

Plant Parts Used: Flowers, leaves, root

Dosages and Routes

Adult
- PO extract: 2-4 ml tid
- PO herb: 5-10 g qd (Blumenthal, 1998)
- PO tea: pour boiling water over 2 tsp herb, let steep 15 min, take tid

Precautionary Information

Contraindications

Because it may cause uterine contractions, lady's mantle should not be used during pregnancy. Until more research is available, this herb should not be used during lactation and should not be given to children. Persons with hypersensitivity to this herb should not use it. Class 1 herb (whole herb).

Continued

🍀 Endangered Herb   Adverse effects: BOLD = life-threatening

> **Precautionary Information—cont'd**
> **Side Effects/Adverse Reactions**
> *Gastrointestinal:* Nausea, vomiting, anorexia, HEPATIC DAMAGE
> *Integumentary:* Hypersensitivity reactions

> **Interactions with Lady's Mantle**
>
> **Drug**
> *Iron salts:* Lady's mantle tea may decrease the absorption of iron salts; separate by 2 hr.
>
> | Food | Herb | Lab Test |
> |------|------|----------|
> | None known | None known | None known |

Client Considerations

Assess

- Assess for hypersensitivity reactions. If present, discontinue use of lady's mantle and administer antihistamine or other appropriate therapy.
 - Assess for hepatic damage including increased liver function studies.

Administer

- Instruct the client to store lady's mantle products in a cool, dry place, away from heat and moisture.

Teach Client/Family

 - Because it may cause uterine contractions, caution the client not to use lady's mantle during pregnancy. Until more research is available, caution the client not to use this herb during lactation and not to give it to children.

Pharmacology

Pharmacokinetics

Pharmacokinetics and pharmacodynamics are unknown.

Primary Chemical Components of Lady's Mantle and Their Possible Actions

Chemical Class	Individual Component	Possible Action
Elligitannin Flavonoid Tannin	Quercetin Pedunculagin; Alchemillin	Antiinflammatory Wound healing; astringent

Actions

Lady's mantle is used primarily for its astringent and antidiarrheal effects. Its astringent effects are responsible for its ability to both lessen bleeding and decrease diarrhea (Bisset, 1994). The high tannin content (pedunculagin and alchemillin) is probably responsible for the wound-healing properties and astringent effects of this herb. The tannins may also inhibit the enzyme elastase (Lamaison, 1990), and the flavonoid components of lady's mantle have been shown to inhibit two other enzymes, trypsin and chymotrypsin. These enzyme inhibitory effects may protect elastic tissues. (Jonadet, 1986).

References

Bisset NG: *Herbal drugs and phytopharmaceuticals,* Stuttgart, 1994, Medpharm.

Blumenthal M, editor: *The complete German Commission E monographs: therapeutic guide to herbal medicines,* Austin, Tex, American Botanical Council; Boston, Integrative Medicine Communication, 1998.

Lamaison JL et al: Tannin content and inhibiting activity of elastase in Rosaceae, *Ann Pharm Fr* 48(6):335, 1990 (review).

Jonadet M et al: Flavonoids extracted from *Ribes nigrum* L. and *Alchemilla vulgaris* L.: in vitro inhibitory activities on elastase, trypsin and chymotrypsin, *J Pharmacol* 17(1):21-27, 1986.

L

Lavender
(la'vuhn-duhr)

Scientific names: *Lavandula officinalis, Lavandula latifolia, Lavandula angustifolia, Lavandula stoechas*

Other common names: Aspic, echter lavendel, English lavender, esplieg, French lavender, garden lavender, lavanda, lavande commun, lavandin, nardo, Spanish lavender, spigo, spike lavender, true lavender **Class 1 (Flower)**

Origin: Lavender is a flowering shrub found in the Mediterranean.

Uses

Reported Uses

Lavender traditionally has been used as a sedative, as an anxiolytic, and to relieve insomnia. It has also been used to increase the appetite and to treat cuts and abrasions and various conditions of the nervous system. It is a common aromatherapeutic agent and is a component in many cosmetic products such as shampoos, conditioners, lotions, and soaps.

Investigational Uses

Initial research studies are available documenting the use of lavender to treat cancer. Lavender may be used to produce diuresis.

Product Availability and Dosages

Available Forms

Candles, flowers, oil, tincture; component of lotions, soaps, shampoos, and conditioners

Plant Parts Used: Flowers

Dosages and Routes

Standardized forms are not available.

Adult

- PO oil: place 2-4 drops on a sugar cube
- PO tea: place 1-2 tsp flowers in 1 cup boiling water (Blumenthal, 1998), steep 10-15 min
- PO tincture: take up to 2 ml tid
- Topical: place 1-2 cups flowers in teapot, heat to boiling, strain, add to bath water (Blumenthal, 1998)

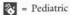 = Pregnancy   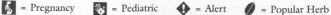 = Pediatric   = Alert   = Popular Herb

Precautionary Information

Contraindications

Until more research is available, lavender should not be used during pregnancy and lactation and should not be given to children. Persons with hypersensitivity to lavender should not use it. Class 1 herb (flower).

Side Effects/Adverse Reactions

Central Nervous System: Headache, drowsiness, dizziness, euphoria, CENTRAL NERVOUS SYSTEM DEPRESSION
Gastrointestinal: Nausea, vomiting, increased appetite, constipation
Integumentary: Hypersensitivity reactions, contact dermatitis

Interactions with Lavender

L

Drug
Alcohol, antihistamines, opioids, and sedative/hypnotics may increase sedation when used with lavender; avoid concurrent use.

Iron salts: Lavender tea may decrease the absorption of iron salts; separate by 2 hr.

Food	Herb	Lab Test
None known	None known	None known

Client Considerations

Assess

- Assess for hypersensitivity reactions such as contact dermatitis. If these are present, discontinue use of lavender and administer antihistamine or other appropriate therapy.
- Assess the client's use of alcohol, antihistamines, opioids, and sedative/hypnotics (see Interactions).

Administer

- Instruct the client to store lavender products in a cool, dry place, away from heat and moisture.
- Lavender oil should be taken internally only under the supervision of a qualified herbalist.

 Endangered Herb   Adverse effects: BOLD = life-threatening

Teach Client/Family

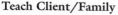

- Until more research is available, caution the client not to use lavender during pregnancy and lactation and not to give it to children.

Pharmacology

Pharmacokinetics

Pharmacokinetics and pharmacodynamics are unknown.

Primary Chemical Components of Lavender and Their Possible Actions		
Chemical Class	**Individual Component**	**Possible Action**
Volatile oil	Linalool; Limonene; Perillyl alcohol	Antitumor
	Linalyl acetate; Cis-ocimene; Beta-caryophyllene; Terpinene	
Coumarin	Umbelliferone	
	Herniarin	
Caffeic acid (derivative)		Bile stimulant
Tannin		Wound healing; astringent

Actions

Research on lavender is limited. However, it is thought that lavender, when inhaled, acts directly on the olfactory nerve in the brain, producing a sedative effect (Buchbauer, 1991). Its antitumor effects may be due to perillyl alcohol and limonene, two chemical components of the herb (Mills, 2000). Several studies have documented the use of lavender for the treatment of different types of cancer (breast, pancreatic, ovarian, liver, breast, and prostate) (Bronfen, 1994; Gould, 1995; Stark, 1995; Haag, 1994). These studies show varying results, but all indicate disease stabilization or tumor regression. The anticancer action of lavender may be due to its ability to produce redifferentiation in cancer cells (Shi, 1995). The diuretic activity of lavender was studied in rats. There was an increase in diure-

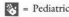 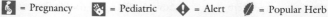

sis that may be attributed to specific chemical components (Elhajili, 2001).

References

Buchbauer G et al: Aromatherapy: evidence for sedative effects of the essential oil of lavender after inhalation, *Z Naturforsch* 46(11-12): 1067-1072, 1991.

Blumenthal M, editor: *The complete German Commission E monographs: therapeutic guide to herbal medicines,* Austin, Tex, American Botanical Council; Boston, Integrative Medicine Communication, 1998.

Bronfen JH et al: Inhibition of human pancreatic carcinoma cell proliferation by perillyl alcohol, *Am Assoc Cancer Res* 35:431, 1994 (proceedings).

Duke J: *CRC handbook of medicinal herbs,* Boca Raton, Fla, 1985, CRC Press, pp 374-375.

Elhajili M et al: Diuretic activity of the infusion of flowers from *Lavandula officinalis, Reprod Nutr Dev* 41(5):393-399, 2001.

Gould M: *J Cell Biochem* 22(suppl):139-144, 1995.

Haag JD, Gould MN: Mammary carcinoma regression induced by perillyl alcohol, a hydroxylated analog of limonene, *Cancer Chemother Pharmacol* 34:477-483, 1994.

Mills S, Bone K: *Principles and practice of phytotherapy,* London, 2000, Churchill Livingstone.

Shi W, Gould MN: Induction of differentiation in neuro-2A cells by the monoterpene perillyl alcohol, *Cancer Lett* 95:1-6, 1995.

Stark M et al: *Cancer Lett* 96(1):15-21, 1995.

L

Lecithin
(leh'suh-thuhn)

Scientific name: 1,2,diacyl-sn-glycero-3-phosphatidycholine

Other common names: Granulestin, kelecin, lecithol, vitellin

Origin: Lecithin is found in foods such as eggs, beef liver, and peanuts. Commercial sources are available.

Uses

Reported Uses

Lecithin is used to reduce cholesterol levels; to treat hepatic diseases including hepatitis, cirrhosis, and liver damage, and prevent the formation of gallstones; to treat diseases of the central nervous system such as Alzheimer's disease, bipolar disorder, and myasthenia gravis; to limit tardive dyskinesia; and to boost the immune system. It is also used as an emulsifier in food and in cosmetics and other pharmaceutical products. It may be used to maintain choline concentration in marathon runners.

Product Availability and Dosages
Available Forms
Capsules, tablets

Dosages and Routes
Adult
All dosages listed are PO.
Alzheimer's Disease
- Capsules/tablets: 100 mg tid (as phosphatidylcholine) (Murray, 1998)

Bipolar Disorder
- Capsules/tablets: 15-30 g (as phosphatidylcholine) (Murray, 1998)

Gallstone Prevention
- Capsules/tablets: 100 mg tid (Murray, 1998)

Precautionary Information
Contraindications
Until more research is available, lecithin should not be used therapeutically during pregnancy and lactation and should not be given therapeutically to children.

Side Effects/Adverse Reactions
Gastrointestinal: Nausea, vomiting, anorexia, gastrointestinal upset, HEPATITIS

Interactions with Lecithin

Drug	Food	Herb
None known	None known	None known

Lab Test
Lecithin may decrease cholesterol results.

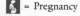 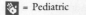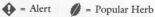

Client Considerations

Assess

- Assess for symptoms of hepatitis (jaundice, clay-colored stools). If these are present, discontinue use of lecithin.
- If the client is taking lecithin long-term, monitor liver function studies (AST, ALT, and bilirubin). If results are elevated, discontinue use of lecithin.

Administer

- Instruct the client to store lecithin products in a sealed container away from heat and moisture.

Teach Client/Family

- Until more research is available, caution the client not to use lecithin therapeutically during pregnancy and lactation and not to give it therapeutically to children.

Pharmacology

Pharmacokinetics

Pharmacokinetics and pharmacodynamics are unknown.

Primary Chemical Components of Lecithin and Their Possible Actions		
Chemical Class	Individual Component	Possible Action
Phosphatide	Phosphatidylcholine	Antidepressant; improved cognition
	Phosphatidyl ethanolamine; Phosphatidyl serine; Phosphatidyl inositol	
Fatty acid	Palmitic acid; Oleic acid; Stearic acid	
Carbohydrate		

Actions

Lecithin is found in food such as meat products, fruits, and vegetables. The best sources are oranges, beef liver, eggs, and some nuts. Lecithin reduces high cholesterol levels, improves memory, decreases tardive dyskinesia, and improves liver function. One of its chemical components, phosphatidylcholine,

🕊 Endangered Herb   Adverse effects: BOLD = life-threatening

is also present in *S*-adenosyl-L-methionine, commonly known as SAM-e, a supplement used to treat depression.

Antihypercholesteremic Action

Both the antihypercholesterolemic effect of lecithin and its ability to prevent atherosclerosis are believed to result from its ability to increase the metabolism of cholesterol in the gastrointestinal system. In one study in which 21 hyperlipidemic clients were given soybeans for 4 months, cholesterol, triglycerides, and total serum lipids were reduced by a statistically significant amount (Saba, 1978). In contrast, many earlier studies showed inconclusive results.

Memory Improvement

Lecithin has been shown to increase acetylcholine at receptor sites in the neurologic system, improving memory. One of the chemical components of lecithin, phosphatidylcholine, is a precursor to acetylcholine. One study demonstrated that memory improved significantly after 4 to 6 weeks of lecithin administration (Murray, 1996).

Other Actions

Phosphatidylcholine is used in Germany to treat cirrhosis of the liver, hepatitis, and toxic liver. One study using baboons showed that lecithin exerted a hepatoprotective effect against cirrhosis when the study animals were fed alcohol along with phosphatidylcholine (Murray, 1996). Lecithin has also been shown to increase immunity and dissolve gallstones.

References

Murray M: *Encyclopedia of nutritional supplements,* Roseville, Calif, 1996, Prima.

Murray M, Pizzarno J: *The encyclopedia of natural medicine,* 2 ed (revised), Roseville, Calif, 1998, Prima.

Saba P et al: *Curr Ther Res Clin Exp* 24:299-306, 1978.

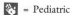 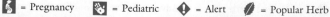

Lemon Balm
(leh'muhn bawlm)

Scientific name: *Melissa officinalis* L.

Other common names: Balm, cure-all, dropsy plant, honey plant, Melissa, sweet balm, sweet Mary

Class 1 (Leaf)

Origin: Lemon balm is a perennial found in the Mediterranean, Asia, Europe, and North America.

Uses

Reported Uses

Lemon balm traditionally has been used orally to treat insomnia, anxiety, gastric conditions, psychiatric conditions including depression and hysteria, migraines, hypertension, and bronchial conditions. It also has been used orally to treat Grave's disease and attention deficit disorder (ADD) and topically to treat cold sores.

Product Availability and Dosages

Available Forms

Comminuted herb, concentrated extract, cream, dry extract, fluid extract, herb powder

Plant Parts Used: Dried leaves, fresh leaves, whole plant

Dosages and Routes

Adult

Canker Sores, Herpes Simplex Type 1, Mouth Ulcers
- Topical concentrated extract: apply prn (dilution of 70:1)
- Topical cream: apply bid (Murray, 1998)
- Topical poultice: apply prn

Other
- PO infusion: pour boiling water over 1.5-4.5 g herb, let set 10 min, strain; usual dose is 8-10 g/day (Blumenthal, 1998)

Precautionary Information

Contraindications

Until more research is available, lemon balm should not be used during pregnancy and lactation and should not be given to children. This herb should not be used by persons with hypothyroidism or by those who are hypersensitive to it. Class 1 herb (leaf).

Side Effects/Adverse Reactions

Gastrointestinal: Nausea, anorexia
Integumentary: Hypersensitivity reactions

Interactions with Lemon Balm

Drug

Barbiturates (amobarbital, aprobarbital, butabarbital, phenobarbital, secobarbital): Lemon balm may potentiate the sedative effects of barbiturates.

Central nervous system depressants (including alcohol): Lemon balm may potentiate the sedative effects of central nervous system depressants.

Iron salts: Lemon balm tea may decrease the absorption of iron salts; separate by 2 hr.

Food	Herb	Lab Test
None known	None known	None known

Client Considerations

Assess

- Assess for hypersensitivity reactions. If present, discontinue use of lemon balm and administer antihistamine or other appropriate therapy.
- Assess for client use of barbiturates, other central nervous system depressants or iron salts.

Administer

- Instruct the client to store lemon balm products in a sealed container, away from heat and moisture. Products may be kept for up to 1 year.

 = Pregnancy    = Pediatric   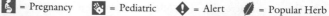 = Alert   = Popular Herb

Teach Client/Family

- Until more research is available, caution the client not to use lemon balm during pregnancy and lactation and not to give it to children.

Pharmacology

Pharmacokinetics

Pharmacokinetics and pharmacodynamics are unknown.

Primary Chemical Components of Lemon Balm and Their Possible Actions		
Chemical Class	**Individual Component**	**Possible Action**
Volatile oil	Geranial; Neral; Citronellal; Linalool; Geraniol; Geranylactetate	
Glycoside	Eugenol	Antioxidant
Flavonoid	Cynaroside; Rhamnocitrin; Isoquercitrin; Cosmosiin; Luteolin, Apigonin	
Triterpene acid	Caffeic acid; Ferulic acid Rosmarinic acid	Bile stimulant

Actions

Lemon balm has been studied for its antimicrobial, antiviral, and sedative actions, and also as a treatment for colitis. Multiple studies are not yet available to confirm any of these proposed actions.

Antimicrobial Actions

One study evaluating the antimicrobial effect of lemon balm found that *Melissa officinalis* exhibited a relatively higher degree of activity against bacteria, fungi, and yeasts than did *Lavandula officinalis* (lavender) (Larrondo, 1995).

Antiviral Action

Researchers have evaluated the virucidal and antiviral effects of *M. officinalis* with respect to herpes simplex virus type 1. The virucidal effect was found to occur within 3 to 6 hours of treatment (Dimitrova, 1993).

L

Sedative Action

The sedative action of lemon balm was identified when the hydroalcoholic extract of *M. officinalis* was given to mice. With high doses, the sedative effect was confirmed by a reduction in acetic acid-induced pain and induced sleep in the mice (Kennedy, 2002; Soulimani, 1991).

Colitis Treatment

Lemon balm was evaluated in combination with *Taraxacum officinale, Hipericum perforatum, Calendula officinalis,* and *Foeniculum vulgare* for the treatment of chronic nonspecific colitis (Chakurski, 1981). Results indicated that all 24 patients in the study experienced the disappearance of pain in the large intestine.

References

Blumenthal M, editor: *The complete German Commission E monographs: therapeutic guide to herbal medicines,* Austin, Tex, American Botanical Council; Boston, Integrative Medicine Communication, 1998.

Chakurski I et al: Treatment of chronic colitis with an herbal combination of *Taraxacum officinale, Hipericum perforatum, Melissa officinalis, Calendula officinalis* and *Foeniculum vulgare, Vutr Boles* 20(6):51-54, 1981.

Dimitrova Z et al: Antiherpes effect of *Melissa officinalis* L. extracts, *Acta Microbiol Bulg* 29:65-72, 1993.

Kennedy DO et al: Modulation of mood and cognitive performance following acute administration of *Melissa officinalis, Pharmacol Biochem Behav* 72(4)953-964, 2002.

Larrondo JV et al: Antimicrobial activity of essences from labiates, *Microbios* 82(332):171-172, 1995.

Murray M, Pizzarno J: *The encyclopedia of natural medicine,* 2 ed (revised), Roseville, Calif, 1998, Prima.

Soulimani R et al: Neurotropic action of the hydroalcoholic extract of *Melissa officinalis* in the mouse, *Planta Med* 57(2):105-109, 1991.

Lemongrass
(leh'muhn-gras)

Scientific name: *Cymbopogon citratus*

Other common names: Capim-cidrao, Guatemala
lemongrass, Madagascar
lemongrass   **Class 2b (Whole Herb)**

Origin: Lemongrass is a perennial grass found in Central
American, South America, the tropics of Asia, and the West
Indies.

Uses
Reported Uses
Lemongrass has been used in traditional herbal medicine to
treat anxiety, insomnia, gastrointestinal complaints, vomiting,
hypertension, and fever. It is also used as an antitussive, antiseptic, and antirheumatic.

Investigational Uses
The antibacterial, antifungal, analgesic, and anticholesteremic
properties of lemongrass are under investigation.

Product Availability and Dosages
Available Forms
Tea

Plant Parts Used: Leaves

Dosages and Routes
Adult
- PO tea: lemongrass tea may be made from fresh or dried
  leaves; no consensus on dosage is available

Precautionary Information
Contraindications
No absolute contraindications have been identified. Class 2b
herb (whole herb).

Side Effects/Adverse Reactions
None known

Interactions with Lemongrass			
Drug	Food	Herb	Lab Test
None known	None known	None known	None known

Client Considerations

Assess

- Determine the reason the client is using lemongrass.

Administer

- Instruct the client to store lemongrass products in a cool, dry place, away from heat and moisture.

Teach Client/Family

- Advise the client that lemongrass has no known toxicity or side effects.

Pharmacology

Pharmacokinetics

Pharmacokinetics and pharmacodynamics are unknown.

Primary Chemical Components of Lemongrass and Their Possible Actions		
Chemical Class	**Individual Component**	**Possible Action**
Essential oil	Myrcene	Analgesic
	Geraniol; Citral	
Diterpene		
Aldehyde		
Alcohol		

Actions

Studies done on lemongrass have focused on its antibacterial, antifungal, analgesic, and anticholesteremic actions. Multiple studies are not yet available to confirm any of the proposed actions.

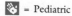 = Pregnancy   = Pediatric   ◆ = Alert   🖋 = Popular Herb

Antibacterial and Antifungal Actions

Lemongrass has been shown to inhibit gram-positive cocci and rods, gram-negative rods, and 12 types of fungi (Pattnaik, 1996). One study has confirmed the bacteriocidal effect of lemongrass on *Escherichia coli* (Pattnaik, 1995b), while a similar study showed a resistance to *Pseudomonas aeruginosa* when combined with lemongrass (Pattnaik, 1995a).

Analgesic Action

One study that tested lemongrass for its analgesic effect supports its use in folk medicine as a sedative. When rats were given an infusion of lemongrass, a dose-dependent analgesia occurred (Lorenzetti, 1991; Viana, 2000).

Anticholesteremic

During a study in which lemongrass was given to 22 hypercholesteremic subjects, serum cholesterol decreased in amounts that approached clinical significance. However, 90 days after completion of the study, cholesterol levels were found to have not remained at the decreased level (Elson, 1989).

References

Elson CE et al: Impact of lemongrass oil, an essential oil, on serum cholesterol, *Lipids* 24(8):677-679, 1989.

Lorenzetti BB et al: Myrcene mimics the peripheral analgesic activity of lemongrass tea, *J Ethnopharmacol* 34(1):43-48, 1991.

Pattnaik S et al: Characterization of resistance to essential oils in a strain of *Pseudomonas aeruginosa*, *Microbios* 81(326):29-31, 1995a.

Pattnaik S et al: Effect of essential oils on the viability and morphology of *Escherichia coli*, *Microbios* 84(340):195-199, 1995b.

Pattnaik S et al: Antibacterial and antifungal activity of ten essential oils in vitro, *Microbios* 86(349):237-246, 1996.

Viana GS et al: Antinociceptive effect of the essential oil from *Cymbopogon citratus* in mice, *J Ethnopharmacol* 70(3):323-327, 2000.

Lentinan
(lehnt'nehn)

Scientific names: *Lentinula edodes, Lentinus edodes*

Other common names: Forest mushroom, hua gu, pasania fungus, shiitake mushroom, snake butter

Origin: Lentinan is found in the shiitake mushroom, which is found in Japan and China.

Endangered Herb   Adverse effects: **BOLD** = life-threatening

Uses

Reported Uses

Lentinan is used as an immune regulator and to treat bacterial and viral infections and cancer.

Investigational Uses

Lentinan has been used in treatment of digestive cancer.

Product Availability and Dosages

Available Forms

Whole mushroom

Plant Parts Used: Fruiting body

Dosages and Routes

No dosage consensus exists.

Precautionary Information

Contraindications

Until more research is available, consumption of lentinan (shiitake mushrooms) is not recommended during pregnancy and lactation or for children. Persons with hypersensitivity to shiitake mushrooms should not consume them. Shiitake mushrooms have been shown to promote severe respiratory, immunologic, and dermatologic reactions (Sastre, 1990; Van Loon, 1992; Nakamura, 1992); however, most of the available studies have focused on farmers who grow shiitake mushrooms or workers who handle them.

Side Effects/Adverse Reactions

Gastrointestinal: Nausea, vomiting, anorexia
Integumentary: Hypersensitivity reactions, contact dermatitis, TOXICODERMIA
Systemic: RESPIRATORY AND IMMUNOLOGIC REACTIONS IN PERSONS WORKING WITH MUSHROOMS

Interactions with Lentinan

Drug	Food	Herb	Lab Test
None known	None known	None known	None known

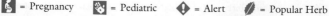

Client Considerations

Assess

- Assess for hypersensitivity reactions, contact dermatitis, toxicodermia. If these are present, discontinue consumption of shiitake mushrooms and administer antihistamine or other appropriate therapy.

Administer

- Instruct the client to store shiitake mushrooms in a cool, dry place, away from moisture and heat.

Teach Client/Family

- Until more research is available, caution the client not to consume shiitake mushrooms during pregnancy and lactation and not to give them to children.

Pharmacology

Pharmacokinetics

Pharmacokinetics and pharmacodynamics are unknown.

Primary Chemical Components of Lentinan and Their Possible Actions		
Chemical Class	**Individual Component**	**Possible Action**
Mannitol Polysaccharide		Diuretic

Actions

Antibacterial and Antiviral Actions

Initial research is available that documents the antibacterial action of lentinan. Lentinan has been shown to be effective against *Streptococcus* sp., *Actinomyces* sp., *Lactobacillus* sp., *Prevotella* sp., and *Porphyromonas* sp., and to promote resistance to *Staphylococcus* sp., *Escherichia* sp., *Bacillus* sp., *Candida* sp., and *Enterococcus* sp. (Hirasawa, 1999). Another study showed that lentinan exerts significant antiviral action against the western equine encephalitis virus in mice (Takehara, 1979).

Antihypertensive Action

An early study indicated that lentinan decreases hypertension in hypertensive rats. Investigators fed mice a diet of 5% mushroom powder and 0.5% NaCl (sodium chloride) solution as drinking water for 9 weeks. At the end of the study, blood pressure and plasma-free cholesterol were reduced (Kabir, 1987).

Hemagglutinin Action

A recent study (Tsivileva, 2000) has identified the hemagglutinating activity (HA) of *Lentinus edodes*. One morphogenetic structure of the mushroom was shown to possess significant hemagglutinating activity.

Other Actions

A study has shown a rebalance of cell-mediated immunity in digestive cancers with use of lentinan (Yoshino, 2000). However, lentinan may cause a worsening of ulcerative colitis as studied in rats (Mitamura, 2000).

References

Hirasawa M et al: Three kinds of antibacterial substances from *Lentinus edodes, Int J Antimicrob Agents* 11(2):151-157, 1999.

Kabir Y et al: Effect of shiitake *(Lentinus edodes)* and maitake *(Grifola frondosa)* mushrooms on blood pressure and plasma lipids of spontaneously hypertensive rats, *J Nutr Sci Vitaminol* 33(5):341-346, 1987.

Mitamura T et al: Effects of lentinan on colorectal carcinogenesis in mice with ulcerative colitis, *Oncol Rep* 7(3):599-601, 2000.

Nakamura T: Shiitake *(Lentinus edodes)* dermatitis, *Contact Dermatitis* 27(2):65-70, 1992.

Sastre J et al: Respiratory and immunological reactions among shiitake *(Lentinus edodes)* mushroom workers, *Clin Exp Allergy* 20(1):13-19, 1990.

Takehara M et al: Antiviral activity of virus-like particles from *Lentinus edodes* (shiitake): brief report, *Arch Virol* 59(3):269-274, 1979.

Tsivileva OM et al: Hemagglutinating activity of *Lentinus edodes* (Berk) Sing [*Lentinula edodes* (Berk) Pegler], *Mikrobiologiia* 69(1):38-44, 2000.

Van Loon PC et al: Mushroom worker's lung: detection of antibodies against Shii-take *(Lentinus edodes)* spore antigens in shii-take workers, *J Occup Med* 34(11):1097-1101, 1992.

Yoshino S et al: Immunoregulatory effects of the antitumor polysaccharide lentinan on Th1/Th2 balance in patients with digestive cancers, *Anticancer Res* 20(6C):4707-4711, 2000.

Licorice
(li'kuh-rish)

Scientific name: *Glycyrrhiza glabra*

Other common names: Chinese licorice, licorice root, Persian licorice, Russian licorice, Spanish licorice, sweet root

Class 2b/2c/2d (Root)

Origin: Licorice is a shrub found in subtropical climates.

Uses

Reported Uses

Licorice has been used as a laxative and as a treatment for asthma, malaria, hepatitis, abdominal pain, gastric disorders, infections, eczema, chronic fatigue syndrome, and sleeplessness. It has also been used as a flavoring and coloring agent and as a component in shampoos.

Investigational Uses

Studies are underway to investigate the estrogenic, antiinflammatory, antiviral (HIV/AIDS), antibacterial, and pseudo-aldosterone actions of licorice, most of which result from the chemical components glycyrrhizin and glycyrrhetinic acid.

Product Availability and Dosages

Available Forms

Candy, capsules, chewable tablets, deglycyrrhizinated licorice (DGL), fluid extract, gum, smoking products, solid extract, tablets, tea, tincture

Plant Parts Used: Rhizome, roots

Dosages and Routes

Adult

All dosages listed are PO.

Asthma
- Fluid extract: 2-4 ml (1:1 dilution) tid (Murray, 1998)
- Powdered root: 1-2 g tid (Murray, 1998)
- Solid extract (dry powdered): 250-500 mg (4:1 dilution) tid (Murray, 1998)

Chronic Fatigue Syndrome
- Fluid extract: 2-4 ml (1:1 dilution) (Murray, 1998)
- Powdered root: 1-2 g tid (Murray, 1998)

 Endangered Herb   Adverse effects: BOLD = life-threatening

- Solid extract (dry powdered): 250-500 mg (4:1 dilution) tid (Murray, 1998)

Gastric Disorders

- Capsules: 200-600 mg/day standardized to glycyrrhizin, taken <6 wk; 400-500 mg up to 6x/day (Foster, 1998)
- DGL: 6-8 250 mg chewable tablets/day (McCaleb, 2000), taken between meals or 20 min ac
- Fluid extract: 2-4 ml (1:1 dilution) tid
- Powdered root: 1 g up to tid (McCaleb, 2000)
- Solid extract (dry powder): 250-500 mg (4:1 concentration) tid
- Tea: place 1 tsp crude herb in 4 oz boiling water, simmer at least 5 min, strain; tea may be taken tid pc
- Tincture: 20-30 drops up to tid (Foster, 1998)

Hepatitis

- Fluid extract: 2-4 ml (1:1 dilution) tid (Murray, 1998)
- Powdered root: 1-2 g tid (Murray, 1998)
- Solid extract (dry powdered): 250-500 mg tid (Murray, 1998)

HIV/AIDS

- Fluid extract: 2-4 ml (1:1 dilution) tid (Murray, 1998)
- Solid extract (dry powdered): 250-500 mg tid (5% glycyrrhetinic acid) (Murray, 1998)

Menopause

- Fluid extract: 4 ml (1 tsp) (1:1 dilution) tid (Murray, 1998)
- Powdered root: 1-2 g tid (Murray, 1998)
- Solid extract (dry powdered): 250-500 mg (4:1 dilution) (Murray, 1998)

Peptic Ulcer Disease, Acute

- Chewable tablets: 2-4 tablets (190-380 mg) 20 min ac (Murray, 1998)

Peptic Ulcer Disease, Maintenance

- Chewable tablets: 1-2 tablets 20 min ac (Murray, 1998)

Precautionary Information

Contraindications

Until more research is available, licorice should not be used during pregnancy and lactation and should not be given to children. Licorice should not be used by persons with liver disease, renal disease, hypokalemia, hypertension, arrhythmias, congestive heart failure, or by those with hypersensitivity to it. Class 2b/2c/2d herb (root).

 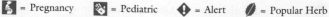

Precautionary Information—cont'd

Side Effects/Adverse Reactions

Cardiovascular: Hypertension, edema, ARREST
Central Nervous System: Headache, weakness
Endocrine: HYPOKALEMIA
Gastrointestinal: Nausea, vomiting, anorexia
Integumentary: Hypersensitivity reactions

Interactions with Licorice

Drug

Antiarrhythmics: Licorice may increase the cardiac effects of antiarrhythmics; do not use concurrently.

Antihypertensives: Use of licorice with antihypertensives may cause increased hypokalemia; do not use concurrently.

Azole antifungals: Licorice may increase the levels of azole antifungals; avoid concurrent use.

Cardiac glycosides (digoxin): Use of licorice with cardiac glycosides may cause increased toxicity and increased hypokalemia; do not use concurrently.

Corticosteroids (betamethasone, dexamethasone, hydrocortisone, methylprednisolone, prednisone, triamcinolone): Licorice may increase the effects of corticosteroids; avoid concurrent use.

Diuretics (amiloride, triamterene): Use of licorice with diuretics may cause increased hypokalemia; avoid concurrent use.

Food

None known

Herb

Licorice may cause hypokalemia when used with aloe (taken internally), buckthorn, cascara sagrada, and Chinese rhubarb; avoid concurrent use.

Continued

 Endangered Herb   Adverse effects: BOLD = life-threatening

Interactions with Licorice—cont'd

Lab Test

Licorice may decrease anion gap, blood; potassium (long-term use); serum prolactin; serum or urine sodium results. Licorice may cause a possible positive test for serum, urine myoglobin.

Client Considerations

Assess

- Assess for hypersensitivity reactions. If present, discontinue use of licorice and administer antihistamine or other appropriate therapy.
- Assess medications and herbs the client may be taking, including cardiac glycosides, antihypertensives, antiarrhythmics, and corticosteroids (see Interactions).

Administer

- Instruct the client to store licorice products in a cool, dry place, away from heat and moisture.
- Instruct the client not to use licorice for longer than 6 weeks.

Teach Client/Family

- Until more research is available, caution the client not to use licorice during pregnancy and lactation and not to give it to children.
- Advise client to increase potassium intake if using licorice for extended periods.

Pharmacology

Pharmacokinetics

Pharmacokinetics and pharmacodynamics are unknown.

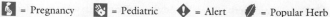

Primary Chemical Components of Licorice and Their Possible Actions

Chemical Class	Individual Component	Possible Action
Saponin	Glycyrrhizin; Glycyrrhetinic acid	Estrogenic; antiinflammatory; antiviral; antibacterial; pseudoaldosterone
Flavonoid	Licoagrodione	Antimicrobial (Li, 1998)
	Liquiritigenin; Isoliquiritigenin; Isolicoflavonol	
Isoflavonoid	Formononetin; Glabren; Glabridin; Glabrol; Hydroxyglabrol; Glycyrrhisoflavone; Isoflavonol; Kumatakenin; Licoricone; Glabrizoflavone, Pinocernbrin; Galangin	
Coumarin	Herniarin; Umbelliferone; Glycocoumarin; Licopyranocoumarin	
Sterol	Stigmasterol; Beta-sitosterol	

Actions

Traditionally, licorice has been used as an expectorant, an antitussive, and a laxative. More recently, studies have begun to focus on its antiinfective, estrogenic, antiinflammatory, and pseudoaldosterone effects.

Antiinfective Action

One study has shown that glycyrrhizin and glycyrrhetinic acid are able to stimulate interferon, which in turn is able to block DNA replication in viruses (Abe, 1982). This action has definite applications for HIV/AIDS patients. Another study focused on 16 hemophilic patients with HIV infection. These patients were given 150 to 225 mg of glycyrrhizin for 3 to 7 years. While immune system results were monitored, none of the patients showed progression of the infection (Ikegami, 1993). Two other studies have reported similar results (Mori, 1989; Hattori, 1989). Glycyrrhiza has also been shown effective against *Staphylococcus aureus, Streptococcus mutans, Mycobacterium,* and *Candida albicans* (Mitscher, 1980).

Estrogenic Action

Glycyrrhizin has been shown to exert estrogenic activity. It is responsible for both increasing estrogen levels that are too low and decreasing those that are too high (Kumagai, 1967a). It is thought that the isoflavone (saponin) content is responsible.

Antiinflammatory Action

Glycyrrhizin and glycyrrhetinic acid are able to bind to glucocorticoid receptors, thus decreasing the inflammatory response. Research has also demonstrated that many enzymes related to the inflammatory response are decreased as well (Kumagai, 1967b).

Pseudoaldosterone Action

Pseudoaldosterone syndrome has been induced when large amounts of glycyrrhiza were taken, resulting in increased blood pressure, electrolyte imbalances, and decreased aldosterone levels. Glycyrrhiza may be helpful in the treatment of Addison's disease.

Other Actions

Glycyrrhetinic acid has been proven useful in the treatment of peptic ulcer, duodenal ulcer, and apthous ulcer disease. Topical application of glycyrrhetinic acid has been shown to be effective against skin disorders such as psoriasis, eczema, and herpes simplex.

References

Abe N et al: Interferon induction by glycyrrhizin and glycyrrhetinic acid in mice, *Microbiol Immunol* 26:535-539, 1982.

Foster S: *101 medicinal herbs,* Loveland, Colo, 1998, Interweave Press.

Hattori T et al: Preliminary evidence for inhibitory effect of glycyrrhizin on HIV replication in patients with AIDS, *Antiviral Res* 11:255-261, 1989.

Ikegami N et al: Prophylactic effect of long-term oral administration of glycyrrhizin on AIDS development of asymptomatic patients, *Int Conf AIDS 1993* 9:234, 1993.

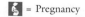 = Pregnancy    = Pediatric   = Alert   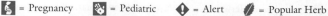 = Popular Herb

Kumagai A et al: Effect of glycyrrhizin on estrogen action, *Endocrinol Jpn* 14:34-38, 1967a.

Kumagai A et al: Effects of glycyrrhizin on thymolytic and immunosuppressive action of cortisol, *Endocrinol Jpn* 14:39-42, 1967b.

Li W et al: Antimicrobial flavonoids from *Glycyrrhiza glabra* hairy root cultures, *Planta Med* 64(8):746-747, 1998.

McCaleb R et al: *The encyclopedia of popular herbs: your complete guide to leading medicinal plants,* Roseville, Calif, 2000, Prima Health.

Mitscher L et al: Antimicrobial agents from higher plants: antimicrobial isoflavonoids from *Glycyrrhiza glabra* L. var. *typica, J Nat Products* 43:259-269, 1980.

Mori K et al: The present status in prophylaxis and treatment of HIV infected patients with hemophilia in Japan, *Rinsho Byhori* 37:1200-1208, 1989.

Murray M, Pizzarno J: *The encyclopedia of natural medicine,* 2 ed (revised), Roseville, Calif, 1998, Prima.

L

Lily of the Valley
(li-lee)

Scientific name: *Convallaria majalis*

Other common names: Jacob's ladder, ladder-to-heaven, lily constancy, lily convalle, male lily, May lily, muguet, our-lady's-tears   **Class 3 (Whole Plant)**

Origin: Lily of the valley is a perennial found in the United States, Canada, and Europe.

Uses

Reported Uses
Lily of the valley has been used as an anticonvulsant, as a cardiotonic, and to treat heart disease. Topically, it has been used to treat burns.

Product Availability and Dosages

Available Forms
Extract, powder

Plant Parts Used: Flowers, leaves, roots

Dosages and Routes
Adult
- PO standardized powder: 0.6 g (Blumenthal, 1998)

 Endangered Herb   Adverse effects: **BOLD** = life-threatening

Precautionary Information

Contraindications

Until more research is available, lily of the valley should not be used during pregnancy and lactation and should not be given to children. Persons with cardiac conditions such as heart failure and arrhythmias should not use this herb. The FDA considers lily of the valley an unsafe herb; therefore it is not recommended for use. Class 3 herb (whole plant).

Side Effects/Adverse Reactions

Cardiovascular: ARRHYTHMIAS, HEART FAILURE, DEATH
Central Nervous System: Headache, dizziness, psychosis, PARALYSIS, COMA
Ear, Eye, Nose, and Throat: Dilated pupils
Gastrointestinal: Nausea, vomiting, anorexia, abdominal pain, diarrhea, increased salivation
Integumentary: Hypersensitivity reactions, clammy skin, dermatitis
Miscellaneous: Hyperkalemia, urinary urgency

Interactions with Lily of the Valley

Drug

Beta-blockers, calcium channel blockers, cardiac glycosides: Lily of the valley used with beta-blockers or calcium channel blockers increases the risk of bradycardia; do not use concurrently. Lily of the valley may increase the effects of digoxin; do not use concurrently.

Food

None known

Herb

Buckthorn, cascara sagrada: Hypokalemia can result from the use of buckthorn or cascara sagrada with lily of the valley; avoid concurrent use. Hawthorn increases the action of lily of the valley when taken concurrently.

Lab Test

None known

 = Pregnancy   = Pediatric  = Alert = Popular Herb

Client Considerations

Assess

- Assess for hypersensitivity reactions and dermatitis. If these are present, discontinue use of lily of the valley and administer antihistamine or other appropriate therapy.
- Assess for use medications and herbs used (see Interactions).
- Determine whether the client is using this herb under the supervision of a qualified herbalist. Lily of the valley is potentially deadly.
- Assess for cardiac conditions such as heart failure and arrhythmias. Because research information is lacking, clients with these conditions should not use lily of the valley.

Administer

- Instruct the client to store lily of the valley in a cool, dry place, away from heat and moisture.

Teach Client/Family

- Until more research is available, caution the client not to use lily of the valley during pregnancy and lactation and not to give it to children.
- Warn the client that the FDA considers lily of the valley unsafe. Advise the client to use this herb only under the supervision of a qualified herbalist.

Pharmacology

Pharmacokinetics

Pharmacokinetics and pharmacodynamics are unknown.

Primary Chemical Components of Lily of the Valley and Their Possible Actions		
Chemical Class	**Individual Component**	**Possible Action**
Glycoside	Convallatoxol; Convallarinycoside; Convallotoxin; Convallamarin; Locundjosid; Convallosid	Cardiac glycoside
Saponin		
Volatile oil		
Asparagin		
Rutin		Antioxidant
Resin		

Endangered Herb   Adverse effects: BOLD = life-threatening

Actions

The cardiac glycoside action of lily of the valley is due to the chemical components convallatoxol, convallarinycoside, convallotoxin, convallamarin, locundjosid, and convallosid. These chemical components are less toxic than those of foxglove, which has been used as a source for digitalis (McGuigan, 1984). Several other actions have been proposed, but to date none is supported by research. Among these proposed actions are hypoglycemic, emetic, and diuretic effects.

References

Blumenthal M, editor: *The complete German Commission E monographs: therapeutic guide to herbal medicines,* Austin, Tex, American Botanical Council; Boston, Integrative Medicine Communication, 1998.
McGuigan MA: Plants—cardiac glycosides, *Clin Toxic Res* 6:1-2, 1984.

Lobelia
(loe-beel′yuh)

Scientific name: *Lobelia inflata*

Other common names: Asthma weed, bladderpod, cardinal flower, emetic herb, gagroot, great lobelia, Indian pink, Indian tobacco, pukeweed, rapuntium inflatum, vomitroot, vomitwort

Class 2b

Origin: Lobelia is found in wooded areas of the United States and Canada.

Uses

Reported Uses

Lobelia traditionally has been used to treat asthma, bronchitis, cough, and pneumonia, usually as an expectorant.

Investigational Uses

Researchers are studying lobelia for its cardiac effects and its antispasmodic effects in the gastrointestinal system. Its use as a smoking deterrent and treatment for psychostimulant abuse is also under investigation.

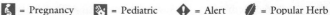

= Pregnancy   = Pediatric   = Alert   = Popular Herb

Product Availability and Dosages

Available Forms

Capsules, fluid extract, lozenges, tablets, tincture; available in combination with cayenne pepper *(Capsicum frutescens)* and lungwort *(Pulmonaria officinalis)*

Plant Parts Used: Dried leaves

Dosages and Routes

Adult

All dosages listed are PO.

Smoking Deterrent

- Tablets: the usual dosage is 2 mg taken with 4 oz water pc for 6 wk

Other

- Dried herb: 0.2-0.6 g tid
- Fluid extract: 8-10 drops tid (Pizzarno, 1999)
- Tincture: 15-30 drops tid

L

Precautionary Information

Contraindications

Until more research is available, lobelia should not be used during pregnancy and lactation, and it should not be given to children in large doses as an emetic. This herb should not be used by elderly persons or by persons with hepatic and renal disorders; pneumonia; cardiovascular disorders such as congestive heart failure, cardiac decompensation, sinus arrhythmias, valvular dysfunction, bundle branch block, or hypertension; nicotine sensitivity; or hypersensitivity to it. Toxicity can result from the use of lobelia. Class 2b herb.

Side Effects/Adverse Reactions

Cardiovascular: Palpitations, HYPOTENSION OR HYPERTENSION
Central Nervous System: Tremors, dizziness, headache, anxiety, insomnia, SEIZURES
Gastrointestinal: Nausea, vomiting, anorexia, pain in abdomen, heartburn
Integumentary: Hypersensitivity reactions
Respiratory: Cough, RESPIRATORY DEPRESSION OR STIMULATION
Toxicity: SEIZURES, NAUSEA, VOMITING, INCREASED SALIVATION, DIARRHEA, MENTAL CONFUSION, WEAKNESS, CHANGE IN VISION AND HEARING, RESPIRATORY DEPRESSION, ARRHYTHMIAS, TREMORS, HYPOTHERMIA, COMA, DEATH

 Endangered Herb   Adverse effects: BOLD = life-threatening

Interactions with Lobelia

Drug
Nicotine: Lobelia increases the effects of nicotine-containing products; do not use concurrently.

Food
None known

Herb
Mayapple: Lobelia may decrease the laxative effect of mayapple; do not use concurrently.

Lab Test
None known

Client Considerations

Assess

- Assess for hypersensitivity reactions. If present, discontinue use of lobelia and administer antihistamine or other appropriate therapy.
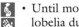 - Assess for symptoms of toxicity: seizures, nausea, vomiting, increased salivation, diarrhea, mental confusion, weakness, change in vision and hearing, respiratory depression, arrhythmias, tremors, hypothermia and coma.
- Assess for the use of nicotine-containing products and mayapple (see Interactions).

Administer

- Instruct the client to store lobelia products in a cool, dry place, away from heat and moisture.
- Instruct the client to use lobelia for no more than 6 weeks for smoking cessation.
- Administer atropine 2 mg SC for acute toxicity.

Teach Client/Family

- Until more research is available, caution the client not to use lobelia during pregnancy and lactation and not to give it to children in large doses as an emetic.
- Because nicotine toxicity can occur, warn the client to stop smoking before using lobelia as a smoking deterrent.

 = Pregnancy    = Pediatric   = Alert   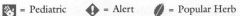 = Popular Herb

Pharmacology

Pharmacokinetics

Chemical components of lobelia may cross the placenta and enter the breast milk. Components are metabolized by the liver and lung and excreted via the kidneys. Lobelia is well absorbed by the mouth and lungs.

Primary Chemical Components of Lobelia and Their Possible Actions		
Chemical Class	**Individual Component**	**Possible Action**
Alkaloid	Lobeline	Nicotine-like, respiratory stimulant
	Lobelanine; Lobelanidine	Emetic, respiratory stimulant

Actions

Lobelia is often used in combination with *Capsicum frutescens* (capsicum peppers) and *Symphlocarpus factida* (skunk cabbage). Studies have focused on its use as a smoking deterrent and its emetic, cardiac, and expectorant properties.

Smoking Deterrent

Three of the chemical components of lobelia, lobeline, lobelanine, and lobelanidine, have properties similar to those of nicotine but generally are considered less potent (Mansuri, 1973). However, toxicity is higher with lobelia than with other traditional smoking deterrents currently on the market, such as nicotine transdermal systems (e.g., Nicoderm and Habitrol). The chemical components of lobelia inhibit smoking by first stimulating nicotine receptors and then inhibiting them (Rapp, 1997).

Emetic Action

The emetic action of lobelia results from stimulation of the chemoreceptor trigger zone. This action is similar to that of other emetics that are available. Lobelia also activates the vagal and afferent neural pathways responsible for vomiting (Laffan, 1957).

Cardiovascular Action

Lobelia's cardiac action results from both positive inotropic and chronotropic effects. Blood pressure and the neurotransmitters epinephrine and norepinephrine are increased in a manner similar to that seen with nicotine usage.

Expectorant Action

Lobelia is considered to be a very effective expectorant and has been used to treat respiratory conditions for many years. In laboratory animals it causes cholinergic effects, including bronchoconstriction and respiratory stimulation (Mitchell, 1983). In humans, bronchodilation occurs.

Other Actions

Lobelia inflata was found to functionally antagonize the neurochemical and behavioral effects of the psychostimulants amphetamine and methamphetamine (Dwoskin, 2002).

References

Dwoskin LP et al: A novel mechanism of action and potential use for lobeline as a treatment for psychostimulant abuse, *Biochem Pharmacol* 63(2):89-98, 2002.

Laffan R et al: Emetic action of nicotine and lobeline, *J Pharmacol Exp Ther* 121:468-476, 1957.

Mansuri S et al: Some pharmacological characteristics of ganglionic activity of lobeline, *Arzneimittelforschung* 23:1271-1275, 1973.

Mitchell W: Naturopathic applications of the botanical remedies, Seattle, Wash, 1983, Mitchell.

Pizzarno J, Murray M: *Textbook of natural medicine,* London, 1999, Churchill Livingstone.

Rapp GW et al: Pharmacology of lobeline, a nicotine receptor ligand, *J Pharmacol Exp Ther* 282:410-419, 1997.

Lovage
(luh'vij)

Scientific names: *Levisticum officinale, Levisticum radix*

Other common names: Maggi plant, sea parsley, smellage   Class 2b (Root)

Origin: Lovage is a perennial found in Europe, the United States, and Canada.

Uses

Reported Uses

Lovage has been used to treat renal disorders as a diuretic, an antilithic, and a renal antiinflammatory. It may also be used as a sedative and to treat gastric conditions and respiratory congestion.

Product Availability and Dosages

Available Forms

Essential oil, tea

Plant Parts Used: Roots, seeds

Dosages and Routes

Adult

- PO tea: place 1.5-3 g finely cut root in 8 oz boiling water, let stand 15 min, strain; up to 8 g herb/day may be used

Precautionary Information

Contraindications

Until more research is available, lovage should not be used during pregnancy and lactation and should not be given to children. This herb should not be used by persons with renal disease or irritation of the kidneys. Lovage should not be used by persons who are hypersensitive to it. Class 2b herb (root).

Side Effects/Adverse Reactions

Gastrointestinal: Nausea, anorexia
Integumentary: Hypersensitivity reactions, photodermatitis

Interactions with Lovage

Drug

Anticoagulants (heparin, warfarin): Lovage may increase the effects of anticoagulants such as heparin, warfarin, and salicylates; avoid concurrent use.

Food	Herb	Lab Test
None known	None known	None known

Client Considerations

Assess

- Assess for hypersensitivity reactions, photodermatitis. If these are present, discontinue use of lovage and administer antihistamine or other appropriate therapy.
- Assess for edema in the feet. If the client is using lovage to treat this condition, advise to use other proven treatments.
- Monitor BUN, creatinine, potassium, sodium, and chloride levels during lovage therapy. If results are elevated, use of lovage should be discontinued.
- Assess the client's use of anticoagulants, which should not be used concurrently with lovage (see Interactions).

Administer

- Instruct the client to store lovage products in a cool, dry place, away from heat and moisture.

Teach Client/Family

- Until more research is available, advise the client not to use lovage during pregnancy and lactation and not to give it to children.

Pharmacology

Pharmacokinetics

Pharmacokinetics and pharmacodynamics are unknown.

Primary Chemical Components of Lovage and Their Possible Actions*		
Chemical Class	**Individual Component**	**Possible Action**
Volatile oil	Ligusticumlactone	Antispasmodic
	Butylphthalide; Citronellal	
Lactone	Phthalide	
Coumarin		
Furocoumarin	Bergaptene; Apterin	
Hydroxycoumarin	Umbelliferone	
Polyyne	Falcarindiol	
Terpenoid		
Volatile acid		

*Investigation of the chemical components of this herb is not complete.

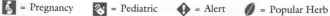

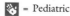

= Pregnancy   = Pediatric   ◆ = Alert   ∥ = Popular Herb

Actions
No well-controlled studies have been carried out on lovage, and at present, none of its uses or actions can be confirmed. For this reason, use of lovage cannot be recommended.

Lungwort
(luhng wawrt)

Scientific name: *Pulmonaria officinalis*

Other common names: Dage of Jerusalem, Jerusalem cowslip, Jerusalem sage, lung moss, lungs of oak, spotted comfrey

Class 1

Origin: Lungwort is found in many parts of Europe.

Uses
Reported Uses
Traditionally, lungwort has been used to treat respiratory conditions including bronchitis, congestion, and cough. It also has been used to treat diarrhea and menstrual irregularities and may be used topically as a compress to promote wound healing.

Investigational Uses
Lungwort has been investigated for use as an anticoagulant.

Product Availability and Dosages
Available Forms
Extract, tablets, tincture

Plant Parts Used: Leaves

Dosages and Routes
Adult
- PO infusion: place 1-2 tsp dried leaves in 8 oz boiling water, let stand 10 min, take tid; alternatively, add 1 g finely cut herb to 8 oz cold water, boil rapidly 5-10 min, strain
- PO tincture: 1-4 ml tid

Precautionary Information
Contraindications

Until more research is available, lungwort should not be used during pregnancy and lactation and should not be given to children. This herb should not be used by persons with hypersensitivity to it. Class 1 herb.

Side Effects/Adverse Reactions

Gastrointestinal: Nausea, anorexia, irritation
Integumentary: Hypersensitivity reactions, contact dermatitis
Systemic: Increased bleeding time

Interactions with Lungwort

Drug
Anticoagulants: Lungwort may increase the effects of anticoagulants such as heparin, warfarin, and salicylates; avoid concurrent use.

Food	Herb	Lab Test
None known	None known	None known

Client Considerations
Assess

- Assess for hypersensitivity reactions, contact dermatitis. If these are present, discontinue use of lungwort and administer antihistamine or other appropriate therapy.
- Assess for bleeding. Monitor anticoagulant studies (see Interactions).
- Assess the client's respiratory status, including rate, character, cough, and congestion.

Administer

- Instruct the client to store lungwort products in a cool, dry place, away from heat and moisture.

Teach Client/Family

- Until more research is available, caution the client not to use lungwort during pregnancy and lactation and not to give it to children.

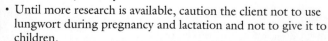 = Pregnancy = Pediatric = Alert = Popular Herb

- Caution the client not to confuse *Pulmonaria officinalis* with *Pulmonaria mollis*.

Pharmacology

Pharmacokinetics

Pharmacokinetics and pharmacodynamics are unknown.

Primary Chemical Components of Lungwort and Their Possible Actions

Chemical Class	Individual Component	Possible Action
Allantoin		Emollient
Flavonoid	Quercetin; Kaempferol	Antiinflammatory
Tannin		Wound healing
Anticoagulant	Glycopeptide	Anticoagulant
Vitamin	C	
Saponin		
Caffeic acid (derivative)	Chlorogenic acid; Rosmarinic acid	
Mucilage	Polygalacturonane; Arabinogalactans; Rhamnogalacturonane	

Actions

Research on any of the uses or actions of lungwort is lacking. To date, no controlled studies have been done on either laboratory animals or humans. The only studies available deal with the chemical composition of lungwort; therefore this herb should be used under the supervision of a qualified herbalist only. The tannins are probably responsible for the wound healing properties; the glycopeptides, for the anticoagulant effect; and allantoin, for the emollient effect.

References

Duke J: *CRC handbook of medicinal herbs,* Boca Raton, Fla, 1985, CRC Press.

L

Lycopene
(like'uh-peen)

Scientific name: ψ-carotene

Origin: Lycopene is a carotenoid that occurs naturally in tomatoes.

Uses
Reported Uses

Lycopene is used as an antioxidant and may protect against cancer of the prostate, pancreas, and stomach.

Product Availability and Dosages
Available Forms

Capsules, tablets

Dosages and Routes

No dosage consensus exists.

Precautionary Information
Contraindications

Until more research is available, lycopene supplements should not be used during pregnancy and lactation and should not be given to children. Lycopene supplements should not be used by persons with hypersensitivity to this product.

Side Effects/Adverse Reactions
Gastrointestinal: Nausea, anorexia

Interactions with Lycopene			
Drug	Food	Herb	Lab Test
None known	None known	None known	None known

= Pregnancy = Pediatric ◆ = Alert ⫽ = Popular Herb

Client Considerations

Assess
- Assess for adequate lycopene in the diet (tomatoes, processed tomato products).

Administer
- Instruct the client to store lycopene products in a cool, dry place, away from heat and moisture.

Teach Client/Family

- Until more research is available, caution the client not to use lycopene supplements during pregnancy and lactation and not to give them to children.

Pharmacology

Pharmacokinetics
Pharmacokinetics and pharmacodynamics are unknown.

Actions

Lycopene naturally occurs in tomatoes, and processing tomatoes increases the lycopene content. Most of the available research has focused on the antioxidant qualities of lycopene. One study of 19 human subjects evaluated lipid peroxidation and low-density lipoprotein (LDL) oxidation. Lycopene supplementation resulted in a reduction of lipids and LDLs and therefore may decrease the risk of coronary heart disease (Agarwal, 1998). Another study showed that lycopene exerts a protective effect against myocardial infarction (Kohlmeier, 1997) and decreased inflammation in colitis (Reifen, 2001).

References
Agarwal S et al: Tomato lycopene and low density lipoprotein oxidation, *Lipids* 33(10):981-984, 1998.

Kohlmeier L et al: Lycopene and myocardial infarction risk in EURAMIC study, *Am J Epidemiol* 146(8):618-626, 1997.

Reifen R et al: Lycopene supplementation attenuates the inflammatory status of colitis in a rat model, *Int J Vitam Nutr Res* 71(6):347-351, 2001.

Lysine
(lise′een)

Scientific name: 2,6-diaminohexanoic acid

Origin: Lysine is an amino acid manufactured by the body. It also can be found in dairy products, brewer's yeast, meats, and wheat germ.

Uses

Reported Uses

Lysine has been used to treat cold sores and other herpes infections, including genital herpes. It has also been used with some success to treat Bell's palsy and rheumatoid arthritis and to detoxify opiates.

Product Availability and Dosages

Available Forms

Capsules, tablets

Dosages and Routes

Adult

PO dosages as high as 4000 mg/day have been reported.

Precautionary Information

Contraindications

Until more research is available, lysine supplements should not be used during pregnancy and lactation and should not be given to children. Lysine supplements should not be used by persons with hypersensitivity to this product.

Side Effects/Adverse Reactions

Gastrointestinal: Nausea, anorexia

Interactions with Lysine

Drug

Aminoglycosides: Use of large amounts of lysine causes increased aminoglycoside toxicity; avoid concurrent use.

Food	Herb	Lab Test
None known	None known	None known

 = Pregnancy  = Pediatric = Alert 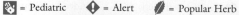 = Popular Herb

Client Considerations

Assess
- Assess for aminoglycoside use. Advise the client to avoid concurrent use with lysine (see Interactions).

Administer
- Instruct the client to store lysine products in a cool, dry place, away from heat and moisture.

Teach Client/Family

- Until more research is available, caution the client not to use lysine supplements during pregnancy and lactation and not to give them to children.

Pharmacology

Pharmacokinetics
Lysine is an amino acid that is naturally present in the body. Its pharmacokinetics and pharmacodynamics are unknown.

Actions
Several reports have shown that lysine improves herpes infections. One study evaluated 1543 participants by questionnaire. More than 80% of those who responded stated that lysine supplements lessened the severity of genital herpes lesions, canker sores, and cold sores (Wash, 1983). Another study evaluating 45 patients taking lysine daily in various doses found a shortened duration of herpes infections and decreased recurrence. The result occurs when the lysine-to-arginine ratio increases (Griffith, 1978). Other studies have refuted these claims, with research showing no reduction in herpes infections (Milman, 1978; Simon, 1985).

References
Griffith R et al: *Dermatologica* 156(5):257-267, 1978.
Milman N et al: *Lancet* 28(2):942, 1978.
Simon C et al: *Arch Dermatol* 121:167, 1985.
Wash D: et al *J Antimicrob Chemother* 12:489-496, 1983.

Madder
(ma'duhr)

Scientific name: *Rubia tinctorum*

Other common names: Dyer's-madder, garance, krapp, madder root, robbia

Origin: Madder is found in Asia, Europe, the Mediterranean, the United States, and Canada.

Uses

Reported Uses
Madder has been used to decrease renal stones. It is also used to treat paralysis, jaundice, and menstrual disorders.

Product Availability and Dosages

Available Forms
Capsules, dried root, fluid extract

Plant Parts Used: Roots

Dosages and Routes
Adult
- PO capsules: 1 dried root cap tid
- PO fluid extract: 20 drops tid

Precautionary Information

Contraindications
Because it may be mutagenic, madder should not be used during pregnancy. Until more research is available, this herb should not be used during lactation and should not be given to children. Madder should not be used by persons with hypersensitivity to it.

Side Effects/Adverse Reactions
Gastrointestinal: Nausea, vomiting, anorexia
Integumentary: Hypersensitivity reactions
Miscellaneous: Red color of secretions, possible liver tumors

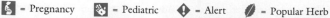
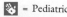

Interactions with Madder			
Drug	Food	Herb	Lab Test
None known	None known	None known	None known

Client Considerations

Assess

- Assess for hypersensitivity reactions. If present, discontinue use of madder and administer antihistamine or other appropriate therapy.

Administer

- Instruct the client to store madder products in a cool, dry place, away from heat and moisture.

Teach Client/Family

- Because it may be mutagenic, caution the client not to use madder during pregnancy. Until more research is available, caution the client not to use this herb during lactation and not to give it to children.
- Inform the client that secretions may turn red while using this herb and that contact lenses may stain.

Pharmacology

Pharmacokinetics

Pharmacokinetics and pharmacodynamics are unknown.

Primary Chemical Components of Madder and Their Possible Actions

Chemical Class	Individual Component	Possible Action
Anthraquinone	Alizarin; Xanthopurparin; Lucidin Hydroxy-anthraquinone; Methylazoxymethyl acetate	Chelating agent; mutagenic; recombinagenic
	Rubiadin; Purpurin; Pseudopurpurin	
Glycoside	Alizarinprimeveroside; Lucidinprimeveroside	
Iridoid	Asperuloside	
Resin		
Electrolyte	Calcium	

🍃 Endangered Herb   Adverse effects: BOLD = life-threatening

Actions

Because research is lacking on any uses or actions of madder, its use cannot be recommended. One study did show the binding of DNA in specific areas of the body, including hepatic, renal, and gastrointestinal systems (Poginsky, 1991). The anthraquinones alizarin and lucidin act as chelating agents with metal ions such as magnesium and calcium (Mills, 2000). The anthraquinones also act as mutagenics and recombinagenics (Tanaka, 2000).

References

Mills S, Bone K: *Principles and practice of phytotherapy,* London, 2000, Churchill Livingstone.

Poginsky B et al: Evaluation of DNA-binding activity of hydroxyanthraquinones occurring in *Rubia tinctorum* L., *Carcinogenesis* 12: 1265-1271, 1991.

Tanaka T et al: Colitis-related rat colon carcinogenesis induced by 1-hydroxy-anthraquinone and methylazoxy-methanol acetate, *Oncol Rep* 7(3):501-508, 2000.

Maitake
(mah-ee-tah'keh)

Scientific name: *Grifola frondosa*

Other common names: Dancing mushroom, king of mushrooms, monkey's bench, shelf fungi

Class 1 (Fruiting Body, Mycelium)

Origin: Maitake is a mushroom found in Japan.

Uses

Reported Uses

Maitake has been used to treat hypertension, diabetes mellitus, cancer, high cholesterol, and obesity.

Product Availability and Dosages

Available Forms

Capsules, extract

Plant Parts Used: Mushroom, whole fungus

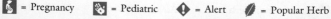

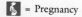 = Pregnancy    = Pediatric   = Alert   💮 = Popular Herb

Dosages and Routes
Adult
- PO: 250-500 mg qd

Precautionary Information
Contraindications

Until more information is available, maitake should not be used during pregnancy and lactation and should not be given to children. Maitake should not be used by persons with hypersensitivity to it. Class 1 herb (fruiting body, mycelium).

Side Effects/Adverse Reactions
None known

Interactions with Maitake

Drug

Immunosuppressants (azathioprine, basiliximab, daclizumab, muromonab, mycophenolate, tacrolimus): Maitake may decrease the effects of immunosuppressant; do not use immediately before, during, or after transplant surgery.

Food	Herb	Lab Test
None known	None known	None known

M

Client Considerations
Assess
- Determine the reason the client is using maitake.
- Assess client for medications taken; do not use with immunosuppressants.

Administer
- Instruct the client to store maitake products in a cool, dry place, away from heat and moisture.

Teach Client/Family

- Until more research is available, caution the client not to use maitake during pregnancy and lactation and not to give it to children.

Pharmacology

Pharmacokinetics

Pharmacokinetics and pharmacodynamics are unknown.

Primary Chemical Components of Maitake and Their Possible Actions		
Chemical Class	**Individual Component**	**Possible Action**
Polysaccharide	Beta-glucan	Antitumor

Actions

Maitake, along with other mushrooms, has been used for thousands of years in Asia for a variety of purposes. It is considered a "miracle herb" by many in the Orient.

Anticancer Action

Maitake is an immune modulator, helping to normalize the immune system. It exerts its anticancer action by activating interleukin-1 and increasing T-cells, both of which inhibit the proliferation of cancers (Adachi, 1987). Multiple studies have identified the cancer-fighting properties of maitake. Besides activating interleukin-1 and increasing T-cells, maitake also increases cytokine production and boosts the action of macrophages. Most studies have identified its anticancer properties as resulting from the polysaccharide beta-glucan.

Antiobesity Action

Although its mechanism of action is unclear, maitake is responsible for weight loss when taken over an extended period of time. In one study, 30 overweight clients were given maitake powder for 2 months. The clients lost between 7 and 26 pounds when taking various dosages ranging from 20 to 500 mg daily (Yokota, 1992). Another study using laboratory animals showed weight loss after 4½ months. The amount of weight lost was significant when compared with that of the control group (Ohtsuru, 1992).

Other Actions

One study has shown that the use of maitake reduces blood pressure and cholesterol and improves diabetes. After hyperten-

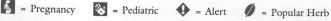

 = Pregnancy   = Pediatric   = Alert   = Popular Herb

sive laboratory animals were fed maitake powder, their blood pressure was evaluated and a small reduction was noted (Kabir, 1989). Other investigators found that maitake inhibits lipid metabolism. Rats given maitake showed a reduction in serum lipids, total cholesterol, and very-low-density lipoprotein (VLDL) (Fukushima, 2001; Kabir, 1987; Kubo, 1996, 1997). The antidiabetic action of maitake is believed to result from its ability to reduce insulin resistance and possibly increase sensitivity to insulin (Horio, 2001; Lieberman, 1997).

References

Adachi K et al: *Chem Pharm Bull* 35(1):262-270, 1987.

Fukushima M et al: Cholesterol-lowering effects of maitake fiber, shiitake fiber, and enokitake, *Exp Biol Med* 226(8):758-765, 2001.

Horio H et al: Maitake improve glucose tolerance of experimental diabetic rats, *J Nutr Sci Vitaminol* 47(1):57-63, 2001.

Kabir Y et al: *J Nutr Sci Vitaminol* 33(1):341-346, 1987.

Kabir Y et al: *J Nutr Sci Vitaminol* 35(1):91-94, 1989.

Kubo K et al: *Altern Ther Health Med* 2(5): 62-66, 1996.

Kubo K et al: *Biol Pharm Bull* 20(7):781-785, 1997.

Lieberman S et al: *Maitake: king of the mushrooms,* New Canaan, Conn, 1997, Keats, pp 7-48.

Ohtsuru M: *Anshin* pp 188-199, July 1992.

Yokota M: *Anshin* pp 202-204, July 1992.

M

Male Fern
(mayl fuhrn)

Scientific name: *Dryopteris filix-mas*

Other common names: Bear's paw, erkek egrelti, helecho macho, knotty brake, marginal shield-fern, shield fern, sweet brake, wurmfarn

Origin: Male fern is a perennial fern found in Asia, Europe, Africa, South America, the United States, and Canada.

Uses

Reported Uses

Male fern has been used primarily as an anthelmintic.

Product Availability and Dosages
Available Forms
Capsules, draught, extract

Plant Parts Used: Dried rhizomes, roots

Dosages and Routes
Use only PO under the supervision of a qualified herbalist.
Adult
- Extract: 3-6 ml

Child

NOTE: Allow 1 week between doses.
- Extract: age 2-12 years: 0.25-0.5 ml/year of age, not to exceed 4 ml in divided doses
- Extract: age <2 years: not to exceed 2 ml in divided doses

Precautionary Information
Contraindications
Because it is an abortifacient, male fern should not be used during pregnancy. Until more research is available, this herb should not be used during lactation and should not be given to infants. Persons with cardiovascular disease, hepatic disease, renal disease, and gastric or duodenal ulcers should not use this herb. Male fern should not be used by persons with hypersensitivity to it.

Side Effects/Adverse Reactions
Central Nervous System: Headache
Gastrointestinal: Nausea, vomiting, anorexia, diarrhea, severe abdominal pain and cramping, HEPATOTOXICITY
Miscellaneous: Albuminuria, shortness of breath, hyperbilirubinemia
Toxicity: SEIZURES, HEART FAILURE, RESPIRATORY FAILURE, COMA, DEATH

Interactions with Male Fern

Drug	Food	Herb	Lab Test
None known	None known	None known	None known

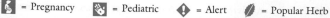

 = Pregnancy   = Pediatric   ◆ = Alert   ∥ = Popular Herb

Client Considerations
Assess
- Assess for hypersensitivity reactions. If these are present, discontinue use of male fern and administer antihistamine or other appropriate therapy.
- Assess for cardiovascular, renal, and liver disease. Clients with these conditions should not use male fern.
- Monitor liver function studies (ALT, AST, bilirubin). Watch for hepatotoxicity.
- Watch for signs of toxicity: seizures, heart failure, respiratory failure, and coma. Death can occur.

Administer
- Instruct the client to use male fern only PO and only under the supervision of a qualified herbalist because it is considered a high-risk herb.
- Instruct the client as follows: The night before treatment, eat only a light meal or no meal, followed by a laxative. The next morning, take male fern with another laxative before breakfast.

Teach Client/Family
- Because it is an abortifacient, caution the client not to use male fern during pregnancy. Until more research is available, caution the client not to use this herb during lactation and not to give it to infants.

Pharmacology
Pharmacokinetics
Pharmacokinetics and pharmacodynamics are unknown.

Primary Chemical Components of Male Fern and Their Possible Actions		
Chemical Class	**Individual Component**	**Possible Action**
Phloroglucinol Filicic acid Flavaspidic acid Volatile oil Tannin		Wound healing; astringent
Albaspidin Desaspidin		

Endangered Herb   Adverse effects: BOLD = life-threatening

Actions

The anthelmintic activity of male fern against tapeworms is well documented (Palva, 1963). This herb is thought to produce fewer side effects than do products containing quinacrine. Male fern should be considered if traditional treatments do not result in complete expulsion of the worms. However, consideration must also be given to the toxicity of this herb, including hepatotoxicity, even though it produces fewer side effects than products with quinacrine. Clients with cardiac, renal, or liver disease should not use male fern.

References

Palva IP et al: The effectiveness of certain drugs in the expulsion of fish tapeworms, *Ann Med Intern Fenn* 52:89-92, 1963.

Mallow
(ma'loe)

Scientific name: *Malva sylvestris*

Other common names: Blue mallow, cheeseflower, cheeseweed, field mallow, fleurs de mauve, high mallow, malve, zigbli

Origin: Mallow is found in subtropical and temperate climates.

Uses

Reported Uses

Mallow has been used to treat respiratory conditions such as cough, tonsillitis, sore throat, bronchitis, and irritation of the respiratory tract. It has also been used to relieve the pain of teething, scratches, and scrapes, and the leaves have been used to treat constipation.

Product Availability and Dosages

Available Forms

Dried herb, fluid extract

Plant Parts Used: Dried flowers, dried leaves

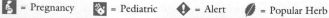

 = Pregnancy    = Pediatric   = Alert   ✔ = Popular Herb

Dosages and Routes
Adult
- PO infusion: mix 5 g dried herb with boiling water, let stand, strain, drink qd

Precautionary Information
Contraindications
Until more research is available, mallow should not be used during pregnancy and lactation and should not be given to children. Mallow should not be used by persons with hypersensitivity to it.

Side Effects/Adverse Reactions
Integumentary: Hypersensitivity reactions

Interactions with Mallow

Drug	Food	Herb	Lab Test
None known	None known	None known	None known

M

Client Considerations
Assess
- Assess for hypersensitivity reactions (rare). If these occur, discontinue use of mallow and administer antihistamine or other appropriate therapy.

Administer
- Instruct the client to store mallow products away from heat, insects, and moisture.

Teach Client/Family
- Until more research is available, caution the client not to use mallow during pregnancy and lactation and not to give it to children.
- Caution the client not to confuse mallow with marshmallow *(Althaea officinalis)* because they are different herbs.
- Because little research is available on mallow, caution the client that this herb should be used only under the supervision of a qualified herbalist.

 Endangered Herb   Adverse effects: BOLD = life-threatening

Pharmacology

Pharmacokinetics

Pharmacokinetics and pharmacodynamics are unknown.

Primary Chemical Components of Mallow and Their Possible Actions		
Chemical Class	**Individual Component**	**Possible Action**
Glycoside		
Tannin		Wound healing; astringent
Mucilage	Galacturonorhamane; Arabinogalactane	
Leukocyanin		
Flavonoid	Hypolaetin; Gossypetin	

Actions

Research is lacking on any uses or actions of mallow. To date, no controlled studies for mallow have been carried out in either laboratory animals or humans. The only studies available deal with its chemical composition; therefore mallow should be used only under the supervision of a qualified herbalist.

Marigold
(mar'uh-goeld)

Scientific name: *Calendula officinalis*

Other common names: Calendula, garden marigold, pot marigold, poet's marigold

Origin: Marigold is an annual found in parts of Europe, the United States, and Canada.

Uses

Reported Uses

Marigold is used topically to treat skin disorders such as venous stasis ulcers, decubitus ulcers, varicose veins, bruises, boils, and

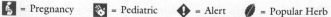

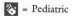 = Pregnancy   = Pediatric   ◆ = Alert   ✔ = Popular Herb

rashes. It also is used topically to help heal chapped, cracked skin and for aromatherapy. Marigold is used internally to treat gastric disorders and promote digestion. It is used both internally and topically to treat inflammation of the oral and pharyngeal mucosa.

Investigational Uses
Studies are underway to determine the antitumor and antiinfective properties of marigold.

Product Availability and Dosages
Available Forms
Mouthwash, ointment, tea, tincture

Plant Parts Used: Flowers

Dosages and Routes
Adult
- PO tea: 1-4 ml tid
- PO tincture: 1-4 ml tid
- Topical ointment: may be applied prn to the affected area

Precautionary Information
Contraindications
Until more research is available, marigold should not be used during pregnancy and lactation and should not be given to children. Persons with hypersensitivity to marigold or other plants of the Compositae family should not use it.

Side Effects/Adverse Reactions
Gastrointestinal: Nausea, vomiting, anorexia
Integumentary: Hypersensitivity reactions

Interactions with Marigold

Drug	Food	Herb	Lab Test
None known	None known	None known	None known

Client Considerations

Assess

- Assess for hypersensitivity reactions. If these are present, discontinue use of marigold and administer antihistamine or other appropriate therapy.
- Determine whether the client is allergic to other members of the Compositae family. If so, marigold should not be used.

Administer

- Instruct the client to store marigold products in a cool, dry place, away from heat and moisture.

Teach Client/Family

- Until more research is available, caution the client not to use marigold during pregnancy and lactation and not to give it to children.
- Inform the client that allergies to this plant can occur and that use of the herb should be discontinued if necessary.

Pharmacology

Pharmacokinetics

Pharmacokinetics and pharmacodynamics are unknown.

Primary Chemical Components of Marigold and Their Possible Actions		
Chemical Class	**Individual Component**	**Possible Action**
Triterpenoid Glycoside	Faradiol	Antiinflammatory
Lutein		Antitumor
Sterol		
Fatty acid		
Carotenoid pigment		
Polysaccharide		
Volatile oil		
Calendulen		
Sesquiterpene Oligoglycosides	Officinosides C, D	
Calendasaponins	A, B, C, D	
Ionone glucosides	Officinosides A, B	

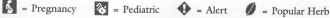

Actions
Antitumor Action
Research is available documenting the use of lutein, a chemical component of marigold, as an antitumor agent. Mice fed a diet of lutein from marigold extract were inoculated after 2 weeks with tumor cells. Cell proliferation was measured for 70 days. Low levels of lutein were found to lower the incidence of mammary tumors, tumor growth, and lipid peroxidation, while higher levels were found to be less effective. Investigators concluded that low levels of dietary lutein can decrease mammary tumor development (Park, 1998). An earlier study showed similar results (Chew, 1996).

Antiinfective Action
One study has evaluated the use of marigold in treating the tick-borne encephalitis virus (Fokina, 1991). In mice inoculated with the virus, marigold was only partly effective in killing the virus. Other herbal preparations exhibited much more antiviral activity. Another study examining the effectiveness of various herbs against dermal staphylococcus found that marigold was one of the most active extracts. This information may be useful for the development products to treat dermal diseases (Molochko, 1990).

References
Chew BP et al: Effects of lutein from marigold extract on immunity and growth of mammary tumors in mice, *Anticancer Res* 16(6B):3689-3694, 1996.

Fokina GI et al: Experimental phytotherapy of tick-borne encephalitis, *Vopr Virusol* 36(1):18-21, 1991.

Molochko VA et al: The antistaphylococcal properties of plant extracts in relation to their prospective use as therapeutic and prophylactic formulations for the skin, *Vestn Dermatol Venerol* (8):54-56, 1990.

Park JS et al: Dietary lutein from marigold extract inhibits mammary tumor development in BALB/c, *J Nutr* 128(10):1650-1656, 1998.

Marjoram
(mahr′juh-ruhm)

Scientific name: *Origanum majorana* L.

Other common names: Garden marjoram, knotted marjoram, oleum majoranae (oil), sweet marjoram

Class 1 (Leaf)

Origin: Marjoram is found throughout the world.

Uses

Reported Uses

Marjoram has been used as a diuretic and to treat bruises, headache, cough, paroxysmal cough, rhinitis, amenorrhea, dysmenorrhea, arthritis, muscle pain and stiffness, insomnia, motion sickness, and snakebite. It is also used as a food flavoring.

Investigational Uses

Marjoram may be used in Alzheimer's disease.

Product Availability and Dosages

Available Forms

Tea, tincture

Plant Parts Used: Dried leaves, flowering tops

Dosages and Routes

Adult

- PO tea: add 1-2 tsp dried leaves and flowering tops to 8 oz boiling water, let stand 10 min, take bid-tid
- PO tincture: 1 tsp qd

Precautionary Information

Contraindications

Until more research is available, marjoram should not be used therapeutically during pregnancy and lactation, and it should not be given therapeutically to children. It should not be used therapeutically by persons with hypersensitivity to this herb or other members of the Labiatae family, including mint, basil, thyme, oregano, hyssop, and sage. Class 1 herb (leaf).

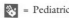 = Pregnancy   = Pediatric   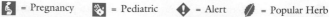 = Alert   = Popular Herb

> **Precautionary Information—cont'd**
> **Side Effects/Adverse Reactions**
> *Gastrointestinal:* Nausea, vomiting, anorexia, diarrhea
> *Integumentary:* Serious hypersensitivity reactions

Interactions with Marjoram			
Drug	Food	Herb	Lab Test
None known	None known	None known	None known

Client Considerations
Assess
 • Assess for hypersensitivity reactions (facial edema, inability to breathe, itching, dysphagia, dysphonia). If these symptoms are present, discontinue use of marjoram and administer antihistamine or other appropriate therapy.

Administer
- Instruct the client not to use marjoram long-term because of its arbutin content.
- Instruct the client not to use the essential oil internally.
- Instruct the client to store marjoram products in a cool, dry place, away from heat and moisture.

Teach Client/Family
- Until more research is available, caution the client not to use marjoram therapeutically during pregnancy and lactation and not to give it to children therapeutically. It should be used as a food flavoring only.
- Inform the client that marjoram is not the same herb as oregano.
- Advise the client that cross-sensitivity may occur with other herbs of the Labiatae family, such as oregano, thyme, hyssop, basil, mint, sage, and lavender (Benito, 1996).

Pharmacology
Pharmacokinetics
Pharmacokinetics and pharmacodynamics are unknown.

Primary Chemical Components of Marjoram and Their Possible Actions		
Chemical Class	**Individual Component**	**Possible Action**
Lactone	Thymol Carvacrol	Antiinfective
Flavonoid	Diosmetin; Luteolin; Apigenin	
Tannin		Astringent; wound healing
Hydroquinone		Cytotoxic
Glycoside	Arbutin; Methylarbutin; Vitexin; Orientin; Thymonin	
Triaconatane		
Sitosterol		
Acid	Oleanolic acid Ursolic acid	Potent acetylcholinesterase inhibitor
	Rosmarinic acid; Caffeic acid; Chlorogenic acid	

Actions

Only a few studies on marjoram have been published. Among them are investigations into the use of marjoram for the treatment of eczema and as an antiinfective.

Eczema Treatment

One investigator evaluated the use of marjoram in the treatment of childhood atopic eczema (Anderson, 2000). In this study, eight children received massage with essential oils (aromatherapy) as part of their medical regimen to control eczema. One of the essential oils preferred by the mothers doing the massage was marjoram. A significant improvement occurred in the eczema in this group.

Other Actions

The ursolic acid in *Origanum majorana* demonstrated a potent acetylcholinesterase inhibitor and therefore should be useful in Alzheimer's disease (Chung, 2001).

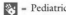 = Pregnancy = Pediatric 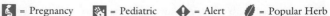 = Alert = Popular Herb

References

Anderson C et al: Evaluation of massage with essential oils on childhood atopic eczema, *Phytother Res* 14(6):452-456, 2000.

Benito M et al: Labiatae allergy: systemic reactions due to ingestion of oregano and thyme, *Ann Allergy Asthma Immunol* 76(5):416-418, 1996.

Chung YK et al: Inhibitory effect of ursolic acid purified from *Origanum majorana* L. on the acetylcholinesterase, *Mol Cell* 11(2):137-143, 2001.

Marshmallow
(mahrsh'meh-low)

Scientific name: *Althaea officinalis*

Other common names: Althaea root, althea, mortification root, sweetweed, wymote

Class 1 (Root, Leaf, Flower)

M

Origin: Marshmallow is a perennial found in Europe and the United States.

Uses

Reported Uses

Marshmallow is used traditionally to suppress cough, to relieve sore throat, and to relieve gastric disorders such as irritable bowel syndrome (IBS), gastritis, and constipation. Topically, it is used to treat minor skin disorders.

Product Availability and Dosages

Available Forms

Capsules, dried flowers, dried leaves, dried whole root, syrup

Plant Parts Used: Dried flowers, dried leaves, dried root

Dosages and Routes

Adult

All dosages listed are PO.

Throat Irritation
• Syrup: 10 ml as a single dose (Blumenthal, 1998)

Other
• Dried leaves: 5 g qd (Blumenthal, 1998)
• Dried root: 6 g crude herb qd (Blumenthal, 1998)
• Powdered, crushed plant: whole or part, 2 g/day

🍀 Endangered Herb   Adverse effects: BOLD = life-threatening

Precautionary Information
Contraindications
Until more research is available, marshmallow should not be used during pregnancy and lactation and should not be given to children. Persons who are hypersensitive to this herb should not use it. Class 1 herb (root, leaf, flower)

Side Effects/Adverse Reactions
Gastrointestinal: Nausea, vomiting, anorexia
Integumentary: Hypersensitivity reactions

Interactions with Marshmallow

Drug
Iron salts: Marshmallow may reduce the absorption of iron salts; separate by 2 hr.
Oral medications: Marshmallow may reduce the absorption of oral medications; do not use concurrently.

Food	Herb	Lab Test
None known	None known	None known

Client Considerations
Assess
- Assess for hypersensitivity reactions. If these are present, discontinue use of marshmallow and administer antihistamine or other appropriate therapy.
- Assess for oral medication use (see Interactions).

Administer
- Instruct the client to store marshmallow products in a cool, dry place, away from heat and moisture.

Teach Client/Family
- Until more research is available, caution the client not to use marshmallow during pregnancy and lactation and not to give it to children.

Pharmacology
Pharmacokinetics
Pharmacokinetics and pharmacodynamics are unknown.

 = Pregnancy   = Pediatric    = Alert   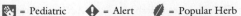 = Popular Herb

Primary Chemical Components of Marshmallow and Their Possible Actions		
Chemical Class	**Individual Component**	**Possible Action**
Polysaccharide	Arabinogalactans; Arabans; Glucans; Galacturonic rhamnans	
Flavonoid	Quercetin; Kaempferol Scopoletin	Antiinflammatory
Pectin		
Starch		
Calcium oxalate		
Sterol		
Fat		
Coumarin		
Phenolic acid	Caffeic acid; Syringic acid; Chlorogenic acid; Ferulic acid	

M

Actions

Very little primary research is available for marshmallow. Existing studies focus primarily on its antitussive and antiinfective properties.

Antitussive Action

One study evaluated the antitussive action of marshmallow and other nonnarcotic antitussives on cats (Nosal'ova, 1992). A nylon fiber was used to mechanically stimulate the mucous area of the respiratory system, and cough was evaluated on the basis of lateral tracheal pressure. The antitussive effect of marshmallow was found to be stronger than that of some of the nonnarcotic antitussives evaluated, which are not available in the United States.

Antiinfective Action

In a study focusing on the antiinfective properties of marshmallow and several other herbs against *Vibrio cholerae*, marshmallow was found to be less effective than some of the other plants evaluated (Guevara, 1994).

References

Blumenthal M, editor: *The complete German Commission E monographs: therapeutic guide to herbal medicines,* Austin, Tex, American Botanical Council; Boston, Integrative Medicine Communication, 1998.

Guevara JM et al: The in vitro action of plants on *Vibrio cholerae, Rev Gastroenterol Peru* 14(1):**27-31**, 1994.

Nosal'ova G et al: Antitussive action of extracts and polysaccharides of marshmallow *(Althea officinalis* L., var. *robusta), Pharmazie* 47(3): 224-226, 1992.

Mayapple
(may′a-puhl)

Scientific name: *Podophyllum peltatum*

Other common names: American mandrake, devil's-apple, duck's foot, ground lemon, hog apple, Indian apple, mandrake, raccoon berry, umbrella plant, wild lemon, wild mandrake

Class 2b/3 (Root)

Origin: Mayapple is a perennial found in the United States and Canada.

Uses
Reported Uses
Mayapple has been used in China to treat snakebites, general weakness, poisoning, lymphadenopathy, condyloma acuminata, and tumors. In Western medicine, mayapple has been used as a laxative. Topically, the concentrated tincture and resin are useful for removing warts and condyloma.

Product Availability and Dosages
Available Forms
Concentrated tincture, dried rhizome, fluid extract (by prescription), resin, tincture

Plant Parts Used: Rhizome

Dosages and Routes
Adult
Wart Removal
- Topical concentrated tincture: apply to wart, leave on for up to 6 hr, wash off; may be used q wk for up to 4 wk

 = Pregnancy    = Pediatric   = Alert   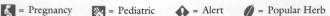 = Popular Herb

- Topical resin: apply to wart bid for 3 days, repeat q wk for 5 wk; do not wash off

Other

- PO fluid extract 1.5-3 g qd (Blumenthal, 1998)
- PO powdered root: 10-30 grains
- PO tincture: 2-10 drops qd-bid; 2.5-7.5 g qd (Blumenthal, 1998)

Precautionary Information

Contraindications

Until more research is available, mayapple should not be used during pregnancy and lactation and should not be given to children. Mayapple should not be used by elderly or debilitated persons, or by those who are hypersensitive to it. Persons with gallbladder disease, intestinal obstruction, or diabetes should avoid its use. All parts of the mayapple plant except the ripe fruit are toxic both orally and topically. Mayapple should not be used topically on large areas or on irritated warts, moles, or birthmarks. Class 2b/3 herb (root).

Side Effects/Adverse Reactions

Central Nervous System: Confusion, dizziness, headache, psychosis, hallucinations, SEIZURES, STUPOR
Gastrointestinal: Nausea, vomiting, anorexia, diarrhea, abdominal pain, HEPATOTOXICITY
Hematologic: LEUKOPENIA, THROMBOCYTOPENIA
Integumentary: Hypersensitivity reactions
Miscellaneous: Weakness, orthostatic hypotension
Podophyllotoxin Intoxication: NAUSEA, VOMITING, DIARRHEA, ABDOMINAL PAIN, THROMBOCYTOPENIA, LEUKOPENIA, ABNORMAL LIVER FUNCTION TESTS, ATAXIA, NUMBNESS, ALTERED CONSCIOUSNESS
Respiratory: Shortness of breath, APNEA

M

Interactions with Mayapple

Drug

Belladonna alkaloids: Belladonna alkaloids may decrease the laxative effects of mayapple; do not use concurrently.
Ipecac: Ipecac may decrease the laxative effects of mayapple; do not use concurrently.

Continued

Interactions with Mayapple—cont'd

Food

Salt: Salt may increase the laxative effect of mayapple; do not use concurrently.

Herb

Hyoscyamus, lobelia, and leptandra may decrease the laxative effect of mayapple; do not use concurrently.

Lab Test

Mayapple may cause decreased red blood cells.

Client Considerations

Assess

- Assess for hypersensitivity reactions. If these are present, discontinue use of mayapple and administer antihistamine or other appropriate therapy.
- Assess for the symptoms of podophyllotoxin intoxication: nausea, vomiting, diarrhea, abdominal pain, thrombocytopenia, leukopenia, abnormal liver function tests, ataxia, numbness, and altered consciousness.
- Assess for the use of medications, herbs, and salt (see Interactions).

Administer

- Instruct the client to treat only 25 cm² at a time. Mayapple is extremely irritating to skin and mucous membranes.
- Instruct the client to store mayapple products in a cool, dry place, away from heat and moisture.

Teach Client/Family

- Until more research is available, caution the client not to use mayapple during pregnancy and lactation and not to give it to children.
- Caution the client that all parts of the mayapple plant except the ripe fruit are toxic, both orally or topically.
- Advise the client that the health care provider may use mayapple to treat genital, vaginal, or perianal warts.

Pharmacology
Pharmacokinetics
Pharmacokinetics and pharmacodynamics are unknown. Mayapple is antimitotic.

Primary Chemical Components of Mayapple and Their Possible Actions		
Chemical Class	**Individual Component**	**Possible Action**
Podophyllotoxin		Antimitotic; toxic
Resin		
Flavonoid	Quercetin	Antiinflammatory
Starch		
Picropodophyllin		

Actions

M

Very few research studies have been done on mayapple. The few that are published deal with the toxicity of podophyllotoxin, one of its chemical components.

Podophyllotoxin Intoxication
One study using rats revealed severe nervous system changes when mayapple was injected. The changes included increased coarseness of nerve fibers in the cerebellum, cerebral cortex, brainstem, and spinal cord. Neuronal swelling also occurred. Although the nervous system was the only system studied, toxicity undoubtedly occurs in other systems as well (Chang, 1992). Another study showed similar results (Kao, 1992).

References

Blumenthal M, editor: *The complete German Commission E monographs: therapeutic guide to herbal medicines,* Austin, Tex, American Botanical Council; Boston, Integrative Medicine Communication, 1998.

Chang LW et al: Experimental podophyllotoxin (bajiaolian) poisoning: I, effects on the nervous system, *Biomed Environ Sci* 5(4):283-292, 1992.

Kao WF et al: Podophyllotoxin intoxication: toxic effect of bajiaolian herbal therapeutics, *Hum Exp Toxicol* 11(6):480-487, 1992.

Meadowsweet
(meh'dow-sweet)

Scientific names: *Filipendula ulmaria, Spiraea ulmaria*

Other common names: Bridewort, dolloff, dropwort, fleur d'ulmaire, flores ulmariae, gravel root, meadow queen, meadwort, mede-sweet, queen of the meadow, spierstaude

Class 1

Origin: Meadowsweet is a perennial shrub found in Europe and North America.

Uses
Reported Uses
Traditionally, meadowsweet has been used to treat gastrointestinal disorders such as gastritis, heartburn, indigestion, irritable bowel syndrome (IBS), and peptic ulcer disease. It has also been used to treat urinary tract infections, joint and rheumatic muscle and joint pains, headache, fever, and colds.

Product Availability and Dosages
Available Forms
Dried flowers, dried herb, fluid extract, infusion, powder, tablets, tincture

Plant Parts Used: Dried flowers, other aboveground parts

Dosages and Routes
Adult
All dosages listed are PO.
- Dried flowers: 2.5-3.5 g qd (Blumenthal, 1998)
- Dried herb: 1.5-5 g bid-tid
- Fluid extract: 2-3 ml tid (1:1 dilution in 25% alcohol)
- Infusion: 100 ml q2h
- Powder: ½ tsp dissolved in 1 oz water
- Tincture: 2-4 ml bid-tid (1:5 dilution in 25% alcohol)

Precautionary Information
Contraindications
Until more research is available, meadowsweet should not be used during pregnancy and lactation and should not be given to children. Meadowsweet should not be used by

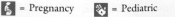 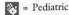 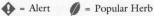

 = Pregnancy   = Pediatric   = Alert   = Popular Herb

Precautionary Information—cont'd

Contraindications—cont'd

persons with asthma or hypersensitivity to salicylates. Class 1 herb.

Side Effects/Adverse Reactions

Gastrointestinal: Nausea, vomiting, anorexia

Integumentary: Hypersensitivity reactions

Respiratory: BRONCHOSPASM

Interactions with Meadowsweet

Drug

Anticoagulants: Anticoagulants such as heparin, warfarin, and salicylates may increase the risk of bleeding when used with meadowsweet; avoid concurrent use (Kudriashowv, 1991; Kudriashowv, 1990; Liapina, 1993).

Iron salts: Meadowsweet may decrease the absorption of iron salts; separate by 2 hr.

Food	Herb	Lab Test
None known	None known	None known

Client Considerations

Assess

- Assess for hypersensitivity reactions. If these are present, discontinue use of meadowsweet and administer antihistamine or other appropriate therapy. Clients with salicylate sensitivity or asthma should not use this herb.
- Assess for anticoagulants taken (heparin, warfarin, salicylates); these drugs should be avoided when using this herb (see Interactions).
- Monitor coagulation studies if the client is taking high doses of meadowsweet over a long period.

Administer

- Instruct the client to store meadowsweet products in a cool, dry place, away from heat and moisture.

M

Teach Client/Family

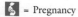

- Until more research is available, caution the client not to use meadowsweet during pregnancy and lactation and not to give it to children.

Pharmacology

Pharmacokinetics

Pharmacokinetics and pharmacodynamics are unknown.

Primary Chemical Components of Meadowsweet and Their Possible Actions		
Chemical Class	**Individual Component**	**Possible Action**
Flavonoid	Quercetin; Naringenin, Flavone	Antimicrobial
	Kaempferol Spiraeoside; Avicularin; Hyperoside	Antiinflammatory
Phenolic glycoside	Spiraein Monotropin; Primaverosides	Antioxidant
Tannin		Wound healing; astringent
Volatile oil	Methylsalicylate Salicylaldehyde; Gaultherin; Isosalicin; Monotropitin; Salicylic acid; Spirein	Anticoagulant
Coumarin Mucilage Ascorbic acid		Anticoagulant

Actions

Anticoagulant Action

In one study focusing on the anticoagulant effects of meadowsweet, extracts were administered orally and anticoagulant levels tested (Liapina, 1993). The flowers and seeds showed a high level of anticoagulant activity. Another study using various methods showed that all components of meadowsweet exhibit heparin-like action (Kudriashowv, 1991). A third study showed similar results (Kudriashowv, 1990).

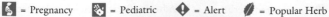

= Pregnancy   = Pediatric   ◆ = Alert   = Popular Herb

Antiinfective Action

A study evaluating the antimicrobial effects of various herbs found that those with the greatest effect against bacteria were meadowsweet, willow herb, cloudberry, and raspberry (Rauha, 2000).

Antioxidant Action

When researchers used spectrometry to evaluate the antioxidative activity of 92 phenolic extracts from plants, meadowsweet showed a high level of antioxidative activity calculated as gallic acid equivalents (Kahkonen, 1999).

Antidiabetic Action

Meadowsweet was tested for possible antidiabetic effects, but results did not confirm its efficacy. In a study evaluating its antidiabetic action in streptozocin-diabetic mice, the mice that received meadowsweet showed no change in diabetes symptoms (Swanston-Flatt, 1989).

Anticancer Action

Another study found that meadowsweet caused a significant decrease in precancerous changes in mice. Mice with cervical dysplasia or carcinoma of the vagina were given meadowsweet prepared from flowers. A 67% drop in dysplasia occurred, and no recurrence was observed in 10 subjects considered completely cured in 1 year (Peresun'ko, 1993).

Antiulcer Action

One foreign study has demonstrated the antiulcer action of meadowsweet. The herb was shown to decrease formation of stomach lesions when reserpine injections were given to rats or mice (Barnaulov, 1980).

References

Barnaulov OD et al: Anti-ulcer action of a decoction of the flowers of the dropwort, *Filipendula ulmaria* (L.) *maxim, Farmakol Toksikol* 43(6): 700-705, 1980.

Blumenthal M, editor: *The complete German Commission E monographs: therapeutic guide to herbal medicines,* Austin, Tex, American Botanical Council; Boston, Integrative Medicine Communication, 1998.

Kahkonen MP et al: Antioxidant activity of plant extracts containing phenolic compounds, *J Agric Food Chem* 47(10):3954-3962, 1999.

Kudriashowv BA et al: The content of a heparin-like anticoagulant in the flowers of the meadowsweet *(Filipendula ulmaria), Farmakol Toksikol* 53(4):39-41, 1990.

Kudriashowv BA et al: Heparin from the meadowsweet *(Filipendula ulmaria)* and its properties, *Izv Akad Nauk SSSR* (6):939-943, 1991.

Liapina LA et al: A comparative study of the action on the hemostatic system of extracts from the flowers and seeds of the meadowsweet *(Filipendula ulmaria* [L.] *maxim), Izv Akad Nauk Ser Biol* (4):625-628, 1993.

Peresun'ko AP et al: Clinical-experimental study of using plant preparations from the flowers of *Filipendula ulmaria* (L.) *maxim* for the treatment of precancerous changes and prevention of uterine cervical cancer, *Vopr Onkol* 39(7-12):291-295, 1993.

Rauha JP et al: Antimicrobial effects of Finnish plant extracts containing flavonoids and other phenolic compounds, *Int J Food Microbiol* 56(1):3-12, 2000.

Swanston-Flatt SK et al: Evaluation of traditional plant treatments for diabetes: studies in streptozotocin diabetic mice, *Acta Diabetol Lat* 26(1):51-55, 1989.

Melatonin

(meh-luh-toe'nuhn)

Scientific name: N-Acetyl-5-methoxytryptamine

Other common name: MEL

Origin: Melatonin is a naturally occurring hormone in the body.

Uses

Reported Uses

Melatonin is used to treat insomnia and to inhibit cataract formation. It is also used to increase longevity, treat jet lag, and prevent weight loss in cancer patients. Because it lowers luteinizing hormone (LH), estradiol, and progesterone levels, melatonin possibly is useful as a contraceptive (Voordouw, 1992).

Product Availability and Dosages

Available Forms

Extended release capsules: 3 mg; injectable; liquid: 500 mcg/ml; tablets: 500 mcg, 1 mg, 1.5 mg, 3 mg

Dosages and Routes

Adult

Cancer (as a single agent)

• 20 mg qd × 2 mo IM (injectable form), then 10 mg PO qd

Cancer (in combination with interleukein-2)

• PO: 40-50 mg hs for 1 wk before interleukin-2

 = Pregnancy  = Pediatric   = Alert 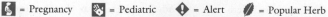 = Popular Herb

Chronic Insomnia
• PO tablets: 75 mg hs (Murray, 1998)
Delayed Sleep-Phase Syndrome
• PO: 5 mg hs
Jet Lag
• PO: 5 mg qd 2-3 days before and 3 days after travel
Elderly
Chronic Insomnia
• PO tablets: er 1-2 mg 2 hr ac

Precautionary Information
Contraindications
Until more research is available, melatonin should not be used during pregnancy and lactation and should not be given to children. Persons with hypersensitivity to melatonin and those with hepatic or cardiovascular disease, central nervous system disorders, or depression should not use it. Persons with renal disease should use melatonin with caution.

Side Effects/Adverse Reactions
Central Nervous System: Headache, change in sleep patterns, confusion, hypothermia, sedation
Cardiovascular: TACHYCARDIA
Gastrointestinal: Nausea, vomiting, anorexia
Integumentary: Hypersensitivity reactions (rash, pruritus)
Reproductive: Decreased progesterone, estradiol, LH levels

M

Interactions with Melatonin

Drug
Benzodiazepines: Melatonin may increase the anxiolytic effects of benzodiazepines; use together cautiously.
Cerebral stimulants: Cerebral stimulants used with melatonin may have a synergistic effect and exacerbate insomnia; avoid concurrent use.
DHEA: DHEA (dehydroepiandrosterone) used with melatonin may decrease cytokine production; avoid concurrent use.
Magnesium: Magnesium used with melatonin increases inhibition of N-methyl-D-aspartate (NMDA) receptors; avoid concurrent use.

Continued

 Endangered Herb   Adverse effects: BOLD = life-threatening

Interactions with Melatonin—cont'd

Drug—cont'd

Succinylcholine: Melatonin increases the blocking properties of succinylcholine; avoid concurrent use.

Zinc: Zinc used with melatonin increases inhibition of NMDA receptors; avoid concurrent use.

Food	Herb	Lab Test
None known	None known	None known

Client Considerations

Assess

- Assess for hypersensitivity reactions. If these are present, discontinue use of melatonin and administer antihistamine or other appropriate therapy.
- Assess sleep patterns: ability to fall asleep, stay asleep, hours slept, and napping, if using for insomnia
- Assess for central nervous system effects: confusion, headache, sedation, and changes in sleeping patterns.
- Assess for medications used (see Interactions).

Administer

- Instruct the client to take melatonin PO to treat insomnia or jet lag. Melatonin is administered both PO and IM to cancer patients.
- Instruct the client to store melatonin products in a sealed container away from heat and moisture.

Teach Client/Family

- Until more research is available, caution the client not to use melatonin during pregnancy and lactation and not to give it to children.
- Advise client to avoid use with magnesium, zinc, and DHEA.
- Advise the client to notify health care provider of all supplements taken.

Pharmacology

Pharmacokinetics

Pharmacokinetics and pharmacodynamics are unknown.

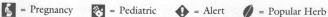

= Pregnancy   = Pediatric   ◆ = Alert   ∅ = Popular Herb

Actions

Melatonin is a hormone produced in the body by the pineal gland. It is an antioxidant and a free-radical scavenger (Reiter, 1995). When tryptophan is converted to serotonin, melatonin results from enzymatic processes in the pineal gland. Melatonin production increases during sleep and decreases during waking hours (James, 1989). Melatonin supplementation has been found to induce and maintain sleep in adults who have low melatonin levels. The most promising use is for the elderly, who typically have low melatonin levels. Melatonin treatment in vivo caused a significant increase in blood glucose and a decreased level of free fatty acids (Fabis, 2002). Parkinson's disease may be treated with melatonin, which lacks any serious side effects (Antolin, 2002).

References

Antolin I et al: Protective effect of melatonin in a chronic experimental model of Parkinson's disease, *Brain Res* 943(2):163-173, 2002.

Fabis M et al: In vivo and in situ action of melatonin on insulin secretion and some metabolic implications in the rats, *Pancreas* 25(2):166-169, 2002.

James SP et al: Melatonin administration in insomnia, *Neuropsychopharacol* 3:19, 1989.

Duke J: *CRC handbook of medicinal herbs,* Boca Raton, Fla, 1985, CRC Press, pp 374-375.

Murray M, Pizzarno J: *The encyclopedia of natural medicine,* 2 ed (revised), Roseville, Calif, 1998, Prima.

Reiter RJ et al: Oxygen radical detoxification processes during aging: the functional importance of melatonin, *Aging Clin Exp Res* 7:340-351, 1995.

Voordouw BCG et al: Melatonin and melatonin-progestin combinations alter pituitary-ovarian function in women and can inhibit ovulation, *J Clin Endocrinol Metab* 74:108, 1992.

M

Milk Thistle
(milk thi'suhl)

Scientific name: *Silybum marianum*

Other common names: Holy thistle, lady's thistle, Marian thistle, Mary thistle, St. Mary thistle

Class 1 (Seed)

Origin: Milk thistle is found in Kashmir, Mexico, Canada, and the United States.

Uses

Reported Uses

Milk thistle has been used to treat hepatotoxicity caused by poisonous mushrooms, cirrhosis of the liver, chronic candidiasis, hepatitis C, exposure to toxic chemicals, and liver transplantation.

Product Availability and Dosages

Available Forms

Tincture, capsule

Plant Parts Used: Seeds

Dosages and Routes

Adult

Alcoholism
- PO tincture: 70-210 mg tid (70%-80% silymarin) (Murray, 1998)

General Dosages
- PO tincture: 200-400 mg qd (dosage standardized to silymarin content) (Blumenthal, 1998)

Hepatitis
- PO tincture: 140-210 mg tid (70%-80% silymarin) (Murray, 1998)

Precautionary Information

Contraindications

Until more research is available, milk thistle should not be used during pregnancy and lactation and should not be given to children. Milk thistle should not be used by persons

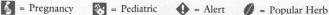

§ = Pregnancy   **☝** = Pediatric   **❶** = Alert   **✿** = Popular Herb

Precautionary Information—cont'd

Contraindications—cont'd

with hypersensitivity to this herb or other plants in the Aster-aceae family. Class 1 herb (seed).

Side Effects/Adverse Reactions

Gastrointestinal: Nausea, vomiting, anorexia, diarrhea
Genitourinary: Menstrual changes
Integumentary: Hypersensitivity reactions

Interactions with Milk Thistle

Drug
Milk thistle should not be used with drugs metabolized by the P-450 enzyme.

Food	Herb	Lab Test
None known	None known	None known

M

Client Considerations

Assess

- Assess for hypersensitivity reactions. If these are present, discontinue use of milk thistle and administer antihistamine or other appropriate therapy.
- Monitor liver function studies (ALT, AST, bilirubin) if the client is using milk thistle to treat hepatic disease.
- Assess medications used (see Interactions).

Administer

- Instruct the client to store milk thistle products in a cool, dry place, away from heat and moisture.

Teach Client/Family

- Until more research is available, caution the client not to use milk thistle during pregnancy and lactation and not to give it to children.

Pharmacology

Pharmacokinetics

Pharmacokinetics and pharmacodynamics are unknown.

Primary Chemical Components of Milk Thistle and Their Possible Actions		
Chemical Class	**Individual Component**	**Possible Action**
Flavonoid	Silybine Isosilybine; Silycristine; Silidianine; Taxifoline (Quaglia, 1999)	Hepatoprotective
Flavonolignan	Dehydrosilybin; Siliandrin; Silyhermin	
Apigenin		
Acid	Linoleic acid; Oleic acid; Palmitic acid	
Tocopherol		
Sterol	Sitosterol; Cholesterol; Campesterol; Stigmasterol	
Mucilage		

Actions

Hepatoprotective Action

Several studies have demonstrated the hepatoprotective action of silymarin, a chemical component of milk thistle (Flora, 1998; Thamsborg, 1996; Feher, 1989). One of these studies noted that silymarin has been used for centuries to treat liver and gall-bladder conditions (Flora, 1998). Silymarin has been found to act as an antioxidant, decreasing free radicals and increasing hepatocyte synthesis as well as exerting other hepatoprotective effects. It has been used to treat acute and chronic liver disease and has been found to inhibit cytochrome P-450 enzymes in liver microsomes (Beckmann-Knopp, 2000). It is possible that drugs metabolized by CYP3A4 or CYP2C9 may interact with this herb. One study using sheep orally infected with sawfly larvae demonstrated a positive response when silymarin was used to treat the resultant hepatotoxicosis (Thamsborg, 1996). Milk thistle has shown promise to treat hepatitis C with few side effects. Silymarin has hepatoprotective, antiinflammatory and regenerative properties (Giese, 2001).

Nephroprotective Action

A study done on African green monkeys confirmed the nephroprotective effects of silibinin and silicristin, two of milk thistle's chemical components (Sonnenbichler, 1999). Kidney cells

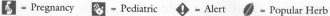 = Pregnancy   = Pediatric   = Alert   = Popular Herb

that had been damaged by cisplatin, vincristine, and paracetamol showed lessened or no nephrotoxic effects.

References

Beckmann-Knopp S et al: Inhibitory effects of silibinin on cytochrome P-450 enzymes in human liver microsomes, *Pharmacol Toxicol* 86(6): 250-256, 2000.

Blumenthal M, editor: *The complete German Commission E monographs: therapeutic guide to herbal medicines,* Austin, Tex, American Botanical Council; Boston, Integrative Medicine Communication, 1998.

Feher J et al: Hepatoprotective activity of silymarin therapy in patients with chronic liver disease, *Orv Hetil* 130:2723-2727, 1989.

Flora K et al: Milk thistle *(Silybum marianum)* for the therapy of liver disease, *Am J Gastroenterol* 93(2):139-143, 1998.

Giese LA: Milk thistle and the treatment of hepatitis, *Gastroenterol Nurs* 24(2):95-97, 2001.

Murray M, Pizzarno J: *The encyclopedia of natural medicine,* 2 ed (revised), Roseville, Calif, 1998, Prima.

Quaglia MG et al: Determination of silymarin in the extract from dried silybum marianum fruits by high performance liquid chromatography and capillary electrophoresis, *J Pharm Biomed Anal* 19(3-4):435-442, 1999.

Sonnenbichler J et al: Stimulatory effects of silibinin and silicristin from the milk thistle *(Silybum marianum)* on kidney cells, *J Pharmacol Exp Ther* 290(3):1375-1383, 1999.

Thamsborg SM et al: Putative effect of silymarin on sawfly *(Arge pullata)*-induced hepatotoxicosis in sheep, *Vet Hum Toxicol* 38(2):89-91, 1996.

Mint
(mint)

Scientific names: *Mentha x piperita* (peppermint), *Mentha spicata* (spearmint)

Other common names: Balm mint, brandy mint, green mint, lamb mint, our lady's mint, peppermint, spearmint

Class 1 (Leaf)

Origin: Mint is found in Europe, the United States, and Canada.

Uses
Reported Uses
Mint has been used internally as an antiseptic and to treat flatulence, vomiting, diarrhea, abdominal pain, indigestion, irritable bowel syndrome (IBS), colic, and gallbladder disorders. It has also been used internally to decrease colonic spasms during endoscopy. Topically, mint has been used to relieve sunburn, arthritis pain, and neuralgia. It is also used in aromatherapy and as a flavoring in liquor, foods, mouthwash, and gum.

Product Availability and Dosages
Available Forms
Enteric-coated capsules (peppermint), fluid extract, gum, liniment, lozenges, mouthwash, oil, ointment, tea, toothpaste

Plant Parts Used: Leaves, oil extracted flowers

Dosages and Routes
Adult
All dosages listed are for peppermint.
Aromatherapy and Congestion Relief
- Inhalant oil: use prn

Irritable Bowel Syndrome
- PO enteric-coated peppermint oil capsules: 2 ml bid between meals (Murray, 1998)

Other
- PO capsules: 2 caps tid
- PO extract: 20 drops with 4 oz of water
- PO oil: 20 drops with 4 oz of water
- PO tea: place 1 tbsp leaves in 2 cups boiling water, steep 15 min; may be taken bid-tid
- Topical ointment: apply prn to affected area up to tid

Precautionary Information
Contraindications

Until more research is available, mint should not be used internally during pregnancy and lactation and should not be given internally to children. Mint should not be used internally by persons with hypersensitivity to it or by those with gallbladder inflammation, severe liver disease, gastroesophageal reflux disease, or obstruction of bile ducts. Mint

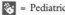

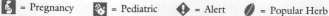
= Pregnancy   = Pediatric   = Alert   = Popular Herb

Precautionary Information—cont'd

Contraindications—cont'd

should not be used topically on the face, particularly near the nose, or on infants or small children. Class 1 herb (leaf).

Side Effects/Adverse Reactions

Gastrointestinal: Nausea, anorexia
Integumentary: Peppermint oil: hypersensitivity reactions (flushing, rash, headache, heartburn, mucous membrane irritation, urticaria, erythema); contact dermatitis (topical)
Systemic: BRONCHOSPASM

Interactions with Mint

Drug	Food	Herb	Lab Test
None known	None known	None known	None known

M

Client Considerations

Assess

- Assess for hypersensitivity reactions (see Side Effects). If these are present, discontinue use of mint and administer antihistamine or other appropriate therapy.

Administer

- Instruct the client to store mint products in a cool, dry place, away from heat and moisture.

Teach Client/Family

- Until more research is available, caution the client not to use mint during pregnancy and lactation and not to give it to children.
- Caution the client to keep mint oil products away from mucous membranes and abrasions.
- Caution clients with gastroesophageal reflux disease not to use mint. It may worsen the condition.
- Caution the client not to use mint oil with a heating pad or near an open flame.

Pharmacology

Pharmacokinetics

Pharmacokinetics and pharmacodynamics are unknown. Carminative action results from esophageal sphincter tone reduction.

Primary Chemical Components of Mint and Their Possible Actions		
Chemical Class	**Individual Component**	**Possible Action**
Peppermint Contains		
Volatile oil	Menthol; Menthone	Counterirritant; spasmolytic; antimicrobial (Iscan, 2002)
Tannin Flavonoid Tocopherol		Choleretic
Spearmint Contains		
Carvone Limonene Phellandrene Pinene		

Actions

Actions for mint are categorized by species (i.e., spearmint, peppermint). Both spearmint and peppermint have similar actions, but research studies tend to focus on one species or the other.

Anti–HIV-1 and Antiviral Actions

One study evaluated the anti–HIV-1 activity of mint using various herbs of the Labiatae family (Yamasaki, 1998). Most of the plants tested showed significant anti–HIV-1 activity, including *Mentha x piperita*. The essential oils in are believed to be responsible for this action. Mint has been shown to also possess antiviral activity against herpes simplex, Newcastle disease, and vaccinia (Leung, 1980).

Antibacterial Action

Other studies have reported on the antibacterial properties of peppermint. It has been shown to decrease *Candida* spp.

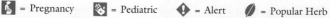

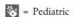 = Pregnancy   = Pediatric   = Alert   = Popular Herb

Irritable Bowel Syndrome

Persons with IBS may find that peppermint oil relieves symptoms. In a placebo-controlled, double-blind study, *Piper x piperita* extract was evaluated for this purpose. Researchers found that peppermint oil decreased IBS symptoms by inhibiting gastrointestinal smooth-muscle action (Pittler, 1998).

References

Iscan G et al: Antimicrobial screening of *Mentha Piperita* essential oils, *J Agric Food Chem* 50(14):3943-3946, 2002.

Leung AY: *Encyclopedia of common natural ingredients in food, drugs and cosmetics,* New York, 1980, Wiley Intersciences.

Murray M, Pizzarno J: *The encyclopedia of natural medicine,* 2 ed (revised), Roseville, Calif, 1998, Prima.

Pittler MH et al: Peppermint oil for irritable bowel syndrome: a critical review and metaanalysis, *Am J Gastroenterol* 93(7):1131-1135, 1998.

Yamasaki K et al: Anti-HIV-1 activity of herbs in Labiatae, *Biol Pharm Bull* 21(8):829-833, 1998.

M

Mistletoe
(mi′suhl-toe)

Scientific names: *Viscum album, Viscum abietis, Viscum austriacum*

Other common names: All heal, birdlime, devil's fuge, European mistletoe, golden bough, mystyldene   **Class 2d** *(Viscum album)*

Origin: Mistletoe is a parasite found in Europe, Asia, and North America depending on species.

Uses

Reported Uses

Mistletoe has been used to treat hypertension, anxiety, seizure disorders, insomnia, depression, infertility, gout, hysteria, internal bleeding, and atherosclerosis.

Investigational Uses

Research is underway to determine the usefulness of mistletoe in the treatment cancer.

Product Availability and Dosages
Available Forms
Capsules, dried leaves, fluid extract, infusion, tablets, tincture, parenterally

Plant Parts Used: Branches, fruit, leaves

Dosages and Routes
Adult
All dosages listed are PO.
- Dried leaves: 3-6 g tid
- Fluid extract: 2-3 ml tid (1:1 dilution in 25% alcohol)
- Tincture: 0.5 ml bid-tid (1:5 dilution in 45% alcohol)

Precautionary Information
Contraindications
Because it is a uterine stimulant, mistletoe should not be used during pregnancy. Until more research is available, this herb should not be used during lactation and should not be given to children. Mistletoe should not be used by persons who are hypersensitive to it. Persons with protein oversensitivity and those with chronic progressive infections should avoid its use. Mistletoe is a toxic plant and should be kept out of the reach of children. Class 2d herb *(Viscum album)*.

Side Effects/Adverse Reactions
Cardiovascular: Bradycardia, hypotension or hypertension, CARDIAC ARREST
Gastrointestinal: Nausea, vomiting, anorexia, diarrhea, gastritis, HEPATITIS, HEPATOTOXICITY
Integumentary: Hypersensitivity reactions
Miscellaneous: Psychosis, mydriasis, myosis, leukocytosis

Interactions with Mistletoe

Drug
Antihypertensives: Mistletoe may increase the hypotensive effect of antihypertensives; avoid concurrent use.
Cardiac glycosides (digoxin): Use of mistletoe with cardiac glycosides such as digoxin, digitoxin, and calcium channel blockers may cause decreased cardiac function; avoid concurrent use.

& = Pregnancy   **&** = Pediatric   **!** = Alert   *//* = Popular Herb

Interactions with Mistletoe—cont'd

Drug—cont'd

Central nervous system depressants: Use of mistletoe with central nervous system depressants such as opiates, benzodiazepines, sedatives, antianxiety drugs, and alcohol may cause increased sedation; avoid concurrent use.

Immunosuppressants: Immunosuppressants such as azathioprine, basiliximab, cyclosporine, muromonab, sirolimus, and tacrolimus may stimulate immunity when used with mistletoe; avoid concurrent use.

Iron salts: Mistletoe may decrease the absorption of iron salts; separate by 2 hr.

Food	Herb
None known	None known

Lab Test

Mistletoe may cause increased ALT, AST, total bilirubin, urine bilirubin, and lymphocyte counts.

Mistletoe may cause decreased red blood cells *(V. album)*.

M

Client Considerations

Assess

- Assess for hypersensitivity reactions. If these are present, discontinue use of mistletoe and administer antihistamine or other appropriate therapy.
- Assess for life-threatening adverse reactions: cardiac involvement, hepatitis.
- Assess for other adverse reactions: chills, fever, headache, angina, orthostatic hypotension, hypertension.
- Assess medication use (see Interactions).

Administer

- Instruct the client to store mistletoe products away from light, heat, and moisture.

Teach Client/Family

- Because it is a uterine stimulant, caution the client not to use mistletoe during pregnancy. Until more research is available, caution the client not to use this herb during lactation and not to give it to children.

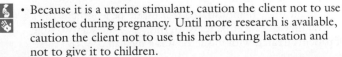 Endangered Herb   Adverse effects: **BOLD** = life-threatening

- Advise the client that mistletoe is a toxic plant and should be kept out of reach of children.

Pharmacology

Pharmacokinetics

Pharmacokinetics and pharmacodynamics are unknown. Stimulates cuti-visceral reflexes following inflammation.

Primary Chemical Components of Mistletoe and Their Possible Actions		
Chemical Class	**Individual Component**	**Possible Action**
Amine	Tyramine	Uterine stimulant
Acetylcholine		
Histamine		
Tyramine		
Phoratoxin		
Choline		
Betaphenylethylamine		
Viscotoxin		
Flavonoid	Quercetin; Kaempferol	Antioxidant
Phenyl alyl alcohol	Syringen	
Lectin		
Sugar alcohol	Mannitol; Quebrachitol; Pinitol; Viscumitol	
Terpenoid		
Alkaloid		
Tannin		Wound healing; astringent

Actions

Mistletoe has been used parenterally for many years in cancer patients. The majority of the research on mistletoe deals with its antineoplastic activity.

Antineoplastic Action

One recent study demonstrated that mistletoe lengthens the survival time of cancer patients. In this study the survival time of patients treated with mistletoe was a median of 9.18 years, compared with 7.54 years for those not treated with mistletoe. However, this difference is not considered statistically significant (Stumpf, 2000). Another study (Stein, 2000) found that mistletoe induces apoptosis in lymphocytes and tumor cells. However, the research on the usefulness of mistletoe for the treatment of cancer has shown inconclusive results.

Anti-HIV Action
Another study showed that mistletoe produces immunomodulatory effects when given to HIV-infected patients and may slow the progression of the disease (Gorter, 1999).

References
Gorter RW et al: Tolerability of an extract of European mistletoe among immunocompromised and healthy individuals, *Altern Ther Health Med* 5(6):37-44, 47-48, 1999.

Stein GM. et al: Toxic proteins from European mistletoe (*Viscum album* L.): increase of intracellular IL-4 but decrease of IFN-gamma in apoptotic cells, *Anticancer Res* 20(3A):1673-1678, 2000.

Stumpf C et al: No title available (in-process citation), *Forsch Komplementarmed Klass Naturheilkd* 7(3):139-146, 2000.

Monascus
(muhn-az'kuhs)

Scientific names: *Monascum purpureus, Monascum anka*
Other common names: Zhi Tai, XueZhiKang

Origin: Monascus is a yeast made by fermentation.

Uses
Reported Uses
Marketed as Cholestin, monascus is used to treat hypercholesteremia. It is also used to treat gastrointestinal upset and circulatory problems.

Investigational Uses
Research is underway to determine the efficacy of monascus as an antimicrobial and antioxidant, as well as for the treatment of liver toxicity.

Product Availability and Dosages
Available Forms
Whole yeast

Plant Parts Used: Whole yeast (mold)

Dosages and Routes
No consensus on dosage exists.

Precautionary Information
Contraindications
Until more research is available, monascus should not be used during pregnancy and lactation and should not be given to children. Monascus should not be used by persons with hypersensitivity to it or by those with hepatic diseases such as cirrhosis or fatty liver.

Side Effects/Adverse Reactions
Gastrointestinal: Nausea, vomiting, anorexia; HEPATOTOXIC-ITY (rare)
Integumentary: Hypersensitivity reactions

Interactions with Monascus			
Drug	Food	Herb	Lab Test
None known	None known	None known	None known

Client Considerations
Assess
- Assess for hypersensitivity reactions. If these are present, discontinue use of monascus and administer antihistamine or other appropriate therapy.
- Monitor liver function studies (AST, ALT, bilirubin) if the client is using high doses of monascus over a long period.

Administer
- Instruct the client to store monascus products in a cool, dry place, away from heat and moisture.

 = Pregnancy = Pediatric = Alert 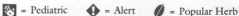 = Popular Herb

Teach Client/Family

- Until more research is available, caution the client not to use monascus during pregnancy and lactation and not to give it to children.

Pharmacology

Pharmacokinetics

Pharmacokinetics and pharmacodynamics are unknown.

Primary Chemical Components of Monascus and Their Possible Actions		
Chemical Class	**Individual Component**	**Possible Action**
Citrinin Monankarins A-F		Nephrotoxic Monoamine oxidase inhibition (Hossain, 1996)

M

Actions

Anticholesterol Action

The anticholesterol action of monascus is well documented. It has been found to inhibit HMG-CoA reductase and to decrease low-density lipoprotein (LDL) and very-low-density lipoprotein (VLDL) cholesterol and plasma triglycerides (Katcher, 1987). This herb has been studied in China for many years, with all studies reporting similar results in the decrease of cholesterol, triglycerides, and LDL cholesterol (Endo, 1979; Wang, 1995; Zhu, 1995).

Antimicrobial Action

One study evaluated the antimicrobial effect of "monascus making" in the open air. In this study, monascus was produced and dried in the open air (Kono, 1999). When the herb was contaminated with *Micrococcus varians* and *Bacillus subtilis*, it was able to inhibit the growth of these two microorganisms.

Antioxidant and Hepatoprotective Actions

Another study reviewed the antioxidant capabilities of monascus (Aniya, 1999) using several types of molds. *Monascus anka* showed the strongest hepatoprotective action in rats. Another study has also confirmed the antioxidant and hepatoprotective actions of monascus (Aniya, 1998).

Monoamine Oxidase Inhibition

A study of the chemical components of *Monascus anka* has identified the presence of monankarins A-F, which inhibit monoamine oxidase (MAO). Investigators found the inhibition of MAO-B to be stronger than that of MAO-A (Hossain, 1996).

References

Aniya Y et al: Protective effect of the mold *Monascus anka* against acetaminophen-induced liver toxicity in rats, *Jpn J Pharmacol* 78(1): 79-82, 1998.

Aniya Y et al: Screening of antioxidant action of various molds and protection of *Monascus anka* against experimentally induced liver injuries or rats, *Gen Pharmacol* 32(2):225-231, 1999.

Endo AJ: *J Antibiot* 32:852-854, 1979.

Hossain CF et al: A new series of coumarin derivatives having monoamine oxidase inhibitory activity from *Monascus anka, Chem Pharm Bull* 44(6):1535-1539, 1996.

Katcher, editor: *Applied therapeutics,* 3 ed, Spokane, Wash, 1987, Applied Therapeutics, pp 651-652.

Kono I et al: Antimicrobial activity of *Monascus pilosus* IFO 4520 against contaminant of Koji, *Biosci Biotechnol Biochem* 63(8):1494-1496, 1999.

Wang Y et al: *Chin J Exp Ther Prepar Chin Med* 1(1):1-5, 1995.

Zhu Y et al: *Chin J Pharmacol* 30(11):4-8, 1995.

Morinda
(mohr-in'duh)

Scientific name: *Morinda citrifolia*

Other common names: Hog apple, Indian mulberry, mengkoedoe, mora de la India, noni, ruibarbo caribe, wild pine

Origin: Morinda is a shrub found in Polynesia, Asia, and parts of Australia.

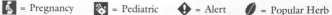

Uses
Reported Uses
Morinda has been used in the South Pacific to treat arthritis, heart disease, diabetes, hypertension, and gastrointestinal disease.

Investigational Uses
Research is underway to determine the anticancer and anthelmintic properties of morinda.

Product Availability and Dosages
Available Forms
Capsules, dried fruit leather, juice, powder

Plant Parts Used: Flowers, fruit, leaves

Dosages and Routes
Adult
No consensus on dosages exists.

Precautionary Information
Contraindications
Until more research is available, morinda should not be used during pregnancy and lactation and it should not be given to children. Morinda should not be use by persons with hyperkalemia or by those with hypersensitivity to it.

Side Effects/Adverse Reactions
Central Nervous System: Sedation (Younos, 1990)
Gastrointestinal: Nausea, vomiting, anorexia
Integumentary: Hypersensitivity reactions
Metabolic: Hyperkalemia (Mueller, 2000)

Interactions with Morinda

Drug	Food	Herb	Lab Test
None known	None known	None known	None known

M

 Endangered Herb   Adverse effects: BOLD = life-threatening

Client Considerations

Assess

- Assess for hypersensitivity reactions. If these are present, discontinue use of morinda and administer antihistamine or other appropriate therapy.

Administer

- Instruct the client to store morinda products in a cool, dry place, away from heat and moisture.

Teach Client/Family

- Until more research is available, caution the client not to use morinda during pregnancy and lactation and not to give it to children.
- Advise the client not to perform hazardous activities such as driving or operating heavy machinery until physical response to the herb can be evaluated.

Pharmacology

Pharmacokinetics

Pharmacokinetics and pharmacodynamics are unknown.

Primary Chemical Components of Morinda and Their Possible Actions		
Chemical Class	Individual Component	Possible Action
Alkaloid	Xeronine	
Glycosides	Glucopyranosyl; Glucopyranose	
Essential oil	Hexoic acid; Octoic acids	
Anthraquinone	Damnacanthal	
Morindone		
Alizarin		
Potassium		
Rutin (Wang, 1999)		
Asperulosidic acid (Wang, 1999)		
Polysaccharide	Noni-ppt (Hirazumi, 1994)	Antitumor

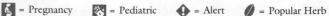

Actions

Very little research is available on morinda. The few studies that have been completed have focused on its anticancer, anthelmintic, and antimalarial effects.

Anticancer Action

One study evaluated the anticancer action of morinda on lung cancer in mice. Morinda was found to increase lifespan in all batches of mice. It is believed to increase immunity by increasing lymphocytes and macrophages (Hirazumi, 1994; Wang, 2001).

Anthelmintic Action

Another study identified the anthelmintic action of morinda (Raj, 1975).

Sedative Action

One older study (Younos, 1990) found morinda to possess sedative effects when administered to mice.

Antimalarial Action

When the antimalarial effects of morinda were tested, researchers noted a 60% inhibition of *Plasmodium falciparum* growth in vitro (Tona, 1999).

M

References

Hirazumi A et al: An immunomodulatory polysaccharide-rich substance from the fruit juice of *Morinda citrifolia* (noni) with antitumor activity, *Proc West Pharmacol Soc* 37:145-146, 1994.

Mueller BA et al: Noni juice *(Morinda citrifolia):* hidden potential for hyperkalemia? *Am J Kidney Dis* 35(2):310-312, 2000.

Raj R: *Indian J Physiol Pharmacol* 19(1):47-49, 1975.

Tona L et al: Antimalarial activity of 20 crude extracts from nine African medicinal plants used in Kinshasa, Congo, *J Ethnopharmacol* 68(1-3): 193-203, 1999.

Wang M et al: Cancer preventive effect of *Morinda citrifolia, Ann NY Acad Sci* 952:161-168, 2001.

Wang M et al: Novel trisaccharide fatty acid ester identified from the fruits of *Morinda citrifolia* (noni), *J Agric Food Chem* 47(12):4880-4882, 1999.

Younos C et al: Analgesic and behavioural effects of *Morinda citrifolia, Planta Med* 56(5):430-434, 1990.

Motherwort
(muh'thur-wawrt)

Scientific name: *Leonurus cardiaca*

Other common names: I-mu-ts'ao, lion's ear, lion's tail, lion's tart, oman, Roman motherwort, throwwort

Class 2b

Origin: Motherwort is found in Europe, Canada, and the United States.

Uses

Reported Uses

Motherwort has been used to treat menstrual disorders and cardiac conditions such as palpitations. It has also been used as an anticoagulant, antiinflammatory, antispasmodic, antianxiety, and anticancer herb, as well as a cardiotonic.

Product Availability and Dosages

Available Forms

Dried leaves, fluid extract, tincture

Plant Parts Used: Leaves, seeds

Dosages and Routes

Adult

All dosages listed are PO.
- 4.5 g qd (Blumenthal, 1998)
- Fluid extract: 4.5 ml (1:1 dilution)
- Tincture: 22.5 ml (1:5 dilution)

Precautionary Information

Contraindications

Because it may cause uterine bleeding, motherwort should not be used during pregnancy. Until more research is available, this herb should not be used during lactation and should not be given to children. Motherwort should not be used by persons with thrombocytopenia or hypersensitivity to this herb or other members of the Labiatae family. Class 2b herb.

 = Pregnancy   = Pediatric   ◆ = Alert   = Popular Herb

Precautionary Information—cont'd

Side Effects/Adverse Reactions

Gastrointestinal: Nausea, vomiting, anorexia, diarrhea, stomach irritation

Hematologic: Increased bleeding time

Integumentary: Hypersensitivity reactions, photosensitivity

Reproductive: Uterine bleeding

Interactions with Motherwort

Drug

Anticoagulants (heparin, warfarin): Use of motherwort with anticoagulants may cause increased risk of bleeding; avoid concurrent use.

Beta-blockers: Use of motherwort with beta-blockers may cause decreased heart rate; avoid concurrent use.

Cardiac glycosides (digoxin): Use of motherwort with cardiac glycosides may cause decreased heart rate; avoid concurrent use.

Iron salts: Motherwort may decrease the absorption of iron salts; separate by 2 hr.

Food	Herb	Lab Test
None known	None known	None known

Client Considerations

Assess

- Assess for hypersensitivity reactions. If these are present, discontinue use of motherwort and administer antihistamine or other appropriate therapy. Check for photosensitivity if the client is taking motherwort in high doses.
- Assess for risks of bleeding: increased bleeding time, bruising, bleeding gums, hematuria, and hematemesis.

Administer

- Instruct the client to store motherwort products in a cool, dry place, away from heat and moisture.

M

🌀 Endangered Herb   Adverse effects: BOLD = life-threatening

Teach Client/Family

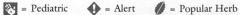

- Because it may cause uterine bleeding, caution the client not to use motherwort during pregnancy. Until more research is available, caution the client not to use this herb during lactation and not to give it to children.
- Because it can cause photosensitivity, advise the client to stay out of the sun or to wear protective clothing while using motherwort.

Pharmacology

Pharmacokinetics

Pharmacokinetics and pharmacodynamics are unknown.

Primary Chemical Components of Motherwort and Their Possible Actions		
Chemical Class	**Individual Component**	**Possible Action**
Alkaloid	Stachydrine; Leonurine	Uterine stimulant
	Betonicine; Turicin; Leunuridin; Leonurinine	
Saponin		
Flavone		
Cardanolide		
Glycoside		
Prehispanolone		Anticoagulant
Iridoid		
Tannin		
Terpenoid		
Triterpene		
Lavandulifolioside		Prolongs P-Q, Q-T intervals, QRS complex; decreases blood pressure (Milkowska, 2002)

Actions

Few research studies have been done on motherwort, although several different actions have been theorized. Traditionally, this herb has been used for its cardiovascular and uterine stimulant actions. A recent study has focused on its chemoprotective action.

Cardiovascular Action

One study (Xia, 1983) has identified the ability of motherwort to inhibit platelets and improve coronary circulation in rats. This herb has also been shown to decrease heart rate and increase the force of myocardial contraction, similar to the action of digoxin.

Anticoagulant Action

The anticoagulant action of motherwort was identified in a study with 105 participants. The anticoagulant effect was found to result from a decrease in fibrinogen and blood viscosity (Zou, 1989). One of the chemical components responsible for this action may be prehispanolone.

Chemoprotective Action

Two studies done by the same group of researchers (Nagasawa, 1990, 1992) demonstrated that motherwort exerts a chemoprotective action in lesions of the breast and uterus. Both studies showed similar results. No effect was seen in pregnancy-dependent mammary tumors, mammary hyperplastic alveolar nodules, or uterine adenomyosis. In fact, motherwort promoted the growth of pregnancy-dependent mammary tumors and inhibited mammary hyperplastic alveolar nodules.

References

Blumenthal M, editor: *The complete German Commission E monographs: therapeutic guide to herbal medicines,* Austin, Tex, American Botanical Council; Boston, Integrative Medicine Communication, 1998.

Milkowska K et al: Pharmacological effects of lavandulifolioside from *Leonurus cardiaca, J Ethnopharmacol* 80(1):85-90, 2002.

Nagasawa H et al: Effects of motherwort (*Leonurus sibiricus* L.) on preneoplastic and neoplastic mammary gland growth in multiparous GR/A mice, *Anticancer Res* 10(4):1019-1023, 1990.

Nagasawa H et al: Further study of the effects of motherwort (*Leonurus sibiricus* L.) on preneoplastic and neoplastic mammary gland growth in multiparous GR/A mice, *Anticancer Res* 12(1):141-143, 1992.

Xia YX et al: The inhibitory effect of motherwort extract on pulsating myocardial cells in vitro, *J Trad Chin Med* 3:185-188, 1983.

Zou QZ et al: Effect of motherwort on blood hyperviscosity, *Am J Chin Med* 17(1-2):65-70, 1989.

Mugwort
(muhg'wawrt)

Scientific name: *Artemisia vulgaris*

Other common names: Ai ye, common mugfelon herb, sailor's tobacco, St. John's plant, wild wormwood, wort

Class 2b (Whole Herb)

Origin: Mugwort is a perennial found in North America.

Uses
Reported Uses
Mugwort has been used as an anthelmintic and as a treatment for menstrual disorders, persistent vomiting, constipation, depression, and anxiety. The roots have been used to treat psychiatric disorders such as psychoneurosis, neurasthenia, depression, and anxiety.

Investigational Uses
Studies are underway to determine the antibacterial and antifungal properties of mugwort.

Product Availability and Dosages
Available Forms
Dried leaves, dried roots, fluid extract, infusion, tincture

Plant Parts Used: Leaves, roots

Dosages and Routes
Adult
- PO tincture: 2-4 ml tid

Precautionary Information
Contraindications
Because it is a uterine stimulant, mugwort should not be used during pregnancy. Until more research is available, this herb should not be used during lactation and should not be given to children. Persons with bleeding disorders or those with hypersensitivity to this herb or other members of the Compositae family should not use mugwort. Class 2b herb (whole herb).

Precautionary Information—cont'd

Side Effects/Adverse Reactions

Gastrointestinal: Nausea, vomiting, anorexia

Integumentary: Hypersensitivity reactions, contact dermatitis

Systemic: ANAPHYLAXIS

Interactions with Mugwort

Drug

Anticoagulants: Use of mugwort with anticoagulants such as heparin and warfarin may cause increased risk of bleeding; do not use concurrently.

Food	Herb
None known	None known

Lab Test

Mugwort may cause an increase in direct bilirubin.

M

Client Considerations

Assess

- Assess for hypersensitivity reactions. If these are present, discontinue use of mugwort and administer antihistamine or other appropriate therapy.
- Assess for the use of anticoagulants (see Interactions).

Administer

- Instruct the client to store mugwort products in a cool, dry place, away from heat and moisture.

Teach Client/Family

- Because it is a uterine stimulant, caution the client not to use mugwort during pregnancy. Until more research is available, caution the client not to use this herb during lactation and not to give it to children
- Advise the client that mugwort and hazelnut can produce cross-sensitivity reactions.
- Caution the client not to use mugwort if he or she is allergic to hazelnut (Caballero, 1997) or other members of the Compositae family.

🍀 Endangered Herb   Adverse effects: BOLD = life-threatening

Pharmacology

Pharmacokinetics

Pharmacokinetics and pharmacodynamics are unknown.

Primary Chemical Components of Mugwort and Their Possible Actions		
Chemical Class	**Individual Component**	**Possible Action**
Volatile oil	Thujone	Uterine stimulant
	Camphor; Linalool; Cineole; Terpineol; Borneol; Monoterpene	
Sesquiterpene lactone		
Glycoside	Quercetin; Rutin	
Coumarin	Aesculetin; Aesculin; Scopoletin; Coumarin; Dioxycoumarin; Umbelliferone	
Polyacetylene		
Triterpene		
Sitosterol		
Stigmasterol		
Carotenoid		

Actions

Little research is available to document the actions of mugwort. A few initial studies have become available on its antiviral and antibacterial actions.

Antiviral Action

One study found mugwort to be active against the herpes simplex virus. Among 78 study participants, a cure occurred in 38, and significant improvement occurred in 37. The remaining three experienced no change in herpetic keratitis caused by HSV-1 (Zheng, 1990).

Antibacterial Action

Another study (Chen, 1989) determined that mugwort exerts a strong antibacterial effect against *Streptococcus mutans*. Several other herbs were tested in this study, with varying results.

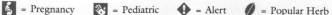

= Pregnancy　　= Pediatric　　= Alert　　= Popular Herb

References

Caballero T et al: IgE crossreactivity between mugwort pollen *(Artemisia vulgaris)* and hazelnut *(Abellana nux)* in sera from patients with sensitivity to both extracts, *Clin Exp Allery* 27(10):1203-1211, 1997.

Chen L et al: Screening of Taiwanese crude drugs for antibacterial activity against *Streptococcus mutans, J Ethnopharmacol* 27(3):285-295, 1989.

Zheng M: Experimental study of 472 herbs with antiviral action against the herpes simplex virus, *Zhong Xi Yi Jie He Za Zhi* 10(1):39-41, 46, 1990.

Mullein
(muh'luhn)

Scientific names: *Verbascum thapsus, Verbasci flos*

Other common names: Aaron's rod, bunny's ears, candle-wick, flannel-leaf, great mullein, Jacob's staff

M

Origin: Mullein is a biennial herb found in Europe, Asia, and the United States.

Uses

Reported Uses

Mullein is used as an expectorant and antitussive to treat cough, the common cold, and upper respiratory conditions. It is often used in combination with other herbs to treat bronchitis and asthma. Mullein is also used to treat urinary tract infections, chronic otitis media, and eczema of the ear.

Product Availability and Dosages

Available Forms

Capsules, fluid extract, oil

Plant Parts Used: Dried leaves, flowers

Dosages and Routes

Adult

All dosages listed are PO.

- Capsules: 580 mg taken bid with meals
- Flowers: 3-4 g qd (Blumenthal, 1998)
- Fluid extract: 1.5-2 ml bid (1:1 dilution)
- Leaves: place 2 tsp dried leaves in 8 oz boiling water, steep 15 min; may be taken tid

🍀 Endangered Herb   Adverse effects: BOLD = life-threatening

- Oil: 5-10 drops qd
- Powdered, crushed, cut, or whole plant: 2 g/day

Precautionary Information

Contraindications

Until more research is available, mullein should not be used during pregnancy and lactation and should not be given to children. This herb should not be used by persons with hypersensitivity to it.

Side Effects/Adverse Reactions

Central Nervous System: Drowsiness
Gastrointestinal: Nausea, anorexia
Integumentary: Hypersensitivity reactions, contact dermatitis

Interactions with Mullein

Drug
Oral Medications: Mullein may decrease the absorption of oral medication; separate by 2 hr.

Food	Herb	Lab Test
None known	None known	None known

Client Considerations

Assess

- Assess for hypersensitivity reactions, contact dermatitis. If these are present, discontinue use of mullein and administer antihistamine or other appropriate therapy.

Administer

- Instruct the client to store mullein products in a cool, dry place, away from heat and moisture.

Teach Client/Family

- Until more research is available, caution the client not to use mullein during pregnancy and lactation and not to give it to children.

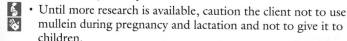
 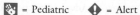

Pharmacology

Pharmacokinetics

Pharmacokinetics and pharmacodynamics are unknown.

Primary Chemical Components of Mullein and Their Possible Actions		
Chemical Class	**Individual Component**	**Possible Action**
Saponin Glycoside	Verbascoside; Forsythoside B	Antiinflammatory; antioxidant; antitumor
Complex carbohydrate	D-galactose; Arabinose; D-xylose; D-glucose	
Flavonoid		
Sterol		
Fructose		
Glucose		

Actions

Very few research studies are available for mullein. Those that have been done focus primarily on its antiviral properties.

Antiviral Action

Two studies have focused on the antiviral action of mullein. In one study, 100 plant extracts were screened for antiviral activity against seven viruses. Mullein was found to be effective against herpesvirus type I (McCutcheon, 1995). A recent study identified mullein's antiviral activity against herpes suis virus (Zanon, 1999).

Other Actions

Another study (Zheng, 1993) showed that verbascoside, a chemical component of mullein, possesses antioxidant, anticancer, and antiinflammatory properties.

References

Blumenthal M, editor: *The complete German Commission E monographs: therapeutic guide to herbal medicines,* Austin, Tex, American Botanical Council; Boston, Integrative Medicine Communication, 1998.

McCutcheon AR et al: Antiviral screening of British Columbian medicinal plants, *J Ethnopharmacol* 499(2):101-110, 1995.

Zanon SM et al: Search for antiviral activity of certain medicinal plants from Cordoba, Argentina, *Rev Latinoam Microbiol* 41(2):59-62, 1999.

Zheng RL et al: Inhibition of autooxidation of linoleic acid by phenylpropanoid glycosides from *Pedicularis* in micelles, *Chem Phys Lipids* 65:151-154, 1993.

Mustard
(muh'stuhrd)

Scientific names: *Brassica nigra, Brassica alba*

Other common names: Black mustard, brown mustard, California rape, charlock, Chinese mustard, Indian mustard, white mustard, wild mustard

Class 1 (Internal)
Class 2d (External, Seed)

Origin: Mustard is found in the Mediterranean region, Europe, and India.

Uses

Reported Uses

Mustard traditionally has been used for diuresis, as an emetic, as an antiflatulent, and to treat inflammation and pain of joints. However, it is better known for its use in "mustard plaster," which is used topically to treat respiratory congestion (bronchial pneumonia, pleurisy).

Product Availability and Dosages

Available Forms

Flour, oil, seeds, tea

Plant Parts Used: Seeds

Dosages and Routes

All dosages listed are topical.

Adult

Decongestant

- Flour poultice: mix 100 g mustard flour with warm water, pack in linen, place on chest 10 min
- Mustard plaster: mix 4 oz ground black mustard seeds with warm water to make a paste, apply to chest area

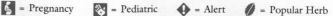

![Pregnancy icon] = Pregnancy   ![Pediatric icon] = Pediatric   ◆ = Alert   ✏ = Popular Herb

Footsoak
- Seeds: place 1 tbsp seeds in 1000 ml hot water, soak feet 15-20 min

Child
Decongestant
- Flour poultice: mix 100 g mustard flour with warm water, pack in linen, place on chest maximum 3-5 min

Precautionary Information
Contraindications
Until more research is available, mustard should not be used therapeutically during pregnancy and lactation and should not be given therapeutically to children younger than 6 years of age. Mustard should not be used therapeutically by persons with hypersensitivity to it or by those with renal disorders, gastrointestinal ulcers, or inflammatory kidney diseases. Do not use mustard on unprotected skin. Class 1 herb (internal); class 2d herb (external, seed).

Side Effects/Adverse Reactions
Endocrine: Goiter
Integumentary: Hypersensitivity reactions, irritation of skin where applied, contact dermatitis

M

Interactions with Mustard			
Drug	**Food**	**Herb**	**Lab Test**
None known	None known	None known	None known

Client Considerations
Assess
- Assess for hypersensitivity reactions or skin irritation where mustard has been applied. Administer antihistamine or other appropriate therapy if necessary. Olive oil may be used to soothe skin after removing mustard plaster.

Administer
- Instruct the client not to use mustard for more than 30 minutes at a time or for longer than 2 weeks.

- Instruct the client to wash hands well with soap and water after use to prevent irritation.
- Instruct the client to store mustard products in a cool, dry place, away from heat and moisture.

Teach Client/Family

- Until more research is available, caution the client not to use mustard therapeutically during pregnancy and lactation and not to give it therapeutically to children younger than 6 years of age.
- Advise the client to keep mustard out of reach of children and to avoid applying it around mucous membranes.
- Inform the client that sneezing, coughing, and possible asthmatic attacks can result from breathing the allylisothiocyanate that arises with preparation and application of mustard poultices.

Pharmacology

Pharmacokinetics

Pharmacokinetics and pharmacodynamics are unknown.

Primary Chemical Components of Mustard and Their Possible Actions		
Chemical Class	**Individual Component**	**Possible Action**
Sinigrin		
Myrosin		
Sinapic acid		
Sinapine		
Fixed oil	Arachic acid; Erucic acid; Eicosenoic acid; Oleic acid; Palmitic acid	
Mucilage		
Globulin		
Volatile oil	Isothiocyanate	Blistering
Protein		

Actions

Very little research has been done on mustard. One study evaluated its anticholesterol action, with negative results. No change occurred in the cholesterol levels of rats fed amounts five times

 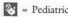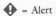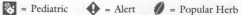

that of normal human consumption (Sambaiah, 1991). Another study showed that mustard oil used in laboratory animals produced an anticancer action (Choudhury, 1997).

References

Choudbury AR et al: Mustard oil and garlic extract as inhibitors of sodium arsenite-induced chromosomal breaks in vivo, *Cancer Lett* 121:45-52, 1997.

Sambaiah K et al: Effect of cumin, cinnamon, ginger, mustard and tamarind in induced hypercholesterolemic rats, *Nahrung* 35(1):47-51, 1991.

Myrrh
(muhr)

Scientific name: *Commiphora molmol*

Other common names: African myrrh, Arabian myrrh, bal, bol, bola, gum myrrh, heerabol, Somali myrrh, Yemen myrrh   **Class 2b/2d (Gum Resin)**

M

Origin: Myrrh is a shrub found in various regions of Africa.

Uses

Reported Uses

Myrrh traditionally has been used internally to treat upper respiratory congestion, pharyngitis, gingivitis, mouth ulcers, stomatitis, and leg ulcers. Topically, it is used to treat wounds, decubitus ulcers, and hemorrhoids. Contemporary use is mostly limited to flavoring in foods and fragrance in cosmetic products.

Investigational Uses

Researchers are experimenting with the use of myrrh in combination with other products to treat colds and infections.

Product Availability and Dosages

Available Forms

Capsules, fluid extract, mouthwash, resin, tincture

Plant Parts Used: Gum, oil, resin

Dosages and Routes
Adult
- PO mouthwash: mix 5-10 drops in glass of water (Blumenthal, 1998)
- PO tea: place 2 tsp resin in 8 oz boiling water, steep 15 min; may be taken tid
- Topical tincture: 1-4 ml may be applied to the affected area bid-tid

Precautionary Information
Contraindications
Until more research is available, myrrh should not be used during pregnancy and lactation and should not be given to children. Myrrh should not be used by persons with hypersensitivity to it or by those with fever, severe uterine bleeding, or tachycardia. Class 2b/2d herb (gum resin).

Side Effects/Adverse Reactions
Central Nervous System: Anxiety, restlessness
Gastrointestinal: Nausea, vomiting, anorexia, diarrhea
Integumentary: Hypersensitivity reactions, dermatitis

Interactions with Myrrh

Drug
Antidiabetics: Use of myrrh with antidiabetics may cause increased hypoglycemic effects; avoid concurrent use.

Food	Herb	Lab Test
None known	None known	None known

Client Considerations
Assess
- Assess for hypersensitivity reactions. If these are present, discontinue use of myrrh and administer antihistamine or other appropriate therapy.
- Assess the client's use of antidiabetics such as insulin. Monitor blood glucose if the client is taking concurrently with myrrh (see Interactions).

= Pregnancy   = Pediatric   = Alert   = Popular Herb

Administer

• Instruct the client to store myrrh products in a cool, dry place, away from heat and moisture.

Teach Client/Family

• Until more research is available, caution the client not to use myrrh during pregnancy and lactation and not to give it to children.

Pharmacology

Pharmacokinetics

Pharmacokinetics and pharmacodynamics are unknown.

Primary Chemical Components of Myrrh and Their Possible Actions		
Chemical Class	**Individual Component**	**Possible Action**
Volatile oil	Cadinene; Dipentene; Heerabolene; Limonene; Pinene; Eugenol; Creosol; Cinnamaldehyde; Cumic alcohol; Cuminaldehyde; Myrcene; Alpha-camphorene	
Resin		
Steroid	Cholesterol; Campesterol; Beta-sitosterol	
Terpenoid	Amyrin; Furanosesquiterpenoid	

Actions

Several studies have focused on the actions of myrrh. Myrrh has been found to decrease cholesterol levels, decrease inflammation, provide analgesia, act as an antiulcer and antitumor agent, and stimulate triiodothyronine production.

Antilipidemic Action

When myrrh was studied along with garlic for reduction of cholesterol, triglycerides, and phospholipids, garlic was found to be far superior to myrrh (Dixit, 1980). However, when myrrh was studied with *Allium sativum* and *Allium cepa,* all three agents were found to prevent a rise in these three indicators (Lata, 1991).

🌱 Endangered Herb   Adverse effects: BOLD = life-threatening

Antiinflammatory and Antipyretic Actions

Three studies have identified the antiinflammatory action of myrrh. One study used laboratory animals that had been injected with liquid paraffin containing killed mycobacterial adjuvant. In this study, phenylbutazone, ibuprofen, and a fraction of myrrh all were shown to provide significant relief of arthritis symptoms (Sharma, 1977). The other studies identified a triterpene with antiinflammatory and analgesic properties (Dolara, 2000; Fourie, 1989). In this study, a significant antiinflammatory effect occurred when myrrh was administered to mice. In another study, an antipyretic action was observed (Tariq, 1986).

Anticancer Action

Myrrh's anticancer action has been demonstrated in a study using mice. The study evaluated results at 25 to 50 days. Anticarcinogenic results were less pronounced after 50 days. The effect was comparable to that of cyclophosphamide (Al-Harbi, 1994). Another study showed similar results, leading researchers to conclude that the use of myrrh for the treatment of cancer is appropriate (Qureshi, 1993).

References

Al-Harbi MM et al: Anticarcinogenic effect of *Commiphora molmol* on solid tumors induced by *Ehrlich carcinoma* cells in mice, *Chemotherapy* 40(5):337-347, 1994.

Blumenthal M, editor: *The complete German Commission E monographs: therapeutic guide to herbal medicines,* Austin, Tex, American Botanical Council; Boston, Integrative Medicine Communication, 1998.

Dixit VP et al: Hypolipidemic activity of guggal resin *(Commiphora mukul)* and garlic *(Alium sativum* linn.) in dogs *(Canis familiaris)* and monkeys *(Presbytis entellus entellus* Dufresne), *Biochem Exp Biol* 16(4): 421-424, 1980.

Dolara P et al: Local anaesthetic, antibacterial, and antifungal properties of sesquiterpenes from myrrh, *Planta Med* 66(4):356-358, 2000.

Fourie TG et al: A pentacyclic triterpene with anti-inflammatory and analgesic activity from the roots of *Commiphora merkeri, J Nat Prod* 52(5):1129-1131, 1989.

Lata S et al: Beneficial effects of *Allium sativum, Allium cepa,* and *Commiphora mukul* on experimental hyperlipidemia and atherosclerosis—a comparative evaluation, *J Postgrad Med* 37(3):132-135, 1991.

Qureshi S et al: Evaluation of the genotoxic, cytotoxic, and antitumor properties of *Commiphora molmol* using normal and Ehrlich ascites carcinoma cell-bearing Swiss albino mice, *Cancer Chemother Pharmacol* 33(2):130-138, 1993.

Sharma JN et al: Comparison of the anti-inflammatory activity of *Commiphora mukul* (an indigenous drug) with those of phenylbuta-

⚕ = Pregnancy   **⚗** = Pediatric   **❗** = Alert   **✐** = Popular Herb

zone and ibuprofen in experimental arthritis induced by mycobacterial adjuvant, *Arzneimittelforschung* 27(7):1455-1457, 1977.

Tariq M et al: Anti-inflammatory activity of *Commiphora molmol*, *Agents Actions* 17(3-4):381-382, 1986.

Myrtle
(muhr'tuhl)

Scientific name: *Myrtus communis*

Other common names: Bridal myrtle, common myrtle, Dutch myrtle, Jew's myrtle, mirth, Roman myrtle

Origin: Myrtle is found in the Middle East and Mediterranean regions.

Uses

Reported Uses

Myrtle traditionally has been used to treat respiratory congestion, gastrointestinal conditions, urinary tract infections, and worm infestations. It is also used topically as an astringent.

Investigational Uses

Initial research is underway to determine the efficacy of myrtle as an antidiabetic agent.

Product Availability and Dosages

Available Forms

Extract, oil

Plant Parts Used: Leaves, seeds

Dosages and Routes

Adult
- PO extract: 0.2 g as a single dose
- PO oil: 2 ml qd

Precautionary Information

Contraindications

Until more research is available, myrtle should not be used during pregnancy and lactation and it should not be given to children. Myrtle should not be used internally by persons

Continued

Precautionary Information—cont'd

Contraindications—cont'd

with inflammation of the gastrointestinal tract or liver disease. Persons with hypersensitivity to this herb should not use it. Clients with diabetes mellitus should use myrtle cautiously.

Side Effects/Adverse Reactions

Endocrine: Hypoglycemia
Gastrointestinal: Nausea, vomiting, anorexia
Integumentary: Hypersensitivity reactions

Interactions with Myrtle

Drug

Antidiabetics: Use of myrtle with antidiabetics such as insulin may cause increased hypoglycemia; do not use concurrently.
Cytochrome P-450: Concurrent use of myrtle with drugs metabolized by cytochrome P-450 should be avoided.

Food	Herb	Lab Test
None known	None known	None known

Client Considerations

Assess

- Assess for hypersensitivity reactions. If these are present, discontinue use of myrtle and administer antihistamine or other appropriate therapy.
- Monitor blood glucose levels in diabetic clients who are taking antidiabetic agents concurrently with myrtle (see Interactions).
- Monitor liver function studies (ALT, AST, bilirubin). If results are elevated, use of myrtle should be discontinued.

Administer

- Instruct the client to store myrtle products in a cool, dry place, away from heat and moisture.

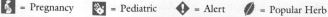

 = Pregnancy   = Pediatric   ◆ = Alert   🖋 = Popular Herb

Teach Client/Family

- Until more research is available, caution the client not to use myrtle during pregnancy and lactation and not to give it to children.
- Advise the client to use the essential oil only under the direction of a qualified herbalist. Overdoses can lead to life-threatening poisoning resulting from high cineol content.

Pharmacology

Pharmacokinetics

Pharmacokinetics and pharmacodynamics are unknown.

Primary Chemical Components of Myrtle and Their Possible Actions		
Chemical Class	Individual Component	Possible Action
Volatile oil	Myrtol; Gelomytrol; Eucalyptol; Pinene; Camphor; Cineol; Myrtenylacetate; Limonene; Alpha-terpineol; Geraniol	
Tannin		Wound healing; astringent
Acylphloroglucinols	Myrtucommulone A	Antibacterial

Actions

Very little research has been done on myrtle, with only one or two research articles at most for any of its actions.

Antihyperglycemic Action

One study older study identified the antihyperglycemic action of myrtle on streptozocin-induced diabetic mice (Elfellah, 1984). Blood glucose levels dropped significantly after administration of myrtle. No effect was observed on normal blood glucose levels.

Hemagglutinin Action

The phytohemagglutinins in myrtle have been found to be useful in the preparation of laboratory samples. Addition of phytohemagglutinins to the samples clarifies the contents and allows for increased visibility (Ortega, 1979).

Antiinflammatory Action

A recent study on laboratory rats has evaluated the antiinflammatory action of myrtle. Rat paws were injected with carrageenan to induce inflammation. When compared with other herbs, *Myrtus communis* was the least effective in the reduction of inflammation (Al-Hindawi, 1989).

Other Actions

One toxicology study using laboratory rats identified the toxicity of myrtle after ingestion of the essential oil from the leaves of *Myrtus communis* (Uehleke, 1979). Interestingly, the rats were able to adapt to myrtle ingestion after repeat dosing. Infections of *Pseudomonas aeruginosa* are susceptible to myrtle (Al-Saimary, 2002).

References

Al-Hindawi MK et al: Anti-inflammatory activity of some Iraqi plants using intact rats, *J Ethnopharmacol* 26(2):163-168, 1989.

Al-Saimary IE et al: Effects of some plant extracts and antibiotics on *Pseudomonas aeruginosa* isolated from various burn cases, *Saudi Med J* 23(7):802-805, 2002.

Elfellah MS et al: Anti-hyperglycaemic effect of an extract of *Myrtus communis* in streptozotocin-induced diabetes in mice, *J Ethnopharmacol* 11(3):275-281, 1984.

Ortega M et al: *Myrtus communis* L. phytohemmagglutinins as a clarifying agent for lipemic sera, *Clin Chim Acta* 92(2):135-139, 1979.

Uehleke H et al: Oral toxicity of an essential oil from myrtle and adaptive liver stimulation, *Toxicology* 12(3):335-342, 1979.

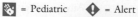

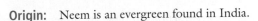

Neem
(neem)

Scientific name: *Azadirachta indica*

Other common names: Margosa, nim, nimba

Origin: Neem is an evergreen found in India.

Uses
Reported Uses
Neem traditionally has been used as an anthelmintic and to treat malaria and diabetes mellitus. It has also been used topically to treat skin conditions. It is an antiinflammatory and antipyretic. Neem has been used intravaginally as a contraceptive.

Investigational Uses
Researchers are experimenting with the use of neem as a contraceptive and an antiinfective.

Product Availability and Dosages
Available Forms
Tincture

Plant Parts Used: Whole plant

Dosages and Routes
No dosage consensus exists.

Precautionary Information
Contraindications
Until more research is available, neem should not be used during pregnancy and lactation and should not be given to children. **Infants have died after ingesting neem oil.** Persons with hypersensitivity to neem should not use it.

Side Effects/Adverse Reactions
Gastrointestinal: Nausea, vomiting, anorexia
Integumentary: Hypersensitivity reactions
Systemic: REYE'S-LIKE SYMPTOMS (infants)

Interactions with Neem			
Drug	**Food**	**Herb**	**Lab Test**
None known	None known	None known	None known

Client Considerations

Assess

- Assess for hypersensitivity reactions. If these are present, discontinue use of neem and administer antihistamine or other appropriate therapy.

Administer

- Instruct the client to store neem in a cool, dry place, away from heat and moisture.

Teach Client/Family

- Until more research is available, caution the client not to use neem during pregnancy and lactation and not to give it to children.

Pharmacology

Pharmacokinetics

Pharmacokinetics and pharmacodynamics are unknown.

Primary Chemical Components of Neem and Their Possible Actions		
Chemical Class	**Individual Component**	**Possible Action**
Triterpenoid	Nimocinol; Meliacinol (Siddiqui, 2000) Odoratone; Trihydroxypregnan; Diacetoxyapotirucall	Insecticide
Mahmoodin	Antibacterial Gedunin; Nimbolide Azadirone; Epoxyazadiradione; Nimbin; Azadiradione; Deacetylnimbin; Hydroxyazadiradione	Antimalarial
Limonoid	Deoxonimbolide Naheedin	Antitumor

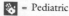 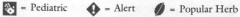

Actions

Several research articles have focused on the actions of neem. Proposed actions include antimalarial, antifertility, immunomodulatory, hypotensive, antiinflammatory, antihyperglycemic, anxiolytic, hepatoprotective, and antimicrobial.

Hepatoprotective, Gastroprotective Action

Hepatotoxicity was induced in rats by using paracetamol. Administration of *Azadirachta indica* significantly reduced liver toxicity as measured by AST, ALT, and histopathologic study of the liver (Bhanwra, 2000). One study (Bandyopadhyay, 2002) identified the gastroprotective effect of neem including control of hyperacidity and ulcer.

Hypoglycemic Action

In one study, diabetic rabbits were given neem leaf extract and seeds. Blood glucose levels were significantly reduced at the end of 4 weeks (Khosla, 2000). When neem was started 2 weeks before the rabbits were diabetically induced, diabetes was partially prevented. This information may be useful for the prevention of, or to delay the onset of, the disease. Another study using rats showed the inhibition of serotonin on insulin secretion that is mediated by glucose (Chattopadhyay, 1999). The leaf extract significantly decreased hyperglycemia.

Antimicrobial and Antimalarial Actions

Neem leaf extract was evaluated for its effects against coxsackievirus B. In an in vitro study of African green monkeys, coxsackie 4 virus was significantly inhibited at levels of 1000 μg/ml at 96 hours (Badam, 1999). Another study identified antiplaque, anticaries, and antimicrobial effects of the neem chewing sticks called Miswak that are used in the Middle East and on the Indian subcontinent (Almas, 1999). The effects were evaluated using blood agar and other methods up to 48 hours after chewing of the sticks. Neem was found to be effective against *Streptococcus mutans* and *Streptococcus faecalis*. A study evaluating the antimalarial action of neem found that the herb is effective even against parasites that are resistant to other antimalarial agents (Dhar, 1998).

Immunomodulatory Action

Immune response was evaluated in laboratory mice and found to be increased after the use of neem. This information corroborates the use of neem for the treatment of many infectious and noninfectious conditions (Nijiro, 1999).

Antifertility Action

Several studies have dealt with the antifertility properties of neem. One study using rats evaluated the effect of neem leaves on the seminal vesicles and ventral prostate. After various oral doses were administered for 24 days, investigators observed a decrease in the weights of the seminal vesicles and ventral prostate. These results suggest that neem exerts an antiandrogenic action (Aladakatti, 2001; Kasutri, 1997). Another study evaluated the occurrence of spontaneous abortion in primates given neem (Mukherjee, 1996). Neem seed extract was given orally for 6 days after pregnancy was confirmed. Termination of pregnancy occurred, as evidenced by a decline in progesterone and chorionic gonadotropin.

References

Aladakatti RH et al: Sperm parameters changes induced by *Azadirachta indica* in albino rats, *J Basic Clin Physiol Pharmacol* 12(1):69-76, 2001.

Almas K: The antimicrobial effects of extracts of *Azadirachta indica* (neem) and *Salvadora persica* (arak) chewing sticks, *Indian J Dent Res* 10(1):23-26, 1999.

Badam L et al: "In vitro" antiviral activity of neem (*Azadirachta indica* A. Juss) leaf extract against group B coxsackieviruses, *J Commun Dis* 31(2):79-90, 1999.

Bandyopadhyay U et al: Gastroprotective effect of neem bark extract: possible involvement of H(+)-K(+)-ATPase inhibition and scavenging hydroxyl radical, *Life Sci* 17(24):2845, 2002.

Bhanwra S et al: Effect of *Azadirachta indica* (neem) leaf aqueous extract on paracetamol-induced liver damage in rats, *Indian J Physiol Pharmacol* 44(1):64-68, 2000 (in-process citation).

Chattopadhyay RR et al: *J Ethnopharmacol* 67(3):373-376, 1999.

Dhar R et al: Inhibition of the growth and development of asexual and sexual stages of drug-sensitive and resistant strains of the human malaria parasite *Plasmodium falciparum* by neem (*Azadirachta indica*) fractions, *J Ethnopharmacol* 61(1):31-39, 1998.

Kasutri M et al: Effects of *Azadirachta indica* leaves on the seminal vesicles and ventral prostate in albino rats, *Indian J Physiol Pharmacol* 41(3):234-240, 1997.

Khosla P et al: A study of hypoglycemic effects of *Azadirachta indica* (neem) in normal and alloxan diabetic rabbits, *Indian J Physiol Pharmacol* 44(1):69-74, 2000 (in-process citation).

Mukherjee S et al: Purified neem (*Azadirachta indica*) seed extracts (praneem) abrogate pregnancy in primates, *Contraception* 53(6):375-378, 1996.

Nijiro SM et al: Effect of an aqueous extract of *Azadirachta indica* on the immune response in mice, *Onderstepoort J Vet Res* 66(1):59-62, 1999.

Siddiqui BS et al: Two insecticidal tetranortriterpenoids from *Azadirachta indica*, *Phytochemistry* 53(3):371-376, 2000.

⑤ = Pregnancy   **✋** = Pediatric   **◆** = Alert   **✦** = Popular Herb

Nettle
(neh'tuhl)

Scientific name: *Urtica dioica*

Other common names: Common nettle, greater nettle, stinging nettle

Class 1 (Leaf)

Origin: Nettle is a perennial found in Europe, the United States, and Canada.

Uses

Reported Uses

Nettle traditionally has been used as a tea to treat cough, tuberculosis, and other respiratory conditions including allergic rhinitis. It is used as an expectorant, an astringent, a diuretic, and as a treatment for urinary tract disorders. Nettle is recognized as a bladder irrigant to reduce blood loss and inflammation in bladder conditions; benign prostatic hypertrophy (BPH). Nettle is also used for arthritis pain, often in conjunction with low doses of NSAIDs. It is used externally as a hair and scalp remedy for oily hair and dandruff.

Investigational Uses

Nettle may be used as a diuretic; to lower blood pressure; and for prostate cancer.

Product Availability and Dosages

Available Forms

Capsules, dried leaves, root extract, root tincture

Plant Parts Used: Leaves, roots, stems

Dosages and Routes

Adult

All dosages listed are PO.
- Capsules: 150-300 mg qd
- Tea: place 2 tsp dried leaves in 8 oz boiling water, steep 15 min; may be taken bid
- Tincture: ½-1 tsp qd-bid

N

Precautionary Information

Contraindications

Until more research is available, nettle should not be used during pregnancy (uterine contractions may occur) and lactation, it should not be given to children younger than 2 years of age, and caution should be used when giving nettle to older children. Elderly persons should use this herb cautiously. Persons with hypersensitivity to nettle should not use it. Class 1 herb (leaf).

Side Effects/Adverse Reactions

Gastrointestinal: Nausea, vomiting, anorexia, diarrhea, gastrointestinal irritation
Integumentary: Hypersensitivity reactions, urticaria
Miscellaneous: Oliguria, edema

Interactions with Nettle

Drug

Anticoagulants (heparin, warfarin): Nettle may decrease the effect of anticoagulants; avoid concurrent use.
Central nervous system depressants (alcohol, barbiturates, sedative/hypnotics, antipsychotics, opiates): Nettle may lead to increased central nervous system depression.
Diuretics: Use of nettle may increase the effects of diuretics, resulting in dehydration and hypokalemia; avoid concurrent use.
Iron salts: Nettle tea may interfere with the absorption of iron salts.
Lithium: Nettle combined with lithium may result in dehydration, lithium toxicity.

Food	Herb	Lab Test
None known	None known	None known

Client Considerations

Assess

- Assess for hypersensitivity reactions. If these are present, discontinue use of nettle and administer antihistamine or other appropriate therapy.

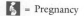 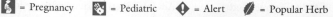

Administer

- Recommend that the client increase his or her intake of potassium-containing foods to prevent hypokalemia.
- Instruct the client to store nettle products in a cool, dry place, away from heat and moisture.

Teach Client/Family

- Until more research is available, caution the client not to use nettle during pregnancy and lactation, not to give it to children younger than 2 years of age, and to use caution when giving nettle to older children.
- Advise the client to use nettle as a urinary tract irrigant only under the supervision of a qualified herbalist.
- Inform the client that stinging and burning will result if the plant is touched.

Pharmacology

Pharmacokinetics

Pharmacokinetics and pharmacodynamics are unknown.

Primary Chemical Components of Nettle and Their Possible Actions		
Chemical Class	Individual Component	Possible Action
Scopoletin		Antiinflammatory
Glucoside		
Flavonoid	Rutin	
Amine	Choline; Histamine; Serotonin; Formic acid	
Volatile oil	Ketones	
Potassium ion		
Pygeum Beta-sitosterol		Improves benign prostatic hypertrophy

Actions

Benign Prostatic Hyperplasia (BPH) Action

Several studies have been performed to confirm the BPH action of nettle. Three double-blind controlled studies showed a considerable improvement in urologic function after nettle was given to 72 men, 40 women, and 50 men, respectively. The change in urination occurred within 4 weeks to 6 months, depending on the study (Dathe, 1987, European-Scientific, 1996-1997, Vontobel, 1985).

Anticancer Action

One recent study has shown that the use of stinging nettle root extract slows the progression of prostate cancer (Konrad, 2000). The rate of slowing observed was statistically significant.

Analgesic and Antiinflammatory Actions

In one study, nettle was shown to be an effective and inexpensive treatment for joint pain (Randall, 1999). (A randomized controlled study with a rheumatology specialist is planned.) In another study with similar results (Riehemann, 1999), nettle decreased the inflammation associated with rheumatoid arthritis.

Other Actions

Nettle was found to possess diuretic and hypotensive effects when a continuous perfusion of the aqueous extract was administered to rats (Tahri, 2000).

References

Dathe G et al: Phytotherapy of benign prostatic hyperplasia (BPH): double-blind study with stinging nettle root extract, *Urolage B,* 27:223-226, 1987.

European-Scientific Cooperative on Phytotherapy: *Urticae radix, Egcop* 2:2-4, 1996-1997.

Konrad L et al: Antiproliferative effect on human prostate cancer cells by a stinging nettle root *(Urtica dioica)* extract, *Planta Med* 66(1):44-47, 2000.

Randall C et al: Nettle sting of *Urtica diocia* for joint pain—an exploratory study of this complementary therapy, *Complement Ther Med* 7(3):126-131, 1999.

Riehemann K et al: Plant extracts from stinging nettle *(Urtica dioica),* an antirheumatic remedy, inhibit the proinflammatory transcription factor NF-kappaB, *FEBS Lett* 442(1):89-94, 1999.

Tahri A et al: Acute diuretic, natriuretic and hypotensive effects of a continuous perfusion of aqueous extract of *Urtica diocia* in the rat, *J Ethnopharmacol* 73(1-2):95-100, 2000.

Vontobel HP et al: Results of a double-blind study on the effectiveness of extracting radicis Urticae capsules as conservative treatment of BPH, *Urologe A,* 49-51, 1985.

New Zealand Green-Lipped Mussel
(new zee'luhnd green lipt muh'suhl)

Scientific name: *Perna canaliculus*

Other common name: NZGLM

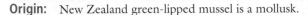

Origin: New Zealand green-lipped mussel is a mollusk.

Uses

Reported Uses

May be used to decrease inflammation and as a treatment for osteoarthritis and rheumatoid arthritis.

Product Availability and Dosages

Available Forms

Capsule

Parts Used: Whole mussel

Dosages and Routes

No dosage consensus exists.

Precautionary Information

Contraindications

Until more research is available, New Zealand green-lipped mussel should not be used during pregnancy and lactation and should not be given to children. Persons with hypersensitivity to shellfish should not use New Zealand green-lipped mussel.

Side Effects/Adverse Reactions

Gastrointestinal: Nausea, vomiting, anorexia
Integumentary: Hypersensitivity reactions

Interactions with New Zealand Green-Lipped Mussel			
Drug	Food	Herb	Lab Test
None known	None known	None known	None known

🍃 Endangered Herb   Adverse effects: **BOLD** = life-threatening

Client Considerations

Assess

- Assess for hypersensitivity reactions. If these are present, discontinue use of New Zealand green-lipped mussel and administer antihistamine or other appropriate therapy.

Administer

- Instruct the client to store New Zealand green-lipped mussel products in a cool, dry place, away from heat and moisture.

Teach Client/Family

- Until more research is available, caution the client not to use New Zealand green-lipped mussel during pregnancy and lactation and not to give it to children.

Pharmacology

Pharmacokinetics

Pharmacokinetics and pharmacodynamics are unknown.

Actions

Antiinflammatory Action

Several studies have evaluated the antiinflammatory action of New Zealand green-lipped mussel. All have shown similar results, with significant antiinflammatory effects documented (Caughey, 1983; Couch, 1982; Halpern, 2001; Miller, 1980, 1993). These studies used various experimental models.

Other Actions

One study (Emelyanov, 2002) identified the positive outcome when New Zealand green-lipped mussel is used for asthma. Since asthma is an inflammatory condition, it was considered appropriate for development of this research model.

References

Caughey DE et al: Perna canaliculus in the treatment of rheumatoid arthritis, *Eur J Rheumatol Inflamm* 6(2):197-200, 1983.

Couch RA et al: Anti-inflammatory activity in fractionated extracts of the green-lipped mussel, *N Z Med J* 95(720):803-806, 1982.

Emelyanov A et al: Treatment of asthma with lipid extract of New Zealand green-lipped mussel: a randomized clinical trial, *Eur Respir J* 20(3): 596-600, 2002.

Halpern GM: Anti-inflammatory effects of stabilized lipid extract of *Perna Canaliculus, Allerg Immunol* 32(7):272-278, 2000.

Miller TE et al: The anti-inflammatory activity of *Perna canaliculus* (New Zealand green lipped mussel), *N Z Med J* 92(667):187-193, 1980.

Miller TE et al: Antiinflammatory activity of glycogen extracted from *Perna Canaliculus* (NZ green-lipped mussel), *Agents Actions* 38(Spec): C139-142, 1993.

Night-Blooming Cereus
(nite blew'ming si'ree-uhs)

Scientific name: *Selenicereus grandiflorus*

Other common names: Large-flowered cactus, queen of the night, sweet-scented cactus, vanilla cactus   **Class 1 (Flower, Stem)**

Origin: Night-blooming cereus is found in the tropics of North America.

Uses
Reported Uses
Night-blooming cereus has been used to treat cardiac conditions such as angina pectoris, endocarditis, myocarditis, and palpitations, as well as urinary tract disorders such as cystitis, irritable bladder, and edema. Other disorders include hyperthyroidism and benign prostatic hypertrophy.

Product Availability and Dosages
Available Forms
Fluid extract, tincture

Plant Parts Used: Flowers, stems

Dosages and Routes
Adult
- PO fluid extract: 0.7 ml q4h
- PO tincture: 1.2-1.8 ml q4h

Precautionary Information
Contraindications
Until more research is available, night-blooming cereus should not be used during the first trimester of pregnancy or during lactation. Persons with hypertension, severe cardiac

Continued

> ## Precautionary Information—cont'd
> ### Contraindications—cont'd
> disorders, or hypersensitivity to this plant should not use it. Class 1 herb (flower, stem).
>
> ### Side Effects/Adverse Reactions
> *Gastrointestinal:* Nausea, vomiting, anorexia, diarrhea, stinging or burning in the oral cavity
> *Integumentary:* Hypersensitivity reactions

Interactions with Night-Blooming Cereus

Drug

Cardiac glycosides: Night-blooming cereus may increase the actions of cardiac glycosides such as digoxin and digitoxin; avoid concurrent use.

MAOIs: Use of MAOIs may increase the cardiac effects of night-blooming cereus; avoid concurrent use. Since tyramine is present in night-blooming cereus, this herb should be avoided with MAOIs (theoretical).

Food	Herb	Lab Test
None known	None known	None known

Client Considerations

Assess

- Assess for hypersensitivity reactions. If these are present, discontinue use of night-blooming cereus and administer antihistamine or other appropriate therapy.
- Assess the cardiac client for use of MAOIs or cardiac drugs; recommend that the client avoid concurrent use of night-blooming cereus with these products (see Interactions).
- Monitor heart rate, rhythm, and character.

Administer

- Instruct the client to store night-blooming cereus products in a cool, dry place, away from heat and moisture.

Teach Client/Family

• Until more research is available, caution the client not to use this herb during the first trimester of pregnancy or during lactation.

Pharmacology

Pharmacokinetics

Pharmacokinetics and pharmacodynamics are unknown.

Primary Chemical Components of Night-Blooming Cereus and Their Possible Actions		
Chemical Class	**Individual Component**	**Possible Action**
Glycoside	Cactine; Hordenine	Cardiac glycoside
Flavonoid	Kaempferitrin; Rutin	Improved capillary function, dilatation
	Narcissin; Cacticine; N-methyl tyramine	
Betacyan	Rutinoside	Improved capillary function
Isorhamnetin		
Betacyanin		
Narcissin		
Grandiflorine		
Hyperoside		
Isorhamnetin		

Actions

Very little research is available for night-blooming cereus, and results of existing studies are inconclusive (Wadworth, 1992; Hapke, 1995). However, two of its chemical components, cactine and hordenine, are known to be cardiac glycosides.

References

Hapke HJ: Pharmacological effects of hordenine, *Dtsch Tierarztl Wochenschr* 102:228-232, 1995 (abstract).

Wadworth NA et al: Hydroxyethylrutosides: a review of pharmacology and therapeutic efficacy in venous insufficiency and related disorders, *Drugs* 44:1013-1032, 1992.

Nutmeg
(nuht'mayg)

Scientific names: *Myristica fragrans*

Other common names: Mace, macis, muscadier, muskat-baum, myristica, noz moscada, nuez moscada, nux moschata   **Class 2b (Seeds, Aril)**

Origin: Nutmeg is a tree found in the West Indies and Sri Lanka.

Uses
Reported Uses
Nutmeg has been used traditionally for gastrointestinal disorders such as gastritis and indigestion; for anxiety, depression, toothache, nausea, and chronic diarrhea; as an antiemetic; as an aphrodisiac; and for joint pain.

Investigational Uses
Research is underway for nutmeg's use as an antimicrobial and anxiogenic.

Product Availability and Dosages
Available Forms
Capsules, essential oil, powder

Plant Parts Used: Dried seeds

Dosages and Routes
Adult
All dosages listed are PO.
Gastrointestinal Disorders
- Capsules: 2 caps as a one-time dose
- Essential oil: 4-5 drops on a sugar cube
- Powder: 4-6 tbsp qd

Precautionary Information
Contraindications

Because it can cause spontaneous abortion, nutmeg should not be used therapeutically during pregnancy. Until more research is available, nutmeg should not be used therapeutically during lactation and should not be given therapeutically

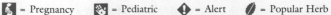

Precautionary Information—cont'd

Contraindications—cont'd

(in doses higher than that found in food) to children. Nutmeg should not be used therapeutically by persons with hypersensitivity to it, and it should be used with caution by persons with major depression and those with anxiety disorders. Class 2b herb (seeds, aril).

Side Effects/Adverse Reactions

Central Nervous System: Confusion, stupor, SEIZURES, DEATH
Gastrointestinal: Nausea, vomiting, anorexia, constipation, dry mouth
Genitourinary: SPONTANEOUS ABORTION
Integumentary: Hypersensitivity reactions

Interactions with Nutmeg

Drug

Antidiarrheals: Antidiarrheals may be potentiated by nutmeg; monitor for constipation.
MAOIs: MAOIs may be potentiated by nutmeg; avoid concurrent use.
Psychotropic agents: Psychotropic agents may be potentiated by nutmeg; avoid concurrent use.

Food	Herb	Lab Test
None known	None known	None known

Client Considerations

Assess

- Assess for hypersensitivity reactions. If these are present, discontinue use of nutmeg and administer antihistamine or other appropriate therapy.
- Assess for the use of antidiarrheals, MAOIs, and psychotropic agents (see Interactions).
- Monitor for central nervous system effects (confusion, stupor, seizures); if these occur, discontinue use of nutmeg and institute supportive measures.

🔆 Endangered Herb   Adverse effects: BOLD = life-threatening

Administer

 • Warn the client that nutmeg is toxic in large doses.
• Instruct the client to store nutmeg products in a cool, dry place, away from heat and moisture.

Teach Client/Family

 • Because it can cause spontaneous abortion, caution the client not to use nutmeg therapeutically during pregnancy. Until more research is available, caution the client not to use nutmeg therapeutically during lactation and not to give it therapeutically to children.
• Advise the client to report central nervous system effects and changes in bowel pattern.

 • Because nutmeg is toxic in large doses, caution the client not to increase the dose and to keep nutmeg out of the reach of children.
• Advise the client not to perform hazardous activities such as driving or operating heavy machinery until physical response to the herb can be evaluated.
• Caution the client not to use nutmeg with psychoactive drugs (see Interactions).

Pharmacology

Pharmacokinetics

Pharmacokinetics and pharmacodynamics are unknown.

Primary Chemical Components of Nutmeg and Their Possible Actions		
Chemical Class	**Individual Component**	**Possible Action**
Fixed oil	Myristic acid; Tridecanoic acid; Lauric acid; Stearic acid; Palmitic acid	
Essential oil	Eugenol; Isoeugenol; Iso-elemicin; Gerianiol; D-pinene; L-pinene; Borneol; Safrole; Limonene; Sabinene; Lysergide	
Resorcinol	Malabaricone B, C	Antimicrobial
Neolignans	A, B, C, dehydroiisoeugenol (Juhasz, 2000)	

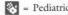 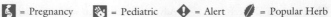

Actions

Nutmeg has been studied for its antimicrobial, antiinflammatory, analgesic, antithrombotic, hypolipidemic, and chemoprotective properties. However, many of these proposed actions are documented by only one study each.

Antimicrobial Actions

Two chemical components of nutmeg known as malabaricones B and C, which are classified as resorcinols, showed powerful antifungal and antibacterial effects when the dried seed covers were evaluated (Orabi, 1991). The volatile oils of several herbs were tested for antibacterial action against 25 types of bacteria. The herbs studied were cloves, black pepper, nutmeg, geranium, oregano, and thyme, and the bacteria tested came from food spoilage, food poisoning, animal pathogens, and plant pathogens. All of the herbs that were tested showed powerful antibacterial effects (Dorman, 2000).

Antiinflammatory, Analgesic, and Antithrombic Actions

A chloroform extract of nutmeg was tested in laboratory rodents. The extract was found to decrease pain in mice and also protect against induced thrombosis (Olajide, 1999). Another study evaluated the antiinflammatory effects of nutmeg by using rats and mice with carrageenan-induced paw edema and acetic acid-induced valcular permeability. At the conclusion of the study, researchers believed myristicin to be the chemical component responsible for the antiinflammatory effect (Ozaki, 1989). An older study showed the analgesic effect of nutmeg on young chickens (Sherry, 1982). An extract of nutmeg was shown to increase both light and deep sleep in these chickens. Anxiogenic activity was identified in nutmeg. The study used mice and several maze-related activities (Sonavane, 2002).

Hypolipidemic Action

In a study of hyperlipidemic rabbits, six rabbits received fluid extract of nutmeg for 60 days at a dose of 500 mg/kg, with the remainder of the rabbits used as the control group. Significantly lower cholesterol levels were found in the hearts and livers of the experimental group, along with platelet antiaggregatory ability (Ram, 1996). Another study using rabbits showed that nutmeg decreased total cholesterol, reduced low-density lipoprotein (LDL) cholesterol, lowered the cholesterol/

N

phospholipid ratio, and increased the high-density lipoprotein (HDL) ratio by significant levels (Sharma, 1995).

Chemoprotective Action

In a study of young mice with induced cancer of the uterine cervix, administration of oral *Myristica fragrans* resulted in a significant reduction of the cancer, with precancerous lesions unaffected (Hussain, 1991). In another study using mice, papilloma was induced before nutmeg was fed to the mice. A significant reduction in papilloma (50%) occurred (Jannu, 1991).

References

Dorman HJ et al: Antibacterial agents from plants: antibacterial activity of plant volatile oils, *J Appl Microbiol* 88(2):308-316, 2000.

Hussain SP et al: Chemoprotective action of mace (*Myristica fragrans* Houtt) on methylcholanthrene-induced carcinogenesis in the uterine cervix in mice, *Cancer Lett* 56(3):231-234, 1991.

Jannu LN et al: Chemoprotective action of mace (*Myristica fragrans* Houtt) on DMBA-induced papillomagenesis in the skin of mice, *Cancer Lett* 56(1):59-63, 1991.

Juhasz L et al: Simple synthesis of benzofuranoid neolignans from *Myristica fragrans, J Nat Prog* 63(6):866-870, 2000.

Olajide OA et al: Biological effects of *Myristica fragrans* (nutmeg) extract, *Phytother Res* 13(4):344-345, 1999.

Orabi KY et al: Isolation and characterization of two antimicrobial agents from mace (*Myristica fragrans*), *J Nat Prod* 54(3):856-859, 1991.

Ozaki Y et al: Antiinflammatory effect of mace, aril of *Myristica fragrans* Houtt and its active principles, *Jpn J Pharmacol* 49(2):155-163, 1989.

Ram A et al: Hyolipidaemic effect of *Myristica fragrans* fruit extract in rabbits, *J Ethnopharmacol* 55(1):49-53, 1996.

Sharma A et al: Prevention of hypercholesterolemia and atherosclerosis in rabbits after supplementation of *Myristica fragrans* seed extract, *Indian J Physiol Pharmacol* 39(4):407-410, 1995.

Sherry CJ et al: The pharmacological effects of the ligroin extract of nutmeg, *J Ethnopharmacol* 6(1):61-66, 1982.

Sonavane GS et al: Anxiogenic activity of Myristica fragrans seeds, *Pharmacol Biochem Behav* 71(1-2):239-244, 2002.

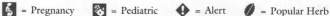

= Pregnancy   = Pediatric   = Alert   = Popular Herb

Oak
(oek)

Scientific names: *Quercus robur, Quercus petraea, Quercus alba*

Other common names: British oak, brown oak, common oak, cortex quercus, ecorce de chene, eichenlohe, eicherinde, encina, English oak, gravelier, nutgall, oak apples, oak bark, oak galls, stone oak, tanner's bark

Class 2d (Bark)

Origin: Oak is a tree found in North America, Australia, Europe, and Asia.

Uses

Reported Uses

Oak bark traditionally has been used for its antiinflammatory and astringent properties. Topically, oak is used to treat skin disorders such as psoriasis, eczema, and contact dermatitis. It has also been used as a gargle and to treat varicose veins, hemorrhoids, and burns. Oak is used internally for diarrhea.

Product Availability and Dosages

Available Forms

Capsules, decoction, extract, gall, ointment, ooze, powder, tincture

Plant Parts Used: Bark, gall

Dosages and Routes

Adult

- PO: 3 g qd (Blumenthal, 1998)
- Rinse/compress/gargle: 20 g/1 L water (Blumenthal, 1998)
- Topical ointment: apply prn to affected area
- Topical powder (bath): 5 g powder/1 L water (Blumenthal, 1998)

O

Precautionary Information

Contraindications

Until more research is available, oak should not be used during pregnancy and lactation and should not be given to children. Oak should not be used by persons with hypersensitivity to it and should not be used topically on large areas of damaged skin. It should not be taken internally in renal or hepatic disease. Class 2d herb (bark).

Side Effects/Adverse Reactions

Gastrointestinal: Nausea, vomiting, anorexia
Integumentary: Hypersensitivity reactions

Interactions with Oak

Drug
Iron salts: Oak bark tea may decrease the absorption of iron salts.

Food	Herb	Lab Test
None known	None known	None known

Client Considerations

Assess

- Assess for hypersensitivity reactions. If these are present, discontinue use of oak and administer antihistamine or other appropriate therapy.
- Assess for renal or hepatic disease if oak is to be taken internally; kidney damage and necrotic liver condition can result.

Administer

- Instruct the client to store oak in a cool, dry place, away from heat and moisture.
- Do not administer PO in large amounts; kidney damage and necrotic liver conditions can result.

Teach Client/Family

- Until more research is available, caution the client not to use oak during pregnancy and lactation and not to give it to children.

 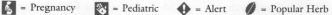

Pharmacology

Pharmacokinetics

Pharmacokinetics and pharmacodynamics are unknown.

Primary Chemical Components of Oak and Their Possible Actions		
Chemical Class	**Individual Component**	**Possible Action**
Tannin	Pedunculagin	Antisecretory; astringent
	Vescalagin; Castalagin; Mongolicanin (bark)	
Flavonoid	Acutissimin A, B; Eugenigrandin A; Guajavin B; Stenophyllanin C	
Calcium oxalate		

Actions

Very little information is available for oak. Its proposed actions include antioxidant, antibacterial, and urolithiasis inhibitor. In one toxicology study evaluating cattle with weakness, diarrhea, and dehydration, one autopsy revealed nephritis and ulceration between the caecum and colon (Neser, 1982).

Antioxidant Action

One study has focused on the antioxidant action of oak (Masaki, 1995). When oak and several other herbs were tested for scavenging activity, its antioxidant properties did not prove significant.

Antibacterial and Urolithiasis Inhibitor Actions

One study of 97 patients with urolithiasis evaluated the ability of oak to inhibit the formation of calculi (Mandana, 1980). Study participants were given doses of 1350 mg/day of oak extract. After 8 to 225 days the kidney stone formation was identified as inhibiting stone growth. Investigators also observed an inhibition of bacteria proliferation.

O

References

Blumenthal M, editor: *The complete German Commission E monographs: therapeutic guide to herbal medicines*, Austin, Tex, American Botanical Council; Boston, Integrative Medicine Communication, 1998.

Mandana R et al: Therapeutic effects of *Quercus* extract in urolithiasis, *Arch Exp Urol* 33(2):205-226, 1980.

Masaki H et al: Active-oxygen scavenging activity of plants extracts, *Biol Pharm Bull* 18(1):162-166, 1995.

Neser JA et al: Oak *(Quercus rubor)* poisoning in cattle, *J S Afr Vet Assoc* 53(3):151-155, 1982.

Oats
(oetz)

Scientific name: *Avena sativa*

Other common names: Groats, haver, haver-corn, haws, oatmeal

Class 1 (Spikelets)

Origin: Oats come from a grain found in North America, Russia, and Germany.

Uses

Reported Uses

Traditionally, oats have been used topically to relieve the itching and irritation of various skin disorders. Taken internally, oats may have sedative properties.

Investigational Uses

Oats are being researched for their antilipidemic, anticholesterol, and antidiabetic effects. Oat green tea may be effective in the treatment of drug, alcohol, and smoking addiction.

Product Availability and Dosages

Available Forms

Bath products, cereal, lotion, powder, tablets, tea, wafers, whole grain

Plant Parts Used: Grain

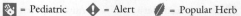

Dosages and Routes
Adult
Skin Irritation
• Topical: apply prn
• Topical (bath): 100 g cut herb/full bathtub of water
To Lower Cholesterol Levels
• PO: 50-100 g qd

Precautionary Information

Contraindications

Oats should not be used by persons with intestinal obstruction, celiac disease, or strangulated bowel. Class 1 herb (spikelets).

Side Effects/Adverse Reactions

Gastrointestinal: Bloating, flatus
Integumentary: Hypersensitivity reactions, contact dermatitis

Interactions with Oats

Drug
Morphine: Oats may decrease the effect of morphine; do not use concurrently.
Nicotine: Oats may decrease the hypertensive effect of nicotine.

Food	Herb	Lab Test
None known	None known	None known

O

Client Considerations

Assess

• Assess for hypersensitivity reactions (rare) and for contact dermatitis from oat flour. If these are present, discontinue use of oats and administer antihistamine or other appropriate therapy.
• Assess for morphine use (see Interactions).

Administer

• Instruct the client to store oats in a cool, dry place, away from heat and moisture.

🌀 Endangered Herb   Adverse effects: BOLD = life-threatening

Teach Client/Family

- Caution the client with bowel obstruction, strangulated bowel, or celiac disease not to use oats.
- Advise client who is using oats to decrease cholesterol to make other prescribed lifestyle changes as well.
- Inform the client that bowel function may change and flatus may occur.

Pharmacology

Pharmacokinetics

Pharmacokinetics and pharmacodynamics are unknown.

Primary Chemical Components of Oats and Their Possible Actions		
Chemical Class	**Individual Component**	**Possible Action**
Saponin	Triterpenoid Furostandl	Fungicidal
Carotenoid		
Polyphenol		
Monosaccharide		
Oligosaccharide		
Gluten		
Mineral	Iron; Manganese; Zinc	
Fiber		
Cellulose		Anticholesterol

Actions

Anticholesterol Action

Most of the research on oats has focused on the anticholesterol effect of oat bran. The bran fiber binds to cholesterol and bile components, thus removing them from the body when the fiber is excreted.

Antioxidant Action

Oats may possess antioxidant properties. Several components in the enrichment process are antioxidants (Emmons, 1999).

Antiaddiction Action

One study has shown that the use of oat tincture can decrease the nicotine cravings of smokers, as well as the pressor effect

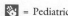 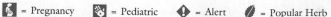

that occurs when nicotine is administered intravenously (Connor, 1975). In another study, 100 smokers with an average consumption of 20 cigarettes a day were treated with an extract of *Avena sativa* for the purpose of disaccustoming them to nicotine. The light smokers showed a positive result, whereas the heavy smokers did not (Schmidt, 1976).

References

Connor J et al: The pharmacology of *Avena sativa, J Pharm Pharmacol* 27(2):92-98, 1975.

Emmons CL et al: Antioxidant capacity of oat (*Avena sativa* L.) extracts, II: in vitro antioxidant activity and contents of phenolic and tocol antioxidants, *J Agric Food Chem* 47(12):4894-4898, 1999.

Schmidt K et al: Pharmacotherapy with *Avena sativa:* a double blind study, *Int J Clin Pharmacol Biopharm* 14(3):214-216, 1976.

Octacosanol
(ahk-tuh-kah′suhn-awl)

Scientific names: Sources include *Eupolyphaga sinensis, Acacia modesta, Serenoa repens,* and others

Other common names: 1-octacosanol, 14c-octacosanol, n-octacosanol, octacosyl alcohol, policosanol

Origin: Octacosanol is developed from wheat germ, sugar cane, or vegetable waxes.

Uses
Reported Uses
Octacosanol is used to increase athletic performance.

Investigational Uses
Researchers are experimenting with the use of octacosanol to treat Parkinson's disease, amyotrophic lateral sclerosis (ALS), hyperlipidemia, and intermittent claudication.

Product Availability and Dosages
Available Forms
Capsules, tablets

Plant Parts Used: Octacosanol is isolated from several different plants.

Dosages and Routes
Adult
• PO capsules/tablets: 40-80 mg qd

Precautionary Information
Contraindications
Until more research is available, octacosanol should not be used during pregnancy and lactation and should not be given to children.

Side Effects/Adverse Reactions
Cardiovascular: Orthostatic hypotension
Central Nervous System: Dyskinesia, restlessness, nervousness
Gastrointestinal: Nausea, vomiting, anorexia

Interactions with Octacosanol

Drug
Carbidopa/levodopa: Octacosanol may cause dyskinesia when used with carbidopa/levodopa; avoid concurrent use.

Food	Herb	Lab Test
None known	None known	None known

Client Considerations
Assess
• Assess clients with Parkinson's disease for increased dyskinesia if taking carbidopa/levodopa concurrently with octacosanol (see Interactions).

Administer
• Instruct the client to store octacosanol in a cool, dry place, away from heat and moisture.

Teach Client/Family
• Until more research is available, caution the client not to use octacosanol during pregnancy and lactation and not to give it to children.
• Advise the client that research is lacking to support any use of octacosanol.

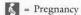 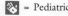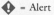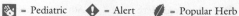

Pharmacology

Pharmacokinetics

Pharmacokinetics and pharmacodynamics are unknown.

Actions

Hyperlipidemia Action

There have been several studies on the use of octacosanol for use in hyperlipidemia. One study has evaluated its use in lipid metabolism. When rats fed a high-fat diet were given octacosanol, triglycerides were reduced significantly and serum fatty acids were increased (Kato, 1995). There have been several studies that confirmed the improvement in total and LDL cholesterol levels, as well as LDL/HDL ratios. All of these studies were double-blind placebo-controlled trials (Castano, 2000; Mas, 1999). In a study using octacosanol to treat ALS, no improvement was observed (Norris, 1986).

References

Castano G et al: Effects of policosanol on post menopausal women with type II hypercholesterolemia, *Gynecol Endocrinol* 14:187-195, 2000.

Kato S et al: Octacosanol affects lipid metabolism in rats fed on a high-fat diet, *Br J Nutr* 73(3):433-441, 1995.

Mas R et al: Effects of policosanol in patients with type II hypercholesterolemia and additional coronary risk factors, *Clin Pharmacol Ther* 65:439-447, 1999.

Norris FH et al: Trial of octacosanol in amyotrophic lateral sclerosis, *Neurology* 36(9):1263-1264, 1986.

Oleander

(oe'lee-an-duhr)

Scientific names: *Nerium oleander, Nerium odoratum*

Other common names: Adelfa, laurier rose, rosa francesa, rosa laurel, rose bay

Origin: Oleander is a shrub found in the southern United States, Indonesia, and the Mediterranean region.

Uses

Reported Uses

Traditionally, oleander has been used to treat cardiac disease, diuresis, and menstrual irregularities. It has also been used as a laxative, an insecticide, an abortifacient, and a parasiticide. In some countries it is used internally as an anthelmintic and topically to treat warts and other skin disorders.

Investigational Uses

New studies have shown a use for oleander in cancer.

Product Availability and Dosages

Available Forms

Extract, tincture

Plant Parts Used: Leaves

Dosages and Routes

No published dosages are available.

Precautionary Information

Contraindications

Because it can cause spontaneous abortion, oleander should not be used during pregnancy. Until more research is available, this herb should not be used during lactation and should not be given to children. Persons with hypersensitivity to oleander should not use it. Because of the toxic nature of this plant, oleander is not recommended for any use.

Side Effects/Adverse Reactions

Central Nervous System: Depression, dizziness, stupor, headache
Cardiac: DYSRHYTHMIAS, VENTRICULAR ECTOPY, BRADYCARDIA, CV COLLAPSE, DEATH
Gastrointestinal: Nausea, vomiting, anorexia, abdominal cramps
Genitourinary: SPONTANEOUS ABORTION
Integumentary: Hypersensitivity reactions, contact dermatitis
Metabolic: Hyperkalemia, peripheral neuritis
Respiratory: Tachypnea

 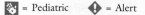

Interactions with Oleander		
Drug		
Cardiac glycosides (digoxin): Use of oleander with cardiac glycosides may cause fatal digitalis toxicity; do not use concurrently.		
Food	Herb	Lab Test
None known	None known	None known

Client Considerations

Assess

- Assess for hypersensitivity reactions and contact dermatitis. If these are present, discontinue use of oleander and administer antihistamine or other appropriate therapy.
- Assess for the use of cardiac glycosides. Fatal digitalis toxicity can result from concurrent use (see Interactions).

Administer

- Instruct the client to store oleander in a cool, dry place, away from heat and moisture.

Teach Client/Family

- Because it can cause spontaneous abortion, caution the client not to use oleander during pregnancy. Until more research is available, caution the client not to use this herb during lactation and not to give it to children.
- Advise the client that oleander is extremely toxic and should not be used except under the supervision of a qualified herbalist. All plant parts are potentially dangerous.

Pharmacology

Pharmacokinetics

Pharmacokinetics and pharmacodynamics are unknown.

O

Primary Chemical Components of Oleander and Their Possible Actions		
Chemical Class	**Individual Component**	**Possible Action**
Glycoside	Nerioside; Oleandrin; Neriin; Oleandroside; Digitoxigenin; Gentiobiosyl-oleandrin; Odoroside A Glucosyl-oleandrin	Cardiac glycoside
Folinerin Rosagenin Rutin Cornerine Oleandromycin		

Actions

Many of the chemical components of oleander are cardiac glycosides (see table). Several studies have investigated the digoxin-like toxicity of this plant. One such study focused on the toxicity of oleander in a guinea pig that experienced seizures and cardiac symptoms after eating dried oleander leaves (Kirsch, 1997). The guinea pig was released after undergoing intensive care for 24 hours. Another study reported complete atrioventricular block in a 33-year-old woman who was self-medicating with oleander (Nishioka, 1995). A third report focused on a 38-year-old woman with poisoning after ingesting oleander leaves. Her symptoms included those of digitalis intoxication. Use of digoxin-specific FAB proved successful (Romano, 1990) in the treatment of the toxicity, as was the case in another reported case of oleander poisoning (Shumaik, 1988). One study (Pathak, 2000) showed a cancer cell death in human, but not murine, cancer cell death. Different concentrations of oleander were used. Canine oral cancer cells treated showed immediate response.

References

Kirsch M: Acute glycoside intoxication from the intake of oleander *(Nerium oleasder)* leaves in a guinea pig, *Tierarztl Prax* 25(4):398-400, 1997.

Nishioka Sd et al: Transitory complete atrioventricular block associated to ingestion of *Nerium oleander, Rev Assoc Med Bras* 41(1):60-62, 1995.

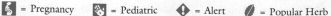

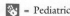 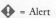

Pathak S et al: Anvirzel, an extract of *Nerium Oleander,* induces cell death in human but not murine cancer cells, *Anticancer Drugs* 11(6):455-463, 2000.

Romano GA et al: Poisoning with oleander leaves, *Schweiz Med Wochenschr* 120(16):596-597, 1990.

Shumaik GM et al: Oleander poisoning: treatment with digoxin-specific FAB antibody fragments, *Ann Emerg Med* 17(7):732-735, 1988.

Oregano
(uh-reh′guh-noe)

Scientific names: *Origanum vulgare, Panax quinquefolis*

Other common names: Mountain mint, origanum

Class 1 (Leaf)

Origin: Oregano is found throughout Asia, Europe, and northern Africa. It is cultivated throughout the world, including the United States.

Uses
Reported Uses
Oregano is best known for its use as a food flavoring used in cooking. Therapeutically, oregano is used internally as an expectorant and to treat respiratory disorders, cough, and bronchial catarrh; for intestine disorders such as dyspepsia and for intestinal parasites. It has also been used as a systemic tonic and diaphoretic, as well as to treat menstrual irregularities. Topically, oregano is used to treat infection. It may also be added to shampoo for its antiseptic action.

Investigational Uses
Initial research supports the use of oregano as an antibacterial, antifungal, and antioxidant.

Product Availability and Dosages
Available Forms
Capsules, dried herb, oil

Plant Parts Used: Aboveground parts (dried)

Dosages and Routes
Adult
- PO capsules: 2 caps qd-bid with meals

- PO dried herb: pour 250 ml boiling water over 1 tsp dried herb, let stand 10 min, strain
- PO oil: 5 drops added to liquid
- PO: tea
- Topical oil: apply to affected area prn as an antiseptic

Precautionary Information
Contraindications
Until more research is available, oregano should not be used therapeutically during pregnancy and lactation and should not be given therapeutically to children. Oregano should not be used therapeutically by persons with hypersensitivity to this herb or other members of the Labiatae family, such as mint, sage, marjoram, thyme, basil, lavender, or hyssop. Class 1 herb (leaf).

Side Effects/Adverse Reactions
Gastrointestinal: Nausea, vomiting, anorexia (large amounts)
Integumentary: Hypersensitivity reactions—facial edema, itching, dysphagia, dysphonia, INABILITY TO BREATHE

Interactions with Oregano

Drug	Food	Herb	Lab Test
None known	None known	None known	None known

Client Considerations
Assess
- Assess for hypersensitivity reactions (facial edema, itching, inability to breathe, dysphonia, dysphagia). If these are present, discontinue use of oregano and administer antihistamine or other appropriate therapy. If client is allergic to other herbs in the Lamiaceae family (basil, marjoram, lavendar, hyssop, mint, sage), cross sensitivity may occur.

Administer
- Instruct the clients to store oregano products in a sealed container away from heat and moisture.

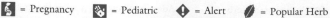

Teach Client/Family

- Until more research is available, caution the client not to use oregano therapeutically during pregnancy and lactation and not to give it therapeutically to children.
- Caution the client not to confuse oregano with marjoram *(Origanum marjorana)*.
- Because cross-sensitivity is possible, advise the client who is allergic to other plants of the Labiatae family (thyme, hyssop, basil, marjoram, mint, sage, and lavender) not to use oregano (Benito, 1996).

Pharmacology

Pharmacokinetics

Pharmacokinetics and pharmacodynamics are unknown.

Primary Chemical Components of Oregano and Their Possible Actions		
Chemical Class	**Individual Component**	**Possible Action**
Tannin		Wound healing; astringent
Acid	Gallic acid	
Tocopherol	Alpha; Beta; Gamma; Delta	Antioxidant
Volatile oil	Carvacrol; Gamma-terpinene; P-cymene; Thymol	

Actions

Little information is available on the actions of oregano. Proposed actions include antioxidant, antibacterial, and antifungal.

Antioxidant Action

Oregano is high in tocopherols, which are responsible for its antioxidant action (Lagouri, 1996). Another study (Nakatani, 2000) identified phenolic antioxidants from several herbs and spices. One of the herbs studied was *Origanum vulgare*.

Antibacterial and Antifungal Actions

Several herbs were evaluated to determine the antibacterial effects of their volatile oils. The volatile oils of black pepper,

O

cloves, geranium, nutmeg, oregano, and thyme all showed significant antibacterial action against the 25 bacteria species tested (Dorman, 2000). Inhibition of *Aspergillus* was evaluated using the essential oils of oregano, mint, basil, sage, and coriander. Oregano and mint completely inhibited the growth of *Aspergillus,* whereas sage and coriander showed no inhibitory effects. Basil was only slightly effective (Basilico, 1999).

References

Basilico MA et al: Inhibitory effects of some spice essential oils on *Aspergillus ochraceus* NRRL 3174 growth and ochratoxin A production, *Lett Appl Microbiol* 29(40):238-241, 1999.

Benito M et al: Labiatae allergy: systemic reactions due to ingestion of oregano and thyme, *Ann Allergy Asthma Immunol* 76(5):416-418, 1996.

Dorman HJ et al: Antimicrobial agents from plants: antibacterial activity of plant volatile oils, *J Appl Microbiol* 88(2):308-316, 2000.

Lagouri V et al: Nutrient antioxidants in oregano, *Int J Food Sci Nutr* 47(6):493-497, 1996.

Nakatani N: Phenolic antioxidants from herbs and spices, *Biofactors* 13(1-4):141-146, 2000.

Oregon Grape
(aw'ri-guhn grayp)

Scientific name: *Mahonia aquifolium*

Other common names: Holly-leaved barberry, mountain grape

Class 2b (Root)

Origin: Oregon grape is a shrub found in the western region of the United States.

Uses

Reported Uses

Different forms of Oregon grape have different uses. The tincture is used to treat skin disorders such as eczema, psoriasis, dandruff, herpes, and acne, as well as hepatitis, upper-respiratory congestion, sexually transmitted diseases, arthritis, and other joint disorders. The root bark is used to treat diarrhea, fever, gallbladder conditions, renal calculi, gastrointestinal upset, and leukorrhea.

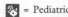 = Pregnancy   = Pediatric   = Alert   = Popular Herb

Investigational Uses

Initial research is available that focuses on the use of Oregon grape as an antioxidant and as a treatment for some skin disorders.

Product Availability and Dosages

Available Forms

Capsules, fluid extract, powder, tincture, topical ointment, topical cream

Plant Parts Used: Bark, roots, stems

Dosages and Routes

Adult
- PO powder: ½-1 g tid
- PO tincture: 2-4 ml tid
- Topical: Apply tid to affected areas.

Precautionary Information

Contraindications

Until more research is available, Oregon grape should not be used during pregnancy and lactation and should not be given to children. Oregon grape should not be used by persons with hypersensitivity to this herb or related herbs. Class 2b herb (root).

Side Effects/Adverse Reactions

Gastrointestinal: Nausea, vomiting, anorexia
Integumentary: Hypersensitivity reactions, burning
Systemic: POISONING, DEATH (high doses)

Interactions with Oregon Grape

Drug	Food	Herb	Lab Test
None known	None known	None known	None known

Client Considerations

Assess

- Assess for hypersensitivity reactions. If these are present, discontinue use of Oregon grape and administer antihistamine or other appropriate therapy.

• Assess for use of excessive doses. Poisoning and death can result.

Administer

• Instruct the client to store Oregon grape products in a cool, dry place, away from heat and moisture.

Teach Client/Family

 • Until more research is available, caution the client not to use Oregon grape during pregnancy and lactation and not to give it to children.

• Advise the client that Oregon grape is not the same as barberry *(Berberis vulgaris)*.

• Inform the client that research is minimal for any uses and actions of Oregon grape.

• Caution the client that poisoning and death may result from high doses.

Pharmacology

Pharmacokinetics

Pharmacokinetics and pharmacodynamics are unknown.

Primary Chemical Components of Oregon Grape and Their Possible Actions		
Chemical Class	**Individual Component**	**Possible Action**
Alkaloid	Berberine; Magnoflorine	Weak antioxidant
	Oxyacanthine; Berbamine; Bisbenzy lisoquinoline alkaloid complex (BBI); Oxyberberine; Corytuberine; Columbamine; Armoline; Baluchistine; Obamegine; Aquifoline; Jatorrhizine	Antioxidant
	Isocorydine; Isothebaine Hydrastine; Canadine; Corypalmine; Mahonine; Isoquinolone	Cardiac relaxant
Tannin		

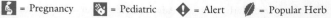
 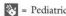

Actions

The possible actions of Oregon grape include antioxidant, antiproliferative, and cardiac relaxant.

Antioxidant Action

Most research studies have focused on the alkaloid components of Oregon grape and their antioxidant actions. Those with the most potent antioxidant actions are isothebaine and isocorydine (Sotnikova, 1997), berbamine and oxyacanthine (Bezakova, 1996), and oxyberberine, corytuberine, and columbamine (Misik, 1995). Other alkaloids have been found to possess only weak antioxidant effects.

Antiproliferative Action

Several studies have demonstrated the antiproliferative action of Oregon grape (Muller, 1994, 1995; Augustin, 1999). All studies have confirmed that Oregon grape decreases the proliferation of psoriasis. Topical application was used to treat psoriasis in a double-blind placebo-controlled study with 82 individuals. Participants rated the effectiveness of Oregon grape as being more effective (Weisenauer, 1996). Another study (Augustin, 1999) compared treatments that differed on each side of participants' body. Skin biopsies were used to compare each sample. There was significant improvement in the Oregon grape group.

Cardiac Relaxant Action

The cardiac relaxant ability of Oregon grape was demonstrated by the use of the alkaloids isothebaine and isocorydine in rats. Both alkaloids showed relaxant effects in the aorta (Sotnikova, 1997).

References

Augustin M et al: Effects of *Mahonia aquifolium* ointment on the expression of adhesion, proliferation, and activation markers in the skin of patients with psoriasis, *Forsch Komplementarmed* 6(suppl 2):19-21, 1999.

Bezakova L et al: Lipoxygenase inhibition and antioxidant properties of bisbenzylisoqunoline alkaloids isolated from *Mahonia aquifolium, Pharmazie* 51(10):758-761, 1996.

Misik V et al: Lipoxygenase inhibition and antioxidant properties of protoberberine and aporphine alkaloids isolated from *Mahonia aquifolium, Planta Med* 61(4):372-373, 1995 (letter).

Muller K et al: The antipsoriatic *Mahonia aquifolium* and its active constituents, I: pro- and antioxidant properties and inhibition of 5-lipoxygenase, *Planta Med* 60(5):421-424, 1994.

Muller K et al: The antipsoriatic *Mahonia aquifolium* and its active constituents, II, antiproliferative activity against cell growth of human keratinocytes, *Planta Med* 61(1):74-75, 1995 (letter).

Sotnikova R et al: Relaxant properties of some aporphine alkaloids from *Mahonia aquifolium, Methods Find Exp Clin Pharmacol* 19(9):589-597, 1997.

Wiesenauer M et al: *Mahonia aquifolium* in patients with psoriasis vulgaris: an intraindividual study, *Phytomedicine* 3:231-235, 1996.

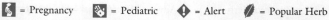

= Pregnancy   = Pediatric   = Alert   = Popular Herb

Pansy
(pan'zee)

Scientific name: *Viola tricolor*

Other common names: Field pansy, heartsease, Johnny-jump-up, jupiter flower, ladies' delight, wild pansy

Origin: Pansy is found throughout the world.

Uses

Reported Uses

Pansy traditionally has been used to treat whooping cough, upper respiratory conditions such as bronchitis, skin cancer, joint pain, and inflammation. Internally it is used as a laxative and to promote metabolism. Externally it is used to treat seborrheic skin diseases, acne, impetigo, pruritus vulvae, and cradle cap in children.

Investigational Uses

Initial research is available documenting the use of pansy in the treatment of heart conditions.

Product Availability and Dosages

Available Forms

Extract, tea, tincture

Plant Parts Used: Flowers

Dosages and Routes

Adult
- PO tea: 2-4 ml tid
- PO tincture: 2-4 ml tid

Precautionary Information

Contraindications

Until more research is available, pansy should not be used during pregnancy and lactation and should not be given to children. Pansy should not be used by persons with hypersensitivity to this herb or salicylates.

Continued

 Endangered Herb   Adverse effects: **BOLD** = life-threatening

Precautionary Information—cont'd

Side Effects/Adverse Reactions

Gastrointestinal: Nausea, vomiting, anorexia, diarrhea (seeds)

Integumentary: Hypersensitivity reactions

Interactions with Pansy

Drug

Salicylates (aspirin): The actions of salicylates may be increased when used with pansy.

Food	Herb	Lab Test
None known	None known	None known

Client Considerations

Assess

- Assess for hypersensitivity reactions. If these are present, discontinue use of pansy and administer antihistamine or other appropriate therapy.

Administer

- Instruct the client to store pansy products away from heat, light, and moisture.

Teach Client/Family

- Until more research is available, caution the client not to use pansy during pregnancy and lactation and not to give it to children.

Pharmacology

Pharmacokinetics

Pharmacokinetics and pharmacodynamics are unknown.

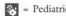 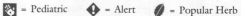

Primary Chemical Components of Pansy and Their Possible Actions		
Chemical Class	Individual Component	Possible Action
Flavonoid	Rutin; Luteolin; Scoparin; Saponarine; Violanthin	
Salicylate		Antiinflammatory; antipyretic
Terpene		
Carbohydrate		
Sterine		
Cyclic peptide	Kalata-peptide B1	Antimicrobial
Tannin		
Hydroxycoumarin	Umbelliferone	Anticoagulant

Actions

Little research has been done on pansy. One study showed a reduction in glucose transport in the rat small intestine (Gurman, 1992). Another demonstrated that one of the chemical components, kalata-peptide B_1, exerts antimicrobial activity (Gran, 2000). All other information available to date is anecdotal and unconfirmed.

References

Gurman EG et al: *Fiziol Zh SSSR Im IM Sechenova* 78(8):109-116, 1992 (abstract).

Gran L et al: *Oldenlandia affinis* (R & S) DC: a plant containing uteroactive peptides used in African traditional medicine, *J Ethnopharmacol* 70(3):197-203, 2000.

P

Papaya
(puh-pai'uh)

Scientific name: *Carica papaya*

Other common names: Melon tree, papain, pawpaw

Origin: Papaya is a tree grown in Mexico, Central America, and many tropical regions.

 Endangered Herb   Adverse effects: BOLD = life-threatening

Uses

Reported Uses

Papaya is used orally for intestinal worms and for gastrointestinal disorders and topically for debridment of wounds such as decubiti and other necrotic ulcers. It is used by intradisk injection in a herniated lumbar intervetebral disk.

Product Availability and Dosages

Available Forms

Tablets

Plant Parts Used: Seeds, pulp, leaves, latex

Dosage and Routes

Adult

- PO: 10 mg qid for 7 days
- Topical: Apply to affected area as needed for debridement
- Intradisk injection

Precautionary Information

Contraindications

Papaya should not be used in hypersensitivity, pregnancy, or lactation; for children; in contact dermatitis; or in bleeding disorders.

Side Effects/Adverse Reactions

Cardiovasular: Hypotension, bradycardia
Central nervous system: Paralysis
Gastrointestinal: Severe gastritis, ESOPHAGEAL PERFORATION
Integumentary: Dermatitis, caroteinemia
Systemic: ANAPHYLAXIS, allergic reactions

Interactions with Papaya

Drug

Anticoagulants (anisindione, dicumarol, heparin): When papaya is given with anticoagulants, there is a greater risk of bleeding and an increase in International Normalized Ratio (INR) and prothrombin time.

Food	Herb	Lab Test
None known	None known	None known

 = Pregnancy  = Pediatric   = Alert 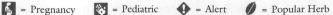 = Popular Herb

Client Considerations
Assess
- Assess the reason client is using papaya.
- Identify if the client is using anticoagulants. There is an increased risk of bleeding when papaya is used with anticoagulants.

Administer
- Keep papaya in a closed container away from excessive heat, light, and moisture.

Teach Client/Family
- Teach the patient that papaya should not be used medicinally in pregnancy, in lactation, or for children until more research is completed with these populations.

Pharmacology
Pharmacokinetics
Pharmacokinetics and pharmacodynamics are unknown.

Primary Chemical Components of Papaya and Their Possible Actions		
Chemical Class	**Individual Component**	**Possible Action**
Proteolytic enzymes	Papain	Debridment enzyme
	Chymopapain	
Alkaloids	Carpaine	
Glycosides	Myrosin; Caricin	

Actions
The primary action of papaya is its use as a debridement enzyme. The proteolytic enzymes papain and chymopapain have been used for centuries as a debridement vehicle for necrotic skin, primarily in decubitus ulcers. A new research study (Rajkapoor, 2002) has shown dried papaya fruits to be hepatoprotective.

References
Rajkapoor B et al: Effect of dried fruits of *Carica papaya* on hepatotoxicity, *Biol Pharm Bull* 25(12):1645-1646, 2002.

 Endangered Herb   Adverse effects: BOLD = life-threatening

Parsley
(pahr'slee)

Scientific name: *Petroselinum crispum*

Other common names: Common
parsley, garden parsley, rock parsley   **Class 2b/2d (Leaf, Root)**

Origin: Parsley is found throughout the world.

Uses

Reported Uses

Traditionally, parsley has been used to treat cough, menstrual irregularities, gastrointestinal upset, dysuria, flatulence, and joint
pain and inflammation. It is also used as a diuretic, antiinfective, and antispasmodic. In the fourteenth century, parsley was
used to treat gastrointestinal conditions, asthma, urinary and
hepatic disease, and the plague.

Investigational Uses

Initial research indicates that parsley may be useful for the treatment of hypertension; urinary tract dysfunction, including urinary tract infection and kidney stones; menopausal as an
antioxidant; and in women for symptoms.

Product Availability and Dosages

Available Forms

Capsules, essential oil, fluid extract, tea

Plant Parts Used: Leaves, oil, roots, seeds

Dosages and Routes

Adult

All dosages listed are PO.

- Crushed herb and root: 6 g/day
- Fluid extract: 2-4 ml (1:1 dilution in 25% alcohol) tid
- Tea: use 2-6 g leaves or roots

Precautionary Information

Contraindications

Until more research is available, parsley should not be used
therapeutically during pregnancy and lactation and should
not be given therapeutically to children. The essential oil

 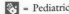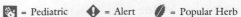

Precautionary Information—cont'd

Contraindications—cont'd

should not be used by persons with renal inflammation, and those with cardiac, renal, or hepatic conditions should avoid the therapeutic use of this herb. Class 2b, 2d herb (leaf, root).

Side Effects/Adverse Reactions

Cardiovascular: Hypotension, ARRHYTHMIAS
Gastrointestinal: Nausea, vomiting, anorexia, GASTROINTESTINAL BLEEDING, HEPATOTOXICITY, FATTY LIVER
Genitourinary: RENAL DAMAGE
Integumentary: Hypersensitivity reactions, contact dermatitis, phototoxicity (Ojala, 2000)
Respiratory: Pulmonary vascular congestion

Interactions with Parsley

Drug

Anticoagulants (heparin, warfarin): Large amounts of parsley may interfere with anticoagulation therapy (theoretical).
Antihypertensives: Parsley may cause increased hypotension when used with antihypertensives; do not use concurrently.
Lithium: Parsley combined with lithium may lead to dehydration, lithium toxicity.
MAOIs: MAOIs used with tricyclics or selective serotonin reuptake inhibitors (SSRIs) may lead to serotonin syndrome when used with parsley; do not use concurrently.
Opiates: Opiates may cause serotonin syndrome when used with parsley; do not use concurrently.

Food	Herb	Lab Test
None known	None known	None known

P

Client Considerations

Assess

- Assess for hypersensitivity reactions. If these are present, discontinue use of parsley and administer antihistamine or other appropriate therapy.

- Assess for cardiac, hepatic, or renal disease. Clients with these conditions should avoid using parsley therapeutically.
- Assess for medications used (see Interactions).

Administer

- Instruct the client to store parsley products in a cool, dry place, away from heat and moisture.

Teach Client/Family

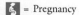

- Until more research is available, caution the client not to use parsley therapeutically during pregnancy and lactation and not to give it therapeutically to children.
- Inform the client that research is lacking for any uses or actions of parsley.
- Advise the client to use sunscreen and wear protective clothing to prevent phototoxic reactions.

Pharmacology

Pharmacokinetics

Pharmacokinetics and pharmacodynamics are unknown.

Primary Chemical Components of Parsley and Their Possible Actions		
Chemical Class	**Individual Component**	**Possible Action**
Mineral	Calcium; Iron	
Vitamin	A; B; C	
Glycoside	Acetylapiin	Estrogenic
	Apigenin; Luteolin	
Glucoside	Petroside	Estrogenic
Protein		
Carbohydrate		
Furanocoumarin	Bergapten	Phototoxicity
	Psoralen; Methoxypsoralen; Oxypeucedanin	
Volatile oil	Myristicin; Apiole; Beta-phellandrene	
Flavonoid	Apiin; Luteolin	

Actions

Researchers have identified that parsley contains phytoestrogens and that it possesses urinary antioxidant, antidiabetic, and an-

 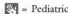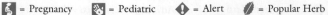

tihypertensive properties. However, little research has been done on any of its proposed actions.

Estrogenic Action

The phytoestrogens in parsley were identified when researchers were screening for an estrogen-sensitive breast cancer cell line. Parsley was shown to exert potent estrogenic activity, equal to that of soybeans (Yoshikawa, 2000).

Antioxidant Action

Parsley's urinary antioxidant action was demonstrated in a study involving seven men and seven women (Nielsen, 1999). Participants began intake of parsley to identify the excretion of flavones and on biomarkers for oxidative stress. Researchers observed an increase in the antioxidant effect. Another earlier study (Fejes, 1998, 2000) produced similar results. The flavonoids present in parsley were shown to exert the strongest antioxidant effect.

References

Fejes S et al: Investigation of the in vitro antioxidant effect of *Petroselinum crispum, Acta Pharm Hung* 68(3):150-156, 1998.

Fejes S et al: Free radical scavenging membrane protective effects of methanol extracts from *Anthriscus cerefolium* L. and *Petroselinum crispum, Phytother Res* 14(5):362-365, 2000.

Nielsen SE et al: Effect of parsley *(Petroselinum crispum)* intake on urinary apigenin excretion, blood antioxidant enzymes and biomarkers for oxidative stress in human subjects, *Br J Nutr* 81(6):447-455, 1999.

Ojala T et al: A bioassay using *Artemia salina* for detecting phototoxicity of plant coumarins, *Planta Med* 65(8):715-718, 2000.

Yoshikawa M et al: Medicinal foodstuffs, XVIII: phytoestrogens from the aerial part of *Petroselinum crispum* MIII (parsley) and structure of 6″-acetylapiin and a new monoterpene glycoside, petroside, *Chem Pharm Bull* 48(7):1039-1044, 2000.

P

Parsley Piert
(pahr'slee)

Scientific name: *Aphanes arvensis*

Other common names: Field lady's mantle, parsley breakstone, parsley piercestone

Origin: Parsley piert is an annual found in North America, Europe, and parts of Africa.

 Endangered Herb   Adverse effects: **BOLD** = life-threatening

Uses
Reported Uses
Parsley piert is used to treat urinary tract disorders such as infections and renal stones. It is also used as a diuretic.

Product Availability and Dosages
Available Forms
Dried herb, fluid extract, tincture

Plant Parts Used: Aerial parts

Dosages and Routes
Adult
All dosages listed are PO.
- Fluid extract: 2 4 ml tid
- Tincture: 2-10 ml tid
- Tea: ½ cup herb in 1 pt boiling water; may be taken tid-qid
- Dried herb: 2-4 g tid
- Infusion: 2-4 g tid

Precautionary Information
Contraindications
Until more research is available, parsley piert should not be used during pregnancy and lactation and should not be given to children. This herb should not be used by persons with hypersensitivity to it.

Side Effects/Adverse Reactions
Gastrointestinal: Nausea, vomiting, anorexia
Integumentary: Hypersensitivity reactions

Interactions with Parsley Piert

Drug	Food	Herb	Lab Test
None known	None known	None known	None known

 = Pregnancy = Pediatric = Alert 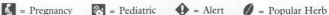 = Popular Herb

Client Considerations

Assess

- Assess for hypersensitivity reactions. If these are present, discontinue use of parsley piert and administer antihistamine or other appropriate therapy.

Administer

- Instruct the client to store parsley piert in a cool, dry place, away from heat and moisture.

Teach Client/Family

- Until more research is available, caution the client not to use parsley piert during pregnancy and lactation and not to give it to children.
- Advise the client that research is lacking for any uses or actions of this herb.

Pharmacology

Pharmacokinetics

Pharmacokinetics and pharmacodynamics are unknown.

Primary Chemical Components of Parsley Piert and Their Possible Actions		
Chemical Class	**Individual Component**	**Possible Action**
Tannin		Wound healing; astringent

Actions

No research studies have been done for parsley piert, although its use continues. This herb is known to contain tannins, which are well known for their wound-healing and astringent properties. These chemicals are thought to act on the genitourinary system to soothe irritation.

Passion Flower
(pa'shuhn flou'uhr)

Scientific name: *Passiflora incarnata*

Other common names: Apricot vine, granadilla, Jamaican honeysuckle, maypop, maypot, passion fruit, passion vine, purple passion flower, water lemon

Class 1

Origin: Passion flower is a perennial found in the tropics of the Americas.

Uses

Reported Uses

Passion flower is used as a sedative and to treat anxiety sleep disorders, neuralgia, nervous tachycardia, restlessness, and opiate withdrawal.

Investigational Uses

Initial research is underway to identify the use of passion flower in the treatment of the symptoms of Parkinson's disease and as an antitussive.

Product Availability and Dosages

Available Forms

Crude extract, dried herb, fluid extract, homeopathic products, tincture

Plant Parts Used: Flowers, fruit

Dosages and Routes

Adult

All dosages listed are PO.

General Dosages

- 10-30 drops tid (0.7% flavonoids)
- Dried herb: 0.25-1 g tid
- Fluid extract: 0.5-1 ml tid
- Tea: 4-6 tsp of herb in three divided doses
- Tincture: 0.5-2 ml tid

Insomnia

- Dried herb/tea: 4-8 g hs (Murray, 1998)
- Dry powdered extract: 300-450 mg hs (2.6% flavonoids) (Murray, 1998)

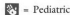

🝖 = Pregnancy   🐾 = Pediatric   ◆ = Alert   🍃 = Popular Herb

- Fluid extract: 2-4 ml (½-1 tsp) hs (1:1 dilution) (Murray, 1998)
- Tincture: 6-8 ml (1½-2 tsp) hs (1:5 dilution) (Murray, 1998)

Precautionary Information

Contraindications

Until more research is available, passion flower should not be used during pregnancy and lactation and should not be given to children. Passion flower should not be used by persons with hypersensitivity to it. Class 1 herb.

Side Effects/Adverse Reactions

Integumentary: Hypersensitivity reactions
Gastrointestinal: Nausea, vomiting, anorexia, LIVER TOXICITY
Central Nervous System: CENTRAL NERVOUS SYSTEM DEPRESSION (high doses)
Toxicity: SEVERE NAUSEA, VOMITING, DROWSINESS, PROLONGED QTC, NONSUSTAINED VENTRICULAR TACHYCARDIA (Fisher, 2000)

Interactions with Passion Flower

Drug

Central nervous system depressants (alcohol, antianxiety agents, antipsychotics, barbiturates, opiates, benzodiazepines, sedative/hypnotics): Use of passion flower with central nervous system depressants may cause increased sedation; avoid concurrent use (theoretical).

MAOIs: Use of passion flower with MAOIs may cause increased MAOI activity; avoid concurrent use (theoretical).

Food	Herb	Lab Test
None known	None known	None known

P

Client Considerations

Assess

- Assess for hypersensitivity reactions. If these are present, discontinue use of passion flower and administer antihistamine or other appropriate therapy.
- Assess for toxicity (see Side Effects) if the client is using high doses of this herb or is taking it for a prolonged period.

 Endangered Herb   Adverse effects: BOLD = life-threatening

Administer

- Instruct the client to store passion flower products in a cool, dry place, away from heat and moisture.

Teach Client/Family

- Until more research is available, caution the client not to use passion flower during pregnancy and lactation and not to give it to children.

Pharmacology

Pharmacokinetics

Pharmacokinetics and pharmacodynamics are unknown.

Primary Chemical Components of Passion Flower and Their Possible Actions		
Chemical Class	**Individual Component**	**Possible Action**
Flavonoid	Vitexin; Isoorientin (Li, 1991); Isovitexin Umbelliferone; Coumarin; Schaftoside; Isoschaftoside	Anxiolytic
Alkaloid	Harman; Harmaline	Uterine stimulant; MAOI action
	Harmine; Harmalol; Harmol	
Pyrone	Maltol	Sedative
Glycoside	Gynocardin	Cyanogenic
Carbohydrate	Sucrose	

Actions

Anxiolytic Action

Research on passion flower is lacking. Initial evidence indicates a possible anxiolytic action. One study using laboratory mice evaluated several herbs for their central nervous system effects: *Crataegus oxyacantha, Valeriana officinalis, Hyoscyamus niger, Matricaria chamomilla, Piscidia erythrina, Atropa bella-donna,* and *Passiflora incarnata. Passiflora incarnata* showed anxiolytic action, whereas *Crataegus oxyacantha* and *Valeriana officinalis* showed sedative effects. The other herbs showed

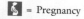 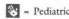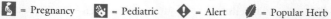

either no action or only limited central nervous system activity (Della Loggia, 1981). Another study (Soulimani, 1997) showed similar results when the chemical components harman, harmine, harmaline, harmol, harmalol, orientin, isoorientin, vitexin, and isovitexin were tested in mice. Sedative effects were confirmed after laboratory testing.

Opiate Withdrawal

One study is available that confirmed the decrease in opiate cravings, restlessness, anxiety, and irritability (Akhond-Zadeh, 2001).

Antitussive Action

The significant antitussive activity of *Passiflora incarnata* was identified when administered to sulfur-dioxide–induced cough in mice (Dhawan, 2002).

References

Akchondzadeh S et al: Passion flower in the treatment of opiate withdrawal: a double-blind randomized controlled trial, *J Clin Pharm Ther* 26:369-373, 2001.

Della Loggia R et al: Evaluation of the activity on the mouse central nervous system of several plant extracts and a combination of them, *Riv Neurol* 51(5):297-310, 1981.

Dhawan K et al: Antitussive activity of the methanol extract of *Passiflora incarnata* leaves, *Fitoterapia* 73(5):397-399, 2002.

Fisher AA et al: Toxicity of *Passiflora incarnata* L., *J Toxicol Clin Toxicol* 38(1):63-66, 2000.

Li QM et al: Mass spectral characterization of C-glycosidic flavonoids isolated from a medicinal plant *(Passiflora incarnata)*, *J Chromatogr* 562(1-2):435-446, 1991.

Murray M, Pizzarno J: *The encyclopedia of natural medicine*, 2 ed (revised), Roseville, Calif, 1998, Prima.

Soulimani R et al: Behavioural effects *Passiflora incarnata* L. and its indole alkaloid and flavonoid derivatives and maltol in the mouse, *J Ethnopharmacol* 57(1):11-20, 1997.

P

Pau D'arco
(pah'ew dahr'koe)

Scientific name: *Tabebuia impetiginosa*

Other common names: Ipe, ipe roxo, ipes, la pacho, lapacho, lapacho colorado, lapacho morado, lapachol, purple lapacho, red lapacho, roxo, taheebo, tajibo, trumpet bush, trumpet tree   Class 1 (Bark)

Origin: Pau d'arco is a tree found in South America, Central America, Mexico, and Florida.

Uses

Reported Uses

Pau d'arco is used in South America and the Caribbean to treat various conditions such as cold and flu, diarrhea, fever, sexually transmitted diseases, candida infection (orally, topically) snakebite, wounds, joint pain, urinary incontinence, psoriasis, and infections. It is also used as an aphrodisiac.

Investigational Uses

Other possible uses for pau d'arco include the treatment of cancer, HIV/AIDS, hepatic disorders, diabetes mellitus, and lupus (systemic lupus erythematosus). It may also show efficacy as an antimicrobial.

Product Availability and Dosages

Available Forms

Capsules, extract, salve, tablets, tea

Plant Parts Used: Bark

Dosages and Routes

Adult

All dosages listed are PO.

- Capsules/tablets: 2 caps/tabs bid with water at meals; may be used as a tea
- Lapachol: 1-2 g qd
- Tea: place 15 g bark in 2 cups water, boil 10 min, strain

🍃 = Pregnancy   🐾 = Pediatric   ❗ = Alert   🌿 = Popular Herb

Precautionary Information

Contraindications

Until more research is available, pau d'arco should not be used during pregnancy and lactation and should not be given to children. It should not be used by persons with hypersensitivity to this herb or those with hemophilia, von Willebrand's disease, or thrombocytopenia. Class 1 herb (bark).

Side Effects/Adverse Reactions

Gastrointestinal: Nausea, vomiting, anorexia
Integumentary: Hypersensitivity reactions
Systemic: BLEEDING; TOXIC REACTIONS (theoretical)

Interactions with Pau D'arco

Drug

Anticoagulants (heparin, salicylates, warfarin): Use of pau d'arco with anticoagulants may result in an increased risk of bleeding; avoid concurrent use (theoretical).

Food	Herb	Lab Test
None known	None known	None known

P

Client Considerations

Assess

- Assess for hypersensitivity reactions. If these are present, discontinue use of pau d'arco and administer antihistamine or other appropriate therapy.
- Determine whether the client is using other anticoagulants (e.g., warfarin, heparin, salicylates) or has a coagulation deficiency. These clients should avoid using this herb (see Interactions).

Administer

- Instruct the client to store pau d'arco in a cool, dry place, away from heat and moisture.

Teach Client/Family

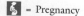

- Until more research is available, caution the client not to use pau d'arco during pregnancy and lactation and not to give it to children.

Pharmacology

Pharmacokinetics

Pharmacokinetics and pharmacodynamics are unknown.

Primary Chemical Components of Pau D'arco and Their Possible Actions		
Chemical Class	**Individual Component**	**Possible Action**
Quinone	Lapachone; Lapachol Tabebuin	Antimicrobial
Dialdehyde	Methoxybenzoyloxy; Dimethoxybenzoyloxy (Koyama, 2000)	

Actions

Antimicrobial Action

The major focus of research for pau d'arco is its antimicrobial effects. One study demonstrated its activity against *Staphylococcus aureus, Escherichia coli,* and *Aspergillus niger.* Of the extracts tested, pau d'arco was one of the most active (Anesini, 1993). Another study demonstrated the remarkable broad-spectrum antimicrobial activity of this herb against many gram-positive and gram-negative bacteria and fungi (Binutu, 1994). The stem bark was shown to be the most active; extracts of leaves were active only against *Candida albicans.*

Antipsoriatic Action

The antipsoriatic activity of pau d'arco was confirmed using compounds available in passion flower (Muller, 1999).

References

Anesini C et al: Screening of plants used in Argentine folk medicine for antimicrobial activity, *J Ethnopharmacol* 39(2):119-128, 1993.

Binutu OA et al: Antimicrobial potentials of some plant species of the Bigoniaceae family, *Afr J Med Sci* 23(3):269-273, 1994.

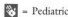 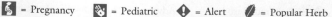

Koyama J et al: Cyclopentene dialdehydes from *Tabebuia impetiginosa*, *Phytochemistry* 53(8):869-872, 2000.

Muller K et al: Potential antipsoriatic agents: lapacho compounds as potent inhibitors of HaCaT cell growth, *J Nat Prod* 62(8):1134-1136, 1999.

Peach
(peech)

Scientific name: *Prunus persica*

Other common names: Amygdalin, laetrile, vitamin B-17

Class 2d (Seed)

Origin: Peach is a tree found throughout the world.

Uses

Reported Uses

Traditionally, the bark and leaves of the peach tree have been used as an anthelmintic, an astringent, and a diuretic, as well as to treat insomnia, cough, and constipation. In the 1970s, peach pits (Laetrile) were a popular but unproved treatment for cancer in other countries. Topically, peach is used to treat minor skin disorders such as burns, abrasions, blisters, scratches, eczema, psoriasis, and warts.

Product Availability and Dosages

Available Forms

Bark, kernel oil, leaves, persic oil, seeds

Plant Parts Used: Bark, kernels, leaves, seeds

Dosages and Routes

Adult PO

- PO tea (bark): boil ½ oz bark in 1 pt water, let stand 15 min, strain; may be taken tid
- PO tea (leaves): boil 1 oz leaves in 1 pt water, let stand 15 min, strain; may be taken tid

Precautionary Information

Contraindications

Until more research is available, peach should not be used therapeutically during pregnancy and lactation and should not be given therapeutically to children. Peach should not be used by persons with hypersensitivity to it. Class 2d herb (seed).

Side Effects/Adverse Reactions

Cyanide poisoning (peach pits): SEVERE VOMITING, ABDOMINAL OR EPIGASTRIC PAIN, DIZZINESS, COMA, SEIZURES, DEATH
Ear, Eye, Nose, and Throat: Optic atrophy, tinnitus
Gastrointestinal: Nausea, vomiting, anorexia
Integumentary: Hypersensitivity reactions

Interactions with Peach			
Drug	**Food**	**Herb**	**Lab Test**
None known	None known	None known	None known

Client Considerations

Assess

- Assess for hypersensitivity reactions. If these are present, discontinue use of peach and administer antihistamine or other appropriate therapy. Advise clients who are hypersensitive to peach skin to wear gloves when handling.
- Assess for chronic cyanide poisoning: vision changes with optic atrophy, dizziness, nerve pain, and nerve deafness. If these are present, discontinue use of peach immediately.

Administer

- Instruct the client to store peach in a cool, dry place, away from heat and moisture.

Teach Client/Family

- Until more research is available, caution the client not to use peach therapeutically during pregnancy and lactation and not to give it therapeutically to children.

 = Pregnancy    = Pediatric   = Alert   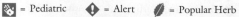 = Popular Herb

- Advise the client to use only the bark, leaves, or seeds—never peach pits—because of the potential for cyanide poisoning.

Pharmacology

Pharmacokinetics

Pharmacokinetics and pharmacodynamics are unknown.

Primary Chemical Components of Peach and Their Possible Actions		
Chemical Class	Individual Component	Possible Action
Bark, Leaves, and Seeds Contain		
Amygdalin		Cyanide poisoning
Bark and Leaves Also Contain		
Phloretin		

Actions

Initial research is available on the use of *Prunus persica* as an antifungal, as an agent to decrease melanin biosynthesis, and in combination to treat platelet aggregation defect and uterine myomas.

Antifungal Action

Peach has been shown to possess antifungal properties. When researchers screened 15 species of leaves for fungitoxic activity, the leaves of *Prunus persica* completely inhibited mycelial growth of *Aspergillus flavus* (Mishra, 1990).

Melanin Biosynthesis Inhibitor

Another study identified the inhibitory properties of peach on melanin biosynthesis (Matsuda, 1994). Investigators collected 38 different herbs and used the dried leaves. Results suggest that dried peach leaves may be used as a whitening agent for the skin.

Platelet Aggregate Action

In a study testing the platelet aggregate properties of *Prunus persica, Carthamus tinctorium,* and *Glycyrrhiza uralensis,* the

P

experimental group experience a significant change in platelet aggregation (Shen, 1994).

Uterine Myoma Inhibitor

In a study testing the effects of peach on uterine myomas, the myomas shrank in 60% of the cases (Sakamoto, 1992).

Anticancer Action

Peach pits (under the product name Laetrile) were used extensively as a cancer treatment in the 1970s, primarily in Mexico. However, Laetrile is not currently used because of the potential for cyanide poisoning.

References

Matsuda H et al: Studies of cuticle drugs from natural sources, II: inhibitory effects of *Prunus* plants on melanin biosynthesis, *Biol Pharm Bull* 17(10):1417-1420, 1994.

Mishra AK et al: Fungitoxic properties of *Prunus persica* oil, *Hindustan Antibiot Bull* 32(3-4):91-93, 1990.

Sakamoto S et al: Pharmacotherapeutic effects of kuei-chih-fu-ling-wan (Keishi-bukuryo-gan) on human uterine myomas, *Am J Chin Med* 20(3-4):314-317, 1992.

Shen D et al: Effect of xiaoyu pian on new platelet aggregation defect, *Chung Kuo Chung Hsi I Chieh Ho Tsa Chih* 14(10):589-591, 1994.

Pectin
(pehk'tuhn)

Origin: Pectin is found in the cell walls of all plants.

Uses

Reported Uses

Traditionally, pectin has been used to treat diarrhea and to reduce blood glucose and high cholesterol levels.

Investigational Uses

Investigators are working to determine whether pectin can help prevent or reduce radiation sickness.

Product Availability and Dosages

Available Forms

Pectin is not commercially available.

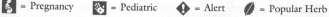

 = Pregnancy   = Pediatric   = Alert   = Popular Herb

Plant Parts Used: Cell walls of all plants, usually obtained from the rind of citrus fruits and apple.

Dosages and Routes
No dosage consensus is available.

Precautionary Information
Contraindications
No absolute contraindications are known.

Side Effects/Adverse Reactions
Gastrointestinal: Nausea, vomiting, anorexia
Integumentary: Hypersensitivity reactions
Respiratory: Asthma (inhalation of pectin dust)

Interactions with Pectin

Drug
Pectin reduces the absorption of all drugs, vitamins, and minerals if taken concurrently. Separate doses by 3 hours to ensure adequate absorption.

Food
None known

Herb
Beta-carotene: Pectin reduces beta-carotene absorption.

Lab Test
None known

Client Considerations
Assess
- Assess for hypersensitivity reactions, such as asthma from the inhalation of pectin dust. If present, discontinue use of pectin and administer antihistamine or other appropriate therapy.

Administer
- Instruct the client to store pectin in a cool, dry place, away from heat and moisture.

Teach Client/Family
- Advise the client not to inhale pectin dust.

🕊 Endangered Herb   Adverse effects: **BOLD** = life-threatening

- Inform the client that it is necessary to separate doses of drugs, vitamins, and minerals from doses of pectin to ensure adequate absorption (see Interactions).

Pharmacology

Pharmacokinetics

Pectin is an adsorbent, a soluble fiber; binds cholesterol and is not metabolized.

Primary Chemical Components of Pectin and Their Possible Actions		
Chemical Class	Individual Component	Possible Action
Polysaccharide Protopectin		Insoluble compound

Actions

Most of the available research focuses on the use of pectin to lower blood glucose levels and cholesterol.

Anticholesterol Action

The addition of pectin and guar to the diet has been shown to reduce total cholesterol and triglycerides (Biesenbach, 1993). Another study showed that pectin decreases the transit time of feces in the colon, possibly reducing the risk of colon cancer (Harris, 1993).

Other Actions

One study (Rabbani, 2001) identified the use of pectin in controlling persistent diarrhea in Bangladeshi children. The diarrhea was significantly decreased by day 4 after green banana or pectin was introduced.

References

Biesenbach G et al: *Leber Magen Darm* 23(5):204, 1993 (abstract).
Harris PJ et al: *Mutat Res* 290(1):97, 1993.
Rabbini GH et al: Clinical studies in persistent diarrhea: dietary management with green banana or pectin in Bangladeshi children, *Gastroenterology* 121(3):554-560, 2001.

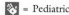 = Pregnancy   = Pediatric   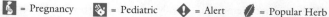 = Alert   = Popular Herb

Pennyroyal
(pehn-ee-rawee'uhl)

Scientific names: *Hedeoma pulegioides* (American pennyroyal), *Mentha pulegium* (European pennyroyal)

Other common names: American pennyroyal, European pennyroyal, mock pennyroyal, mosquito plant, pudding grass, squawbalm, squawmint, tickweed

Class 2b

Origin: American pennyroyal is found throughout North America in wooded regions.

Uses
Reported Uses
Traditionally, pennyroyal has been used as an abortifacient and to treat digestive, liver, and gallbladder disorders; gout; menstrual ailments; uterine fibroids; colds; fevers; flu; chest congestion; and colic. Externally, it is used to treat skin diseases. Some herbalists recommend its use for treating tumors. It may also be used as an insect repellant.

Product Availability and Dosages
Available Forms
Dried herb, dried leaves, flowers, oil

Plant Parts Used: Flowering tops, leaves

Dosages and Routes
Adult
All dosages listed are PO. NOTE: Pennyroyal is extremely toxic and should not be ingested.
- Tea (dried herb): place 1 tbsp dried herb in 8 oz warm water; may be taken bid
- Tea (dried leaves): place 2 tsp dried leaves in 8 oz boiling water, let stand 15 min, strain; may be taken bid

P

Precautionary Information

Contraindications

Because it is an abortifacient, pennyroyal should not be used during pregnancy. Pennyroyal should not be used during lactation and should not be given to children. Persons with seizure disorders, renal disease, or hepatic disease, or those with hypersensitivity to this herb, should not use it. Pennyroyal oil is extremely toxic and should not be ingested. Dried leaf tea is safe to drink. Class 2b herb.

Side Effects/Adverse Reactions

Cardiovascular: Hypertension
Central Nervous System: Fatigue, confusion, dizziness, hallucinations, malaise, SEIZURES, RIGORS, COMA, DEATH
Gastrointestinal: Nausea, vomiting, anorexia, abdominal pain and cramping, HEPATOTOXICITY
Genitourinary: NEPHROTOXICITY
Integumentary: Hypersensitivity reactions
Reproductive: ABORTION
Respiratory: RESPIRATORY DEPRESSION

Interactions with Pennyroyal

Drug

Cytochrome P-450: Concurrent use of pennyroyal with drugs metabolized by cytochrome P-450 should be avoided.

Food
None known

Herb
None known

Lab Test

Pennyroyal may cause increased ALT, AST, total bilirubin, and urine bilirubin. Pennyroyal may cause decreased red blood cells.

Client Considerations

Assess

- Assess for hypersensitivity reactions. If these are present, discontinue use of pennyroyal and administer antihistamine or other appropriate therapy.

 = Pregnancy    = Pediatric   = Alert   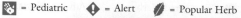 = Popular Herb

• Assess for symptoms of toxicity: lethargy, malaise, fatigue, oliguria, jaundice, seizures. If these are present, discontinue use of pennyroyal immediately and administer supportive measures.

Administer

 • Instruct the client to use pennyroyal only under the supervision of a qualified herbalist. This herb can be toxic.
• Instruct the client to store pennyroyal products in a cool, dry place, away from heat and moisture.

Teach Client/Family

 • Caution the client not to use pennyroyal during pregnancy and lactation and not to give it to children.
• Caution the client to avoid self-administration of this herb because of its toxicity.

Pharmacology

Pharmacokinetics

Pharmacokinetics and pharmacodynamics are unknown.

Primary Chemical Components of Pennyroyal and Their Possible Actions		
Chemical Class	**Individual Component**	**Possible Action**
Monoterpene	Pulegone	Abortifacient
Hedeomal		
Tannin	Rosmarinic acid	
Alpha-pinene		
Beta-pinene		
Octanone		
Limonene		
Cymene		
Octanol		
Octylacetate		
Methylcyclohexanone		
Methone		
Piperitenone		
Paraffin		
Volatile oil	Isomenthone; D-pulegone; Menthone	
Flavonoid	Diosmin; Hesperidin	

P

Actions

Little scientific research has been done on any uses or actions of pennyroyal. This herb is used as an insect repellent and has been used in the food and cosmetic industry for years. Most of the available information comes from anecdotal reports. Pennyroyal oil is extremely toxic and should not be ingested for any use.

Perilla
(puh-ri′luh)

Scientific name: *Perilla frutescens* L.

Other common names: Beefsteak plant, wild coleus

Origin: Perilla is found in the Orient.

Uses

Reported Uses

Perilla is used to treat allergic reactions. It is also used as a flavoring. Traditionally, perilla has been used as an antispasmodic, as well as to treat nausea, vomiting, and upper-respiratory conditions.

Investigational Uses

Initial research is available that documents the use of perilla as a hyperlipidemic antiasthma and a cancer protectant.

Product Availability and Dosages

Available Forms

Expressed oil of the seed, tea

Plant Parts Used: Dried leaves, seeds

Dosages and Routes

Asthma
• PO: seed oil: 10-20 g
No other published dosages are available.

🔥 = Pregnancy   ✋ = Pediatric   ◆ = Alert   🍃 = Popular Herb

Precautionary Information

Contraindications

Until more research is available, perilla should not be used during pregnancy and lactation and should not be given to children. Persons with hypersensitivity to perilla should not use it.

Side Effects/Adverse Reactions

Gastrointestinal: Nausea, vomiting, anorexia
Integumentary: Hypersensitivity reactions

Interactions with Perilla

Drug
Corticosteroids (betamethasone, dexamethasone, hydrocortisone, methylprednisolone, prednisolone, prednisone, triamcinolone): Perilla may augment the effect of corticosteroids; avoid concurrent use.

Food	Herb	Lab Test
None known	None known	None known

Client Considerations

Assess

- Assess for hypersensitivity reactions. If these are present, discontinue use of perilla and administer antihistamine or other appropriate therapy.

Administer

- Instruct the client to store perilla in a cool, dry place, away from heat and moisture.

Teach Client/Family

- Until more research is available, caution the client not to use perilla during pregnancy and lactation and not to give it to children.

Pharmacology

Pharmacokinetics

Pharmacokinetics and pharmacodynamics are unknown.

Primary Chemical Components of Perilla and Their Possible Actions

Chemical Class	Individual Component	Possible Action
Benzoxepin	Perilloxin; Dehydroperilloxin (Liu, 2000)	
Essential oil	Perillaldehyde; Perilla alcohol	Dermatitis
	Perilla ketone	Lung toxin
	Trans-caryophyllene; Hexadecanoic acid; Alpha-pinene; Citral; Limonene	
Flavone	Apigenin; Shishonin	
	Luteolin	Inhibitor of arachidonic-acid, tumor necrosis factor-α, oxazolone-induced allergic edema

Actions

Most of the research on perilla has focused on its ability to inhibit allergic reactions. Initial research has also begun to determine its hyperlipidemic and cancer protectant actions.

Antiallergy Action

One study tested the ability of perilla to inhibit induced systemic allergic reactions. Perilla was found to inhibit mast cell-mediated immediate-type allergic reactions (Shin, 2000). Other studies have also confirmed the use of perilla for the inhibition of allergic reactions (Ishihara, 1999; Imaoka, 1993). Luteolin, one of perilla's chemical components, showed a potent inhibitor of tumor necrosis factor-α, inhibitor of oxazolone-induced allergic edema and an inhibitor of arachidonic acid (Ueda, 2002).

References

Imaoka K et al: Effects of *Perilla frutescens* extract on anti-DNP IgE antibody production in mice, *Arerugi* 42(1):74-80, 1993.
Ishihara T et al: Inhibition of antigen-specific T helper type 2 responses by *Perilla frutescens* extract, *Arerugi* 48(4):443-450, 1999.

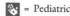 = Pregnancy   = Pediatric 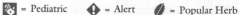 = Alert = Popular Herb

Liu J et al: Two new prenylated 3-benzoxepin derivatives as cyclooxygenase inhibitors from *Perilla frutescens* var. *acuta, J Nat Prod* 63(3):403-405, 2000.

Shin TY et al: Inhibitory effect of mast cell-mediated immediate-type allergic reactions in rats by *Perilla frutescens, Immunopharmacol Immunotoxicol* 22(3):489-500, 2000 (in-process citation).

Ueda H et al: Luteolin as an anti-inflammatory and anti-allergic constituent of *Perilla frutescens, Biol Pharm Bull* 25(9):1197-1202, 2002.

Peyote
(pay-oe′tay)

Scientific name: *Lophophora williamsii*

Other common names: Anhalonium, big chief, buttons, cactus, mesc, mescal, mescal buttons, mescaline, mexc, moon, pan peyote, peyote button

Controlled Substance: Schedule I

Origin: Peyote is found in Mexico and the southwestern region of the United States.

Uses
Reported Uses
Traditionally, peyote has been used in Indian culture during religious activities. Other traditional uses include treatment for arthritis, rheumatism, snakebite, burns, cardiac ailments, addiction, and paralysis. Peyote is also used as a hallucinogenic, an antimicrobial, and a sedative. Its use is illegal in the United States and most European countries.

Product Availability and Dosages
Available Forms
Basic pan peyote, button, mescaline hydrochloride, mescaline sulfate, soluble peyote, tincture

Plant Parts Used: Dried tops, whole plant

Dosages and Routes
No published dosages are available.

P

Precautionary Information

Contraindications

Peyote should not be used during pregnancy and lactation and should not be given to children. Persons with hypersensitivity to this herb should not use it. Physical dependence and death can result from the use of peyote.

Side Effects/Adverse Reactions

Cardiovascular: HYPERTENSION, TACHYCARDIA
Central Nervous System: Anxiety, paranoia, hallucinations, tremors, ataxia
Gastrointestinal: Nausea, vomiting, anorexia
Integumentary: Hypersensitivity reactions

Interactions with Peyote

Drug

Central nervous system drugs (alcohol, opiates, marijuana, LSD, angel dust): Peyote may increase the effects of other central nervous system drugs; avoid concurrent use.

Food	Herb	Lab Test
None known	None known	None known

Client Considerations

Assess

- Assess for the client's use of this drug or other hallucinogens (see Interactions).

Administer

- Peyote should not be administered for any reason. Use of this herb is illegal in the United States and most European countries. Physical dependence and death can occur from its use.

Teach Client/Family

- Caution the client not to use peyote during pregnancy and lactation and not to give it to children.
- Advise the client that peyote is illegal and is not considered useful for any condition.

 = Pregnancy    = Pediatric   = Alert   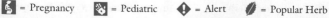 = Popular Herb

- Inform the client that physical dependence and death can result from peyote use.

Pharmacology
Pharmacokinetics
Peak 4-6 hours; duration 14 hours.

Primary Chemical Components of Peyote and Their Possible Actions		
Chemical Class	**Individual Component**	**Possible Action**
Alkaloid	Mescaline Formylmescaline; Acetylmescaline; Methylmescaline; Demethylmescaline; Dimethoxyphenylethylamine; Tyramine; Hordenine; Candicine; Anhalamine; Anhaladine; Anhalanine; Formylanhalamine	Hallucinogenic

P

Actions
Hallucinogenic Action
Research studies to date have focused on the hallucinogenic effects of peyote. One study (Keller, 1980) identified the ability of this herb to promote catecholamine metabolism. This research compared normal brain catecholamine formation with catecholamine metabolism that causes mind-altering effects. Results of these studies may eventually be useful in identifying a use for peyote in the treatment of mental illness.

References
Keller WJ et al: Catecholamine metabolism in a psychoactive cactus, *Clin Toxicol* 16(2):233-243, 1980.

Pill-Bearing Spurge
(pil beh'ring spuhrj)

Scientific names: Euphorbia pilulifera; also known as *Euphorbia hirta, Euphorbia capitata*

Other common names: Asthma weed, catshair, euphorbia, garden spurge, milkweed, queensland asthmaweed, snake weed

Origin: Pill-bearing spurge is an annual found in India, Australia, and the southwestern region of the United States.

Uses
Reported Uses
Pill-bearing spurge is used to treat respiratory conditions such as asthma, bronchitis, and allergies. It is also used to treat colds, diarrhea, amebiasis, sexually transmitted diseases, snake bite, and ophthalmic conditions.

Product Availability and Dosages
Available Forms
Capsules, fluid extract, powder, tablets, tincture

Plant Parts Used: Dried whole plant

Dosages and Routes
Adult
All dosages listed are PO.
- Fluid extract: 0.2-0.3 ml tid (1:1 dilution in 45% alcohol)
- Infusion: 120-300 mg tid
- Powder: 120-300 mg tid
- Tincture: 0.5-2 ml tid (1:5 dilution in 60% alcohol)

Precautionary Information
Contraindications
Until more research is available, pill-bearing spurge should not be used in during pregnancy and lactation and should not be given to children. Persons with hemophilia, von Willebrand's disease, or other bleeding disorders should not use this herb. Persons with hypersensitivity to pill-bearing spurge should not use it.

= Pregnancy   = Pediatric   = Alert   = Popular Herb

Precautionary Information—cont'd

Side Effects/Adverse Reactions

Gastrointestinal: Nausea, vomiting, anorexia, gastric symptoms

Integumentary: Hypersensitivity reactions, contact dermatitis

---

Interactions with Pill-Bearing Spurge

Drug

ACE inhibitors: ACE inhibitors may increase hypotension when used with pill-bearing spurge; avoid concurrent use (theoretical).

Anticholinergics (atropine, belladonna, scopolamine): Pill-bearing spurge may decrease the effects of anticholinergics; avoid concurrent use (theoretical).

Anticoagulants (heparin, salicylates, warfarin): Pill-bearing spurge may increase the effects of anticoagulants; avoid concurrent use (theoretical).

Barbiturates (phenobarbital): Pill-bearing spurge may increase the effects of barbiturates; avoid concurrent use (theoretical).

Cholinesterase inhibitors (edrophonium, donepezil, physostigmine): Pill-bearing spurge may increase the effects of cholinesterase inhibitors (theoretical).

Disulfiram: Reaction may occur when disulfiram is used with pill-bearing spurge; do not use concurrently (theoretical).

Food	Herb	Lab Test
None known	None known	None known

P

Client Considerations

Assess

- Assess for hypersensitivity reactions. If present, discontinue use of pill-bearing spurge and administer antihistamine or other appropriate therapy.
- Assess all medications used by the client. Several theoretical drug interactions may occur (see Interactions).

Administer

- Instruct the client to store pill-bearing spurge in a cool, dry place, away from heat and moisture.

Teach Client/Family

- Until more research is available, caution the client not to use pill-bearing spurge during pregnancy and lactation and not to give it to children.
- Give the client a written list of medications that should not be taken with this herb.
- Advise the hypersensitive client to avoid even touching this herb.

Pharmacology

Pharmacokinetics

Pharmacokinetics and pharmacodynamics are unknown.

Primary Chemical Components of Pill-Bearing Spurge and Their Possible Actions

Chemical Class	Individual Component	Possible Action
Choline		Antispasmodic
Shikimic acid		Antispasmodic
Flavonoid	Quercitrin; Quercetin; Leuocyanidin	
Triterpene	Taraxerone; Taraxerol; Alpha-amyrin; Beta-amyrin	
Sterol	Campesterol; Sitosterol	
Alkane	Hentriacontane	
Phenol	Sinapylglutathione	
Resin		
Tannin		

Actions

Very little primary research has been done on pill-bearing spurge. Most research or literature identifies the toxicity of the plant. One study identifies the cancer risk for humans who consume products from livestock fed species of spurge (Zayed, 1998). Iranians who consumed milk from goats and sheep fed spurge showed a high local incidence of esophageal cancer.

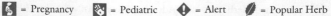

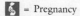 = Pregnancy    = Pediatric   = Alert   = Popular Herb

Another earlier study discusses the tumor-producing action of spurge (Hergenhahn, 1984).

One study identified the antidiarrheal action of spurge resulting from quercetin, one of its chemical components (Galvez, 1993). Another study has shown the sedative actions of this herb, with lower doses producing an anxiolytic action (Lanhers, 1991).

References

Galvez J et al: Antidiarrheic activity of *Euphorbia hirta* extract and isolation of an active flavonoid constituent, *Planta Med* 59:333-336, 1993.

Hergenhahn M et al: On the active principles of the spurge family (Euphorbiaceae), V: extremely skin-irritant and moderately tumor-promoting diterpene esters from *Euphorbia resinifera* Berg, *J Cancer Res Clin Oncol* 108(1):98-109, 1984.

Lanhers MC et al: Analgesic, antipyretic and anti-inflammatory properties of *Euphorbia hirta*, *Planta Med* 57:225-231, 1991.

Zayed SM et al: Dietary cancer risk from conditional cancerogens in produce of livestock fed on species of spurge (Euphorbiaceae), III: milk of lactating goats fed on the skin irritant herb *Euphorbia peplus* is polluted by tumor promoters of the ingenane diterpene ester type, *J Cancer Res Clin Oncol* 124(6):301-306, 1998.

P

Pineapple
(pine'a-puhl)

Scientific name: *Ananas comosus*

Other common names: Ananas, golden rocket, smooth cayenne

Origin: Pineapple is found in South America, Thailand, and Hawaii.

Uses

Reported Uses

Pineapple is used therapeutically to treat obesity and constipation. Topically, pineapple may be used to treat wounds and inflammation.

Product Availability and Dosages

Available Forms

Candy, extract, flavorings, juice, syrups, whole fruit

 Endangered Herb   Adverse effects: **BOLD** = life-threatening

Plant Parts Used: Fruit

Dosages and Routes
Adult
No published dosages are available

Precautionary Information

Contraindications

Until more research is available, pineapple should not be used therapeutically during pregnancy and lactation and should not be given therapeutically to children. Pineapple should not be used therapeutically by persons with coagulation disorders. Persons with hypersensitivity to pineapple should not use it.

Side Effects/Adverse Reactions

Gastrointestinal: Nausea, vomiting, anorexia, diarrhea, stomatitis
Genitourinary: Uterine contractions
Integumentary: Hypersensitivity reactions, rash

Interactions with Pineapple

Drug
ACE inhibitors: Pineapple may antagonize the action of ACE inhibitors; avoid concurrent use.
Anticoagulants (heparin, salicylates, warfarin): Pineapple may increase bleeding time when used with anticoagulants; avoid concurrent use.

Food	Herb	Lab Test
None known	None known	None known

Client Considerations

Assess

- Assess for hypersensitivity reactions. If present, discontinue use of pineapple and administer antihistamine or other appropriate therapy.
- Assess for the use of ACE inhibitors and anticoagulants (see Interactions).

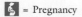 = Pregnancy    = Pediatric   = Alert   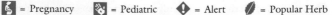 = Popular Herb

Administer
- Instruct the client to store pineapple in a cool, dry place, away from heat and moisture.

Teach Client/Family
- Until more research is available, caution the client not to use pineapple therapeutically during pregnancy and lactation and not to give it therapeutically to children.
- Advise the client not to use large amounts of pineapple; gastrointestinal upset may occur.

Pharmacology

Pharmacokinetics
Pharmacokinetics and pharmacodynamics are unknown.

Primary Chemical Components of Pineapple and Their Possible Actions		
Chemical Class	Individual Component	Possible Action
Proteolytic enzyme	Bromelain	Wound healing; antiinflammatory; antitumor
Acid	Malic acid; Citric acid	
Vitamin	A; C	

P

Actions

Antifungal Action
One study found that the chemical components of pineapple stems possess antifungal effects against *Pythium* sp. (Tawata, 1996).

Other Actions
Bromelain, a chemical component of pineapple, has shown promise as a platelet aggregation inhibitor. Bromelain also possesses fibrinolytic, antiinflammatory, antitumor, and skin debridement actions (Taussig, 1988). Another study (Rowan, 1990) showed rapid debridement of wounds using enzyme fractions from the pineapple stem. Debridement occurred within 4 hours.

🝿 Endangered Herb   Adverse effects: BOLD = life-threatening

References

Rowan AD et al: Debridement of experimental full-thickness skin burns of rats with enzyme fractions derived from pineapple stems, *Burns* 16(4):243-246, 1990.

Taussig SJ et al: Bromelain, the enzyme complex of pineapple *(Ananas comosus)* and its clinical application: an update, *J Ethnopharmacol* 22(2):191-203, 1988.

Tawata S et al: Synthesis and antifungal activity of cinnamic acid ester, *Biosci Biotechnol Biochem* 60(5):909-910, 1996.

Pipsissewa
(pip-si′suh-wah)

Scientific name: *Chimaphila umbellata*

Other common names: Ground holly, prince's pine, spotted wintergreen, wintergreen

Origin: Pipsissewa is a perennial found in North America, Europe, and Asia.

Uses

Reported Uses

Pipsissewa is used as an astringent and antispasmodic, as well as to treat anxiety, seizures, gastrointestinal disorders, and kidney stones. The most common use is as a urinary antiseptic. It is used topically to treat decubitus ulcers, venous statis ulcers, and superficial wounds.

Investigational Uses

Pipsissewa is used experimentally as a treatment for diabetes and urinary tract infections.

Product Availability and Dosages

Available Forms

Crude extract

Plant Parts Used: Dried herb

Dosages and Routes

No published dosages are available.

Precautionary Information

Contraindications

Until more research is available, pipsissewa should not be used during pregnancy and lactation and should not be given to children. Persons with peptic or duodenal ulcers, ulcerative colitis, Crohn's disease, diabetes mellitus, gastroesophageal reflux disease (GERD), or iron deficiency should not use this herb. Persons who are hypersensitive to pipsissewa should not use it.

Side Effects/Adverse Reactions

Gastrointestinal: Nausea, vomiting, anorexia, diarrhea, gastrointestinal irritation
Integumentary: Hypersensitivity reactions

Interactions with Pipsissewa

Drug
Minerals: Minerals should be taken 2 hours before or after this herb.

Food	Herb	Lab Test
None known	None known	None known

P

Client Considerations

Assess

• Assess for hypersensitivity reactions and contact dermatitis. If present, discontinue use of this herb and administer antihistamine or other appropriate therapy.

Administer

• Instruct the client to store pipsissewa in a cool, dry place, away from heat and moisture.
• Instruct the client to take mineral supplements 2 hours before or after this herb.
• Not for long-term use because of hydroquinine content; can cause hydroquinone toxicity (tinnitus, nausea, vomiting, convulsions, collapse).

 Endangered Herb   Adverse effects: **BOLD** = life-threatening

Teach Client/Family

• Until more research is available, caution the client not to use pipsissewa during pregnancy and lactation and not to give it to children.

Pharmacology

Pharmacokinetics

Pharmacokinetics and pharmacodynamics are unknown.

Primary Chemical Components of Pipsissewa and Their Possible Actions		
Chemical Class	Individual Component	Possible Action
Arbutin		Urinary antiseptic
Naphthoquinone	Chimaphilin	Contact dermatitis; urinary antiseptic
Hydroquinone		
Ericolin		
Chlorophyll		
Urson		
Isohomarbutin		
Reinfolin		
Homogentisic acid		
Toluquinol		
Hyperoside		
Taraxasterol		
Nonacosane		
Methyl salicylate		
Mineral		
Pectic acid		
Tannin		
Resin		
Gum		
Starch		
Sugar		

Actions

Very little information is available for pipsissewa. One study (Hausen, 1988) identified a naturally occurring quinone present in pipsissewa. Chimaphilin, a naphthoquinone, was found to cause contact dermatitis. Another older study (Segelman, 1969) found pipsissewa to possess hypoglycemic properties.

 = Pregnancy    = Pediatric   = Alert   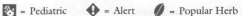 = Popular Herb

References

Hausen BM et al: The sensitizing capacity of chimaphilin, a naturally-occuring quinone, *Contact Dermatitis* 19(3):180-183, 1988.

Segelman AB et al: Biological and phytochemical evaluation of plants, IV: a new rapid procedure for the simultaneous determination of saponins and tannins, *Lyoydia* 32(1):59-65, 1969.

Plantain
(plan'tuhn)

Scientific names: *Plantago lanceolata, Plantago major, Plantago psyllium, Plantago ovata*

Other common names: Blond plantago, broadleaf plantain, buckhorn, cart tract plant, common plantain, English plantain, flea seed, French psyllium, greater plantain, Indian plantago, lanten, narrowleaf plantago seed, plantain seed, psyllium, ribwort, ripple grass, snakeweed, Spanish psyllium, tract plant, way-bread, white man's foot, wild plantain, wild saso

Origin: Plantain is found worldwide.

Uses

Reported Uses

Several different products are derived from plantain. Psyllium is used as a bulk laxative. Other internal uses include treatment for cough, urinary tract conditions, and diarrhea. Two plantain species are used to treat inflammation from burns and wounds. Plantain leaves are used topically for wound healing.

Investigational Uses

Plantain is used experimentally for the treatment of cancer and immunosuppressive disorders.

Product Availability and Dosages

Available Forms

Fluid extract; psyllium seeds, powder, tablets; tincture

Plant Parts Used: Husks, leaves, and seeds depending on product

Dosages and Routes
Adult
- PO fluid extract: 2-4 ml tid (1:1 dilution)
- PO seeds: 7.5 g with several glasses of water

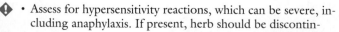

Precautionary Information
Contraindications

Until more research is available, plantain should not be used during pregnancy and lactation. It should not be used by persons with intestinal obstruction. Persons who are hypersensitive to plantain should not use it.

Side Effects/Adverse Reactions
Gastrointestinal: Nausea, vomiting, anorexia, flatus, diarrhea, bloating, obstruction
Integumentary: Hypersensitivity reactions, dermatitis
Systemic: ANAPHYLAXIS

Interactions with Plantain

Drug
Carbamazepine: Plantain may decrease the effects of carbamazepine; avoid concurrent use.
Cardiac agents (beta-blockers, calcium channel blockers, cardiac glycosides): Plantain may increase the effects of cardiac tracts; avoid concurrent use.
Iron salts: Plantain tea may decrease the absorption of iron salts.
Lithium: Plantain may decrease the effects of lithium; avoid concurrent use.

Food	Herb
None known	None known

Lab Test
Plantain may cause a false increase in serum digoxin.

Client Considerations
Assess
- Assess for hypersensitivity reactions, which can be severe, including anaphylaxis. If present, herb should be discontin-

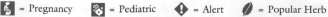
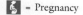 = Pregnancy   = Pediatric  = Alert = Popular Herb

ued and antihistamines or other appropriate therapy administered immediately.

- Assess bowel pattern if using as a bulk laxative.
- Assess medication use (see Interactions).

Administer

- Instruct the client to store plantain in a cool, dry place, away from heat and moisture.
- Instruct the client to take all other medications 2 hours before or 2 hours after this herb to ensure proper absorption.

Teach Client/Family

- Until more research is available, caution the client not to use plantain during pregnancy and lactation.

Pharmacology

Pharmacokinetics

Pharmacokinetics and pharmacodynamics are unknown.

Primary Chemical Components of Plantain and Their Possible Actions

Chemical Class*	Individual Component	Possible Action
Alkaloid		
Flavonoid	Verbascoside; Homoplantaginin (Kunvari, 1999)	Possible antitumor
Amino acid		
Tannin		
Mucilage		
Polysaccharide		
Lipid		
Glycoside		
Terpenoid		
Polyholozidic		Gastroprotective
Phenylethanoid	Acteoside; Plantamajoside Cistanoside; Lavandulifolioside; Isoacetoside (Murai, 1995)	Inhibits arachidonic acid

*Varies depending on species

 Endangered Herb   Adverse effects: BOLD = life-threatening

Actions

Two chemical components of *Plantago media,* verbascoside and homoplantaginin, have shown variable antiproliferative actions (Kunvari, 1999). *Plantago lanceolata* has been shown to decrease inflammation in the respiratory tract and may be recommended as a treatment for moderate chronic cough, especially for children (Wegener, 1999). Another study showed the gastroprotective action of the chemical component polyholozide. This chemical component also has laxative action at higher doses (Hriscu, 1990). A new study (Rezaeipoor, 2000) has shown suppression of the humoral immune response in rabbits given *Plantago ovato.*

References

Hriscu A et al: A pharmacodynamic investigation of the effect of polyholozidic substances extracted from *Plantago* sp. on the digestive tract, *Rev Med Chir Soc Med Nat Iasi* 94(1):165-170, 1990.

Kunvari M et al: Biological activity and structure of antitumor compounds from *Plantago media* L., *Acta Pharm Hung* 69(5):232-239, 1999.

Murai M et al: Phenylethanoids in the herb of *Plantago lanceolata* and inhibitory effect on arachidonic acid-induced mouse ear edema, *Planta Med* 61(5):479-480, 1995 (letter).

Rezaeipoor R et al: The effect of *Plantago ovata* on humoral immune responses in experimental animals, *J Ethnopharmacol* 72(1-2):283-286, 2000.

Wegener T et al: Plantain (*Plantago lanceolata* L.): anti-inflammatory action in upper respiratory tract infections, *Wien Med Wochenschr* 149(8-10):211-216, 1999.

Pokeweed
(poek′weed)

Scientific name: *Phytolacca americana*

Other common names: Cancer jalap, cancer root, changras, coakum, crowberry, garget, pigeonberry, pocon, pokeberry, poke salad, redink plant, redwood, scoke, txiu kub nyug, Virginia poke

Origin: Pokeweed is a perennial found in the eastern region of North America.

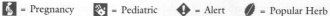

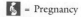 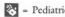

Uses

Reported Uses

Pokeweed has been used as a laxative and an emetic, as well as to treat pruritus; rheumatic disorders; and upper respiratory infections including cough, sore throat, and pharyngitis.

Investigational Uses

Pokeweed is being investigated for its antifungal, antiviral, flu, HSV-1, polio, and antitumor uses.

Product Availability and Dosages

Available Forms

Dried root, extract, powder, tincture

Plant Parts Used: Fruit, leaves, roots, stems

Dosages and Routes

Adult

Emesis
- PO dried root: 60-300 mg

Other
- PO extract: 0.2-0.5 ml

Precautionary Information

Contraindications

Because it is teratogenic, pokeweed should not be used during pregnancy, and until more research is available, it should not be used during lactation. Pokeweed should not be given to children; deaths have been reported. Persons who are hypersensitive to pokeweed should not use it.

Side Effects/Adverse Reactions

Cardiovascular: Hypotension, tachycardia (rare)

Central Nervous System: Confusion, ataxia, dizziness, headache, weakness, sweating, tremors; SEIZURES, COMA (rare)

Ear, Eye, Nose, and Throat: Blurred vision, eye itching and irritation, sneezing

Gastrointestinal: Nausea, vomiting, anorexia, diarrhea

Integumentary: Hypersensitivity reactions, contact dermatitis

Respiratory: RESPIRATORY DEPRESSION (rare)

P

 Endangered Herb   Adverse effects: BOLD = life-threatening

Interactions with Pokeweed

Drug

Central nervous system depressants (alcohol, benzodiazepines, opiates, sedative/hypnotics): Pokeweed may increase the action of central nervous system depressants; avoid concurrent use.

Food	Herb	Lab Test
None known	None known	None known

Client Considerations

Assess

- Assess for hypersensitivity reactions. If present, discontinue use of this herb and administer antihistamine or other appropriate therapy.
- Assess for the use of central nervous system depressants (see Interactions).
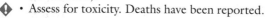 • Assess for toxicity. Deaths have been reported.

Administer

- Instruct the client to store the dried root of pokeweed in a paper or cloth sack, away from heat and moisture.

Teach Client/Family

- Until more research is available, caution the client not to use pokeweed during pregnancy and lactation and not to give it to children.
- Warn the client to store pokeweed out of the reach of children and pets. Poisoning can occur.
- Instruct the client to institute emergency poison treatment in small children who consume even one berry.
- Advise the client not to perform hazardous activities such as driving or operating heavy machinery until physical response to the herb can be evaluated.

Pharmacology

Pharmacokinetics

Pharmacokinetics and pharmacodynamics are unknown.

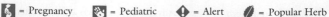

⚕ = Pregnancy   **✋** = Pediatric   **❶** = Alert   **✿** = Popular Herb

Primary Chemical Components of Pokeweed and Their Possible Actions

Chemical Class	Individual Component	Possible Action
Saponin	Phytolaccigenin Phytolaccoside A-G	Toxic
Glycoprotein	Phytolaccatoxin; Asparagine; Oxalic acid	
Triterpene glycosides	1, 2, 3, 4, 5, 6 (Takahashi, 2001)	
Tannin		
Resin		
Betacyanin	Betanin	
Neo-lignan	Isoamericanol A; Americanol A	
Ferredoxin	Ferredoxin I, II	
Lectin		
Lignan		
Flavonoids	Kaempferol; Quercetin	Antioxidant (Bylka, 2001)

Actions

Most research available for pokeweed focuses on the antifungal or antiviral actions.

References

Bylka W et al: Flavonoids and free phenolic acids from *Phytolacca Americana* L. leaves, *Acta Pol Pharm* 58(1):69-72, 2001.

Duke J: *CRC handbook of medicinal herbs,* Boca Raton, Fla, 1985, CRC Press.

Takahashi H et al: Triterpene glycosides from the cultures of *Phytolacca Americana, Chem Pharm Bull* 49(2):246-248, 2001.

Pomegranate
(pahm'uh-gra-nuht)

Scientific name: *Punica granatum*

Other common name: Granatum

Origin: Pomegranate is found throughout the world.

Uses

Reported Uses

Pomegranate is used as an anthelmintic for tapeworm and opportunistic intestinal worms, as well as to treat diarrhea. It is also used to treat hemorrhoids, as a gargle for sore throat, and as an abortifacient. Pomegranate may be effective as an antimicrobial, in the treatment of diabetes, and antioxidant.

Product Availability and Dosages

Available Forms

Crude herb

Plant Parts Used: Bark, fruit, pell, roots, stem

Dosages and Routes

No published dosages are available.

Precautionary Information

Contraindications

Because it is an abortifacient, pomegranate should not be used therapeutically during pregnancy. Until more research is available, pomegranate should not be used therapeutically during lactation and should not be given therapeutically to children. Pomegranate should not be used therapeutically by persons with hepatic disease or asthma. Persons who are hypersensitive to pomegranate should not use it.

Side Effects/Adverse Reactions

Gastrointestinal: Nausea, vomiting, anorexia, HEPATOTOXICITY

Integumentary: Hypersensitivity reactions

Miscellaneous: CARCINOGENIC

Overdose: HEMATEMESIS, VISION DISTURBANCE, ACIDOSIS, CARDIOVASCULAR SHOCK, DEATH

 = Pregnancy   = Pediatric   ❶ = Alert   ⫻ = Popular Herb

Interactions with Pomegranate			
Drug	Food	Herb	Lab Test
None known	None known	None known	None known

Client Considerations

Assess

- Assess for hypersensitivity reactions. If present, discontinue use of this herb and administer antihistamine or other appropriate therapy.
 · Monitor liver function studies (ALT, AST, bilirubin) for hepatotoxicity; herb should be discontinued if liver function studies are elevated.
· Monitor for overdose symptoms (see Side Effects).

Administer

- Instruct the client to store pomegranate in a sealed container, away from heat and moisture.

Teach Client/Family

- Because it is an abortifacient, caution the client not to use pomegranate therapeutically during pregnancy. Until more research is available, caution the client not to use pomegranate therapeutically during lactation and not to give it therapeutically to children.

P

Pharmacology

Pharmacokinetics

Pharmacokinetics and pharmacodynamics are unknown.

Primary Chemical Components of Pomegranate and Their Possible Actions		
Chemical Class	Individual Component	Possible Action
Alkaloid	Pelletierine; Methylpelletierine; Pseudopelletierine; Isopelletierine	Anthelmintic; hypoglycemic; antidiarrheal

Continued

 Endangered Herb   Adverse effects: BOLD = life-threatening

Primary Chemical Components of Pomegranate and Their Possible Actions—cont'd		
Chemical Class	**Individual Component**	**Possible Action**
Phenol Acid Monoacylglycerol	Gallic acid; Ellagic acid	
Bark and Rinds Also Contain		
Tannin	Punicalin; Punicalagin; Granatins A, B; Gallaglydilactone; Casuarinin; Tellimagrandin; Corilagin	Antimicrobial

Actions

The proposed actions for pomegranate include hypoglycemic, antidiarrheal, antimicrobial, and anthelmintic. Blood glucose levels were reduced when the extract was given to hyperglycemic rats (Jafri, 2000). Diarrhea was reduced significantly when the extract of pomegranate seeds was given to rats induced with diarrhea by castor oil (Das, 1999).

Antimicrobial, Amebicide, and Anthelmintic Actions

Effective antiviral action was shown against genital herpes virus (HSV-2) in cell cultures when pomegranate was used (Zhang, 1995). Many herbs grown in Peru were tested against *Vibrio cholerae*, which is prevalent in that part of the world. Tea infusions and decoction of pomegranate showed the best action against this organism (Guevara, 1994). Another study evaluated the use of pomegranate root against *Entamoeba histolytica* and *Entamoeba invadens.* The alkaloids of the root showed no amebicide action; however, the tannic acid showed high inhibition of these organisms (Segura, 1990). Many herbs have been studied for their anthelmintic action against human *Ascaris lumbricoides.* However, only moderate inhibition has been shown when pomegranate is used in vitro (Raj, 1975).

Other Actions

Pomegranate peel extract has been shown to possess significant antioxidant activity in various in vitro models (Chidambara,

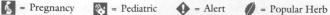

= Pregnancy   = Pediatric   = Alert   = Popular Herb

2002). One study (Kim, 2002) identified the chemoprotective potential of pomegranate for human breast cancer.

References

Chidambara KN et al: Studies in antioxidant activity of pomegranate *(Punica granatum)* peel extract using in vivo models, *J Agric Food Chem* 50(17):4791-4795, 2002.

Das AK et al: Studies on antidiarrhoeal activity of *Punica granatum* seed extract in rats, *J Ethnopharmacol* 58(1-2):205-208, 1999.

Guevara JM et al: The in vitro action of plants of *Vibrio cholerae, Rev Gastroenterol Peru* 14(1):27-31, 1994.

Jafri MA et al: Effect of *Punica granatum* Linn (flowers) on blood glucose level in normal and alloxan-induced diabetic rats, *J Ethnopharmacol* 70(3):309-314, 2000.

Kim ND et al: Chemopreventive and adjuvant therapeutic potential of pomegranate for human breast cancer, *Breast Cancer Res Treat* 71(3): 203-217, 2002.

Raj RK: Screening of indigenous plants for anthelmintic action against human *Ascaris lumbricoides,* part II, *Indian J Physiol Pharmacol* 19(1), 1975.

Segura JJ et al: Growth inhibition of *Entamoeba histolytica* and *E. invadena* produced by pomegranate root (*Punica granatum* L.), *Arch Invest Med (Mex)* 21(3):235-239, 1990.

Zhang J et al: Antiviral activity of tannin from the pericarp of *Punica granatum* L. against genital Herpes virus in vitro, *Chung Kuo Chung Yao Tsa Chih* 20(9):556-558, 576, inside back cover, 1995.

P

Poplar
(pahp′luhr)

Scientific names: *Populus alba, Populus tremuloides, Populus nigra*

Other common names: American aspen, black poplar, quaking aspen, white poplar

Origin: Poplar is a tree found in the United States.

Uses

Reported Uses

Poplar is used to treat arthritis and other joint conditions, diarrhea, urinary tract infections, colds, flu, and gastrointestinal disorders.

🌀 Endangered Herb   Adverse effects: BOLD = life-threatening

Product Availability and Dosages

Available Forms

Dried bark, fluid extract

Plant Parts Used: Bark

Dosages and Routes

Adult

All dosages listed are PO.

- Decoction: 2-5 g powdered bark, decocted, tid
- Fluid extract: 2-5 ml tid (1:1 dilution in 25% alcohol)
- Powdered bark: 2-5 g tid

Precautionary Information

Contraindications

Until more research is available, poplar should not be used during pregnancy and lactation and should not be given to children younger than 12 years of age. Persons with hypersensitivity to salicylates, peptic ulcer disease, gastrointestinal bleeding, coagulation disorders, nasal polyps, or asthma should use this herb cautiously. Persons who are hypersensitive to poplar should not use it.

Side Effects/Adverse Reactions

Ear, Eye, Nose, and Throat: Tinnitus
Gastrointestinal: Nausea, vomiting, anorexia, GASTROINTESTINAL BLEEDING, HEPATOTOXICITY
Integumentary: Hypersensitivity reactions, pruritus, rash; contact dermatitis (propolis only)

Interactions with Poplar

Drug

Anticoagulants (heparin, salicylates, warfarin): Poplar may increase bleeding time when used with anticoagulants; avoid concurrent use.
Iron salts: Poplar tea may decrease the absorption of iron salts; separate by 2 hr.

Food	Herb	Lab Test
None known	None known	None known

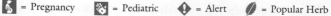

Client Considerations

Assess

- Assess for hypersensitivity reactions. If present, discontinue use of this herb and administer antihistamine or other appropriate therapy.
- Assess for anticoagulants use (heparin, warfarin, salicylates). Concurrent poplar use should be avoided (see Interactions).

Administer

- Instruct the client to store poplar in a cool, dry place, away from heat and moisture.

Teach Client/Family

- Until more research is available, caution the client not to use poplar during pregnancy and lactation.
- Advise client not to give poplar to children younger than 12 years of age. Reye's syndrome may occur with viral infections (theoretical).

Pharmacology

Pharmacokinetics

Pharmacokinetics and pharmacodynamics are unknown.

Primary Chemical Components of Poplar and Their Possible Actions		
Chemical Class	Individual Component	Possible Action
Glycoside	Salicin	Salicylate
	Populin; Tremuloidin; Tremulacin	
Tannin		
Triterpene		
Alpha-amyrin		
Beta-amyrin		
Sugar		

Actions

Very little information on the therapeutic actions of poplar is available. Most studies focus on agricultural rather than medicinal use of the tree. Because of the presence of salicin, a salicylate, many of the actions and uses are the same as commer-

 Endangered Herb   Adverse effects: BOLD = life-threatening

cially prepared salicylates. Only one study could be found for any other actions. In this study the antiviral actions of the poplar tree leaf buds were identified (Amoros, 1994).

References

Amoros M et al: Comparison of the anti-herpes simplex virus activities of propolis and 3-methyl-but-2-enyl caffeate, *J Nat Prod* 57(5):644-647, 1994.

Poppy
(pah'pee)

Scientific names: *Papaver somniferum, Papaver bracteatum*

Other common names: Great scarlet poppy, opium poppy, poppyseed, thebaine poppy

Origin: Poppy is an annual found throughout the world.

Uses

Reported Uses

Poppy is used as a treatment for diarrhea, as a sedative, as an antitussive, and to relax gastrointestinal and smooth muscles. It is also used as an analgesic to treat colic and painful wounds.

Product Availability and Dosages

Available Forms

None available commercially

Plant Parts Used: Seeds are used in bread and confections

Dosages and Routes

No dosage consensus exists.

Precautionary Information

Contraindications

Until more research is available, poppy should not be used during pregnancy and lactation and should not be given to children. Persons who are hypersensitive to poppy should not use it.

 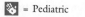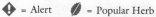

Precautionary Information—cont'd

Side Effects/Adverse Reactions

Central Nervous System: Clonic twitching, dizziness, weakness, headache, tremors, CENTRAL NERVOUS SYSTEM DEPRESSION

Gastrointestinal: Nausea, vomiting, anorexia, abdominal contractions

Integumentary: Hypersensitivity reactions, pruritis, rash

Respiratory: RESPIRATORY DEPRESSION

Interactions with Poppy

Drug

Central nervous system depressants (alcohol, barbiturates, benzodiazepines, other opiates, sedative/hypnotics): Poppy increases central nervous system depression when used with central nervous system depressants; do not use concurrently.

Food   **Herb**

None known   None known

Lab Test

Poppy may cause a false positive result in urine heroine and urine morphine tests.

Client Considerations

Assess

- Assess for hypersensitivity reactions. If present, discontinue use of this herb and administer antihistamine or other appropriate therapy.
- Assess for the use of central nervous system depressants (see Interactions).

Administer

- Instruct the client to take poppy PO.

Teach Client/Family

- Until more research is available, caution the client not to use poppy during pregnancy and lactation and not to give it to children.

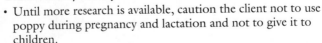

Pharmacology
Pharmacokinetics

Very little is known about the pharmacokinetics in humans except when synthetic forms such as morphine are used.

Primary Chemical Components of Poppy and Their Possible Actions		
Chemical Class	**Individual Component**	**Possible Action**
Opiate Narcotine Papaverine Thebaine	Codeine; Morphine	Opiate analgesic

Actions

Poppy is used as an illicit drug and to manufacture opiates. It is able to decrease pain impulse transmission at the spinal cord level by interacting with opiate receptors. Although most opiates are now synthetically manufactured, *Papaver somniferum* is still used in some parts of the world for opiate production. One study identified three compounds present in poppy: narcotine, papaverine, and thebaine (Paul, 1996). In the event of testing for the use of illicit drugs, the presence of these three chemicals confirms ingestion of the poppy plant.

References

Paul BD et al: Gas chromatographic/mass spectrometric detection of narcotine, papaverine, and thebaine in seeds of *Papaver somniferum, Planta Med* 62(6):544-547, 1996.

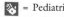 = Pregnancy   = Pediatric   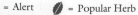 = Alert   = Popular Herb

Prickly Ash
(prik'lee ash)

Scientific names: *Zanthoxylum americanum, Zanthoxylum clava-herculis*

Other common names: Angelica tree, Hercules' club, northern prickly ash, southern prickly ash, suterberry, toothache tree, yellow wood

Origin: Prickly ash is a tree found in the United States.

Uses
Reported Uses
Prickly ash is used to treat flatulence, fever, and circulatory disorders such as low blood pressure. Traditionally, prickly ash has been used to treat gastrointestinal disorders and to decrease inflammation resulting from arthritis and rheumatism.

Product Availability and Dosages
Available Forms
Bark, fluid extract, tincture

Plant Parts Used: Bark

Dosages and Routes
Adult
- PO decoction: 15 g bark in ½ L water
- PO tincture: 5 ml tid (1:5 dilution in 45% alcohol)

P

Precautionary Information
Contraindications
Until more research is available, prickly ash should not be used during pregnancy, during lactation, or for children. Persons with peptic or duodenal ulcers, inflammatory conditions of the gastrointestinal tract, or hypersensitivity to this or related herbs should not use prickly ash.

Side Effects/Adverse Reactions
Cardiovascular: HYPOTENSION (Bowen, 1996)
Gastrointestinal: Nausea, vomiting, anorexia
Integumentary: Hypersensitivity reactions, photosensitivity
Systemic: BLEEDING

Endangered Herb   Adverse effects: BOLD = life-threatening

Interactions with Prickly Ash

Drug

Anticoagulants (heparin, salicylates, warfarin): Prickly ash may increase bleeding when used with anticoagulants; avoid concurrent use.

Iron salts: Prickly ash tea may decrease the absorption of iron salts; separate by 2 hr.

Food	Herb	Lab Test
None known	None known	None known

Client Considerations

Assess

- Assess for hypersensitivity reactions. If present, discontinue use of this herb and administer antihistamine or other appropriate therapy.
- Assess for the use of anticoagulants (heparin, warfarin, salicylates). These drugs should not be used with prickly ash (see Interactions).

Administer

- Instruct the client to store prickly ash in a cool, dry place, away from heat and moisture.

Teach Client/Family

- Until more research is available, caution the client not to use prickly ash during pregnancy, lactation, or for children.

Pharmacology

Pharmacokinetics

Pharmacokinetics and pharmacodynamics are unknown.

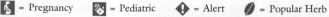

Primary Chemical Components of Prickly Ash and Their Possible Actions

Chemical Class	Individual Component	Possible Action
Coumarin	Xanthyletin; Xanthoxyletin; Allo-xanthoxyletin; Dipetaline	Anticoagulant
Ligans	Sesamin; Asarinin (Ju, 2001)	Cytotoxic
Tannin		
Resin		
Alkaloid	Nitidine; Laurifoline	
Volatile oil		
Isoquinoline alkaloid	Berberine	

Actions

There are very few research studies on prickly ash. One study (Gessler, 1994) identified the antimalarial action of *Zanthoxylum chalybeum*. Forty-three different herbs were tested for their antimalarial activity against *Plasmodium falciparum*. Of these 43 herbs, several plant parts were studied. The four most active herbs in the study were *Cissampelos mucronata, Maytenus senegalensis, Salacia madagascariensis,* and *Zanthoxylum chalybeum*. Another study identified hepatic carcinogen-metabolizing enzymes, among them cytochrome P-450 (Banerjee, 1994). Researchers concluded that essential oils from prickly ash affect the enzymes present for activation and detoxication of certain antibiotics that use these enzymes in metabolism. Another study identified the reason for toxicity in cattle (Bowen, 1996). Toxicity was found to be due to an inhibitory reaction, resulting in hypotension that could be antagonized by calcium and neostigmine.

References

Banerjee S et al: Influence of certain essential oils on carcinogen-metabolizing enzymes and acid-soluble sulfhydryls in mouse liver, *Nutr Cancer* 21(3):263-269, 1994.

Bowen JM et al: Neuromuscular effects of toxins isolated from southern prickly ash *(Zanthoxylum clava-herculis)* bark, *Am J Vet Res* 57(8): 1239-1244, 1996.

P

 Endangered Herb   Adverse effects: BOLD = life-threatening

Gessler MC et al: Screening Tanzanian medicinal plants for antimalarial activity, *Acta Trop* 56(1):65-77, 1994.
Ju Y et al: Cytotoxic coumarins and lignans from extracts of the northern prickly ash, *Phytother Res* 15(5):441-443, 2001.

Propolis
(prah′puh-luhs)

Scientific names: Propolis balsam, propolis resin, propolis wax

Other common names: Bee glue, hive dross

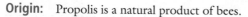

Origin: Propolis is a natural product of bees.

Uses

Reported Uses
Traditionally, propolis has been used to treat inflammation and to promote wound healing.

Investigational Uses
Propolis may have antioxidant and antitumor uses. It may also be used as an antiinflammatory to treat a variety of conditions.

Product Availability and Dosages

Available Forms
Tablets 600 mg; capsules 200, 500, 600 mg; topical cream, fluid extract, lozenges, gum, jelly

Plant Parts Used: Buds of conifers

Dosages and Routes

Adult
- PO capsules or tablets: 600 mg qd
- Fluid extract: 15-30 gtt mixed in 3-4 oz warm water tid
- Topical cream: apply to affected area prn

Precautionary Information

Contraindications

Until more research is available, propolis should not be used during pregnancy and lactation and should not be given to

---

 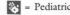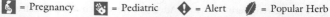

children. Persons who are hypersensitive to propolis should not use it.

Side Effects/Adverse Reactions
Gastrointestinal: Nausea, anorexia, oral mucositis, stomatitis
Integumentary: Hypersensitivity reactions, dermatitis, eczema

Interactions with Propolis			
Drug	Food	Herb	Lab Test
None known	None known	None known	None known

Client Considerations

Assess
- Assess for hypersensitivity reactions, contact dermatitis, and oral mucositis. If present, discontinue use of this herb and administer antihistamine or other appropriate therapy.

Administer
- Instruct the client to store propolis in a cool, dry place, away from heat and moisture.

Teach Client/Family

- Until more research is available, instruct the client not to use propolis during pregnancy and lactation and not to give it to children.

Pharmacology

Pharmacokinetics
Pharmacokinetics and pharmacodynamics are unknown.

Primary Chemical Components of Propolis and Their Possible Actions		
Chemical Class	Individual Component	Possible Action
Resin Wax Essential oil Pollen		
Flavonoid	Pinocembrin; Pinobanksin; Galangin; Chrysin	Antimicrobial
Prenyl esters	Caffeic acid, Ferulic acid (Bankova, 2002)	Antimicrobial
P-coumaric acid		Antimicrobial

Actions

Most of the information on propolis focuses on contact dermatitis, which is quite common. Several articles have been published since 1976 on this hypersensitivity reaction. Most other research focuses on the antimicrobial actions of propolis. Studies have shown antiviral action against herpes simplex virus type I (Amoros, 1992); antiinfluenza action (Serkedjieva, 1992); and antibacterial actions that are significant and nonspecific (Dimov, 1992). Propolis has also been effective against *Streptococcus mutans* present in the mouth (Park, 1998). Another proposed action has been antiinflammation (Khayyal, 1993).

References

Amoros M et al: Synergistic effect of flavones and flavonols against herpes simplex virus in cell culture: comparison with antiviral activity of propolis, *J Nat Prod* 55(12):1732-1740, 1992.

Bankova V et al: Chemical composition of European propolis: expected and unexpected results, *Z Naterforsch* 57(5-6):530-533, 2002.

Dimov V et al: Immunomodulatory action of propolis, IV: prophylactic activity against gram-negative infections and adjuvant effect of the water-soluble derivative, *Vaccine* 10(12):817-823, 1992.

Khayyal MT et al: Mechanisms involved in the antiinflammatory effect of propolis extract, *Drugs Exp Clin Res* 19(5):197-203, 1993.

Park YK et al: Antimicrobial activity of propolis on oral microorganisms, *Curr Microbiol* 36(1):24-28, 1998.

Serkedjieva J et al: Anti-influenza virus effect of some propolis constituents and their analogues (esters of substituted cinnamic acids), *J Nat Prod* 55(3):294-302, 1992.

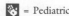 = Pregnancy   = Pediatric   ◆ = Alert   ✐ = Popular Herb

Pulsatilla
(puhl-suh-til'uh)

Scientific name: *Anemone pulsatilla*

Other common names: Crowfoot, Easter flower, kubjelle, meadow anemone, meadow windflower, pasque flower, prairie anemone, smell fox, stor, wind flower

Origin: Pulsatilla is a perennial found in Europe.

Uses
Reported Uses
Pulsatilla traditionally has been used as a sedative and diuretic, as well as to treat insomnia; cough; genitourinary disorders; menstrual irregularities; otitis media; and eye conditions including cataract, glaucoma, iritis, and scleritis.

Product Availability and Dosages
Available Forms
Dried herb, fluid extract, homeopathic products, tincture

Plant Parts Used: Dried leaves, flowers, stems

Dosages and Routes
Adult
All dosages listed are PO.
- Fluid extract 0.1-0.3 ml tid (1:1 dilution in 25% alcohol)
- Infusion: 0.1-0.3 g dried herb infusion tid
- Tea: ½ tsp dried herb in 1 cup boiling water, let stand 15 min, drink tid
- Tincture 0.5-3 ml tid (1:10 dilution in 25% alcohol)

P

Precautionary Information
Contraindications
Because it is an abortifacient, pulsatilla should not be used during pregnancy. Until more research is available, this herb should not be used during lactation. Persons who are hypersensitive to pulsatilla should not use it.

Side Effects/Adverse Reactions
Gastrointestinal: Nausea, vomiting, anorexia; burning of the tongue, throat (chewing)

Continued

 Endangered Herb   Adverse effects: **BOLD** = life-threatening

> **Precautionary Information—cont'd**
> **Side Effects/Adverse Reactions—*cont'd***
> *Genitourinary:* ALBUMINURIA, HEMATURIA (irrigation)
> *Integumentary:* Hypersensitivity reactions
> *Toxicity:* SEIZURES, DIZZINESS, BLURRED VISION, SNEEZING PARALYSIS, IRRITATION OF NASAL PASSAGES AND THROAT, VOMITING, ABDOMINAL CRAMPING AND PAIN, DIARRHEA, NEPHROTOXICITY

Interactions with Pulsatilla			
Drug	**Food**	**Herb**	**Lab Test**
None known	None known	None known	None known

Client Considerations

Assess

- Assess for hypersensitivity reactions. If present, discontinue use of this herb and administer antihistamine or other appropriate therapy.

- Assess for toxicity: seizures, dizziness, blurred vision, sneezing paralysis, irritation of nasal passages and throat, vomiting, abdominal cramping and pain, diarrhea, and nephrotoxicity.

Administer

- Instruct the client to store pulsatilla in a cool, dry place, away from heat and moisture.

Teach Client/Family

- Because it is an abortifacient, caution the client not to use pulsatilla during pregnancy. Until more research is available, caution the client not to use this herb during lactation.
- Because of its toxicity, advise the client not to touch the pulsatilla plant.

Pharmacology

Pharmacokinetics

Pharmacokinetics and pharmacodynamics are unknown.

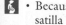

Primary Chemical Components of Pulsatilla and Their Possible Actions		
Chemical Class	Individual Component	Possible Action
Glucoside	Protoanemonin	Central nervous system depression; abortifacient
Saponin		
Tannin		
Volatile oil		
Acid	Chelidonic acid; Succinic acid	
Flavonoid		
Glucose		

Actions

Pulsatilla has shown promise in the treatment of otitis media in children. Herbalists have used this plant for many years to treat this condition (Friese, 1997). However, little primary research is available to support this use. Protoanemonin is known to be a central nervous system depressant and to induce abortions.

References

Friese KH et al: The homeopathic treatment of otitis media in children—comparisons with conventional therapy, *Int J Clin Pharmacol Ther* 35:296-301, 1997.

P

Pumpkin
(puhmp′kuhn)

Scientific names: *Cucurbita pepo, Cucurbita maxima, Cucurbita moschata*

Other common names: Cucurbita, pumpkinseed, vegetable marrow

Origin: Pumpkin is found in Canada and the United States.

Uses
Reported Uses
Pumpkin is used as an anthelmintic, primarily for tapeworms; to treat benign prostatic hypertrophy (BPH); and to treat childhood enuresis and irritable bladder.

Product Availability and Dosages
Available Forms
Seed extract, seed oil, seeds, tablets, tea

Plant Parts Used: Seeds

Dosages and Routes
Adult
Anthelmintic
• PO: 20-150 g tid
Other
• PO seeds: 10 g/day coarsely ground seeds taken with fluids

Precautionary Information
Contraindications
Until more research is available, pumpkin should not be used therapeutically during pregnancy and lactation. Persons who are hypersensitive to pumpkin should not use it.

Side Effects/Adverse Reactions
Endocrine: Electrolyte loss (sodium, potassium chloride)
Gastrointestinal: Nausea, vomiting, anorexia
Integumentary: Hypersensitivity reactions

Interactions with Pumpkin		

Drug
Diuretics: Pumpkin may increase the action of diuretics; use together cautiously.

Food	Herb	Lab Test
None known	None known	None known

Client Considerations

Assess

- Assess for hypersensitivity reactions. If present, discontinue use of this herb and administer antihistamine or other appropriate therapy.
- Assess electrolytes levels (sodium, potassium, chloride) if client is using pumpkin for an extended period to treat BPH.
- Assess for expulsion of worms if client is using pumpkin as an anthelmintic.

Administer

- Instruct the client to store pumpkin in a cool, dry place, away from heat and moisture.

Teach Client/Family

- Until more research is available, caution the client not to use pumpkin therapeutically during pregnancy and lactation.

Pharmacology

Pharmacokinetics

Pharmacokinetics and pharmacodynamics are unknown.

Primary Chemical Components of Pumpkin and Their Possible Actions		
Chemical Class	**Individual Component**	**Possible Action**
Amino acid	Cucurbitin	
Fatty acid	Oleic acid; Linoleic acid; Palmitic acid; Stearic acid	
Mineral	Calcium; Selenium; Zinc; Copper; Iron; Manganese; Phosphorous; Potassium	
Tocopherol		
Carotenoid		

Actions

Pumpkin has been shown to reduce benign prostatic hypertrophy and to decrease human tapeworms, although no studies for either use are available.

References

Duke J: *CRC handbook of medicinal herbs,* Boca Raton, Fla, 1985, CRC Press, pp 374-375.

Pycnogenol

Scientific names: Procyanidol oligomers from *Pinus maritima;* also known as *Pinus nigra* var. *maritima*

Other common names: Pine Bark

Origin: Pycnogenol is a mixture of bioflavonoids found in pine bark.

Uses

Reported Uses

Pycnogenol is used to treat hypoxia in cardiac or cerebral infarction. It is also used as an antioxidant, as an antitumor, and to treat inflammation. It is often used in place of grape seed extract.

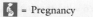 = Pregnancy    = Pediatric   = Alert   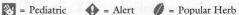 = Popular Herb

Investigational Uses

Research is underway for the uses of pycnogenol in melasma, attention deficit hyperactivity disorder (ADHD), gingival bleeding, plaque formation, chronic venous insufficiency, reduction of platelet aggregation, systemic lupus erythematous, and vascular retinopathies.

Product Availability and Dosages

Available Forms

Capsules, tablets

Plant Parts Used: Water-soluble bioflavonoids from pine

Dosages and Routes

No published dosages are available.

Precautionary Information

Contraindications

Until more research is available, pycnogenol should not be used during pregnancy and lactation and should not be given to children.

Side Effects/Adverse Reactions

None known

P

Interactions with Pycnogenol

Drug	Food	Herb
None known	None known	None known
Lab Test		

Pycnogenol may cause reduced blood platelet aggregation.

Client Considerations

Assess

• Assess for reason client is taking this supplement.

Administer

• Instruct the client to store pycnogenol in a cool, dry place, away from heat and moisture.

 Endangered Herb   Adverse effects: BOLD = life-threatening

Teach Client/Family

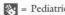

- Until more research is available, caution the client not to use pycnogenol during pregnancy and lactation and not to give it to children.

Pharmacology

Pharmacokinetics

Pharmacokinetics and pharmacodynamics are unknown.

Primary Chemical Components of Pycnogenol and Their Possible Actions		
Chemical Class	**Individual Component**	**Possible Action**
Bioflavonoid	Proanthocyanidins	Antioxidant; antitumor

Actions

Pycnogenol is a mixture of bioflavonoids found in pine. Preliminary research suggests antioxidant and antitumor actions, inhibition of tumor necrosis factor (TNF)-alpha, and inhibition of smoking-induced platelet aggregation. The antioxidant effect, including antiaging, has been evaluated and shown to be significant (Liu, 1998). Two studies show the antitumor properties of pycnogenol (Huynh, 1999, 2000). In both studies pycnogenol was able to induce death in cancer cells, although one study showed healthy cells intact. There was inhibition of TNF-alpha in human vascular endothelial cells (Peng, 2000). In another study, smoking-induced platelet aggregation was inhibited by the use of either 500 mg of aspirin or 125 mg of pycnogenol. Aspirin increased bleeding time; pycnogenol did not (Putter, 1999).

Gingival and Antiplaque Actions

One study (Kimbrough, 2002) identified the antiplaque action and the minimization of gingival bleeding in participants using chewing gum with pycnogenol. Those subjects using this type of gum showed no increase in plaque formation in 2 weeks.

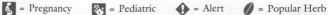

Attention Deficit Hyperactivity Disorder

One small study with 24 individuals age 24-53 years old were studied in a double-blind, placebo-controlled crossover study with pycnogenol, and methylphenidate, and placebo. The placebo ranked higher on a self-reporting scale (Tenenbaum, 2002).

References

Huynh HT et al: Effects of intragastrically administered pycnogenol on NNK metabolism in F344 rats, *Anticancer Res* 19(3A):2095-2099, 1999.

Huynh HT et al: Selective induction of apoptosis in human mammary cancer cells (MCF-7) by pycnogenol, *Anticancer Res* 20(4):2417-2420, 2000 (in-process citation).

Kimbrough C et al: Pycnogenol chewing gum minimizes gingival bleeding and plaque formation, *Phytomedicine* 9(5):410-413, 2002.

Liu FJ et al: Pycnogenol enhances immune and haemopoietic functions in senescene-accelerated mice, *Cell Mol Life Sci* 54(10):1168-1172, 1998.

Peng Q et al: Pycnogenol inhibits tumor necrosis factor-alpha–induced nuclear factor kappa B activation and adhesion molecule expression in human vascular endothelial cells, *Cell Mol Life Sci* 57(5):834-841, 2000.

Putter M et al: Inhibition of smoking-induced platelet aggregation by aspirin and pycnogenol, *Thromb Res* 95(4):155-161, 1999.

Tenenbaum S et al: An experimental comparison of pycnogenol and methylphenidate in adults with attention deficit/hyperactivity disorder (ADHD), *J Atten Disord* 6(2):49-60, 2002.

P

Pygeum
(pie-jee'uhm)

Scientific name: *Pygeum africanum*

Other common name: African plum tree

Origin: Pygeum is an evergreen found in Africa.

Uses

Reported Uses

Pygeum had been used to treat urinary tract infections and benign prostatic hypertrophy (BPH), as well as to increase prostatic secretions that may cause sterility.

Product Availability and Dosages

Available Forms

Powder; standardized extract (14% triterpenoids, 0.5% N-docosanol)

Plant Parts Used: Bark

Dosages and Routes

BPH

Adult PO: 75-200 mg qd may be combined with nettle for increased effectiveness.

Precautionary Information

Contraindications

Until more research is available, pygeum should not be used during pregnancy and lactation and should not be given to children. Persons who are hypersensitive to pygeum should not use it.

Side Effects/Adverse Reactions

Gastrointestinal: Nausea, vomiting, anorexia, gastrointestinal irritation

Integumentary: Hypersensitivity reactions

Interactions with Pygeum

Drug	Food	Herb	Lab Test
None known	None known	None known	None known

Client Considerations

Assess

• Assess for hypersensitivity reactions. If present, discontinue use of this herb and administer antihistamine or other appropriate therapy.

Administer

• Instruct the client to store pygeum in a cool, dry place, away from heat and moisture.

Teach Client/Family

• Until more research is available, caution the client not to use pygeum during pregnancy and lactation and not to give it to children.

 = Pregnancy   = Pediatric   ◆ = Alert   ∥ = Popular Herb

Pharmacology
Pharmacokinetics
Pharmacokinetics and pharmacodynamics are unknown.

Primary Chemical Components of Pygeum and Their Possible Actions		
Chemical Class	**Individual Component**	**Possible Action**
Triterpene	Urolic acids; Oleanolic acid; Crataegolic acid	Prostatic antiinflammatory
Fatty acid		
Tannin		
Phytosterol	Beta-sitosterol	Competes with cholesterol; inhibits arachidonic acid metabolites
	Beta-sitosterone; Campesterol	

Actions
BPH Action
Studies have focused on the use of pygeum as a treatment for BPH. Pygeum both decreases inflammation and gland size and increases prostatic secretions and urinary flow (Levin, 1997). Rabbits given pygeum showed a significant decrease in the partial outlet obstruction that occurs with BPH.

Other Actions
Pygeum may be useful for male sexual dysfunction related to the BPH (Carani, 1991). It may also be useful in chronic prostatitis (Del Vaglio, 1974). However, more research will be necessary to confirm these results.

References
Carani C et al: Urological and sexual evaluation of treatment of benign prostatic disease using *Pygeum africanum* at high doses, *Arch Ital Urol Nefrol Androl* 63:341-345, 1991.
Del Vaglio B: Use of a new drug in the treatment of chronic prostatitis, *Minerva Urol* 26:81-94, 1974.
Levin R et al: *Eur Urol* 32(suppl):15-21, 1997.

Queen Anne's Lace
(kween anz lays)

Scientific name: *Daucus carota*

Other common names: Bee's nest, bird's nest, carrot, devil's plague, mother's die, oil of carrot, philatron, wild carrot

Origin: Queen Anne's lace is found in North America.

Uses

Reported Uses

Queen Anne's lace has been used to protect the liver and for hypertension. It has also been used as an antibacterial, antispasmodic, and antisteroidogenic. In children, Queen Anne's lace is used to treat tonsillitis, intestinal parasites (as a tea), and dermatologic conditions such as photodermatosis.

Product Availability and Dosages

Available Forms

Crude extract, tea

Plant Parts Used: Leaves, roots, seeds

Dosages and Routes

No published dosages are available

Precautionary Information

Contraindications

Until more research is available, Queen Anne's lace should not be used during pregnancy and lactation. Persons who are hypersensitive to Queen Anne's lace should not use it.

Side Effects/Adverse Reactions

Cardiovascular: Hypotension, CARDIAC DEPRESSION
Central Nervous System: Central nervous system depression, sedation, drowsiness
Gastrointestinal: Nausea, vomiting, anorexia
Integumentary: Hypersensitivity reactions, contact dermatitis, photosensitivity

 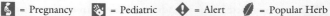

Interactions with Queen Anne's Lace

Drug

Antihypertensives: Queen Anne's lace increases hypotension when used with antihypertensives; use together cautiously.

Cardiac glycosides (digoxin, digotoxin): Queen Anne's lace used with cardiac glycosides may increase cardiac depression; avoid concurrent use.

Central nervous system depressants (alcohol, analgesics, anti-anxiety agents, sedatives): Queen Anne's lace increases the action of central nervous system depressants; use together cautiously.

Diuretics: Queen Anne's lace used with diuretics causes increased hypotension; use together cautiously.

Food	Herb	Lab Test
None known	None known	None known

Client Considerations

Assess

- Assess for hypersensitivity reactions. If present, discontinue use of this herb and administer antihistamine or other appropriate therapy.
- Assess for medication use (see Interactions).

Administer

- Instruct the client to store Queen Anne's lace in a cool, dry place, away from heat and moisture.

Teach Client/Family

- Until more research is available, caution the client not to use Queen Anne's lace during pregnancy and lactation.
- Because this herb causes increased photosensitivity, advise client to stay out of the sun or to use protective clothing.
- Advise the client not to perform hazardous activities such as driving or operating heavy machinery until physical response to the herb can be evaluated.

Pharmacology

Pharmacokinetics

Pharmacokinetics and pharmacodynamics are unknown.

 Endangered Herb   Adverse effects: BOLD = life-threatening

Primary Chemical Components of Queen Anne's Lace and Their Possible Actions		
Chemical Class	**Individual Component**	**Possible Action**
Flavonoid	Apigenin; Chrysin; Luteolin	
Porphyrin		
Furanocoumarin	DC-2,3	Calcium channel blocker (Gilani, 2000)
Volatile oil	Pinene; Geraniol; Limonene; Terpinen; Carophyllene; Carotol; Daucol; Asarone; Dipentin; P-cymene	
Seeds Also Contain		
Fatty acid	Oleic acid; Linolenic acid; Palmitic acid	

Actions

Queen Anne's lace has shown to be antihypotensive, antispasmodic, antisteroidogenic, hepatoprotective, and bacteriosorbent. The antispasmodic effect was evaluated in different species of animals on smooth muscles of the uterus, blood vessels, ileum, and trachea. It was found to be a smooth muscle relaxant (nonspecific) similar to papaverine, but only one-tenth as potent (Gambhirr, 1979). The antisteroidogenic action was studied using carrot seeds, which were able to arrest the development of the ovaries and reduce weight in the mouse (Majumder, 1997). The hepatoprotective action of carrot was evaluated against carbon tetrachloride intoxication in mouse liver (Bishayee, 1995). Liver function study results were lowered, and carrot provided significant protection against liver damage. The bacteriosorbent action has been shown by induction of agglutination (Bratthall, 1978).

References

Bishayee A et al: Hepatoprotective activity of carrot (*Daucus carota* L.) against carbon tetrachloride intoxication in mouse liver, *J Ethnopharmacol* 47(2):69-74, 1995.

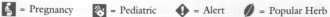 = Pregnancy   = Pediatric   = Alert   = Popular Herb

Bratthall D: *Daucus carota* (carrot)—a selective bacteriosorbent, *Adv Exp Med Biol* 107:327-333, 1978.

Gambhirr SS et al: Antispasmodic activity of the tertiary base of *Daucus carota* Linn seeds, *Indian J Physiol Pharmacol* 23(3):225-228, 1979.

Gilani AH et al: Hypotensive action of coumarin glycosides from *Daucus Carota, Phytomedicine* 7(5):423-426, 2000.

Majumder PK et al: Anti-steroidogenic activity of the petroleum ether extract and fraction 5 (fatty acids) of carrot (*Daucus carota* L.) seeds in mouse ovary, *J Ethnopharmacol* 57(3):209-212, 1997.

Quince
(kwins)

Scientific name: *Cydonia oblonga*

Other common names: Common quince, golden apple

Origin: Quince is found in Southwest and Central Asia and in Europe.

Uses

Reported Uses

Quince traditionally has been used to treat diarrhea, gonorrhea, dysentery, *Candida* infections of the mouth, and sore throat. It is also a component in lotions, creams, and mouthwash. It is used topically to treat canker sores and gum disease.

Investigational Uses

Researchers are experimenting with the use of quince as an antibacterial and to treat cancer.

Product Availability and Dosages

Available Forms

Decoction, fruit syrup, mucilage of seeds

Plant Parts Used: Fruit, seeds

Dosages and Routes

Adult

Diarrhea, Thrush, Gonorrhea
- PO seeds: boil 2 drams in 1 pt water for 10 min; strain
- Topical seeds: apply poultice of ground seeds to affected area prn

Q

Precautionary Information

Contraindications

Until more research is available, quince should not be used during pregnancy and lactation. Persons who are hypersensitive to quince should not use it.

Side Effects/Adverse Reactions

Integumentary: Hypersensitivity reactions
Systemic: TOXICITY (seeds)

Interactions with Quince			
Drug	Food	Herb	Lab Test
None known	None known	None known	None known

Client Considerations

Assess

- Assess for hypersensitivity reactions. If present, discontinue use of this herb and administer antihistamine or other appropriate therapy.
- Assess for toxicity.

Administer

- Instruct the client to store quince in a cool, dry place, away from heat and moisture.

Teach Client/Family

- Until more research is available, caution the client not to use quince during pregnancy and lactation.
- Advise the client to store quince out of the reach of children and pets.

Pharmacology

Pharmacokinetics

Pharmacokinetics and pharmacodynamics are unknown.

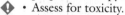

Primary Chemical Components of Quince and Their Possible Actions		
Chemical Class	**Individual Component**	**Possible Action**
Seeds Contain		
Fixed oil		
Protein		
Amygdalin		Toxicity

Actions

The variety of quince that is common in Peru has been shown to be effective against *Vibrio cholerae* when tested with several other herbs (Guevara, 1994). Traditional literature shows actions for cardiac and renal effects. Most of this literature is based on anecdotal reports. Primary research is lacking for this herb.

References

Guevara JM et al: The in vitro action of plants on *Vibrio cholerae*, *Rev Gastroenterol Peru* 14:27-31, 1994.

Q

Quinine
(kwy'nine)

Scientific name: *Cinchona succirubra*

Other common names: Cinchona, Jesuit's bark, Peruvian bark

Origin: Quinine is a tree found in mountainous tropical regions of the United States.

Uses

Reported Uses

Quinine has been used to treat malaria. It has been used in mainstream medicine to treat *Plasmodium falciparum* and nocturnal leg cramps.

Product Availability and Dosages

Available Forms

Capsules, tablets

Plant Parts Used: Bark of 6- to 8-year-old trees

Dosages and Routes

Adult

Leg Cramps

- PO capsules/tablets: 250-300 mg hs

Other

- PO capsules/tablets: 650 mg q8h × 10 days, given with pyrimethamine 25 mg q12h × 3 days and sulfadiazine 500 mg qid × 5 days

Child

- PO capsules/tablets: 25 mg/kg/day divided q8h × 3-7 days

Precautionary Information

Contraindications

Quinine should not be used during pregnancy and lactation. It should not be used by persons with G6PD deficiency and retinal field changes. Caution should be exercised by persons with blood dyscrasias, severe gastrointestinal disease, neurologic disease, severe hepatic disease, psoriasis, cardiac arrhythmias, and tinnitus. Persons who are hypersensitive to quinine should not use it.

Side Effects/Adverse Reactions

Cardiovascular: ANGINA, ARRHYTHMIAS, TACHYCARDIA, HYPOTENSION, ACUTE CIRCULATORY FAILURE

Central Nervous System: Headache, stimulation, fatigue, irritability, SEIZURES, bad dreams, dizziness, fever, confusion, anxiety

Ear Eye Nose Throat: BLURRED VISION, CORNEAL CHANGES, DIFFICULTY FOCUSING, tinnitus, deafness, photophobia, diplopia, night blindness

Endocrine: Hypoglycemia

Gastrointestinal: Nausea, vomiting, anorexia, diarrhea, epigastric pain

Genitourinary: RENAL TUBULE DAMAGE, ANURIA

Hematologic: THROMBOCYTOPENIA, PURPURA, HYPOTHROMBINEMIA, HEMOLYSIS

[S] = Pregnancy   **[P]** = Pediatric   **◆** = Alert   **[leaf]** = Popular Herb

Precautionary Information—cont'd

Side Effects/Adverse Reactions—cont'd

Integumentary: Hypersensitivity reactions, pruritus, pigmentary changes, skin eruptions, lichen planus-like eruptions, flushing, facial edema sweating

Respiratory: Dyspnea

Interactions with Quinine

Drug

Acetazolamide: Quinine used with acetazolamide may lead to toxicity; do not use concurrently.

Aluminum salts: Aluminum salts may caused decreased absorption of quinine; separate doses by 3 hours.

Anticoagulants (heparin, salicylates, warfarin): Quinine may increase the action of anticoagulants; avoid concurrent use.

Cardiac glycosides (digoxin): Quinine may increase the action of cardiac glycosides; avoid concurrent use.

Magnesium: Magnesium may cause decreased absorption of quinine; separate doses by 3 hours.

Neuromuscular blockers: Quinine may increase the action of neuromuscular blockers; avoid concurrent use.

Sodium bicarbonate: Quinine used with sodium bicarbonate may lead to toxicity; do not use concurrently.

Food	Herb	Lab Test
None known	None known	None known

Q

Client Considerations

Assess

- Assess for hypersensitivity reactions, itching and skin eruptions. If present, quinine use should be discontinued and antihistamine or other appropriate therapy administered.
- Monitor liver function studies every week (ALT, AST, bilirubin). If elevated, herb use should be discontinued.
- Assess for cinchonism: nausea, blurred vision, tinnitus, headache, and difficulty focusing.

🌀 Endangered Herb   Adverse effects: BOLD = life-threatening

- Monitor blood pressure and pulse. Watch for hypotension and tachycardia.
- Monitor blood studies and CBC. Blood dyscrasias can occur.
- Assess for medications used (see Interactions).

Administer

- Instruct the client to store quinine in a sealed, light-resistant container, away from heat and moisture.
- Instruct the client to take quinine 2 hr before or after meals at the same time of day to maintain blood level.

Teach Client/Family

- Caution the client not to use quinine during pregnancy and to avoid its use during lactation.
- Advise the client to avoid the concurrent use of quinine and over-the-counter cold preparations.

Pharmacology

Pharmacokinetics

PO: Peak 1 to 3 hours, metabolized in the liver, excreted in the urine, half-life is 4 to 5 hours.

Primary Chemical Components of Quinine and Their Possible Actions		
Chemical Class	**Individual Component**	**Possible Action**
Quinine		Parasitic

Actions

Quinine inhibits parasite replication and transcription of DNA to RNA by forming complexes with the DNA of the parasite.

References

Skidmore-Roth: *Mosby's 2001 nursing drug reference*, St Louis, 2001, Mosby.

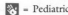 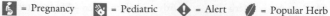

Ragwort
(rag′wawrt)

Scientific name: *Senecio jacoboea*

Other common names: Cankerwort, cocashweed, cough-weed, dog standard, false valerian, golden ragwort, golden senecio, liferoot, ragweed, St. James wort, staggerwort, stammerwort, stinking nanny, squaw weed, squawroot

Origin: Ragwort is found in North America.

Uses

Reported Uses

Ragwort has been used internally to treat menstrual irregularities. Ragwort can be applied topically to stings, leg ulcers, and ulcers of the oral cavity. Only external use is recommended.

Product Availability and Dosages

Available Forms

Dried herb, fresh herb

Plant Parts Used: Flowers, leaves, seeds

Dosages and Routes

Adult

- Gargle: soak dried herb in warm water, strain, gargle prn
- Topical: make poultice from bruised fresh herb added to a little water; apply to affected area prn
- Topical: soak dried herb in warm water; apply to affected area prn

Precautionary Information

Contraindications

Until more research is available, ragwort should not be used internally during pregnancy and lactation and it should not be given internally to children. Persons who are hypersensitive to ragwort and those with hepatic disease should not use it. Internal use of ragwort is not recommended.

Continued

> **Precautionary Information—cont'd**
> **Side Effects/Adverse Reactions**
> *Gastrointestinal:* Nausea, vomiting, anorexia, HEPATOTOXIC-
> ITY, LIVER FAILURE (internal use)
> *Integumentary:* Hypersensitivity reactions

Interactions with Ragwort			
Drug	**Food**	**Herb**	**Lab Test**
None known	None known	None known	None known

Client Considerations
Assess
- Assess for hypersensitivity reactions. If present, herb use
  should be discontinued and antihistamine or other appropriate
  therapy administered.

- Monitor liver function studies (ALT, AST, bilirubin) if
  ragwort is taken internally. If results are elevated, herb use
  should be discontinued.

Administer
- Instruct the client to store ragwort in a cool, dry place, away
  from heat and moisture.

Teach Client/Family

- Until more research is available, caution the client not to use
  ragwort internally during pregnancy and lactation and not to
  give it internally to children.

Pharmacology
Pharmacokinetics
Pharmacokinetics and pharmacodynamics are unknown.

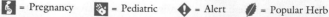

= Pregnancy   = Pediatric   = Alert   = Popular Herb

Primary Chemical Components of Ragwort and Their Possible Actions		
Chemical Class	Individual Component	Possible Action
Pyrrolizidine alkaloid	Floridanine; Florosenine; Senecionine; Otosenine	Toxic

Actions

The only documented studies of ragwort focus on its toxicity. Ragwort should not be taken internally for any reason.

References

Duke J: *CRC handbook of medicinal herbs,* Boca Raton, Fla, 1985, CRC Press, pp 374-375.

Raspberry
(raz′beh-ree)

Scientific name: *Rubus idaeus*

Other common names: Bramble, bramble of Mount Ida, hindberry, red raspberry

R

Origin: Raspberry is found in Europe, North America, and Asia.

Uses

Reported Uses

Raspberry leaves are used to promote diuresis and to treat inflammation and cough. Raspberry may be used topically to treat wounds. Raspberry, like cranberry, is considered useful for the prevention of urinary tract infections and renal calculi. There may be an antimicrobial action in raspberry roots; therefore they are used to promote wound healing and to treat sore throats and canker sores. Raspberry tea is used during pregnancy to relieve morning sickness and to speed and ease labor.

Investigational Uses
Research is underway to confirm the antioxidant use of raspberry and as a gastrointestinal relaxant.

Product Availability and Dosages
Available Forms
Capsules, fluid extract, powder, tablets

Plant Parts Used: Berries, leaves, roots

Dosages and Routes
Adult
- PO fluid extract: 4-8 ml tid (1g leaves/ml 25% alcohol)
- PO powder/tablets: 4-8 g tid

Precautionary Information
Contraindications
Until more research is available, raspberry should not be used therapeutically during pregnancy and lactation. Persons who are hypersensitive to raspberry should not use it.

Side Effects/Adverse Reactions
Integumentary: Hypersensitivity reactions

Interactions with Raspberry

Drug
Antidiabetics (acetohexamide, chlorpropamide, glipizide, insulin, metformin, tolazamide, tolbutamide, troglitazone): Antidiabetics may increase hypoglycemia when used with this herb; monitor blood glucose levels (theoretical).
Iron salts: Raspberry tea may decrease the absorption of iron salts; separate by 2 hr.

Food	Herb	Lab Test
None known	None known	None known

Client Considerations
Assess
- Assess for hypersensitivity reactions. If present, herb use should be discontinued and antihistamine or other appropriate therapy administered.

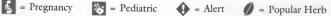
 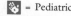

- Monitor blood glucose levels in diabetic clients (see Interactions).

Administer
- Instruct the client to store raspberry in a cool, dry place, away from heat and moisture.

Teach Client/Family
- Until more research is available, caution the client not to use raspberry therapeutically during pregnancy and lactation.

Pharmacology

Pharmacokinetics

Pharmacokinetics and pharmacodynamics are unknown.

Primary Chemical Components of Raspberry and Their Possible Actions

Chemical Class	Individual Component	Possible Action
Leaves Contain		
Flavonoid		
Tannin		Astringent
Fragarin		Mild oxytocic
Acid	Gallic acid; Ellagic acid	
Vitamin	C	
Fruit Contains		
Pectin		
Fructose		
Vitamin	C	

Actions

Raspberry shows antidiabetic and antimicrobial effects. Raspberry is commonly used during pregnancy to relieve morning sickness and as an aid to childbirth.

Antimicrobial Action

Twenty-nine Finnish plants were evaluated for their antimicrobial effects. Raspberry was shown to be effective against bacteria only (Rauha, 2000). The microbes used in this study were *Aspergillus niger, Bacillus subtilis, Candida albicans, Escherichia coli, Micrococcus luteus, Pseudomonas aeruginosa, Saccharomyces cerevisiae, Staphylococcus aureus,* and *Staphylococcus epidermis.*

Antidiabetic Action

One study evaluated raspberry for use as a treatment for diabetes. In this study, blood glucose levels were reduced significantly in laboratory animals (Briggs, 1997).

Antioxidant

One small study identified the antioxidant content of five types of berries by measuring their oxygen radical absorbance capacity. All berries had high antioxidant properties (Wada, 2002).

References

Briggs CJ et al: Raspberry, *Can Pharmaceutical* 130:41-43, 1997.
Rauha JP et al: Antimicrobial effects of Finnish plant extracts containing flavonoids and other phenolic compounds, *Int J Food Microbiol* 56(1):3-12, 2000.
Wada L et al: Antioxidant activity and phenolic content of Oregon caneberries, *J Agric Food Chem* 50(12):3495-3500, 2002.

Rauwolfia
(rau-wul'fee-uh)

Scientific name: *Rauvolfia serpentina*
Other common names: Indian snakeroot, snakeroot

Origin: Rauwolfia is found in the Far East, India, and South America.

Uses

Reported Uses

Rauwolfia is most often used to treat hypertension. Reserpine, one of its chemical components, is used in mainstream pharmacology, although newer synthetic drugs for hypertension are thought to be more effective. Traditional uses of rauwolfia include treatment for snake bite, insect bites, fever, and dropsy. It is also used to treat nervousness and insomnia.

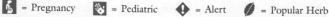

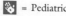

Product Availability and Dosages
Available Forms
Crude herb, fluid extract, injectable (reserpine), powdered extract, suppositories (reserpine), tablets, tea

Plant Parts Used: Root

Dosages and Routes
Adult
- PO: 200-400 mg qd in divided doses; maintenance 50-300 mg qd or in two divided doses (available from a pharmacy with a prescription
- PO tablets: 600 mg qd (equivalent to 6 mg alkaloids)

Precautionary Information
Contraindications
Rauwolfia should not be used during pregnancy and lactation and should not be given to children. Persons who are hypersensitive to rauwolfia or those with depression, suicidal tendencies, active peptic ulcer disease, ulcerative colitis, Parkinson's disease, or pheochromocytopenia should not use it. Clients with seizure disorders or renal disease should use rauwolfia with caution.

Side Effects/Adverse Reactions
Cardiovascular: Chest pain, BRADYCARDIA, ARRHYTHMIAS
Central Nervous System: Drowsiness, fatigue, lethargy, dizziness, depression, anxiety, headache, seizures, parkinsonism
Gastrointestinal: Nausea, vomiting, anorexia
Hematologic: Purpura, INCREASED BLEEDING TIME, THROMBOCYTOPENIA
Integumentary: Hypersensitivity reactions, bruising, purpura, ecchymosis

Interactions with Rauwolfia

Drug
Amphetamines: Use of rauwolfia with amphetamines may cause decreased pressor effects; avoid concurrent use.
Cardiac drugs (beta-blockers, diuretics): Use of rauwolfia with cardiac drugs may result in increased hypotension; avoid concurrent use.

Continued

 Endangered Herb   Adverse effects: BOLD = life-threatening

Interactions with Rauwolfia—cont'd

Drug—cont'd

Cardiac glycosides (digoxin): Use of rauwolfia with cardiac glycosides will cause severe bradycardia, do not use together.

Central nervous system depressants (alcohol, barbiturates, opioids): Use of rauwolfia with central nervous system depressants may cause increased central nervous system depression; avoid concurrent use.

Ephedrine: Use of rauwolfia with ephedrine may cause decreased pressor effects; avoid concurrent use.

Epinephrine: Use of rauwolfia with epinephrine may cause decreased pressor effects; avoid concurrent use.

Isoproterenol: Use of rauwolfia with isoproterenol may cause decreased pressor effects; avoid concurrent use.

L-dopa: Use of rauwolfia reduces the effect of L-dopa, with increased extrapyramidal motor symptoms.

MAOIs: Use of rauwolfia with MAOIs may cause excitation and/or hypertension; avoid concurrent use.

Norepinephrine: Use of rauwolfia with norepinephrine may cause decreased pressor effects; avoid concurrent use.

Sympathomimetics: Use of rauwolfia with sympathomimetics will increase blood pressure; avoid concurrent use.

Food

None known

Herb

Ephedra: Use of rauwolfia with ephedra may result in decreased pressor effects; avoid concurrent use.

Lab Test

Rauwolfia may cause increased gastric analysis, basal nocturnal acid output, and serum or urine sodium. It may cause decreased red blood cells, urine vanillylmandelic acid (VMA), and serum gastrin.

Client Considerations

Assess

- Assess for hypersensitivity reactions. If these are present, discontinue use of rauwolfia and administer antihistamine or other appropriate therapy.

 = Pregnancy = Pediatric = Alert 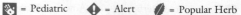 = Popular Herb

- Monitor cardiac status including blood pressure and pulse; watch for hypotension and bradycardia.
- Assess for bleeding, bruising, ecchymosis, and purpura.
- Assess medications and herbs used. Rauwolfia interacts with many drugs (see Interactions).

Administer

- Instruct the client to store rauwolfia products in a cool, dry place, away from heat and moisture.

Teach Client/Family

- Caution the client not to use rauwolfia during pregnancy and lactation and not to give it to children.
- Caution clients with depression, peptic ulcer disease, ulcerative colitis, Parkinson's disease, or seizure disorders not to use rauwolfia.
- Advise the client not to perform hazardous activities such as driving or operating heavy machinery until physical response to the herb can be evaluated.
- To avoid orthostatic hypotension, advise the client to rise slowly to a standing position.

Pharmacology

Pharmacokinetics

Reserpine peaks in 4 hours; duration 2 to 6 weeks; half-life 50 to 100 hours. It is metabolized by the liver, excreted by the kidneys, crosses the blood-brain barrier, and enters breast milk.

R

Primary Chemical Components of Rauwolfia and Their Possible Actions		
Chemical Class	**Individual Component**	**Possible Action**
Indole alkaloid	Reserpine	Antihypertensive
	Serpentinine; Rescinnamine; Raubasine; Raupine	
Starch		

Actions

Rauwolfia inhibits the release of norepinephrine, depleting norepinephrine stores in adrenergic nerve endings (Skidmore-

 Endangered Herb   Adverse effects: BOLD = life-threatening

Roth, 2001). It has been available in mainstream pharmacology as reserpine for many years. Rauwolfia is used rarely today, except in herbal practice.

References

Skidmore-Roth L: *Mosby's nursing drug reference,* St Louis, 2001, Mosby.

Red Bush Tea
(rehd bewsh tee)

Scientific names: *Aspalathus linearis;* also known as *Borbonia pinifolia* and *Aspalathus contaminata*

Other common name: Rooibos tea

Origin: Red bush is a bush found in South Africa.

Uses

Reported Uses

Red bush tea is used as a beverage in place of caffeinated teas.

Investigational Uses

Preliminary research is exploring the antitumor properties of red bush tea and its ability to combat aging in brain tissue. Also being researched is the antihemolytic use.

Product Availability and Dosages

Available Forms

No commercial products are available.

Plant Parts Used: Leaves

Dosages and Routes

No published dosages are available.

Precautionary Information

Contraindications

No absolute contraindications are known.

Side Effects/Adverse Reactions

None known

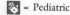 = Pregnancy   = Pediatric   ◆ = Alert   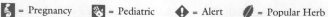 = Popular Herb

Interactions with Red Bush Tea			
Drug	Food	Herb	Lab Test
None known	None known	None known	None known

Client Considerations

Assess
- Identify the reason the client is using this product.

Administer
- Instruct the client to store red bush tea in a cool, dry place, away from heat and moisture.

Teach Client/Family
- Advise the client that red bush tea may be used as a beverage at any time, that it contains no caffeine, and that it is high in vitamin C.

Pharmacology

Pharmacokinetics
Pharmacokinetics and pharmacodynamics are unknown.

Primary Chemical Components of Red Bush Tea and Their Possible Actions		
Chemical Class	Individual Component	Possible Action
Vitamin	C	Antioxidant

R

Actions
Very little research is available for red bush tea. It is known to be high in vitamin C and to contain no caffeine. Initial research is available documenting the antioxidant and antiaging properties of this tea (Sasaki, 1993; Shimoi, 1996). In addition, one study showed that suppression of cancerous cells occurred in mice given *Aspalathus linearis* (Komatsu, 1994). Another study showed that red bush tea suppresses HIV infections (Nakano, 1997). A more recent study (Simon, 2000) has identified the

antihemolytic effect on red blood cells. The degree of inhibition of hemolysis was comparable with the effect of vitamin C.

References

Komatsu K et al: Inhibitory effects of rooibos tea, *Aspalathus linearis,* on x-ray–induced C3H10T1/2 cell transformation, *Cancer Lett* 77(1):33-38, 1994.

Nakano M et al: Anti-human immunodeficiency virus activity of oligosaccharides from rooibus tea *(Aspalathus linearis)* extracts in vitro, *Leukemia* 11(suppl 3):128-130, 1997.

Sasaki Y et al: *Mutat Res* 286(2):221-232, 1993.

Shimoi K et al Radioprotective effects of antioxidative plant flavonoids in mice, *Mutat Res* 350(1):153-161, 1996.

Simon M et al: Antihemolytic effect of Rooibos tea on red blood cells of Japanese quails, *Gen Physiol Biophys* 19(4):365-371, 2000.

Rose Hips
(roez hips)

Scientific name: *Rosa canina*

Other common names: Dog brier fruit, dog rose fruit, hipberries, wild brier berries, brier hip, hip, brier rose, eglantine gall, hog seed, dog berry, sweet brier, witches brier, hip tree, hip fruit, hop fruit

Origin: Rose hips is found in Europe, Asia, the United States, and Canada.

Uses

Reported Uses

Rose hips is usually taken for its vitamin C content. It is used internally as a diuretic and to relieve constipation, increase immunity, and increase capillary strength. It is also used internally to prevent and treat colds and flu and to treat vitamin C deficiency, kidney and urinary tract disorders, arthritic conditions, rheumatism, gout, and sciatica. Topically, the leaves may be used as a poultice to promote wound healing.

Product Availability and Dosages

Available Forms

Capsules, cream, extracts (usually in combination with other products), syrup, tablets, tea, tincture

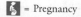 = Pregnancy    = Pediatric   = Alert   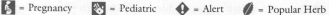 = Popular Herb

Plant Parts Used: Fruit

Dosages and Routes

Adult

- PO infusion: scald 1-2 g powdered herb and steep 10-15 min, strain

Precautionary Information

Contraindications

Until more research is available, rose hips should not be used during pregnancy and lactation. Persons with hypersensitivity to rose hips should not use it.

Side Effects/Adverse Reactions

Gastrointestinal: Nausea, vomiting, anorexia, diarrhea
Integumentary: Hypersensitivity reactions

Interactions with Rose Hips

Drug	Food	Herb	Lab Test
None known	None known	None known	None known

Client Considerations

Assess

- Assess for hypersensitivity reactions. If these are present, discontinue use of rose hips and administer antihistamine or other appropriate therapy.

Administer

- Instruct the client to store rose hips in a cool, dry place, away from heat and moisture.

Teach Client/Family

- Until more research is available, caution the client not to use rose hips during pregnancy and lactation.

Pharmacology

Pharmacokinetics

Pharmacokinetics and pharmacodynamics are unknown.

Primary Chemical Components of Rose Hips and Their Possible Actions

Chemical Class	Individual Component	Possible Action
Tannin		
Carotenoid		
Pectin		
Vitamin	C	Antioxidant
	A; B_1; B_2; B_3; E; K	
Acid	Mallic acid; Citric acid	
Flavonoid		
Phenol		
Volatile oil		
Vanillin		
Sugar	Invert sugar; Saccharose	

Actions

Very little scientific research is available for rose hips. In one study that identified its allergic properties (Kwaselow, 1990), workers exposed to the dust of rose hips developed asthma, rhinitis, and urticaria. Two other studies evaluated the effect of rose hips on cholesterol and triglyceride levels. Hamsters and mice fed rose hips and other fatty acids showed little or no change in the blood levels of these lipids (Lutz, 1993; Gonzalez, 1997).

References

Gonzalez I et al: Plasma lipids of golden Syrian hamsters fed dietary rose hip, sunflower, olive and coconut oils, *Rev Esp Fisiol* 53(2):199-204, 1997.

Kwaselow A et al: Rose hips: a new occupational allergen, *J Allergy Clin Immunol* 83(4):704-708, 1990.

Lutz M et al: Comparative effects of rose hip and corn oils on biliary and plasma lipids in rats, *Arch Latinoam Nutr* 43(1):23-27, 1993.

Rue
(rew)

Scientific name: *Ruta graveolens*

Other common names: Herb-of-grace,
herbygrass, rutae herba, vinruta **Class 2b/2d (Whole Herb)**

Origin: Rue is found in the Mediterranean, the Americas, Asia, Africa, and Europe.

Uses

Reported Uses

Rue traditionally has been used as a sedative and an anthelmintic; to induce abortion; to reduce inflammation in joint disease; to relieve menstrual and gastrointestinal disorders; and to treat earaches, snake bite, and insect stings. It may also be used as an abortive agent for contraception. However, supporting evidence for many of these uses is lacking.

Product Availability and Dosages

Available Forms

Capsules, creams, crude herb, extract, oil

Plant Parts Used: Leaves, roots

Dosages and Routes

Adult

Earache
• Topical oil: pour oil on cotton and insert into affected ear
Toothache
• Topical leaves: may be used to fill hollow teeth
Other
• PO capsules: 1 capsule with meals tid
• PO extract: ½-1 tsp with meals tid
• Topical cream: apply prn to affected area.

Precautionary Information

Contraindications

Because it can cause spontaneous abortion, rue should not be used during pregnancy. Until more research is available, this herb should not be used during lactation and should not

Continued

R

Precautionary Information—cont'd

Contraindications—cont'd

be given to children. Persons with hypersensitivity to rue should not use it. Persons with cardiac disease should use rue with caution. Class 2b/2d herb (whole herb).

Side Effects/Adverse Reactions

Cardiovascular: Hypotension
Genitourinary: SPONTANEOUS ABORTION
Integumentary: Hypersensitivity reactions, photosensitivity, rash, erythema, blisters (topical)

Interactions with Rue

Drug
Antihypertensives: Use of rue with antihypertensives may cause increased vasodilation; avoid concurrent use.
Cardiac glycosides (digoxin): Use of rue with cardiac glycosides may cause increased inotropic effects; avoid concurrent use.

Food	Herb	Lab Test
None known	None known	None known

Client Considerations

Assess

- Assess for hypersensitivity reactions. If these are present, discontinue use of rue and administer antihistamine or other appropriate therapy.
- Determine whether the client is taking other antihypertensives and/or cardiac glycosides (see Interactions).
- Monitor cardiac status periodically, including blood pressure and pulse.

Administer

- Instruct the client to store rue in a cool, dry place, away from heat and moisture.

Teach Client/Family

- Because it can cause spontaneous abortion, caution the client not to use rue during pregnancy. Until more research is avail-

 = Pregnancy   = Pediatric   = Alert   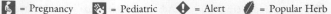 = Popular Herb

able, caution the client not to use rue during lactation and not to give it to children.
- Caution the client to avoid using antihypertensives and cardiac glycosides concurrently with this herb (see Interactions).
- Warn the client that rue is toxic at high doses.

Pharmacology

Pharmacokinetics

Pharmacokinetics and pharmacodynamics are unknown.

Primary Chemical Components of Rue and Their Possible Actions		
Chemical Class	Individual Component	Possible Action
Alkaloid	Quinoline; Acridine; Quinazoline	
Coumarin	Isogravacridonchlorine; Bergapten	Mutagenic
Volatile oil		
Psoralen		
Gamma-fagarine		
Furoquinoline	Dictamnine	
Glycosides	Feruloylsucrose; Methylcnidioside A; Methylpicraquassioside A; Rutin; Picraquassioside (Chen, 2001)	

R

Actions

Cardiovascular Action

Rue has been found to produce cardiovascular effects, including hypotension (Chiu, 1997). Investigators studied the effects of green beans, common rue, and kelp used concurrently. When rue was tested alone, it was found to exert positive chronotropic and inotropic effects on the right atrium but no effect on atrial tension. This study demonstrates the principle that herbs used in combination often are more potent than a single herb used alone.

Antifertility Action

Rue's postcoital antifertility action was demonstrated in a study using rats and hamsters (Gandhi, 1991). Different preparations of *Ruta graveolens* were given orally. The powdered root, aerial parts, and extract of the aerial parts all showed anticonceptive action. None of these was found to be effective in hamsters. However, another study using the roots, stems, and leaf extracts found that all three preparations showed significant antifertility action in rats (Kong, 1989).

Antiinflammatory and Analgesic Actions

In a recent study, plants indigenous to Jordan were studied for their antiinflammatory and analgesic actions. Rue was found to decrease pain in mice (Atta, 1998).

References

Atta AH et al: Anti-nociceptive and anti-inflammatory effects of some Jordanian medicinal plant extracts, *J Ethnopharmacol* 60(2):117-124, 1998.

Chen CC et al: Water-soluble glycosides from *Rutagraveolens, J Nat Prod* 64(7):990-992, 2001.

Chiu KW et al: The cardiovascular effects of greens beans *(Phaseolus aureaus),* common rue *(Ruta graveolens),* and kelp *(Laminaria japonica)* in rats, *Gen Pharmacol* 29(5):859-862, 1997.

Gandhi M et al: Post-coital antifertility action of *Ruta graveolens* in female rats and hamsters, *J Ethnopharmacol* 34(1):49-59, 1991.

Kong YC et al: Antifertility principle of *Ruta graveolens, Planta Med* 55(2):176-178, 1989.

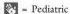 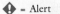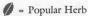

Safflower
(sa'flau-uhr)

Scientific name: *Carthamus tinctorius*

Other common names: American saffron, azafran, bastard saffron, benibana, dyer's saffron, fake saffron, false saffron, zaffer   **Class 2b/2d (Flower)**

Origin: Safflower is found in the Mediterranean, Europe, and the United States.

Uses

Reported Uses

Safflower traditionally has been used to treat constipation and fever. Chinese herbalists use it to treat cough, dysmenorrhea, amenorrhea, and other menstrual irregularities. It has also been used as a component in products such as massage oil.

Investigational Uses

Safflower is being tested for its ability to decrease lipids, to treat fatty acid deficiency and as a COX-2 and prostaglandin inhibitor.

Product Availability and Dosages

Available Forms

Capsules, dried flowers, fluid extract, fresh flowers, tea

Plant Parts Used: Flowers, seeds

Dosages and Routes

Adult

All dosages listed are PO.

- Dried flowers: 3 g tid
- Extract: 3 g dried flowers/15 ml alcohol/15 ml water, take tid
- Fresh flowers: 2 tbsp tid

Precautionary Information

Contraindications

Because it is a uterine stimulant, safflower should not be used during pregnancy. Until more research is available, this herb should not be used during lactation. Persons with

Continued

Precautionary Information—cont'd

Contraindications—cont'd

hypersensitivity to safflower should not use it. Persons with HIV/AIDS, lupus, decreased immunity, burns, or sepsis should avoid its use. Class 2b/2d herb (flower).

Side Effects/Adverse Reactions

Gastrointestinal: Nausea, vomiting, anorexia
Integumentary: Hypersensitivity reactions

Interactions with Safflower

Drug

Anticoagulants (heparin, salicylates, warfarin): Safflower may potentiate anticoagulant action; avoid concurrent use (theoretical).

Immune serums, immunosuppressants, toxoids, vaccines: Use of safflower with immune serums, immunosuppressants, toxoids, and vaccines may cause increased immunosuppression; avoid concurrent use (theoretical).

Food	Herb	Lab Test
None known	None known	None known

Client Considerations

Assess

- Assess for hypersensitivity reactions. If these are present, discontinue use of safflower and administer antihistamine or other appropriate therapy.
- Assess for immunosuppressant medications the client may be taking, such as vaccines, immune serums, toxoids, and immunosuppressants (see Interactions).

Administer

- Instruct the client to store safflower in a cool, dry place, away from heat and moisture.

Teach Client/Family

 • Because it is a uterine stimulant, caution the client not to use safflower during pregnancy. Until more research is available, caution the client not to use this herb during lactation.

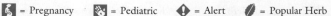

= Pregnancy   = Pediatric   = Alert   = Popular Herb

- Caution the client to avoid taking immunosuppressants concurrently with safflower (see Interactions).

Pharmacology

Pharmacokinetics

Pharmacokinetics and pharmacodynamics are unknown.

Primary Chemical Components of Safflower and Their Possible Actions		
Chemical Class	**Individual Component**	**Possible Action**
Glycosides	Kaempferol; Acacetin	
Fatty Acid	Linoleic acid; Linolenic acid; Oleic acid; Palmitic acid; Steric acid	
Triterpene	Heliaol; Taraxasterol; Psi-taraxasterol; Alpha-amyrin; Beta-amyrin; Lupeol; Taraxerol; Cycloartenol; Enecycloartanol; Tirucalla; Dienol Dammaradienol	Antiinflammatory
Serotonin derivative	Ferulamide; P-coumaramide; Di-p-coumaramide; Diferulamide	Antioxidant Anticoagulant
Cyclohiptenone Oxide derivative	Cartorimine	

S

Actions

The studies done on safflower focus on its antiinflammatory, antioxidant, antimycotic, and antihypertensive actions.

Antiinflammatory Action

The antiinflammatory actions of safflower were evaluated by identifying its triterpene content (Akihisa, 1996). Significant antiinflammatory properties were found in all flower species evaluated from the Compositae family. Cox-2 and prostaglandins are inhibited; this herb may be useful in elevated bone loss (Yuk, 2002).

🌀 Endangered Herb   Adverse effects: BOLD = life-threatening

Antioxidant Action

Antioxidant components were isolated from safflower (see chemical properties table) (Zhang, 1997).

Antimycotic Action

Researchers screened 56 Chinese herbs for their antimycotic action against *Aspergillus fumigatus, Candida albicans, Geotrichum candidum,* and *Rhodotorul rubra.* Safflower exerted the strongest action against *Aspergillus fumigatus* (Blaszczyk, 2000).

Antihypertensive Action

Safflower has been shown to lower blood pressure in hypertensive rats. It is believed to do so by acting on the renin-angiotensin system. Researchers observed a decrease in plasma renin activity and angiotensin II activity (Liu, 1992).

References

Akihisa T et al: Triterpene alcohols from the flowers of compositae and their anti-inflammatory effect, *Phytochemistry* 43(6):1255-1260, 1996.

Blaszczyk T et al: Screening for antimycotic properties of 56 traditional Chinese drugs, *Phytother Res* 14(3):210-212, 2000.

Liu F et al: Hypotensive effects of safflower yellow in spontaneously hypertensive rats and influence on plasma renin activity and angiotensin II level, *Yao Hsueh Hsueh Pao* 27(10):785-787, 1992.

Yuk TH et al: Inhibitory effect of *Carthamus tinctorius* L. seed extracts on bone resorption mediated by tyrosine kinase, COX-2, PG E2, *Am J Chin Med* 30(1):95-108, 2002.

Zhang HL et al: Antioxidative compounds isolated from safflower (*Carthamus tinctorius* L.) oil cake, *Chem Pharm Bull* 45(12):1910-1914, 1997.

Saffron
(sa'-fruhn)

Scientific name: *Crocus sativus*

Other common names: Indian saffron, keser, kum kuma, true saffron, Spanish saffron, zaffron

Origin: Saffron is found in Europe and Asia.

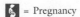 = Pregnancy  = Pediatric = Alert 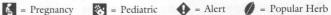 = Popular Herb

Uses

Reported Uses

Saffron is primarily used as a flavoring in food. It is used, traditionally, as a sedative, as an expectorant, and topically to treat skin disorders.

Product Availability and Dosages

Available Forms

Powder

Plant Parts Used: Dried tops

Dosage and Routes

No published dosages are available. Lethal dose is 20 g.

Precautionary Information

Contraindications

Saffron should not be used in hypersensitivity, pregnancy (abortifactant), or lactation or for children.

Side Effects/Adverse Reactions

Cardiovascular: Bradycardia
Central nervous system: Dizziness
Eye, Ear, Nose, and Throat: Epistaxis
Gastrointestinal: Anorexia, nausea, vomiting
Integumentary: Flushing of head and face
Reproductive: SPONTANEOUS ABORTION

Interactions with Saffron

Drug	Food	Herb	Lab Test
None known	None known	None known	None known

S

Client Considerations

Assess

• Assess the reason client is using saffron.

Administer

• Keep saffron in a cool, dry area, away from excessive light.

 Endangered Herb   Adverse effects: BOLD = life-threatening

Teach Client/Family

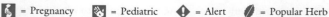

- Teach the patient that saffron should not be used in pregnancy, because spontaneous abortion may occur, and should not be used in lactation until more research is completed with these populations.

Pharmacology

Pharmacokinetics

Pharmacokinetics and pharmacodynamics are unknown.

Primary Chemical Components of Saffron and Their Possible Actions		
Chemical Class	**Individual Component**	**Possible Action**
Carotenoids	Crocine; Crocetin; Picrocrocin; Safranal Dimethyl-crocetin	Cytotoxic

Actions

Cytotoxic Action

Very little supporting evidence is available for the claims that saffron's chemical components crocine, picrocrocin, and safranal are cytotoxic. However, two studies have shown promise in this area (Escribano, 1996; Nair, 1995).

References

Escribano J et al: Crocin, safranal, and pitrocrocin from saffron inhibit the growth of cancer cell in vitro, *Cancer Lett* 100:23-30, 1996.
Nair SC et al: Saffron chemoprevention in biology and medicine: a review, *Cancer Biother* 10:257-264, 1995.

Sage
(sayj)

Scientific name: *Salvia officinalis*

Other common names: Dalmatian, garden sage, meadow sage, scarlet sage, tree sage, common sage, true sage, broad-leafed sage

Class 2b/2d (Leaf)

Origin: Sage is a perennial found in Europe, Canada, and the United States.

Uses

Reported Uses

Sage has been used to treat menstrual disorders, diarrhea, sore throat, gastrointestinal disorders, and gum disease. It is also used as a food flavoring and in cosmetics.

Product Availability and Dosages

Available Forms

Extract

Plant Parts Used: Whole plant

Dosages and Routes

Adult

Menstrual Irregularities
• PO extract: 1-4 ml (1:1 dilution in 45% alcohol) tid
Sore Throat
• PO extract: 1-4 g as a gargle prn

Precautionary Information

Contraindications

Because it is a uterine stimulant, sage should not be used therapeutically during pregnancy. Until more research is available, this herb should not be used during lactation and should not be given to children. Persons with hypersensitivity to sage should not use it, and those with diabetes mellitus and seizure disorders should avoid its use. Class 2b/2d herb (leaf).

Continued

Precautionary Information—cont'd

Side Effects/Adverse Reactions

Central Nervous System: SEIZURES
Gastrointestinal: Nausea, vomiting, anorexia, stomatitis, cheilitis, dry mouth, oral irritation
Integumentary: Hypersensitivity reactions

Interactions with Sage

Drug

Anticonvulsants: Sage may decrease the action of anticonvulsants; avoid concurrent use (theoretical).
Iron salts: Sage tea may decrease the absorption of iron salts; separate by 2 hr.

Food	Herb	Lab Test
None known	None known	None known

Client Considerations

Assess

• Assess for hypersensitivity reactions. If these are present, discontinue use of sage and administer antihistamine or other appropriate therapy.

Administer

• Instruct the client to store sage in a sealed container away from heat and moisture.

Teach Client/Family

• Because it is a uterine stimulant, caution the client not to use sage therapeutically during pregnancy. Until more research is available, caution the client not to use this herb during lactation and not to give it to children.

Pharmacology

Pharmacokinetics

Pharmacokinetics and pharmacodynamics are unknown.

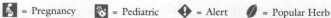

Primary Chemical Components of Sage and Their Possible Actions

Chemical Class	Individual Component	Possible Action
Volatile oil Glycosides	Labiatic acid; Carnosic acid; *CIS*-P-coumaric acid; *Trans*-P-coumaric acid; Luteolin; Hydroxyluteolin; Vicenin-2; Carnosol; Rosmanol; Epirosmanol; Guldosol; Isorosmanol (Miura, 2002)	Antioxidant
Tannin	Phenolic acid	Antimicrobial

Actions

Few studies have been done on the therapeutic uses of sage. Two of its chemical components, labiatic and carnosic acid, have been identified as having antioxidant properties (Leung, 1980). Another study found that sage exerts bactericidal action against a wide range of bacteria (Koga, 1999). Gram-negative bacteria death occurred when sage was used.

References

Koga T et al: Bactericidal activities of essential oils of basil and sage against a range of bacteria and the effect of these essential oils on *Vibrio parahaemolyticus. Microbiol Res* 154(3):267-273, 1999.

Leung AY: Encyclopedia of common natural ingredients used in food, drugs, and cosmetics, New York, 1980, J Wiley & Sons.

Miura K et al: Antioxidant activity of chemical components from sage and thyme measured by the oil stability index method, *J Agric Food Chem* 50(7):1845-1851, 2002.

S

SAM-e

Scientific name: S-adenosylmethionine

Origin: SAM-e is found in all living cells and is a precursor in some amino acids.

🍂 Endangered Herb   Adverse effects: BOLD = life-threatening

Uses

Reported Uses

SAM-e is used to treat depression, Alzheimer's disease, migraine headache and pain in fibromyalgia. It is also used as an antiinflammatory in osteoarthritis.

Product Availability and Dosages

Available Forms

Capsules, tablets

Dosages and Routes

Adult

Migraine

• PO capsules/tablets: 200-400 mg bid

Precautionary Information

Contraindications

Until more research is available, SAM-e supplements should not be used during pregnancy and lactation and should not be given to children. Persons with bipolar disorder should not use SAM-e supplements.

Side Effects/Adverse Reactions

Gastrointestinal: Nausea, vomiting, anorexia

Interactions with SAM-e

Drug

Antidepressants (amitriptyline, amoxapine, citalopram, desipramine, doxepin, fluoxetine, fluvoxamine, imipramine, isocarboxazide, naratriptan, nefazodone, nortriptyline, paroxetine, phenelzine, protroptyline, sertraline, sumatriptan, tramadol, tranylcypromine, trimipramiine, venlafaxine, zolmitriptan): Combining SAM-e with antidepressants may lead to serotonin syndrome; do not use concurrently.

Food	Herb	Lab Test
None known	None known	None known

Client Considerations

Assess

- Assess for client's reason for taking SAM-e.
- Assess for depression or bipolar disorder; SAM-e should not be used in these clients, may precipitate manic episode.

Administer

- Instruct the client to store SAM-e in a cool, dry place, away from heat and moisture.

Teach Client/Family

- Until more research is available, caution the client not to use SAM-e supplements during pregnancy and lactation and not to give them to children.

Pharmacology

Pharmacokinetics

Pharmacokinetics and pharmacodynamics are unknown.

Primary Chemical Components of SAM-e and Their Possible Actions		
Chemical Class	Individual Component	Possible Action
Converted to Cysteine		

Actions

SAM-e plays an important role in normal cell function and survival and is present naturally in the human body. It is necessary for adequate functioning of the central nervous system. SAM-e is considered to be hepatoprotective, as well as an antioxidant and antidepressant. It may also play a role in decreasing *Pneumocystis carinii*, improving cognition in Alzheimer's disease, and protecting against coronary artery disease (CAD).

Antidepressant and Central Nervous System Actions

SAM-e has been shown to be effective in the treatment of depressive disorders by acting on the methylation process in the brain (Bressa, 1994). It also has been shown to be effective in the treatment of Alzheimer's disease, HIV-associated neurop-

 Endangered Herb   Adverse effects: BOLD = life-threatening

athies, and spinal cord degeneration. Deficiencies of certain vitamins, such as folate and B_{12}, decrease levels of SAM-e. Lowered levels of SAM-e are accompanied by a decrease in serotonin levels, which can lead to depression (Young, 1993). It is thought to increase dopamine and serotonin, as well as other neurotransmitters. Because levels of SAM-e in the cerebrospinal fluid are low in those with neurologic disorders, supplementation may decrease central nervous system symptoms. Initial research has shown positive results in clients with Alzheimer's disease (Lamango, 2000; Morrison, 1996), *Pneumocystis carinii* (Merali, 2000), and spinal cord degeneration.

Antiinflammatory Action

The antiinflammatory and analgesic effects of SAM-e have been found to be equal to those of NSAIDs, with many fewer side effects than NSAIDs (Di Padova, 1987). A study using rabbits showed that the addition of SAM-e prevented osteoarthritis (Moskowitz, 1973). SAM-e is thought to protect cartilage and to assist in the repair of cartilage.

Hepatoprotective Action

Studies have found that SAM-e decreases hepatic injury associated with alcoholic cirrhosis (Mato, 1999). The addition of SAM-e allowed liver transplantation to be delayed in alcoholic cirrhosis.

Other Actions

SAM-e has been found to decrease the intensity of migraine headaches at dosages of 200 to 400 mg twice daily (Gatto, 1986).

References

Bressa G: S-adenosyl-l-methionine (SAM-e) as antidepressant: meta-analysis of clincial studies, *Acta Neurol Scand* 154(suppl):7-14, 1994.

Di Padova C: S-adenosylmethionine in the treatment of osteoarthritis, *Am J Med* 83(5A):60-65, 1987.

Gatto G et al: Analgesizing effect of a methyl donor (S-adenosylmethionine) in migraine: an open clinical trial, *Int J Clin Pharmacol Res* 6:15-17, 1986.

Lamango NS et al: Quantification of S-adenosylmethionine-induced tremors: a possible tremor model for Parkinson's disease, *Pharmacol Biochem Behav* 65(3):523-529, 2000.

Mato JM et al: S-adenosylmethionine in alcoholic liver cirrhosis: a randomized, placebo-controlled, double-blind, multicenter clinical trial, *J Hepatol* 30(6):1081-1089, 1999.

Merali S et al: S-adenosylmethionine and *Pneumocystis carinii*, *J Biol Chem* 275(2):14958-14963, 2000.

Morrison LD et al: Brain S-adenosylmethionine levels are severely decreased in Alzheimer's disease, *J Neurochem* 67(3):1328-1331, 1996.

Moskowitz R et al: Experimentally induced degenerative joint lesions following partial meniscectomy in the rabbit, *Arthritis Rheum* 16:397-405, 1973.

Young S: The use of diet and dietary components in the study of factors controlling affect in humans: a review, *J Psychiatry Neurosci* 18(5):235-244, 1993.

Santonica
(san-tahn'ik-uh)

Scientific name: *Artemisia cina*

Other common names: Levant wormseed, sea wormwood, semen cinae, semen sanctum, wormseed

Origin: Santonica is found throughout Asia.

Uses
Reported Uses
Santonica is used, traditionally, as an anthelmintic for children and adults.

Product Availability and Dosages
Available Forms
Tablets, powder, dried herb, lozenges

Plant Parts Used: Flowers, seeds

Dosage and Routes
Adult
PO: 2-4 grains

Precautionary Information
Contraindications
Santonica should not be used in hypersensitivity, pregnancy, or lactation or for children.

Side Effects/Adverse Reactions
Central nervous system: SEIZURES, headache

Continued

 Endangered Herb   Adverse effects: BOLD = life-threatening

Precautionary Information—cont'd

Side Effects/Adverse Reactions—cont'd

Eye, Ear, Nose, and Throat: Blurred vision
Gastrointestinal: Anorexia, nausea, vomiting
Integumentary: Rash

Interactions with Santonica

Drug

Anticonvulsants: Santonica may lower the seizure threshold; do not use concurrently.

Food	Herb	Lab Test
None known	None known	None known

Client Considerations

Assess

- Assess the reason client is using santonica.

Administer

- Keep santonica in a cool, dry area, away from excessive light.

Teach Client/Family

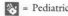 • Teach the patient that santonica should not be used in pregnancy or lactation until more research is completed with these populations.

Pharmacology

Pharmacokinetics

Pharmacokinetics and pharmacodynamics are unknown.

Primary Chemical Components of Santonica and Their Possible Actions

Chemical Class	Individual Component	Possible Action
Glycoside Volatile oil	Santonin	Anthelmintic

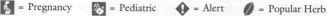

 = Pregnancy   = Pediatric   ◆ = Alert   ⬮ = Popular Herb

Actions

Most of the information on the action and uses for santonica come from anecdotal reports. Research is lacking.

Sassafras
(sa'suh-fras)

Scientific name: *Sassafras albidum*

Other Common Names: Ague tree, Bois De sassafras, cinnamon wood, Fenchelholz, *Lignum floridum, Lignum sassafras,* root bark, saloop, sassafrasholz, saxifras   Class 2d

Origin: Sassafras grows wild in the eastern portion of the United States.

Uses

Reported Uses

Sassafras has been used, traditionally, for integumentary conditions as an antiseptic, to treat syphilis, and as a tonic.

Product Availability and Dosages

Available Forms

Liquid extract, oil, tea, powder, crude bark

Plant Parts Used: Bark

Dosages and Routes

Adult

- PO Infusion: Use 2-4 g bark tid
- Tea: Use ¼ tsp of powder to 1 cup boiling water; infuse for 15 min
- Liquid extract: 2-4 ml tid (1:1 in 25% alcohol)
- Topical: Apply oil topically to area

S

Precautionary Information
Contraindications

Until more research is available, sassafras should not be used in pregnancy, in lactation, or for children; death may occur with only a few drops in children. Use is discouraged because the plant is so toxic. Class 2d (herb).

Side Effects/Adverse Reactions

Cardiovascular: CV COLLAPSE
Central nervous system: CNS DEPRESSION, ataxia, dizziness, hallucinations, paralysis, confusion, stupor, spasms, hypothermia
Gastrointestinal: Nausea, vomiting, anorexia, HEPATIC INJURY/CARCINOMA
Integumentary: Dermatitis, hypersensitivity to touch
Reproductive: SPONTANEOUS ABORTION

Interactions with Sassafras			
Drug	Food	Herb	Lab Test
None known	None known	None known	None known

Client Considerations
Assess

• Assess the reason client is taking this herb.

Administer

• Sassafras should be administered only by a qualified herbalist. Most herbalists do not use this herb because of toxicity.

Teach Client/Family

• Instruct client never to use this herb in pregnancy, in lactation, or for children. The plant is extremely toxic.
• Do not exceed recommended dosage; do not use long-term.

Pharmacology
Pharmacokinetics

Pharmacokinetics and pharmacodynamics are unknown.

 = Pregnancy   = Pediatric   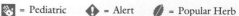 = Alert   = Popular Herb

Primary Chemical Components of Sassafras and Their Possible Actions

Chemical Class	Individual Component	Possible Action
Essential oils	Safarole	Hepatotoxic
	Methyleugenol	
Quinones		Hepatotoxic

Actions

Very little research is available. The few studies that are available focus on sassafras's toxicity. Death can occur with minor amounts of safarole or the quinones, the chemical components of this herb (Craig, 1953; Johneson, 2001; Updyke, 1974).

References

Craig IO: Poisoning by the volatile oils in sassafras in childhood, *Arch Dis Child* 28:475-483, 1953.

Johnson BM et al: Screening botanical extracts for quinoid metabolities, *Chem Res Toxicol* 14(11):1546-1551, 2001.

Updyke DI: Safrole, *Food Cosmet Toxicol* 12:983-986, 1974.

Savory
(say'vree)

Scientific name: *Satureja hortensis L.*

Other common names: Bean herb, white thyme

S

Origin: Savory is found in Europe and is cultivated in North America.

Uses

Reported Uses

Savory is used to treat indigestion, diarrhea, and other GI disorders. Traditionally, savory has also been used to stimulate the libido.

Product Availability and Dosages

Available Forms

Leaves (fresh, dried)

Plant Parts Used: Leaves

Dosage and Routes
Adult
- PO Tincture 1 tsp tid
- Infusion 4 tsp of herb in 8 oz of water
Child
- PO Tincture ½ tsp tid
- Infusion 1 tsp of herb in 8 oz of water

Precautionary Information

Contraindications

Savory should not be used in pregnancy or lactation until more research is available in these populations. The FDA considers savory to be safe.

Side Effects/Adverse Reactions
Gastrointestinal: Anorexia

Interactions with Savory			
Drug	Food	Herb	Lab Test
None known	None known	None known	None known

Client Considerations

Assess
- Assess the reason client is using savory.

Administer
- Keep savory in a cool, dry area, away from excessive light.

Teach Client/Family
- Teach the client that savory should not be used in pregnancy and lactation until more research is available with these populations.

Pharmacology

Pharmacokinetics

Pharmacokinetics and pharmacodynamics are unknown.

🜂 = Pregnancy   🐾 = Pediatric   ❗ = Alert   🪶 = Popular Herb

Primary Chemical Components of Savory and Their Possible Actions		
Chemical Class	**Individual Component**	**Possible Action**
Volatile oils		Antibacterial
Tannin		Astringent
Cineole		Expectorant

Actions

From research with other herbs, it can be deduced that the chemical components of savory may have the following actions: volatile oil (antibacterial), tannin (astringent), cineole (expectorant), although there is a lack of research to confirm this.

Saw Palmetto
(saw pal-meh'toe)

Scientific names: *Serenoa repens, Sabul serrulata*

Other common names: American dwarf palm tree, cabbage palm, fan palm, IDS 89, LSESR, sabal, scrub palm

Origin: Saw palmetto is a palm found in the United States.

Uses

Reported Uses

Saw palmetto is primarily used to treat benign prostatic hypertrophy (BPH). It is also used as a mild diuretic; to treat chronic and subacute cystitis; and to increase breast size, sperm count, and sexual potency.

Investigational Uses

Research is underway to confirm the use in prostate cancer.

Product Availability and Dosages

Available Forms

Berries, capsules, fluid extract, tablets, tea

Plant Parts Used: Fruit

 Endangered Herb   Adverse effects: ʙᴏʟᴅ = life-threatening

Dosages and Routes
Adult
Saw palmetto is standardized to 85% to 95% fatty acids and sterols. All dosages listed are PO.
Benign Prostatic Hypertrophy
- Capsules/tablets: 585 mg up to tid for 4-6 months (Foster, 1998)
- Fluid extract, standardized: 160 mg bid, or 320 mg qd (Braeckman, 1997)
- Tincture: 20-30 drops up to qid (1:2 dilution) (Foster, 1998)

Other
- Decoction: 0.5-1 g dried berries tid
- Decoction: 1-2 g fresh berries tid

Precautionary Information
Contraindications
Because it is an antiandrogen herb that is usually given to men, saw palmetto should not be used during pregnancy. Until more research is available, this herb should not be used during lactation and should not be given to children. Persons with hypersensitivity to saw palmetto should not use it.

Side Effects/Adverse Reactions
Central Nervous System: Headache
Gastrointestinal: Nausea, vomiting, anorexia, constipation, diarrhea, abdominal pain and cramping
Genitourinary: Dysuria, urine retention, impotence
Integumentary: Hypersensitivity reactions
Musculoskeletal: Back pain

Interactions with Saw Palmetto

Drug
Anticoagulants (anisindione, ardeparin, dalteparin, dicumarol, heparin, warfarin): Saw palmetto may potentiate the anticoagulant effects of salicylates; avoid concurrent use.
Antiplatelets: Saw palmetto may lead to increased bleeding; avoid concurrent use.
Hormones (estrogens, oral contraceptives, and androgens): Saw palmetto may antagonize hormone therapy; avoid concurrent use (theoretical).

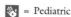 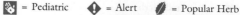

Interactions with Saw Palmetto—cont'd

Drug—cont'd

Immunostimulants: Saw palmetto may increase or decrease the effect of immunostimulants; avoid concurrent use (theoretical).

NSAIDs (bromfenac, diclofenac, etodolac, fenoprofen, flurbiprofen, ibuprofen, indomethacin, ketoprofen, ketorolac, meclofenamate, mefenamic acid, nabumetone, naproxen, oxaprozin, piroxicam, sulindac, tolmetin): Saw palmetto may lead to increased bleeding time; avoid concurrent use.

Food
None known

Herb
None known

Lab Test
Saw palmetto may cause metabolic changes in specimen semen analysis.

Client Considerations

Assess

- Assess for hypersensitivity reactions. If these are present, discontinue use of saw palmetto and administer antihistamine or other appropriate therapy.
- Assess the client's urinary patterns, including retention, frequency, pain, urge, residual urine, and nocturia.
- Assess for the use of antiinflammatories, hormones, and immunostimulants (see Interactions).

Administer

- Instruct the client to store saw palmetto products in a cool, dry place, away from heat and moisture.
- Saw palmetto should be taken with meals to minimize gastrointestinal symptoms.

Teach Client/Family

- Because it is an antiandrogen herb that is usually given to men, caution the client not to use saw palmetto during pregnancy. Until more research is available, caution the client not to use this herb during lactation and not to give it to children.
- Advise the client who is taking saw palmetto for BPH to consult a qualified herbalist for supervision.

 Endangered Herb   Adverse effects: **BOLD** = life-threatening

• Advise the client to obtain a prostate-specific antigen (PSA) before using this herb.

Pharmacology

Pharmacokinetics

Pharmacokinetics and pharmacodynamics are unknown.

Primary Chemical Components of Saw Palmetto and Their Possible Actions		
Chemical Class	**Individual Component**	**Possible Action**
Fatty acid	Lauric acid; Myristic acid; Myristolenic acid	Cytotoxic
Phytosterol		
Polysaccharide	Invert sugar; Galactose; Arabinose	
Steroid		
Flavonoid		
Tannin		
Volatile oil		
Acylglyceride	Monolaurin; Monomyristin (Shimada, 1997)	

Actions

Benign Prostatic Hyperplasia Action

Saw palmetto has been studied extensively for its use in the treatment of BPH. The herb has been found to decrease both the symptoms of BPH and the swelling of the prostate. A new study of a saw palmetto herbal blend versus a placebo noted a decrease in the symptoms and swelling in moderately symptomatic clients with BPH in the experimental group (Marks, 2000). Saw palmetto extract was shown to inhibit alpha 1-adrenoceptors, which may be involved in the production of urinary tract symptoms of BPH (Goepel, 1999). A recent study has found that saw palmetto exerts a significant effect on urine flow rates and that it is able to control symptoms effectively (Gerber, 2000).

Cytotoxicity in Prostate Cancer

One study (Iguchi, 2001) found *Serenoa repens* to be cytotoxic to prostate cancer cells. The chemical component responsible

for the cytotoxic action is myristoleic acid. Further research may confirm the use in prostate cancer.

References

Braeckman J et al: Efficacy and safety of the extract of *Serenoa repens* in the treatment of benign prostatic hyperplasia: therapeutic equivalence between twice and once daily dosage forms, *Phytother Res* 11:558-563, 1997.

Foster S: *101 medicinal herbs*, Loveland, Colo, 1998, Interweave Press.

Gerber GS: Saw palmetto for the treatment of men with lower urinary tract symptoms, *J Urol* 163(5):1408-1412, 2000.

Goepel M et al: Saw palmetto extracts potently and noncompetitively inhibit human alpha 1-adrenoceptors in vitriol, *Prostate* 38(3):208-215, 1999.

Iguchi K et al: Myristoleic acid, a cytotoxic component in the extract from *Serenoa repens*, induces apoptosis and necrosis in human prostatic L NCaP cells, *Prostate* 47(1):59-65, 2001.

Marks LS et al: Effects of saw palmetto herbal blend in men with symptomatic benign prostatic hyperplasia, *J Urol* 163(5):1451-1456, 2000.

Shimada H et al: Biologically active acylglycerides from the berries of saw-palmetto *(Serenoa repens)*, *J Nat Prod* 60(4):417-418, 1997.

Schisandra
(shi-sahn'druh)

Scientific name: *Schisandra chinesis*

Other common names: Gomishi, omicha, schizandra, TJN-101, wu-wei-zu

Class 1 (Fruit)

S

Origin: Schisandra is found in the Far East and Russia.

Uses

Reported Uses

Schisandra has been used in Chinese medicine for the treatment of respiratory, hepatic, and renal disorders. It is thought to possess both antioxidant and immunostimulant properties. It may also be used to enhance athletic performance and energy.

Product Availability and Dosages

Available Forms

Capsules, dried fruit, extract, liquid, tincture, tablets, powder

Plant Parts Used: Fruit, kernel, stems

 Endangered Herb   Adverse effects: **BOLD** = life-threatening

Dosages and Routes
Adult
- PO extract: 100 mg bid

Precautionary Information
Contraindications
Until more research is available, schisandra should not be used during pregnancy and lactation and should not be given to children. Persons with hypersensitivity to schisandra should not use it. Class 1 herb (fruit)

Side Effects/Adverse Reactions
Central Nervous System: CENTRAL NERVOUS SYSTEM DEPRESSION (rare)
Gastrointestinal: Nausea, vomiting, anorexia
Integumentary: Hypersensitivity reactions

Interactions with Schisandra

Drug
Immunosuppressants (azathioprine, basiliximab, corticosteroids, daclizumab, muromonab, mycophenolate, tacrolimus): Schisandra may decrease the effectiveness of immunosuppressants, avoid use before, during or after transplant surgery.

Food
None known

Herb
None known

Lab Test
Schisandra may cause decreased ALT and AST.

Client Considerations
Assess
- Assess for hypersensitivity reactions. If these are present, discontinue use of schisandra and administer antihistamine or other appropriate therapy.

Administer
- Instruct the client to store schisandra products in a cool, dry place, away from heat and moisture.

 = Pregnancy    = Pediatric   = Alert   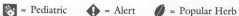 = Popular Herb

Teach Client/Family

- Until more research is available, caution the client not to use schisandra during pregnancy and lactation and not to give it to children.

Pharmacology
Pharmacokinetics
Metabolized by the liver.

Primary Chemical Components of Schisandra and Their Possible Actions		
Chemical Class	**Individual Component**	**Possible Action**
Triterpenoids	Manwuweizic acids; Nigranoic acid; Schisandronic acid	Cytotoxic
Schizandrin B		Hepatoprotective
Schisantherin		
Schizandrol		
Sterol		
Vitamin	A; C; E	
Tannin		
Acid	Malic acid; Tartaric acid; Citric acid	
Resin		

Actions
Hepatoprotective and Regenerative Actions
Most of the research on schisandra focuses on its hepatoprotective and regenerative functions. Two studies have focused on rats with carbon tetrachloride–induced hepatotoxicity (Zhu, 1999, 2000). One study evaluated results of liver function studies and pharmacokinetics, and both documented significant improvement in damaged livers after administration of schisandra. Another older study showed that lignan, a compound found in schisandra fruits, was able to stimulate partial liver regeneration after rats were given carbon tetrachloride (Takeda, 1987).

S

References

Takeda S et al: Effects of TJN-101, a lignan compound isolated from *Schisandra* fruits, on liver fibrosis and on liver regeneration after partial hepatectomy in rats with chronic liver injury induced by CC14, *Nippon Yakurigaku Zasshi* 90(1):51-65, 1987.

Zhu M et al: Evaluation of the protective effects of *Schisandra chinensis* on phase I drug metabolism using a CC14 intoxication model, *J Ethnopharmacol* 67(1):61-68, 1999.

Zhu M et al: Improvement of phase I drug metabolism with *Schisandra chinensis* against CC14 hepatotoxicity in a rat model, *Planta Med* 66(6):521-525, 2000 (in-process citation).

Senega
(seh'ni-guh)

Scientific name: *Polygala senega*

Other common names: Milkwort, mountain flax, northern senega, polygala root, rattlesnake root, seneca, seneca root, seneca snakeroot, senega root, senega snakeroot, seneka

Origin: Senega is a perennial found in the United States and Canada.

Uses

Reported Uses

Senega has widely varied uses, including treatment for snakebite, cough, bronchitis, asthma, croup, pharyngitis, and other respiratory conditions. It is also used to induce vomiting and to treat skin disorders.

Product Availability and Dosages

Available Forms

Dried powdered root, extract, syrup, tea, tincture

Plant Parts Used: Dried root

Dosages and Routes

Adult

All dosages listed are PO.

Expectorant
- Tea: 1 cup bid-tid

Other
- Dried powdered root: 0.5-1 g tid

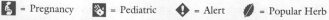

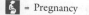 = Pregnancy   = Pediatric   = Alert   = Popular Herb

- Extract: 0.3-1ml q4h prn
- Syrup: 2 tbsp q4h prn
- Tincture: 2.5-5 ml q4h prn

Precautionary Information

Contraindications

Until more research is available, senega should not be used during pregnancy and lactation and should not be given to children. It should not be used by persons with hypersensitivity to this herb or salicylates. Clients with peptic or duodenal ulcers or gastritis also should not use this senega.

Side Effects/Adverse Reactions

Central Nervous System: Dizziness, lethargy, anxiety
Ear, Eye, Nose, and Throat: Blurred vision
Gastrointestinal: Nausea, vomiting, anorexia, abdominal pain, diarrhea
Integumentary: Hypersensitivity reactions

Interactions with Senega

Drug

Anticoagulants (heparin, warfarin, salicylates): Senega may increase bleeding time when used with anticoagulants; avoid concurrent use.
Antidiabetics (insulin): Senega may decrease the effects of antidiabetics; avoid concurrent use.
Central nervous system depressants (alcohol, barbiturates, benzodiazepines, opiates, sedatives/hypnotics): Use of senega with central nervous system depressants may cause increased central nervous system effects; avoid concurrent use.

Food	Herb	Lab Test
None known	None known	None known

S

Client Considerations

Assess

- Assess for hypersensitivity reactions. If these are present, discontinue use of senega and administer antihistamine or other appropriate therapy.

 Endangered Herb   Adverse effects: BOLD = life-threatening

- Determine whether the client is taking anticoagulants, antidiabetics, or central nervous system depressants. Drugs in these classes should not be taken concurrently with this herb (see Interactions).

Administer

- Instruct the client to store senega products in a cool, dry place, away from heat and moisture.

Teach Client/Family

- Until more research is available, caution the client not to use senega during pregnancy and lactation and not to give it to children.

Pharmacology

Pharmacokinetics

Pharmacokinetics and pharmacodynamics are unknown.

Primary Chemical Components of Senega and Their Possible Actions		
Chemical Class	**Individual Component**	**Possible Action**
Saponin	Presenegin; Polygalic acid	
	Senegin	
Salicylate	Methyl salicylate	Hypoglycemia
		Anticoagulant; antiinflammatory
	Salicylic acid	
Resin		
Carbohydrate		
Polygalitol		
Alpha-spinasterol		

Actions

Hypoglycemic Action

The hypoglycemic action of senega results from the chemical component senegin, a saponin (Kako, 1996). The rhizomes appear to contain the chemical responsible for the hypoglycemic action.

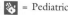

Increased Immune Response

One study determined that the saponins in senega increase specific immune responses and act as vaccine adjuvants (Estrada, 2000).

Sedative Action

Sedative-like effects observed in laboratory animals may be due to the actions of the saponins found in senega (Carretero, 1986).

References

Carretero ME et al: Etudes pharmacodymiques preliminaires de *Polygala microphylla* L. sur le systeme nerveux central, *Planta Med Phytother* 20:148-154, 1986.

Estrada A et al: Isolation and evaluation of immunological adjuvant activities of saponins from *Polygala senga* L., *Comp Immunol Microbiol Infect Dis* 21(1):27-43, 2000.

Kako M et al: Hypoglycemic effect of rhizomes of *Polygala senega* in normal and diabetic mice and its main component, the triterpenoid glycoside senegin-II, *Planta Med* 62(5):440-443, 1996.

Senna
(seh'nuh)

Scientific names: *Cassia* spp., *Senna alexandrina*

Other common names: Alexandrian senna, black draught, Dr. Calwell dosalax, Fletcher's Castoria, Gentlax, Khartoum senna, tinnevelly senna   **Class 2b/2c/2d (Leaf)**

Origin: Senna is found throughout the world.

Uses

Reported Uses

Senna is used to treat acute constipation and for bowel preparation before surgery.

Product Availability and Dosages

Available Forms

Comminuted herb, decoction, dried extract, elixir, granules (pharmaceutical), oral solution, powder, suppositories, tablets

Plant Parts Used: Leaves

Dosages and Routes

Adult

All dosages listed except suppository are PO.

Preparation for Surgery

- Black draught: dissolve ¾ oz in 2.5 oz liquid; take between 2 and 4 PM the day before the procedure

Other

- Cold infusion, comminuted herb: pour cold water over 0.1-0.2 g herb, let stand 10 hr, strain; 1 × dose
- Granules: add ½-4 tsp granules to water or juice
- Infusion, comminuted herb: pour hot water over 0.1-0.2 g herb, let stand 10 min, strain; 1 × dose
- Suppositories: insert 1-2 suppositories hs
- Syrup: 1-4 tsp hs (7.5-15 ml)
- Tablets (Senokot): 1-8 tabs/day

Child

NOTE: Do not give black draught to children.

- PO syrup: >27 kg use ½ adult dose
- PO syrup: 1 mo-1 yr use 1.25-2.5 ml Senokot hs

Precautionary Information

Contraindications

Senna should not be used during pregnancy and lactation and should not be given to children younger than 12 years of age unless prescribed by a physician. Senna should not be used by persons with intestinal obstruction, ulcerative colitis, gastrointestinal bleeding, appendicitis, an acute condition in the abdomen caused by surgery, nausea, vomiting, or congestive heart failure. Persons with hypersensitivity to senna should not use it. This herb should not be used for longer than 1-2 weeks without medical advice. Class 2b/2c/2d herb (leaf).

Side Effects/Adverse Reactions

Gastrointestinal: Nausea, vomiting, anorexia, cramping, diarrhea, flatulence
Genitourinary: Pink, red, brown, or black urine
Integumentary: Hypersensitivity reactions
Metabolic: Hypocalcemia, enteropathy, alkalosis, hypokalemia, TETANY

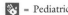

Interactions with Senna

Drug
Cardiac glycosides (digoxin): Chronic use of senna may potentiate cardiac glycosides
Disulfiram: Do not use senna with disulfiram (Antabuse).
Laxatives: Avoid the concurrent use of senna with other laxatives; additive effect can occur.

Food
None known

Herb
Jimsonweed: The action of jimsonweed is increased in cases of chronic use or abuse of senna.

Lab Test
Senna may cause decreased serum and 24-hr urine estriol.

Client Considerations

Assess
- Assess for hypersensitivity reactions. If these are present, discontinue use of senna and administer antihistamine or other appropriate therapy.
- Assess stools for color, consistency, character, and presence of blood and mucus.
- Monitor blood and urine electrolytes if the client is using this product often.
- Determine the cause of constipation (e.g., fluids, bulk, and/or exercise missing from lifestyle).
- Assess for cramping, rectal bleeding, nausea, and vomiting. If these are present, discontinue use of senna.
- Assess medication and herb use (see Interactions).

Administer
- Instruct the client to store senna products in a sealed container away from heat and moisture.
- Instruct the client to dissolve granules in water or juice before use.
- Instruct the client to shake oral solution before use.

S

🌀 Endangered Herb   Adverse effects: **BOLD** = life-threatening

Teach Client/Family

- Caution the client not to use senna during pregnancy and lactation and not to give it to children younger than 12 years of age.
- Advise the client that use of laxatives on a regular basis leads to loss of bowel tone.
- Advise the client that the urine and feces may turn yellow, brown, or red.
- Advise the client not to use senna if abdominal pain, nausea, or vomiting are present.

Pharmacology

Pharmacokinetics

Onset of action 6 to 24 hours; metabolized by the liver; excreted in the feces.

Primary Chemical Components of Senna and Their Possible Actions

Chemical Class	Individual Component	Possible Action
Anthracene	Sennoside A, A$_1$, B, C, D	Laxative
Sugar	Glucose; Fructose; Sucrose	

Actions

Senna stimulates peristalsis by acting on Auerbach's plexus. It softens the feces by increasing the flow of water and electrolytes into the large intestine. Senna has been used for many years in mainstream pharmacology.

References

Skidmore-Roth L: *Mosby's nursing drug reference,* St Louis, 2001, Mosby.

 = Pregnancy   = Pediatric   ◆ = Alert   ∦ = Popular Herb

Shark Cartilage
(shahrk kahr'tuhl-ij)

Scientific names: *Squalus acanthias* (dogfish shark), *Sphyrna lewini* (hammerhead shark), and others

Origin: Shark cartilage is obtained from the hammerhead and spiny dogfish sharks.

Uses

Investigational Uses
Shark cartilage is primarily used to treat cancer, although research attempting to confirm this use has produced mixed results.

Product Availability and Dosages

Available Forms
Capsules, concentrate, injectable, tablets

Parts Used: Cartilage from the dogfish and hammerhead sharks

Dosages and Routes
Adult
- Injectable ampules: 1 qd
- PO capsules/tablets: 1000-4500 mg qd, usually in divided doses
- PO concentrate: 2 tbsp qd

Precautionary Information

Contraindications
Until more research is available, shark cartilage should not be used during pregnancy and lactation and should not be given to children. Shark cartilage should not be used by persons with hepatic disease or by persons who are hypersensitive to it.

Side Effects/Adverse Reactions
Gastrointestinal: Nausea, vomiting, anorexia, HEPATITIS

 Endangered Herb   Adverse effects: BOLD = life-threatening

Interactions with Shark Cartilage		
Drug		
Calcium supplements: Shark cartilage combined with calcium may cause increased calcium levels.		
Food	**Herb**	**Lab Test**
None known	None known	None known

Client Considerations

Assess

- Monitor liver function studies periodically (AST, ALT, bilirubin).

Administer

- Instruct the client to store shark cartilage in a cool, dry place, away from heat and moisture.

Teach Client/Family

- Until more research is available, caution the client not to use shark cartilage during pregnancy and lactation and not to give it to children.

Pharmacology

Pharmacokinetics

Pharmacokinetics and pharmacodynamics are unknown.

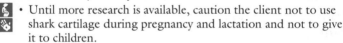

Primary Chemical Components of Shark Cartilage and Their Possible Actions		
Chemical Class	**Individual Component**	**Possible Action**
Glycoprotein	Squalamine Sphyrnastatin 1, 2	Antimicrobial

Actions

Shark cartilage has been investigated for its use in the treatment of cancer. However, the only study professing the usefulness of shark cartilage for this purpose has never been replicated. One of the chemical components in the cartilage of the dogfish shark, squalamine, has been shown to possess antibiotic properties (Moore, 1993). It is effective against both gram-negative and gram-positive organisms.

References

Moore KS et al: Squalamine: an aminosterol antibiotic from the shark, *Proc Natl Acad Sci USA* 90(4):1354, 1993.

Siberian Ginseng
(sy-beer'ee-uhn jehn-sing)

Scientific name: *Acanthopanax senticosus, Eleutherococcus senticosus, Hedera senticosa*

Other common names: Devil's
shrub, shigoka, touch-me-not   **Class 1 (Root, Root Bark)**

Origin: Siberian ginseng is a shrub found throughout the world. It is primarily found in Russia and China.

Uses

Reported Uses

Siberian ginseng has been used to increase immunity, energy and performance and to decrease inflammation and insomnia.

Product Availability and Dosages

Available Forms

Capsules, oil, powder, root, tablets, tea, tincture

Plant Parts Used: Root, root bark

Dosages and Routes

Adult

Some products are standardized to total eleutheroside content or eleutherosides B, D, and E. All dosages listed are PO.
Chronic Fatigue Syndrome
• Dried root: 2-4 g tid (Murray, 1998)
• Tincture: 10-20 ml tid (1:5 dilution) (Murray, 1998)
• Fluid extract: 2-4 ml (1:1 dilution) (Murray, 1998)
• Solid (dry powdered) extract: 100-200 mg (20:1 dilution) standardized to contain >1% eleutheroside E (Murray, 1998)

General Dosages
- Capsules/tablets: 500 mg to 2 g qd
- Extract: 2-12 ml qd (35% alcohol) (McCaleb, 2000)
- Powdered root: 2-8 g (McCaleb, 2000)

Precautionary Information

Contraindications

Until more research is available, Siberian ginseng should not be used during pregnancy and lactation and should not be given to children. Siberian ginseng should not be used by persons with hypersensitivity to this or other ginseng products or persons with hypertension. Siberian ginseng should not be used for longer than 90 days without a rest period. Class 1 herb (root, root bark).

Side Effects/Adverse Reactions

Cardiovascular: Increased blood pressure (high doses)
Central Nervous System: Stimulation, insomnia, dizziness, anxiety, agitation (high doses)
Gastrointestinal: Nausea, vomiting, anorexia
Genitourinary: Increased vaginal bleeding, increased estrogen levels
Integumentary: Hypersensitivity reactions, rash

Interactions with Siberian Ginseng

Drug

Antidiabetics (acetohexamide, chlorpropamide, glipizide, insulin, metformin, tolazumide, tolbutamide, troglitazone): Siberian ginseng may increase levels of antidiabetics; avoid concurrent use.

Cardiac glycosides (digoxin): Siberian ginseng may increase levels of cardiac glycosides; do not use concurrently.

Kanamycin: Siberian ginseng may increase the action of kanamycin.

Stimulants (xanthines): Concurrent use of stimulants with Siberian ginseng is not recommended; overstimulation may occur.

Food

None known

 = Pregnancy    = Pediatric   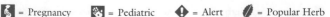 = Alert   = Popular Herb

Interactions with Siberian Ginseng—cont'd

Herb

Ephedra: Concurrent use of ephedra with Siberian ginseng may increase hypertension and central nervous system stimulation; avoid concurrent use.

Lab Test

Siberian ginseng may cause increase in serum androstenedione.

Client Considerations

Assess

- Assess for hypersensitivity reactions, rash. If these are present, discontinue use of the herb and administer antihistamine or other appropriate therapy.
- Assess for use of antidiabetics, cardiac glycosides, kanamycin, stimulants, and ephedra (see Interactions).

Administer

- Instruct the client to store Siberian ginseng products in a cool, dry place, away from heat and moisture.
- Instruct healthy clients to use Siberian ginseng for 6 weeks with a 2-week break before repeating (Mills, 2000), or use for 3 months, then repeat at a later time (German Federal Minister of Justice, 1991).

Teach Client/Family

- Until more research is available, caution the client not to use Siberian ginseng during pregnancy and lactation and not to give it to children.

Pharmacology

Pharmacokinetics

Pharmacokinetics and pharmacodynamics are unknown.

Primary Chemical Components of Siberian Ginseng and Their Possible Actions		
Chemical Class	**Individual Component**	**Possible Action**
Saponin	Protoprimulagenin A	
Glycan	Eleutherane A-G	
Eleutheroside	I, K, L, M	Binds to estrogen receptors
Steroid glycoside	Eleutheroside A	
Lignan	Sesamine; Eleutheroside D	
Hydroxycoumarin	Isofraxidin	
Resin		
Vitamin	E	

Actions

As with ginseng, most of the available research on Siberian ginseng comes from Asia, where it has been studied extensively. In particular, Siberian ginseng has been studied for its adaptogenic, radioprotective, and anticancer actions.

Adaptogenic Action

Siberian ginseng has been found to normalize biologic functioning in a variety of body organs and systems, including the adrenal gland, thyroid, kidneys, white and red blood cells, and blood pressure. The herb also decreases stress reactions in the alarm phase, as seen in stress-induced biologic changes in rats (Brekham, 1969).

Radioprotective Action

Siberian ginseng has exhibited protective and therapeutic effects when laboratory animals are exposed to x-ray radiation. In one study in which rats were exposed to prolonged radiation, lifespans were more than doubled. Some investigators have suggested that Siberian ginseng may be useful in oncologic treatment to protect patients from the ill effects of radiation therapy (Ben-Hur, 1981).

Anticancer Action

In animals, *Eleutherococcus* has decreased thyroid tumors, lung adenomas, and myeloid leukemia. The anticancer action of

 = Pregnancy   = Pediatric   ◆ = Alert   ∅ = Popular Herb

this herb may be due to its immunostimulant properties
(Wagner, 1985).

References

Ben-Hur E et al: Effect of *P. ginseng* saponins and *Eleutherococcus* sp. on survival of cultured mammalian cells after ionizing radiation, *Am J Chin Med* 9:48-56, 1981.

Brekham IL et al: Pharmacological investigation of glycosides from ginseng and *Eleutherococcus, Lloydia* 32:46-51, 1969.

German Federal Minister of Justice: German Commission E for human medicine monograph, *Bundes-Anzeiger (German Federal Gazette)* 17(11):1, 1991.

McCaleb R et al: *The encyclopedia of popular herbs: your complete guide to leading medicinal plants,* Roseville, Calif, 2000, Prima Health.

Mills Simon, Bone K: *Principles and practice of phytotherapy,* London, 2000, Churchill Livingstone.

Murray M, Pizzarno J: *The encyclopedia of natural medicine,* 2 ed (revised), Roseville, Calif, 1998, Prima.

Wagner H et al: Immunostimulating action of polysaccharides (heteroglycans) from higher plants, *Arzneimittelforschung* 35:1069-1075, 1985.

Skullcap
(skuhl'kap)

Scientific names: *Scutellaria laterifolia, Scutellaria baicalensis*

Other common names: Blue pimpernel, helmet flower, hoodwort, huang-qin, mad-dog weed, madweed, Quaker bonnet, scullcap

Class 1 (Root)

S

Origin: Skullcap is found in North America.

Uses

Reported Uses

Skullcap traditionally has been used to treat seizure disorders, inflammation, spastic disorders, and high cholesterol.

Investigational Uses

Initial research is available for the use of skullcap as an antiviral and as a treatment for lung cancer, cerebrovascular accident (CVA), and embolism.

🌀 Endangered Herb   Adverse effects: BOLD = life-threatening

Product Availability and Dosages

Available Forms

Capsules, dried herb tea, fluid extract, tincture

Plant Parts Used: Leaves, roots

Dosages and Routes

Adult

All dosages listed are PO.

- Dried herb tea: 2 g tid
- Fluid extract: 2-4 ml tid (1:1 dilution in 25% alcohol)
- Tincture: 1-2 ml tid (1:5 dilution in 45% alcohol)

Precautionary Information

Contraindications

Until more research is available, skullcap should not be used during pregnancy and lactation and should not be given to children. Persons with hypersensitivity to skullcap should not use it. Class 1 herb (root).

Side Effects/Adverse Reactions

Cardiovascular: ARRHYTHMIAS (overdose of tincture only)
Central Nervous System: TREMORS, CONFUSION, EUPHORIA, SEIZURES, STUPOR (overdose of tincture only)
Gastrointestinal: Nausea, vomiting, anorexia, HEPATOTOXICITY
Integumentary: Hypersensitivity reactions

Interactions with Skullcap

Drug

Central nervous system depressants (alcohol, barbiturates): Skullcap may potentiate sedation of central nervous system depressants; avoid concurrent use.

Immunosuppressants (cyclosporine): Use of skullcap may decrease the effects of immunosuppressants; avoid concurrent use.

Food	Herb
None known	None known

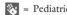 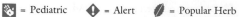

Interactions with Skullcap—cont'd
Lab Test
Skullcap may cause increased ALT, AST, total bilirubin, and urine bilirubin.

Client Considerations

Assess

- Assess for hepatotoxicity, central nervous system overdose symptoms, and cardiovascular overdose symptoms (see Side Effects).
- Assess for hypersensitivity reactions. If these are present, discontinue use of skullcap and administer antihistamine or other appropriate therapy.
- Assess for the use of immunosuppressants (see Interactions).

Administer

- Instruct the client to store skullcap products in a cool, dry place, away from heat and moisture.

Teach Client/Family

- Until more research is available, caution the client not to use skullcap during pregnancy and lactation and not to give it to children.

Pharmacology

Pharmacokinetics

Pharmacokinetics and pharmacodynamics are unknown.

S

Primary Chemical Components of Skullcap and Their Possible Actions

Chemical Class	Individual Component	Possible Action
Flavonoid	Baicalin	Anti-HIV (Li, 1993)
	Luteolin; Apigenin; Hispidulin; Baicalein; Scutellarin; Scutellarein	
Iridoid	Catalpol	

Continued

 Endangered Herb   Adverse effects: **BOLD** = life-threatening

Primary Chemical Components of Skullcap and Their Possible Actions—cont'd		
Chemical Class	Individual Component	Possible Action
Sesquiterpene	Terpineol; Limonene; Caryophyllene; Cadinene	
Tannin		
Resin		
Lignin		
Wogonin		

Actions

Anticancer Action

Skullcap has been shown to normalize platelet-mediated hemostasis in rats with lymphosarcoma (Razina, 1989). This action may be responsible for the antitumor effects of skullcap. Another study documented antitumor action and antineoplastic toxicity in mice (Razina, 1987).

Sleep Disorder Treatment

Epidemiologic studies have shown the use of skullcap for the treatment of sleep disorders (Cauffield, 1999). Skullcap has been shown to decrease interleukin-1 and prostaglandin synthesis (Chung, 1995).

References

Cauffield JS et al: Dietary supplements used in the treatment of depression, anxiety, and sleep disorders, *Lippincotts Prim Care Pract* 3(3):290-304, 1999.

Chung CP et al: Pharmacological effects of methanolic extract from the root of *Scutellaria baicalensis* and its flavonoids on human fibroblasts, *Planta Med* 61:150-153, 1995.

Li BQ et al: Inhibition of HIV infection by baicalin—a flavonoid compound purified from Chinese herbal medicine, *Cell Mol Biol Res* 39:119-124, 1993.

Razina TG et al: Enhancement of the selectivity of the action of the cytostatics cyclophosphamide and 5-fluorouracil by using an extract of the Baikal skullcap in an experiment, *Vopr Onkol* 33:80-84, 1987.

Razina TG et al: The role of thrombocyte aggregation function in the mechanism of the antimetastic action of an extract of Baikal skullcap, *Vopr Onkol* 35(3):331-335, 1989.

Slippery Elm
(sli'puh-ree ehlm)

Scientific names: *Ulmus rubra, Ulmus fulva*

Other common names: American elm, Indian elm, moose elm, red elm, sweet elm

Class 1 (Bark)

Origin: Slippery elm is found in North America.

Uses

Reported Uses
Slippery elm is taken internally to treat cough and gastrointestinal conditions including gastritis and gastric or duodenal ulcers. Topically, it is used for its skin smoothing effect and as a poultice to treat skin inflammation, wounds, and burns.

Product Availability and Dosages

Available Forms
Fluid extract, powdered bark

Plant Parts Used: Inner bark

Dosages and Routes
Adult
- PO: place 4 g in ½ L boiling water; may be taken tid
- PO fluid extract: 5 ml tid
- PO powdered bark decoction: 4-16 ml tid
- Topical poultice: mix boiling water with coarse powdered bark to make a poultice; apply to affected area prn

S

Precautionary Information

Contraindications
Because it may cause spontaneous abortion, slippery elm should not be used during pregnancy. Until more research is available, this herb should not be used during lactation and should not be given to children. Persons with hypersensitivity to slippery elm should not use it. Class 1 herb (bark).

Side Effects/Adverse Reactions
Gastrointestinal: Nausea, vomiting, anorexia
Genitourinary: SPONTANEOUS ABORTION (whole bark)
Integumentary: Hypersensitivity reactions

Interactions with Slippery Elm		
Drug		
Iron salts: Slippery elm tea may decrease the absorption of iron salts; separate by 2 hr.		
Food	Herb	Lab Test
None known	None known	None known

Client Considerations

Assess

- Assess for hypersensitivity reactions. If these are present, discontinue use of slippery elm and administer antihistamine or other appropriate therapy.

Administer

- Instruct the client to store slippery elm products in a cool, dry place, away from heat and moisture.

Teach Client/Family

Because it may cause spontaneous abortion, caution the client not to use slippery elm during pregnancy. Until more research is available, caution the client not to use this herb during lactation and not to give it to children.

Pharmacology

Pharmacokinetics

Pharmacokinetics and pharmacodynamics are unknown.

Primary Chemical Components of Slippery Elm and Their Possible Actions		
Chemical Class	**Individual Component**	**Possible Action**
Tannin		Wound healing; astringent
Hexose		
Pentose		
Methylpentose		
Polyuronide		
Sterol	Citrostandienol; Dolichol; Phytositosterol	
Sesquiterpene		
Mineral	Calcium oxalate	

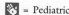 = Pregnancy   = Pediatric   ♦ = Alert   🌿 = Popular Herb

Actions

Very little information is available for slippery elm, other than anecdotal reports. Herbalists continue to use this product to treat cough and gastrointestinal conditions, and for wound healing.

Sorrel
(saw'ruhl)

Scientific name: *Rumex acetosa*. Do not confuse with yellow dock *(Rumex crispus)*

Other common names: Cuckoo's meate, cuckoo sorrow, dock garden sorrel, green sorrel, sour dock

Origin: Sorrel is found in Europe and Asia.

Uses

Reported Uses

Sorrel is used as an antiseptic to treat skin infections. It has been used traditionally to treat scurvy.

Product Availability and Dosages

Available Forms

Liquid, tea, fresh juice

Plant Parts Used: Flowers, leaves

Dosage and Routes

No published dosages are available

S

Precautionary Information

Contraindications

Sorrel should not be used in hypersensitivity, pregnancy, or lactation or for children.

Side Effects/Adverse Reactions

Gastrointestinal: Anorexia, nausea, gastritis, abdominal cramps, HEPATIC DYSFUNCTION

Cardiovascular: CV DAMAGE

Continued

 Endangered Herb   Adverse effects: BOLD = life-threatening

Precautionary Information—cont'd
Side Effects/Adverse Reactions—cont'd
Eye, Ear, Nose, and Throat: Stomatitis
Genitourinary: RENAL DAMAGE
Integumentary: Rash, contact dermatitis

Interactions with Sorrel

Drug
Diuretics: Sorrel combined with diuretics will lead to an additive diuretic effect; avoid concurrent use.

Food	Herb	Lab Test
None known	None known	None known

Client Considerations
Assess
• Assess the reason client is using sorrel.

Administer
• Keep sorrel in a cool, dry area, away from excessive light.

Teach Client/Family

• Teach the patient that sorrel should not be used in pregnancy, in lactation, or for children until more research is completed with these populations.
• Sorrel is fatal at levels over 5 g. Keep from children or pets.

Pharmacology
Pharmacokinetics
Pharmacokinetics and pharmacodynamics are unknown.

Primary Chemical Components of Sorrel and Their Possible Actions

Chemical Class	Individual Component	Possible Action
Oxalates	Potassium	Hepatotoxic
Tannin		Astrigent, wound healing
Anthracene		
Oxymethyl-anthraquinone		

Actions

Research regarding sorrel's actions is lacking. This herb is not used commonly, because it is considered toxic to the liver and renal system with the presence of potassium oxalates.

Soy
(sawee)

Scientific name: *Glycine max*

Other common names: Soya, soybean, soy lecithin

Origin: Soy is a bean found throughout the world.

Uses

Reported Uses

Soy has been used for thousands of years in China. Currently it is used to lower cholesterol and to treat hyperactivity, fever, headache, anorexia, chronic hepatitis, and other hepatic disease.

Investigational Uses

Research supports the use of soy for the treatment of the symptoms of menopause, as well as for the prevention of osteoporosis and various types of cancer (primarily uterine, breast, prostate, and colon cancers).

S

Product Availability and Dosages
Available Forms
Bean curd, capsules, seitan, soy milk, tofu

Plant Parts Used: Bean (seed)

Dosages and Routes
Adult
All dosages listed are PO.
Menopause Symptom Relief
• 50-75 mg isoflavones qd (Murray, 1998)
Osteoporosis Prevention
• 55-100 mg isoflavones qd (Murray, 1998)
Reduction of Cholesterol
• 25-50 g qd (Murray, 1998)

Precautionary Information
Contraindications
No absolute contraindications are known.

Side Effects/Adverse Reactions
Integumentary: Hypersensitivity reactions
Gastrointestinal: Nausea, bloating, diarrhea, abdominal pain

Interactions with Soy

Drug
Thyroid agents (dextrothyroxine, levothyroxine, liothyronine, liotrix, thyroglobulin): Soy may interfere with thyroid hormone absorption; avoid concurrent use.

Food
None known

Herb
None known

Lab Test
Soy may cause increased HDL cholesterol. Soy may cause decreased LDL cholesterol, triglycerides, and total cholesterol.

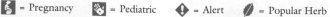

= Pregnancy   = Pediatric   = Alert   = Popular Herb

Client Considerations

Assess

- Assess for hypersensitivity reactions. If these are present, discontinue use of soy and administer antihistamine or other appropriate therapy.

Administer

- Instruct the client to store soy products in a cool, dry place, away from heat and moisture.

Pharmacology

Pharmacokinetics

Pharmacokinetics and pharmacodynamics are unknown.

Primary Chemical Components of Soy and Their Possible Actions		
Chemical Class	**Individual Component**	**Possible Action**
Isoflavone	Daidzein Genistein	Phytoestrogen Antitumor; impairs thyroid function
Phospholipid	Phosphatidylcholine; Phosphatidyleth- anolamine; Phosphatidylinositol	
Sterol		
Protein		
Saponin		
Fatty acid	Palmitic acid; Palmitoleic acid; Linoleic acid; Linolenic acid; Steric acid; Oleic acid	
Oxalates		

Actions

Soy is one of the few natural products that have been researched extensively. Although originally used as a food source, in the last few years soy has been found to possess medicinal properties.

🌀 Endangered Herb   Adverse effects: BOLD = life-threatening

Phytoestrogen Action

The isoflavones in soy are chemically similar to estradiol in the female human body. Research has shown that soy is useful for the prevention of symptoms of menopause in perimenopausal women. Studies document that soy lessens these symptoms and provides an alternative to hormone replacement therapy. A recent study also shows that bone loss in the spine decreases with the addition of soy-rich products to the diets of perimenopausal women (Alekel, 2000).

Anticancer Action

Several studies have evaluated the use of soy for treatment of cancer of the breast, prostate, and colon. Populations in Asia with high-soy diets have been found to have a significantly lower incidence of these cancers than other populations. Genistein, one of the chemical components of soy, has been found to decrease the growth of tumors implanted in mice (Record, 1997). Soy has been found to lengthen the menstrual cycle by prolonging the follicular phase, which may protect against breast cancer. A recent study postulates that the isoflavones and other chemical constituents of soy may lower the cancer risk of postmenopausal women by altering estrogen metabolism such that genotoxic metabolites are converted to inactive metabolites (Xu, 2000). In addition, genistein has been shown to decrease prostatic cancer and to increase the immune response in laboratory animals (Zhang, 1997).

Antilipidemia Action

Most of the research on soy deals with its anticholesterol effects. Soy has been found to lower both low-density lipoprotein (LDL) and total cholesterol levels, with total cholesterol reduction as much as 20% (Anderson, 1995). Investigators have documented a slight increase in high-density lipoprotein (HDL) levels, but not significant. In another study, 32 clients with coronary artery disease discontinued their antilipidemic medication and began a vegetarian diet containing soy-based products. LDL levels dropped significantly, with those who stayed on the diet longer experiencing more significant results (Medkova, 1997).

References

Alekel DL et al: Isoflavone-rich soy protein isolate attenuates bone loss in the lumbar spine of perimenopausal women, *Am J Clin Nutr* 72(3): 844-852, 2000 (in-process citation).

 = Pregnancy   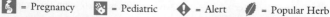 = Pediatric   = Alert   ⫽ = Popular Herb

Anderson JW et al: Meta-analysis of the effects of soy protein intake on serum lipids, *New Engl J Med* 333:276-282, 1995.

Duke J: *CRC handbook of medicinal herbs,* Boca Raton, Fla, 1985, CRC Press, pp 374-375.

Medkova I et al: *Ter Arkh* 69(9):52-55, 1997.

Murray M, Pizzarno J: *The encyclopedia of natural medicine,* 2 ed (revised), Roseville, Calif, 1998, Prima.

Record I et al: *Int J Cancer* 72(5):860-864, 1997.

Xu X et al: Soy consumption alters endogenous estrogen metabolism in postmenopausal women, *Cancer Epidemiol Biomarkers Prev* 9(8):781-786, 2000 (in-process citation).

Zhang R et al: *Nutr Cancer* 29(1):24-28, 1997.

Spirulina
(speer-ew-leen'uh)

Scientific name: *Spirulina* spp. (approximately 35 species)

Other common names: Blue-green algae, DIHE, tecuitlatl

Origin: Spirulina is an alga found in oceans in the tropics and subtropics.

Uses
Reported Uses
Because of its high nutritional value, spirulina has been used both to promote weight gain in malnourished clients and to promote weight loss.

Investigational Uses
Initial research supports the use of spirulina as an antiviral, for fibromyalgia, to decrease cholesterol, and as a chemoprotective agent.

Product Availability and Dosages
Available Forms
Capsules, component in drinks, fresh plant, powder, tablets

Plant Parts Used: Whole plant

Dosages and Routes
Adult
• PO: 3-5 g qd ac

S

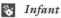 *Infant*
Malnourishment
• PO: 3-15 g qd

Precautionary Information
Contraindications
Until more research is available, spirulina should be used
with caution during pregnancy and lactation, and caution
should be used when giving spirulina products to children.
Clients with thyroid conditions should not use spirulina.
Heavy metal poisoning may result from high mercury
content in some spirulina products.

Side Effects/Adverse Reactions
Gastrointestinal: Nausea, vomiting, anorexia
Integumentary: Hypersensitivity reactions

Interactions with Spirulina

Drug
Thyroid hormones: The high iodine content of spirulina may
decrease the action of thyroid hormones; avoid concurrent use
(theoretical).

Food	Herb	Lab Test
None known	None known	None known

Client Considerations
Assess
• Assess for hypersensitivity reactions. If these are present, discontinue use of spirulina and administer antihistamine or
other appropriate therapy.
• Assess nutritional status if the client is using spirulina to treat
malnourishment.

Administer
• Instruct the client to store spirulina products in a cool, dry
place, away from heat and moisture.

Teach Client/Family

- Until more research is available, advise the client to use spirulina with caution during pregnancy and lactation and to use caution when giving spirulina products to children.
- Advise the client that some spirulina products may have a high mercury and radioactive ion content.
- Inform the client that the protein content of spirulina is higher than the protein content of evening primrose oil and that the iron content of spirulina is more easily absorbed than that of many other iron products.

Pharmacology

Pharmacokinetics

Pharmacokinetics and pharmacodynamics are unknown.

Primary Chemical Components of Spirulina and Their Possible Actions		
Chemical Class	**Individual Component**	**Possible Action**
Amino acid	Phenylalanine	
Fat		
Carbohydrate		
Mineral	Calcium; Potassium; Magnesium; Iron	
Trace element	Selenium; Manganese; Zinc	
Vitamin	B_1; B_{12}; E	
Fatty acid	Gamma-linolenic acid (GLA)	
Nucleic acid		Increased uric acid levels

S

Actions

Spirulina has been used for centuries in South America and Africa. It has been found to possess antiviral, antitumor, anticholesterol, and immunologic properties. Very little research has been done with humans, but animal studies show little toxicity, even at very high amounts (Chamorro, 1996).

Antiallergy Action

One study evaluated the use of spirulina for the treatment of allergic reactions. Spirulina was found to decrease mast cell mediated allergic reactions (Kim, 1998).

Antitumor Action

Spirulina has also been shown to decrease induced tumor necrosis factor (TNF)-alpha.

Iron Storage During Pregnancy

Another study using laboratory rats has shown that a diet of spirulina or spirulina plus wheat gluten promoted greater iron storage and a higher hemoglobin content during pregnancy (Kapoor, 1998).

References

Chamorro G et al: Pharmacology and toxicology of *Spirulina alga*, *Rev Invest Clin* 48(5):389-399, 1996.

Kapoor R et al: Supplementary effect of spirulina on hematological status of rats during pregnancy and lactation, *Plant Foods Hum Nutr* 52(4):315-324, 1998.

Kim HM et al: Inhibitory effect of mast cell-mediated immediate-type allergic reactions in rats by spirulina, *Biochem Pharmacol* 55(7):1071-1076, 1998.

Squill
(skwil)

Scientific names: *Urginea maritima, Drimia maritima*

Other common names: European squill, Indian squill, Mediterranean squill, red squill, scilla, sea onion, sea squill, white squill

Origin: Squill is found in Europe and Mediterranean regions.

Uses

Reported Uses

Traditionally, squill has been used for its cardiac glycoside effect in the treatment of cardiac conditions such as congestive heart failure. It is also used to treat cough and to promote diuresis.

Product Availability and Dosages

Available Forms

Dried bulb, extract, tincture

Plant Parts Used: Bulb

Dosages and Routes

Adult
- PO decoction: pour 8 oz boiling water over 1 tsp dried bulb, let stand 15 min, allow to cool; may be taken tid
- PO tincture: ½-1 ml tid

Precautionary Information

Contraindications

Until more research is available, squill should not be used during pregnancy and lactation and should not be given to children. This herb should not be used by persons with hypokalemia, hypertropic cardiomyopathy, sick sinus syndrome, ventricular tachycardia, or second or third degree heart block. Persons who are hypersensitive to squill should not use it.

Side Effects/Adverse Reactions

Cardiovascular: ARRHYTHMIAS, HEART BLOCK, ASYSTOLE
Central Nervous System: Anxiety, headache, tremors, central nervous system stimulation, SEIZURES
Gastrointestinal: Nausea, vomiting, anorexia
Integumentary: Hypersensitivity reactions

Interactions with Squill

Drug

Cardiac agents (beta-blockers, cardiac glycosides, calcium channel blockers, antiarrhythmics): Squill may increase the effects of cardiac agents, causing life-threatening toxicity; do not use concurrently.
Central nervous system stimulants (amphetamines, cerebral stimulants): Squill may increase the effects of central nervous system stimulants; avoid concurrent use.
Glucocorticoids: Squill may increase the effects of glucocorticoids; avoid concurrent use.

Continued

S

🌀 Endangered Herb   Adverse effects: BOLD = life-threatening

> ## Interactions with Squill—cont'd
>
> ### Drug—cont'd
> *Iron salts:* Squill may decrease the absorption of iron salts; separate by 2 hr.
> *Laxatives:* Squill may increase the effects of laxatives, avoid concurrent use.
>
> | Food | Herb |
> |------|------|
> | None known | None known |
>
> ### Lab Test
> Squill may cause a decrease in red blood cells.

Client Considerations

Assess

- Assess for hypersensitivity reactions. If these are present, discontinue use of squill and administer antihistamine or other appropriate therapy.
- Assess cardiac status (blood pressure, pulse, possibly EKG) if the client is taking squill over an extended period of time.
- Monitor electrolytes and watch for decreasing potassium levels.
- Determine whether the client is taking other cardiac medications such as beta-blockers, calcium channel blockers, cardiac glycosides, and antidysrhythmics. This herb should not be used with these medications (see Interactions).
- Assess for the use of central nervous system stimulants, glucocorticoids, and laxatives (see Interactions.)

Administer

- Instruct the client to store squill products in a cool, dry place, away from heat and moisture.

Teach Client/Family

- Until more research is available, caution the client not to use squill during pregnancy and lactation and not to give it to children.
- Advise the client that other, more mainstream agents are available and are preferred to squill.

 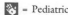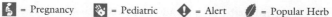

Pharmacology

Pharmacokinetics

Pharmacokinetics and pharmacodynamics are unknown.

Primary Chemical Components of Squill and Their Possible Actions		
Chemical Class	**Individual Component**	**Possible Action**
Cardiac glycoside	Proscillaridin A; Scillaren A, B; Glucoscillaren; Scillaridin A; Scilliroside	Inotropic; Chronotropic
Flavonoid Bufadienolides Ligan		

Actions

In North Africa, squill has been found to be poisonous to live-stock, with ingestion of the plant leading to cardiac toxicity (El Bahri, 2000). Toxicity was also reported in a 55-year-old woman with *Hashimoto thyroiditis* who was taking squill to treat arthritis. Her symptoms were those of cardiac glycoside toxicity (Tuncok, 1995). Squill has exerted cardiac glycoside effects in humans but is considered to be milder than current cardiac glycoside prescription drugs (Stauch, 1977).

S

References

El Bahri L et al: *Urginea maritima* L. (squill): a poisonous plant of North Africa, *Vet Hum Toxicol* 42(2):108-110, 2000.

Stauch M et al: Effect of proscillaridin-4i-methylether on pressure rise velocity in the left ventricle of patients with coronary heart disease, *Klin Wochenschr* 55:705-706, 1977.

Tuncok Y et al: *Urginea maritima* (squill) toxicity, *J Toxicol Clin Toxicol* 33(1):83-86, 1995.

St. John's Wort
(saynt jahnz wawrt)

Scientific name: *Hypericum perforatum* L

Other common names: Amber, goatweed, hardhay, John's wort, klamath weed, mellipertuis, rosin rose, witches' herb

Class 2d (Flowering Tops)

Origin: St. John's wort is found in Europe, Asia, and the United States.

Uses

Reported Uses

St. John's wort is used to treat mild to moderate depression and anxiety. It may be used topically as an antiinflammatory to relieve hemorrhoids, as well as to treat vitiligo and burns.

Investigational Uses

St. John's wort is used experimentally to treat warts, Kaposi's sarcoma, cutaneous T-cell lymphoma, and other viruses such as influenzae. It is also used experimentally as an antiretroviral in the treatment of HIV, as an antiinfective against methicillin-resistant strains of *Staphylococcus aureus,* and for phytotherapy in the treatment of psoriasis. Studies are underway to confirm St. John's Wort's use in menopausal symptoms, and seasonal affective disorder.

Product Availability and Dosages

Available Forms

Cream; sublingual capsules; solid forms: 100, 300, 500 (0.3% hypericin), 250 (0.14% hypericin) mg; tincture

Plant Parts Used: Flowers

Dosages and Routes

Adult

- PO: 300 mg hypericum extract, standardized to 0.3% hypericin, tid
- Topical: apply prn

Precautionary Information
Contraindications
Until more research is available, St. John's wort should not be used during pregnancy and lactation and should not be given to children. Persons who are hypersensitive this herb should not use it. Class 2d herb (flowering tops).

Side Effects/Adverse Reactions
Central Nervous System: Dizziness, insomnia, restlessness, fatigue (PO)
Gastrointestinal: Constipation, abdominal cramps (PO)
Integumentary: Photosensitivity, rash, hypersensitivity

Interactions with St. John's Wort

Drug
ACE inhibitors, loop diuretics, thiazide diuretics: St. John's wort combined with these drugs may lead to severe photosensitivity; avoid concurrent use.

Alcohol: St. John's wort may increase MAO inhibition (suggested by early studies); do not use alcohol and St. John's wort concurrently until research is conclusive.

Amphetamines: St. John's wort used with amphetamines may cause serotonin syndrome.

Antidepressants, tricyclics: St. John's wort used with tricyclics may cause serotonin syndrome.

Antiretrovirals, protease inhibitors: New studies indicate that St. John's wort taken PO in combination with indinavir may decrease the antiretroviral action of this drug.

Immunosuppressants: Rejection of transplanted hearts has occurred when St. John's wort was taken PO with cyclosporine, an immunosuppressant. Other immunosuppressants may have the same drug interaction in heart transplants, as well as other transplants.

MAOIs: St. John's wort may increase MAO inhibition (suggested by early studies); do not use MAOIs and St. John's wort concurrently until research is conclusive.

NSAIDs: St. John's Wort combined with NSAIDs may lead to severe photosensitivity; avoid concurrent use.

Continued

S

 Endangered Herb   Adverse effects: BOLD = life-threatening

Interactions with St. John's Wort—cont'd

Drug—cont'd

Oral contraceptives: St. John's Wort combined with oral contraceptives may lead to severe photosensitivity; avoid concurrent use.

Paroxetine: Increased sedation may result when paroxetine is combined with St. John's wort (Gordon, 1998).

SSRIs: Serotonin syndrome and an additive effect may occur when SSRIs are combined with St. John's wort. Concurrent use may lead to coma. Do not use concurrently.

Sulfonamides, sulfonylureas, tetracyclines: St. John's Wort combined with these drugs leads to severe photosensitivity; avoid concurrent use.

Trazodone: St. John's wort used with trazodone may cause serotonin syndrome.

Food

Limit foods high in tyramine or catecholamines until further research confirms or denies the MAOI action of St. John's wort taken PO.

Herb

None known

Lab Test

St. John's Wort may cause increased growth hormone (somatotropin, GH). It may cause decreased serum prolactin, theophylline (aminophylline), serum iron, and digoxin (peak and trough concentrations).

Client Considerations

Assess

Antidepressant Use

- Assess the client's mental status: mood, sensorium, affect, memory (long, short), change in depression or anxiety levels.
- Assess for the use of MAOIs and SSRIs, which should not be used with St. John's wort (taken PO) until further research is conclusive.
- Assess for other drugs, foods, and herbs the client uses on a regular basis (see Interactions).

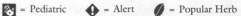

Antiretroviral Use
- Assess for signs of infection.
- Assess CBC, blood chemistry, plasma HIV, RNA, absolute CD4/CD8$^+$/cell counts/%, serum b-2 microglobulin, and serum ICD$^+$ 24 antigen levels.

Administer
- PO: use 2 tsp herb in 150 ml boiling water. Steep 15 minutes to create infusion.
- Topical: use oily hypericum preparations to treat inflammation or burns. Apply as needed.

Teach Client/Family
- Until more research is available, caution the client not to use St. John's wort during pregnancy and lactation and not to give it to children.
- Advise the client to avoid high tyramine foods such as aged cheese, sour cream, beer, wine, pickled products, liver, raisins, bananas, figs, avocados, meat tenderizers, chocolate, and yogurt and to avoid increased caffeine intake when using this herb PO.
- Inform the client that therapeutic effect may take 4 to 6 weeks for the treatment of depression. If no improvement occurs in that time, another therapy should be considered.
- Advise the client to avoid the use of alcohol or over-the-counter products that contain alcohol when using this herb PO.
- Advise the client to avoid the sun or use sunscreen or protective clothing to prevent photosensitivity when using this herb.

Pharmacology

Pharmacokinetics
Very little is known about the pharmacokinetics in humans. St. John's wort is thought to cross the blood-brain and placental barriers and possibly enter breast milk.

Primary Chemical Components of St. John's Wort and Their Possible Actions

Chemical Class	Individual Component	Possible Action
Naphthodianthrone	Hypericin; Pseudohypericin	Antiinflammatory; antitumor; antiviral (Raffa, 1998; Yip, 1996)
	Hyperforin	Antidepressant
Phenol	Caffeic acid; Chlorogenic acid *p*-Coumaric acids; Hyperforin	Antiseptic; disinfectant
Flavonoid	Hyperin; Hyperoside; Isoquercitrin; Kaempferol; Luteolin; Quercetin, Quercitrin, Rutin	
Bioflavonoid	Amenotoflavone; Biapigenin	Antiinflammatory; antiulcergenic
Phloroglucinol	Adhyperforin	Inhibits serotonin, dopamine, norepinephrine; antidepressant
Aboveground Parts Also Contain		
Tannin		Wound healing

Actions

Several different possible actions have been researched in the United States and abroad, primarily in the 1980s and 1990s.

Antidepressant Action

The inhibition of MAO (monoamine oxidase) and COMT (catechol-O-methyl-transferase) by *Hypericum* extracts and hypericin was researched (Suzuki, 1984; Thiede, 1994; Bladt, 1994). Hypericin was found to inhibit in vitro type A and B MAOs. In rats, MAO-A inhibition was greater than MAO-B inhibition (Suzuki, 1984). No relevant MAO inhibitory effect

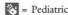

🐾 = Pregnancy   🐾 = Pediatric   ❗ = Alert   🌿 = Popular Herb

could be shown from the results of (Bladt, 1994), and no MAOI reactions have ever been found with St. John's wort. The inhibition of MAO was determined to be the result of flavonoids in the hypericin. Later studies could not confirm the MAOI effect (Muller, 1994). Other studies (Muller, 1998) reported an inhibition of the reuptake of norepinephrine and serotonin by *Hypericum* extract, which is the same mechanism of action as the tricyclics and SSRIs (selective serotonin reuptake inhibitors). Much of the antidepressant action may be attributed to hyperforin and adhyperforin (Chatterjee, 1998a, 1998b). These two constituents are found in the reproductive parts of the plant.

Antiretroviral/Antimicrobial Action

Investigation is underway into the possible antiretroviral action of St. John's wort and its use in the treatment of HIV infections (Chavez, 1997). Antiretroviral action may be due to protein-kinase-C–mediated phosphorylation. However, in one study, significant cutaneous phototoxicity resulted during the study, with no antiretroviral action found in the 30 participants (Gulick, 1999). One study (Reichling, 2001) found *Hypericum perforatum* tea effective against methicillin-resistant strains of *Staphylococcus aureus* with an MIC value of 1.0 μg/ml.

References

Bladt S, Wagner H: Inhibition of MAO by fractions and constituents of *Hypericum* extract, *J Geriatr Psychiatry Neurol* 7(suppl 1):s57-59, 1994.

Chatterjee SS et al: Antidepressant activity of *Hypericum perforatum* and hyperforin: the neglected possibility, *Pharmacopsychiat* 31:7-15, 1998a.

Chatterjee SS et al: Hyperforin as a possible antidepressant component of *Hypericum* extracts, *Life Sci* 63:499-510, 1998b.

Chavez ML: Saint John's wort, *Hosp Pharm* 32:1621-1632, 1997.

Gordon JB: SSRIs and St. John's wort: possible toxicity? *Am Fam Physician* 57:950-953, 1998.

Gulick RM et al: Phase I studies of hypericin, the active compound in St. John's wort, as an antiretroviral agent in HIV-infected adults, *Ann Int Med* 130:510-514, 1999.

Muller WE et al: Effects of *Hypericum* extract on the expression of serotonin receptors, *J Ger Psych Neuro* 7(suppl 1):63-64, 1994.

Muller WE et al: Hyperforin represents the neurotransmitter reuptake inhibiting constituent of *Hypericum* extract, *Pharmacopsychiat* 31(suppl):16-21, 1998.

Raffa, RB: Screen of receptor and uptake-site activity of hypericin component of St. John's wort reveals sigma receptor binding, *Life Sci* 62:265-270, 1998.

Reichling J et al: A current review of the antimicrobial activity of *Hypericum perforatum* L. *Pharmaco/psychiatry* 34(suppl1):S116-S118, 2001.

Suzuki O et al: Inhibition of monoamine oxidase by hypericin, *Planta Med* 50:272-274, 1984.

Thiede HM et al: Inhibition of MAO and COMT by *Hypericum* extracts and hypericin, *J Geriatr Psychiatry Neurol* 7(suppl 1):s54-56, 1994.

Yip L et al: Antiviral activity of a derivative of the photosensitive compound of hyperican, *Phytomed* 3:185-190, 1996.

Storax
(stoe′raks)

Scientific name: *Liquidambar orientalis*

Other common names: Alligator tree, star-leaved gum, sweet gum tree, balsam styracis, liquid amber, opossum tree, red gum, white gum

Origin: Storax is a tree found in Turkey.

Uses

Reported Uses

Traditionally, storax has been used in warm-mist vaporizers and as an expectorant. It is used as a diuretic and to treat diarrhea and sore throat. In addition, it is used in the furniture, cosmetic, and food industries. Externally, storax is used to treat wounds and ulcers.

Product Availability and Dosages

Available Forms

Crude balsam; no medicinal commercial preparations are available

Plant Parts Used: Bark, gum, leaves

Dosages and Routes

No dosage consensus exists.

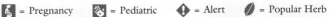

🝤 = Pregnancy   🔲 = Pediatric   ◆ = Alert   ∥ = Popular Herb

Precautionary Information

Contraindications

Until more research is available, storax should not be used during pregnancy and lactation and should not be given to children. Persons with hypersensitivity to storax should not use it.

Side Effects/Adverse Reactions

Gastrointestinal: Nausea, vomiting, anorexia, diarrhea
Integumentary: Hypersensitivity reactions, contact dermatitis

Interactions with Storax			
Drug	Food	Herb	Lab Test
None known	None known	None known	None known

Client Considerations

Assess

- Assess for hypersensitivity reactions. If these are present, discontinue use of storax and administer antihistamine or other appropriate therapy.

Administer

- Instruct the client to store storax in a cool, dry place, away from heat and moisture.
- Instruct the client to use storax externally on small areas only. External administration over large areas can lead to absorptive poisonings resulting in kidney damage.

Teach Client/Family

- Until more research is available, caution the client not to use storax during pregnancy and lactation and not to give it to children.

Pharmacology

Pharmacokinetics

Pharmacokinetics and pharmacodynamics are unknown.

 Endangered Herb   Adverse effects: **BOLD** = life-threatening

Primary Chemical Components of Storax and Their Possible Actions		
Chemical Class	**Individual Component**	**Possible Action**
Cinnamic acid Phenylethylene Vanillin		

Actions

Very little research is available to document any uses or actions of storax. Some investigators have proposed that storax may possess antimicrobial properties similar to those of tea tree (Wyllie, 1989).

References

Wyllie SG et al: The leaf oil of *Liquidambar styraciflua*, *Planta Med* 55:316, 1989.

Tea Tree Oil

Scientific name: *Melaleuca alternifolia*

Other common names: Australian tea tree oil, melaleuca oil, tea tree

Origin: Tea tree is found in Australia.

Uses

Reported Uses

Tea tree oil traditionally has been used to clean superficial wounds and to treat insect bites and other skin conditions. All applications of this herb are topical.

Investigational Uses

Initial evidence is available documenting the use of tea tree oil for the treatment of eczema; psoriasis; acne vulgaris; and bacterial, viral, and fungal infections.

Product Availability and Dosages

Available Forms

Cream, lotion, ointment, soap (5%-100%); component in many other commercial products

Plant Parts Used: Branches, leaves

Dosages and Routes

Adult

- Topical: apply any available form prn (usually 70%-100% used for fungal infections, 5%-15% used for acne)

Precautionary Information

Contraindications

Until more research is available, tea tree oil should not be used during pregnancy and lactation. Persons with hypersensitivity to the tea tree plant should not use tea tree oil.

Side Effects/Adverse Reactions

External Use

Integumentary: Hypersensitivity reactions, contact dermatitis

Continued

 Endangered Herb   Adverse effects: BOLD = life-threatening

Precautionary Information—cont'd
Side Effects/Adverse Reactions—cont'd
Internal Use
Central Nervous System: Depression, dizziness, drowsiness
Gastrointestinal: Nausea, vomiting, anorexia, diarrhea, gastrointestinal upset, irritation

---

Interactions with Tea Tree Oil			
Drug	**Food**	**Herb**	**Lab Test**
None known	None known	None known	None known

Client Considerations

Assess

- Assess for hypersensitivity reactions. If these are present, discontinue use of tea tree oil and administer antihistamine or other appropriate therapy
- If the client is using tea tree to treat skin disorders, assess the client's skin condition, including redness and pustules.

Administer

- Instruct the client to store tea tree oil in a sealed container away from heat and moisture.
- Instruct the client that tea tree oil is for external use only. It should not be taken internally.

Teach Client/Family

- Until more research is available, caution the client not to use tea tree oil during pregnancy and lactation.
- Advise the client that worsening skin conditions should be treated with more conventional therapy.

Pharmacology

Pharmacokinetics

Pharmacokinetics and pharmacodynamics are unknown.

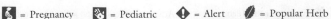

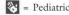

Primary Chemical Components of Tea Tree Oil and Their Possible Actions		
Chemical Class	**Individual Component**	**Possible Action**
Coumarin	Dihydrocoumarin; Melilotic acid; Methyl melilotate; Ethyl melilotate; Coumaric acid (Ehlers, 1995)	Anticoagulant
Hydrocarbon	Terpinene Pinene; Cymene	Antimicrobial
Cineol		

Actions

Antimicrobial Action

Tea tree oil has been tested for its antimicrobial properties. The essential oil shows broad-spectrum activity against *Escherichia coli, Staphylococcus aureus,* and *Candida albicans.* The antimicrobial activity of tea tree oil may result from its ability to disrupt the cell membrane (Cox, 2000). Another study (Hammer, 1998) demonstrated activity against *Candida* spp. Tea tree oil may also be useful for the treatment of yeast and fungal infections of the skin and mucosa. It has been shown to be effective against *C. albicans, Trichophyton rubrum, Trichophyton mentagrophytes, Trichophyton tonsurans, Aspergillus niger, Penicillium* sp., and *Microsporum gypsum* (Concha, 1998). *Pseudomonas aeruginosa* has been shown to be less susceptible than other species to the antimicrobial action of tea tree oil (Mann, 2000).

References

Concha JM et al: 1998 William J Stickel Bronze Award: antifungal activity or *Melaleuca alternifolia* (tea-tree) oil against various pathogenic organisms, *J Am Podiatr Med Assoc* 88(10):489-492, 1998.

Cox SD et al: The mode of antimicrobial action of the essential oil of *Melaleuca alternifolia* (tea tree oil), *J Appl Microbiol* 88(1):170-175, 2000.

Ehlers D et al: HPLC analysis of tonka bean extracts, *Z Lebensm Unters Forsch* 201(3):278-282, 1995.

Hammer K et al: In-vitro of essential oils, in particular *Melaleuca alternifolia* (tea tree) oil and tea tree oil products, against *Candida* spp., *J Antimicrob Chemother* 42(5):591-595, 1998.

T

Mann CM et al: The outer membrane of *Pseudomonas aeruginosa* NCTC 6749 contributes to its tolerance to the essential oil of *Melaleuca alternifolia* (tea tree oil), *Lett Appl Microbiol* 30(4):294-297, 2000.

Tonka Bean
(tawng'kuh been)

Scientific name: *Dipteryx odorata*

Other common names: Cumaru, tonka seed, tonquin bean, torquin bean

Class 3 (Seed)

Origin: Tonka bean is a legume found in South America.

Uses

Reported Uses

Tonka bean is used to decrease nausea and vomiting. Traditionally used as an aphrodisiac, it is now considered by many to be an obsolete herb.

Investigational Uses

Initial research has begun on the use of tonka bean for the treatment of cancer and lymphedema.

Product Availability and Dosages

Available Forms

No commercially prepared forms are available.

Plant Parts Used: Fruit, seeds

Dosages and Routes

Adult
• PO: 60 mg qd (coumarin content)

Precautionary Information

Contraindications

Until more research is available, tonka bean should not be used during pregnancy and lactation and should not be given to children. Persons with hypersensitivity to tonka bean should not use it. The FDA classifies tonka bean as unsafe. Class 3 herb (seed).

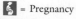 = Pregnancy   = Pediatric   = Alert   ⫝ = Popular Herb

Precautionary Information—cont'd

Side Effects/Adverse Reactions

Gastrointestinal: Nausea, vomiting, anorexia, HEPATOTOXICITY

Integumentary: Hypersensitivity reactions

Interactions with Tonka Bean

Drug

Anticoagulants (heparin, salicylates, warfarin): Use of tonka bean with anticoagulants may result in an increased risk of bleeding; avoid concurrent use.

Food	Herb	Lab Test
None known	None known	None known

Client Considerations

Assess

- Assess for hypersensitivity reactions. If these are present, discontinue use of tonka bean and administer antihistamine or other appropriate therapy.
- Assess for right upper-quadrant pain and assess liver functions studies (AST, ALT, bilirubin) for increased levels. If results are elevated, discontinue use of tonka bean.

Administer

- Instruct the client to store tonka bean in a cool, dry place, away from heat and moisture.

Teach Client/Family

- Until more research is available, caution the client not to use tonka bean during pregnancy and lactation and not to give it to children.
- Advise the client that the FDA classifies tonka bean as unsafe.

Pharmacology

Pharmacokinetics

Pharmacokinetics and pharmacodynamics are unknown.

🌀 Endangered Herb   Adverse effects: BOLD = life-threatening

Primary Chemical Components of Tonka Bean and Their Possible Actions		
Chemical Class	**Individual Component**	**Possible Action**
Coumarin	Coumaric acid; Dihydrocoumarin; Methyl melilotate; Ethyl melilotate; Melilotic acid	Anticoagulant
Hydroxymethylfurfural **Fat**		

Actions

Very few studies on tonka bean are available other than those done to determine its chemical components. The coumarins are known to produce an anticoagulant effect. One study evaluated the use of tonka bean in combination with gingko biloba and *Melilotus officinalis* to treat the functional symptoms of lymphedema. It was found that the use of these three herbs together provided significant improvement after the third month of treatment (Vettorello, 1996).

References

Vettorello G et al: Contribution of a combination of alpha and beta benzopyrones, flavonoids and natural terpenes in the treatment of lymphedema of the lower limbs at the 2d stage of the surgical classification, *Minerva Cardioangiol* 44(9):447-455, 1996.

 = Pregnancy   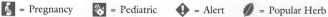 = Pediatric   ◆ = Alert   = Popular Herb

Turmeric
(tuhr′muh-rik)

Scientific name: *Curcuma longa*

Other common names: Curcuma, Indian saffron, Indian valerian, jiang huang, kyoo, radix, red valerian, tumeric, ukon

Class 1 (Root, Rhizome)

Origin: Turmeric is found in the Far East and tropical regions.

Uses

Reported Uses

Turmeric traditionally has been used in both Chinese and Ayurvedic medicine to treat menstrual disorders, colic, inflammation, bruising, dyspepsia, hematuria, and flatulence.

Investigational Uses

Research has begun to focus on the use of turmeric for the treatment of lung, gastrointestinal, oral, and breast cancers; viruses such as HIV/AIDS; cholecystitis; and joint pain associated with arthritis and other joint disorders.

Product Availability and Dosages

Available Forms

Capsules, dried rhizome, fluid extract, oil, spice, tincture

Plant Parts Used: Rhizome

Dosages and Routes

Adult

All dosages listed are PO.

- 400-600 mg tid (standardized to curcumin content)
- Cut root: 1.5-3 g/day
- Fluid extract: 1.5-3 ml (1:1 dilution)
- Tincture: 10 ml (1:5 dilution)

Precautionary Information

Contraindications

Until more research is available, turmeric should not be used therapeutically during pregnancy and lactation. This herb should not be used therapeutically by persons with bile duct

Continued

 Endangered Herb

Precautionary Information—cont'd

Contraindications—cont'd

obstruction, peptic ulcer, hyperacidity, gallstones, bleeding disorders, or hypersensitivity to it. Class 1 herb (root, rhizome).

Side Effects/Adverse Reactions

Gastrointestinal: Nausea, vomiting, anorexia, GASTROINTESTINAL ULCERATION (high doses)

Integumentary: Hypersensitivity reactions

Interactions with Turmeric

Drug

Anticoagulants (heparin, salicylates, warfarin): Use of turmeric with anticoagulants may result in an increased risk of bleeding; avoid concurrent use.

Immunosuppressants (cyclosporine): Turmeric may decrease the effectiveness of immunosuppressants; avoid concurrent use.

NSAIDs (bromfenac, diclofenac, etodolac, fenoprofen, flurbiprofen, ibuprofen, indomethacin, ketoprofen, ketorolac, meclofenamate, mefenamic acid, nabumetone, naproxen, oxaprozin, piroxicam, sulindac, tolmetin): Use of turmeric with NSAIDs may result in an increased risk of bleeding; avoid concurrent use.

Food	Herb	Lab Test
None known	None known	None known

Client Considerations

Assess

- Assess for hypersensitivity reactions, including contact dermatitis. If these are present discontinue use of turmeric and administer antihistamine or other appropriate therapy.
- Assess for the use of anticoagulants, NSAIDs, and immunosuppressants (see Interactions).
- Monitor coagulation studies if the client is using turmeric for long-term treatment.

🔥 = Pregnancy   🔯 = Pediatric   ◆ = Alert   🖋 = Popular Herb

Administer

- Instruct the client to store turmeric in a cool, dry place, away from heat and moisture.
- Instruct the client to take turmeric on an empty stomach.

Teach Client/Family

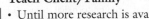 - Until more research is available, caution the client not to use turmeric during pregnancy and lactation.
- Advise the client to report bleeding gums, blood in the urine or stool, and bruising.

Pharmacology

Pharmacokinetics

Pharmacokinetics and pharmacodynamics are unknown.

Primary Chemical Components of Turmeric and Their Possible Actions		
Chemical Class	**Individual Component**	**Possible Action**
Volatile oil	Curcumin I, II, III	Anticancer; antioxidant (Ramsewak, 2000)
	Sesquiterpenes	
Diferuloylmethane		Tissue necrosis factor (TNF)-alpha inhibition
Sugar	Polysaccharides	
Resin		
Vitamin	C	
Mineral	Potassium	
Carotene		

Actions

A recent study (Ramsewak, 2000) has demonstrated the anticancer and antioxidant actions of three chemical components of turmeric, curcumins I, II, and III, on leukemia, central nervous system disorders, renal cancer, breast cancer, colon cancer, and melanoma. Turmeric is also known to inhibit tissue necrosis factor (TNF)-alpha. The chemical component diferuloylmethane has been shown to cause the most significant inhibition (Gupta, 1999). Turmeric may also exert hepatoprotective, antiinflammatory, antispasmodic, and hypolipidemic effects.

References

Gupta B et al: Curcuma longa inhibits TNF-alpha induced expression of adhesion molecules on human umbilical vein endothelial cells, *Int J Immunopharmacol* 21(11):745-757, 1999.

Ramsewak RS et al: Cytotoxicity, antioxidant and anti-inflammatory activities of curcumins I-III from *Curcuma longa, Phytomedicine* 7(4):303-308, 2000 (in-process citation).

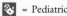

Valerian
(vuh-lir'ee-uhn)

Scientific name: *Valeriana officinalis*

Other common names: All heal, amantilla, baldrianwurzel, capon's tail, great wild valerian, herba benedicta, katzenwurzel, phu germanicum, phu parvum, setewale, setwell, theriacaria, valeriana

Class 1 (Root)

Origin: Valerian is a perennial that is now cultivated throughout the world.

Uses
Reported Uses
Valerian is used to treat nervous disorders such as anxiety, restlessness, and insomnia.

Product Availability and Dosages
Available Forms
Capsules, crude herb, extract, tablets, tea, tincture; combination products containing other herbs

Plant Parts Used: Rhizomes, roots

Dosages and Routes
Adult
All dosages listed are PO.
Insomnia
- Extract: 400-900 mg ½-1 hr before hs (standardized)
- Tea (crude herb): 1 tsp crude herb qid
- Tincture: 3-5 ml qid (standardized)

Precautionary Information
Contraindications

Until more research is available, valerian should not be used during pregnancy and lactation, and caution should be used when giving valerian to children. Persons with hepatic disease and those with hypersensitivity to valerian should not use it. Class 1 herb (root)

Continued

V

Precautionary Information—cont'd

Side Effects/Adverse Reactions

Central Nervous System: Insomnia, headache, restlessness

Gastrointestinal: Nausea, vomiting, anorexia, HEPATOTOXIC-ITY (overdose)

Integumentary: Hypersensitivity reactions

Miscellaneous: Vision changes, palpitations

Interactions with Valerian

Drug

Central nervous system depressants (alcohol, barbiturates, opiates, sedatives/hypnotics): Valerian may increase the effects of central nervous system depressants; avoid concurrent use.

Iron salts: Valerian may interfere with the absorption of iron salts; separate by 2 hr.

MAOIs: Valerian may negate the therapeutic effects of MAOIs; do not use concurrently (Tumova, 2000).

Phenytoin: Valerian may negate the therapeutic effects of medications containing phenytoin; do not use concurrently (Tumova, 2000).

Warfarin: Valerian may negate the therapeutic effects of warfarin; do not use concurrently (Tumova, 2000).

Food

None known

Herb

None known

Lab Test

Valerian may cause increased ALT, AST, total bilirubin, and urine bilirubin.

Client Considerations

Assess

- Assess for hypersensitivity reactions. If these are present, discontinue use of valerian and administer antihistamine or other appropriate therapy.

 • Assess liver function studies (AST, ALT, bilirubin) if the client is using valerian for long-term treatment. If results are elevated, discontinue use of the herb.

- Assess medications used (see Interactions).

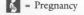 = Pregnancy    = Pediatric   = Alert   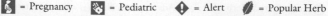 = Popular Herb

Administer

- Valerian products should be kept away from heat and moisture.

Teach Client/Family

- Until more research is available, caution the client not to use valerian during pregnancy and lactation and to use caution when giving this herb to children.
- Because valerian causes sedation and dizziness, advise the client not to perform hazardous activities such as driving or operating heavy machinery until physical response to the herb can be evaluated.
- Advise the client to discontinue use of valerian if symptoms worsen.

Pharmacology

Pharmacokinetics

Pharmacokinetics and pharmacodynamics are unknown.

Primary Chemical Components of Valerian and Their Possible Actions		
Chemical Class	**Individual Component**	**Possible Action**
Volatile oil **Valepotriates** **Alkaloid** **Amino acid** **Flavonoid** **Phenol** **Fatty acid** **Aliphatic** **Resin** **Tannin**	Monoterpene; Sesquiterpene	Increase GABA

V

Actions

Antianxiety Action

Valerian has been studied almost as extensively as St. John's wort. Its effects are primarily neurochemical, acting on gamma-aminobutyric acid A (GABAA) receptors and possibly also with other presynaptic components (Ortiz, 1999). Other studies

 Endangered Herb   Adverse effects: **BOLD** = life-threatening

support this action (Sakamoto, 1992; Cavadas, 1995; Simmen, 1999).

Antiinsomnia Action

The largest study included 121 patients with severe insomnia (Vorbach, 1996). They saw significant improvement within 28 days. This may indicate valerian is most effective in long-term treatment.

Other Actions

Valerian has shown positive results in the treatment of angina, decreasing the frequency and shortening the duration of anginal attacks (Yang, 1994).

References

Cavadas C et al: In vitro study on the interaction of *Valeriana officinalis* L. extracts and their amino acids on GABAA receptor in rat brain, *Arzneimittelforschung* 45(7):753-755, 1995.

Ortiz JG et al: Effects of *Valeriana officinalis* extracts on [3H] flunitrazepam binding, synaptosomal [3H] GABA uptake, and hippocampal [3H] GABA release, *Neurochem Res* 34(11):1373-1378, 1999.

Sakamoto T et al: Psychotropic effects of Japanese valerian root extract, *Chem Pharm Bull* 40:758-761, 1992.

Simmen U et al: Extracts and constituents of *Hypericum perforatum* inhibit the binding of various ligands to recombinant receptors expressed with the Semliki Forest virus system, *J Recept Signal Transduct Res* 19(1-4):59-74, 1999.

Tumova L et al: No title available, *Ceska Slov Farm* 49(4):162-167, 2000 (in-process citation).

Vorbach EU et al: Therapy for insomniacs: effectiveness and tolerance of valerian preparations, *Psychopharmakotherapie* 3:109-115, 1996.

Yang GY et al: Clinical studies on the treatment of coronary heart disease with *Valeriana officinalis* var. *latifolia*, *Chung Kuo Chung Hsi I Chieh Ho Tsa Chih* 14(9):540-542, 1994 (abstract in English).

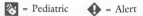 = Pregnancy   = Pediatric   = Alert   = Popular Herb

White Cohosh
(wite koe'hawsh)

Scientific name: *Actaea alba*

Other common names: Baneberry, snakeberry, coralberry, doll's eye

Origin: White cohosh is a perennial found on the west coast of North America and in the eastern region of the United States.

Uses

Reported Uses

Traditionally, white cohosh has been used during childbirth and to treat menstrual disorders, much like black or blue cohosh. Several Native American tribes have used white cohosh to treat colds, cough, gastrointestinal disorders, and urinary tract disorders.

Product Availability and Dosages

Available Forms

This herb is used by homeopaths. No commercial products are available.

Dosages and Routes

No published dosages are available.

Precautionary Information

Contraindications

White cohosh should never be used during pregnancy and lactation and should never be given to children. This is a toxic plant and should never be consumed, especially the fruit and roots. Because if its toxicity, white cohosh is not recommended for use except under the supervision of a qualified herbalist.

Side Effects/Adverse Reactions

Cardiovascular: TACHYCARDIA, CIRCULATORY FAILURE
Central Nervous System: Delirium

Continued

W

 Endangered Herb   Adverse effects: BOLD = life-threatening

> **Precautionary Information—cont'd**
> **Side Effects/Adverse Reactions—cont'd**
> *Gastrointestinal:* Nausea, vomiting, anorexia, severe abdominal cramps
> *Integumentary:* Hypersensitivity reactions

Interactions with White Cohosh			
Drug	**Food**	**Herb**	**Lab Test**
None known	None known	None known	None known

Client Considerations

Assess

 • Assess for symptoms of toxicity: delirium, severe abdominal cramping, headache, tachycardia, and circulatory collapse.

Administer

• Perform lavage or induce vomiting if the client has ingested this herb

Teach Client/Family

 • Warn the client never to use white cohosh during pregnancy and lactation and never to give it to children. Toxicity may result.

• Warn the client not to use white cohosh for any purpose. This plant is too toxic for any use.

Pharmacology

Pharmacokinetics

Pharmacokinetics and pharmacodynamics are unknown.

Primary Chemical Components of White Cohosh and Their Possible Actions		
Chemical Class	**Individual Component**	**Possible Action**
Essential oil Protoanemonin		Severe irritant

 = Pregnancy   = Pediatric   = Alert   = Popular Herb

Actions

Very little information is available for white cohosh, and what information is available is mostly anecdotal. Although the entire white cohosh plant is toxic, the fruit and roots are the most toxic parts (Duke, 1985). Homeopaths have used this herb, but it not recommended for any use.

References

Duke J: *CRC handbook of medicinal herbs,* Boca Raton, Fla, 1985, CRC Press, p 16.

Wild Cherry

Scientific names: *Prunus virginiana, Prunus serotina*

Other common names: Black cherry, black choke, choke cherry, rum cherry, Virginia prune   **Class 2d**

Origin: Wild cherry is found in the United States.

Uses

Reported Uses

Traditionally, wild cherry has been used to treat hot, dry, percussive coughs; colds; respiratory symptoms; and diarrhea. It has also been used as an astringent and bronchial sedative. Wild cherry is typically combined with other supportive lung herbs in formula.

Investigational Uses

Research is underway to determine possible uses for wild cherry as a cancer treatment.

Product Availability and Dosages

Available Forms

Fluid extract, syrup, tea, tincture

Plant Parts Used: Bark

Dosages and Routes

Adult

All dosages listed are PO.

- Syrup: 1-2 g in 8 oz boiling water, tid (whole syrup recipe)
- Tea: 3 tsp dry bark in 8 oz cold water, let stand 8 hr, strain
- Tincture: 1-5 ml qid (1:5 dilution) (Moore, 1995)

W

🌱 Endangered Herb   Adverse effects: **BOLD** = life-threatening

Precautionary Information

Contraindications

Until more research is available, wild cherry should not be used during pregnancy and lactation and should not be given to children. Persons with respiratory or cardiovascular depression or hypotension should not use this herb (Moore, 1995). Class 2d herb.

Side Effects/Adverse Reactions

Central nervous system: Headache, tremors, stupor, COMA, DEATH

Gastrointestinal: Nausea, vomiting, anorexia, constipation, ulcer

Musculoskeletal: Muscle weakness

Respiratory: RESPIRATORY FAILURE

Interactions with Wild Cherry

Drug

CYP3A4 enzyme substrate agents (astemizole, azole antifungals, benzodiazepines, buspirone, calcium channel blockers, cyclosporine, estrogens, statins): Use with wild cherry may slow the metabolism; avoid concurrent use.

Food	Herb	Lab Test
None known	None known	None known

Client Considerations

Assess

- Assess for changes in respiration (decreased or labored breathing, shortness of breath). If these symptoms are present, discontinue use of wild cherry.

Administer

- Instruct the client to store wild cherry in a cool, dry place, away from heat and moisture.

Teach Client/Family

- Because wild cherry is a known teratogen, caution the client not to use it during pregnancy. Until more research is avail-

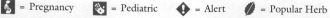

able, caution the client not to use this herb during lactation and not to give it to children.

- Warn the client that overdose can be fatal as a result of cyanide poisoning. If poisoning does occur, an antidote of thiosulfate or ethylenediaminetetraacetic acid (EDTA) may be necessary.

 • Caution the client to store all wild cherry products in a locked cabinet, out of the reach of children.

- Inform the client that no proven uses or actions exist for this herb and that other herbs or medications are safer options.

Pharmacology

Pharmacokinetics

Pharmacokinetics and pharmacodynamics are unknown.

Primary Chemical Components of Wild Cherry and Their Possible Actions		
Chemical Class	Individual Component	Possible Action
Cyanogenic glycoside	Amygdalin	Poison
	Prunasin	
Acid	Phytosterol; Emulsin; Oleic acid; *p*-Coumaric acid; Trimethyl gallic acid	
Ipuranol		
Dextrose		
Tannin		Wound healing; antiinflammatory
Starch		
Calcium oxalate		

Actions

Almost no research exists regarding the actions or uses of wild cherry. The available studies have tended to focus on its toxic effects. Because cyanide is present in the bark, seeds, and leaves, wild cherry should be used only under the direction of a qualified herbalist. If used properly, and for a few days only, this

🌀 Endangered Herb   Adverse effects: BOLD = life-threatening

herb is considered safe. Wild cherry prepared as a cold infusion has a much lower cyanide content than when prepared as a decoction.

References

Moore M: *Materia medica*, Bisbee, Ariz, 1995, Author.

Wild Yam

Scientific name: *Dioscorea villosa* L.

Other common names: Colic root, Mexican wild yam, rheumatism root

Class 1 (Rhizome)

Origin: Wild yam is a vine found in the United States and Central America.

Uses

Reported Uses

Wild yam is used to treat gallbladder disease, dysmenorrhea, menopausal symptoms, rheumatic conditions, and cramps.

Product Availability and Dosages

Available Forms

Fluid extract, oil, powder, tea, tincture; also available as DHEA (see pages 348-351)

Plant Parts Used: Rhizome

Dosages and Routes

Adult

NOTE: See also dosages for DHEA on page 348.
- PO fluid extract: 2-4 ml (5-30 drops) tid
- PO tincture: 2-10 ml tid (1:5 dilution in 45% alcohol)
- Topical oil: may be applied to affected area prn

Precautionary Information

Contraindications

Until more research is available, wild yam should not be used during pregnancy and lactation and should not be given to children. This herb should not be used by persons with hepatic disease or by those with a family history of

---

 = Pregnancy   = Pediatric   ◆ = Alert   ∥ = Popular Herb

Precautionary Information—cont'd
Contraindications—cont'd
breast, uterine, ovarian, or prostate cancer. Persons with hypersensitivity to wild yam should not use it. Class 1 herb (rhizome).

Side Effects/Adverse Reactions
Central Nervous System: Headache
Gastrointestinal: Nausea, vomiting, anorexia
Genitourinary: Menstrual changes, POSSIBILITY OF STIMULATING HORMONE-RELATED CANCERS
Integumentary: Hypersensitivity reactions, acne, alopecia, hirsutism, oily skin

Interactions with Wild Yam

Drug	Food	Herb	Lab Test
None known	None known	None known	None known

Client Considerations
Assess
- Assess for hypersensitivity reactions. If these are present, discontinue use of wild yam and administer antihistamine or other appropriate therapy.
- Assess the client's family history of hormone-induced cancers (breast, ovarian, uterine, prostatic). If these are present, the client should avoid the use of wild yam.

Administer
- Instruct the client to store wild yam products in a cool, dry place, away from heat and moisture.

Teach Client/Family
- Until more research is available, caution the client not to use wild yam during pregnancy and lactation and not to give it to children.
- Advise the client that high doses of wild yam (>25 mg DHEA/day) may cause irreversible voice change and hirsutism.

W

Pharmacology

Pharmacokinetics

Pharmacokinetics and pharmacodynamics are unknown.

Primary Chemical Components of Wild Yam and Their Possible Actions		
Chemical Class	**Individual Component**	**Possible Action**
Steroidal saponin	Dioscin; Diosgenin; Dioscenin; Dioscin	
Sterol	Beta-sitosterol	
Alkaloid		
Tannin		Antiinflammatory
DHEA		Steroid

Actions

Hormone Supplementation/Menopausal Symptoms

DHEA is synthesized from a precursor steroid, pregnenolone, then converted into estrogens and testosterone in both men and women (Baulieu, 1996). Levels of DHEA are reported to decline significantly after age 40; however, supplementation should not be started before a thorough evaluation of hormone-sensitive tumors is performed. Some researchers suspect that the decline in DHEA may be associated with insulin resistance, increased weight gain, and cardiovascular conditions (Sahelian, 1997). DHEA supplementation may be an alternative to hormone replacement therapy in women. Wild yam had little effect on menopausal symptoms when 23 symptomatic women used wild yam cream for 4 weeks (Komesaroff, 2001).

Cancer Stimulant/Cancer Inhibitor

Conflicting studies have reported increased tumor flare of prostate cancer in patients. However, in one study, when antihormone therapy was initiated, the flare retreated (Jones, 1997).

Cardiovascular Action

One study evaluated DHEA levels in patients with congestive heart failure. The results showed that levels of DHEA are lower in patients with congestive heart failure in proportion to the severity of disease (Moriyama, 2000).

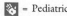 = Pregnancy   = Pediatric   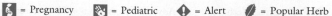 = Alert   = Popular Herb

Immunoregulator Action

A recent study using laboratory mice (Cheng, 2000) evaluated the effects of DHEA and DHEA sulfate on interleukin-10 (IL-10). The results indicated an increase in interleukin-10 (IL-10) and that DHEA may be able affect the functioning of B-lymphocytes.

Cognitive Function Enhancer

DHEA levels have been found to be significantly lower in persons with Alzheimer's disease and vascular dementia than in the general population, whereas the opposite is true for cortisol levels. The applicability of this information in the treatment of clients with cognitive function impairment is unknown at this time (Bernardi, 2000).

References

Baulieu E et al: *J Endocrinol* 150:s221-s239, 1996.

Bernardi F et al: Allopregnanolone and dehydroepiandrosterone response to corticotropin-releasing factor in patients suffering from Alzheimer's disease and vascular dementia, *Eur J Endocrinol* 142(5):466-471, 2000 (in-process citation).

Cheng GF et al: Regulation of murine interleukin-10 production by dehydroepiandrosterone, *J Interferon Cytokine Res* 20(5):471-478, 2000 (in-process citation).

Jones et al: Use of DHEA in a patient with advanced prostate cancer: a case report and review, *Urology* 50(5):784-788, 1997.

Komesaroff PA et al: Effects of wild yam extract on menopausal symptoms, lipids and sex hormones in healthy menopausal women, *Climacteric* 4(2):144-150, 2001.

Moriyama Y et al: The plasma levels of dehydroepiandrosterone sulfate are decreased in patients with chronic heart failure in proportion to severity, *J Clin Endocrinol Metab* 85(5):1834-1840, 2000 (in-process citation).

Sahelian R: New supplements and unknown, long-term consequences, *Am J Nat Med* 4(8):8-9, 1997.

W

Wintergreen
(win'tuhr-green)

Scientific name: *Gaultheria procumbens*

Other common names: Boxberry, Canada tea, checkerberry, deerberry, gaultheria oil, mountain tea, oil of wintergreen, partridgeberry, teaberry   Class 1 (Leaf)

Origin: Wintergreen is a shrub found in North America.

Uses

Reported Uses

Traditionally, wintergreen has been used topically to treat sore, inflamed muscles and joints, often after exercise. It may also be useful in the treatment of neuralgia. Wintergreen is used internally to treat bladder inflammation and urinary tract diseases, as well as diseases of the prostate and kidney.

Product Availability and Dosages

Available Forms

Cream, lotion, lozenges, oil, ointment, tea

Plant Parts Used: Bark, leaves

Dosages and Routes

Adult

- Topical cream/ointment: apply to affected area tid-qid prn (10%-30% strength)

Precautionary Information

Contraindications

Until more research is available, wintergreen should not be used during pregnancy and lactation and should not be given to children. It should not be used internally by persons with gastroesophageal reflux disease (GERD). Persons with hypersensitivity to wintergreen should not use it. Because of its hydroquinone glycoside content, this herb is not recommended for long-term use. Class 1 herb (leaf).

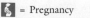 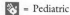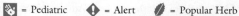

Precautionary Information—cont'd

Side Effects/Adverse Reactions

Internal Use

Gastrointestinal: Nausea, vomiting, anorexia, gastrointestinal irritation

Integumentary: Hypersensitivity reactions

Miscellaneous: Hyperpnea, lethargy

Internal or Topical Use

Systemic: SALICYLATE TOXICITY—TINNITUS, NAUSEA AND VOMITING, ELECTROLYTE IMBALANCES, CENTRAL NERVOUS SYSTEM TOXICITY, BLEEDING, HEPATITIS, ENDOCRINE CHANGES, RHABDOMYOLYSIS, DEATH

Interactions with Wintergreen

Drug

Anticoagulants (heparin, warfarin, salicylates): Use of wintergreen with anticoagulants may cause an increased risk of bleeding; avoid concurrent use.

Food	Herb	Lab Test
None known	None known	None known

Client Considerations

Assess

- Assess for hypersensitivity reactions. If these are present, discontinue use of wintergreen and administer antihistamine or other appropriate therapy. Clients who are hypersensitive to salicylates should not use this product.
- Assess for symptoms of salicylate toxicity (tinnitus, nausea, vomiting) if the client is using high doses of wintergreen over a prolonged period.
- Assess for the use of anticoagulants (see Interactions). Monitor coagulation studies if the client is taking wintergreen internally.

Administer

- Instruct the client to store wintergreen products in a sealed container away from heat and moisture.

W

 Endangered Herb   Adverse effects: BOLD = life-threatening

Teach Client/Family

 • Until more research is available, caution the client not to use wintergreen during pregnancy and lactation.

• Caution the client not to give wintergreen to children. Deaths have been reported. If viral symptoms are present in children, Reye's syndrome may occur if wintergreen is used.

• If the client is using wintergreen topically, advise the client to leave the affected area open to air or to wrap only in material with no heating capability.

• Caution the client not to use wintergreen oil internally.

• Advise the client to avoid use of topical wintergreen products during hot or humid weather.

Pharmacology

Pharmacokinetics

Pharmacokinetics and pharmacodynamics are unknown.

Primary Chemical Components of Wintergreen and Their Possible Actions		
Chemical Class	**Individual Component**	**Possible Action**
Salicylate	Methylsalicylate	Antiinflammatory; anticoagulant
Gaultherin		
Carbohydrate		
Tannin		
Hydroquinone derivative	Isohomoarbutin; Arbutin	

Actions

As is the case with other salicylates, the chemical component methylsalicylate is responsible for the antiinflammatory and anticoagulant properties of wintergreen. It is reported to act as a counterirritant. Oral ingestion stimulates gastric function.

References

Duke JA, *Handbook of medicinal herbs,* Boca Raton, Fla, 1985, CRC Press.

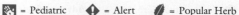

Witch Hazel
(wich hayz'uhl)

Scientific name: *Hamamelis virginiana*

Other common names: Snapping hazel, spotted alder, tobacco wood, winterbloom

Class 1 (Bark, Leaf)

Origin: Witch hazel is a bush found in North America.

Uses

Reported Uses

Traditionally, witch hazel has been used to relieve hemorrhoidal, vaginal, and anal itching; to decrease inflammation; and to promote the healing of bruises, varicose veins, and other local inflammation. It is also used as a gargle to decrease oral irritation and inflammation and may be used as a tea for diarrhea.

Product Availability and Dosages

Available Forms

Cream, dried leaves, fluid extract, pads, rectal suppositories, vaginal suppositories, witch hazel water

Plant Parts Used: Bark, leaves

Dosages and Routes

Adult

- PO dried leaf gargle: 2 g tid
- PO fluid extract: 2-4 ml tid (1:1 dilution in 45% alcohol)
- Topical witch hazel water: apply to affected area tid-qid prn

Precautionary Information

Contraindications

Until more research is available, witch hazel should not be used during pregnancy and lactation. Persons who are hypersensitive to witch hazel should not use it. Witch hazel should not be ingested. Class 1 herb (bark, leaf).

W

Continued

 Endangered Herb   Adverse effects: BOLD = life-threatening

Precautionary Information—cont'd

Side Effects/Adverse Reactions

Gastrointestinal: Nausea, vomiting, anorexia, constipation, HEPATOTOXICITY

Integumentary: Hypersensitivity reactions, contact dermatitis

---

Interactions with Witch Hazel

Drug

Iron salts: Witch hazel leaf, bark tea may decrease the absorption of iron salts; separate by 2 hr.

Food	Herb	Lab Test
None known	None known	None known

Client Considerations

Assess

- Assess for hypersensitivity reactions, including contact dermatitis. If these are present, discontinue use of witch hazel and administer antihistamine or other appropriate therapy.
- ◆ Assess for right upper-quadrant pain. Assess liver function studies (AST, ALT, bilirubin). If results are elevated, discontinue use of witch hazel.

Administer

- Advise the client to use witch hazel topically or as gargle only; it should not be taken internally.
- Instruct the client to store witch hazel products in a sealed container away from heat and moisture.

Teach Client/Family

- ⚘ Caution the client not to use witch hazel during pregnancy and lactation until more research is available.

Pharmacology

Pharmacokinetics

Pharmacokinetics and pharmacodynamics are unknown.

⚘ = Pregnancy   ☼ = Pediatric   ◆ = Alert   ⬦ = Popular Herb

Primary Chemical Components of Witch Hazel and Their Possible Actions		
Chemical Class	**Individual Component**	**Possible Action**
Flavonoid	Quercetin; Kaempferol	
Volatile oil	Eugenol; Safrole	
Saponin		
Tannin		
Calcium oxalate		
Resin		
Gallic acid		

Actions

Witch hazel has been evaluated for its antiinflammatory, antiviral, and antiaging actions.

Antiinflammatory Action

One study evaluated the antiinflammatory action of *Polygonum bistorta, Guaiacum officinale,* and *Hamamelis virginiana* in rats. Witch hazel did not act as an antiinflammatory in the acute stages of inflammation but did show antiinflammatory properties in the chronic phase (Duwiejua, 1994). Another study documented the antiinflammatory properties of witch hazel when used as an after-sun lotion (Hughes-Formella, 1998).

Antiviral Action

The antiviral action of witch hazel was shown against herpes simplex virus type 1 (HSV-1). Its antioxidative qualities were demonstrated by its radical-scavenging ability (Erdelmeier, 1996).

Antiaging Action

The active-oxygen scavenging action of witch hazel has been documented. This action may help to delay aging of the skin (Masaki, 1995).

W

References

Duwiejua M et al: Anti-inflammatory activity of *Polygonum bistorta, Guaiacum officinale* and *Hamamelis virginiana* in rats, *J Pharm Pharmacol* 46(4):286-290, 1994.

Erdelmeier CA et al: Antiviral and antiphlogistic activities of *Hamamelia virginiana* bark, *Planta Med* 62(3):241-245, 1996.

Hughes-Formella BJ et al: Anti-inflammatory effect of hamamelis lotion in UVB erythema test, *Dermatology* 196(3):316-322, 1998.

Masaki H et al: Active-oxygen scavenging activity of plants extracts, *Biol Pharm Bull* 18(1):162-166, 1995.

 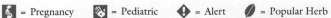

= Pregnancy   = Pediatric   = Alert   = Popular Herb

Yarrow
(ya-row)

Scientific name: *Achillea millefolium*

Other common names: Bloodwort, gordaldo, milfoil, nose-bleed, old man's pepper, sanguinary, soldier's woundwort, stanchgrass, thousand-leaf

Class 2b

Origin: Yarrow is found in Asia, Europe, and North America.

Uses

Reported Uses

Yarrow is used internally to treat respiratory, gastrointestinal, urinary tract, and reproductive conditions. It is used topically to promote wound healing and to treat eczema and other skin disorders.

Product Availability and Dosages

Available Forms

Capsules, fluid extract, powder, tea, tincture

Plant Parts Used: Dried leaves, flowering tops

Dosages and Routes

Adult

- PO fluid extract: 1-2 ml tid (1:1 dilution in 25% alcohol)
- PO tea: 2-4 g tid
- PO tincture: 2-4 ml tid (1:5 dilution in 45% alcohol)
- Topical sitz bath: 100 g herb/5 gal hot water, soak 10-20 min, rinse

Precautionary Information

Contraindications

Until more research is available, yarrow should not be used during pregnancy and lactation. It should not be used by persons with hypersensitivity to this plant or other members of the Compositae family, such as *Chamomilla recutita*, *Tanacetum parthenium*, or *Tanacetum vulgare*. Class 2b herb.

Continued

Y

 Endangered Herb   Adverse effects: **BOLD** = life-threatening

Precautionary Information—cont'd

Side Effects/Adverse Reactions

Central Nervous System: Drowsiness, sedation
Gastrointestinal: Nausea, vomiting, anorexia
Genitourinary: Uterine stimulation
Integumentary: Hypersensitivity reactions, contact dermatitis, photosensitivity

Interactions with Yarrow

Drug

Anticoagulants (heparin, warfarin, salicylates): Use of yarrow with anticoagulants may result in an increased risk of bleeding; do not use concurrently.

Antihypertensives: Use of yarrow with antihypertensives may result in increased hypotension; do not use concurrently.

Central nervous system depressants (sedatives/hypnotics, alcohol, opiates, barbiturates): Use of yarrow with central nervous system depressants may cause increased sedation; avoid concurrent use.

Iron salts: Yarrow tea may decrease the absorption of iron salts; separate by 2 hr.

Food	Herb	Lab Test
None known	None known	None known

Client Considerations

Assess

- Assess for hypersensitivity reactions, including contact dermatitis. If these are present, discontinue use of yarrow and administer antihistamine or other appropriate therapy.
- Determine whether the client is taking anticoagulants, antihypertensives, or central nervous system depressants (see Interactions).

Administer

- Instruct the client to store yarrow products in a cool, dry place, away from heat and moisture.

 = Pregnancy   = Pediatric   ◆ = Alert   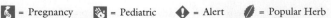 = Popular Herb

Teach Client/Family

- Until more research is available, caution the client not to use yarrow during pregnancy and lactation.
- Advise the client who is allergic to other plants of the Compositae herb family not to use yarrow.
- Inform the client to monitor for bleeding and bruising and to discontinue use of yarrow if these are present.
- Advise the client not to perform hazardous activities such as driving or operating heavy machinery until physical response to the herb can be evaluated.
- Because yarrow may cause photosensitivity, advise the client to use sunscreen and wear protective clothing, or to stay out of the sun, while using yarrow.

Pharmacology

Pharmacokinetics

Pharmacokinetics and pharmacodynamics are unknown.

Primary Chemical Components of Yarrow and Their Possible Actions		
Chemical Class	**Individual Component**	**Possible Action**
Tannin		Astringent; wound healing
Fatty acid	Linoleic acid; Palmitic acid; Oleic acid	
Amino acid	Alanine; Histidine; Leucine; Lysine	
Sesquiterpene Peroxide	Achimillic acids A, B, C	Antitumor
Volatile oil	Linalool; Borneol; Camphor; Cineole	

Actions

Several actions have been proposed for yarrow, including contraceptive, antitumor, and antiplaque actions.

Contraceptive Action

One study showed that antispermatogenesis occurred in mice when an extract of yarrow was given at 200 mg/kg/day intraperitoneally for 20 days (Montanari, 1998).

Y

🌸 Endangered Herb   Adverse effects: BOLD = life-threatening

Antitumor Action

One group of investigators who were observing cell division noted that an increase in tumor growth occurred during metaphase that may be due to the cytotoxic effects of yarrow (Montanari, 1998). Another study evaluated the antitumor properties of yarrow (Tozyo, 1994). The sesquiterpenoids were found to be active against leukemia in the mouse.

Antiplaque Action

One study has proposed that the use of yarrow slows plaque formation and the development of gingivitis; however, no changes were noted in the control group (Van der Weijden, 1998).

References

Montanari T et al: Antispermatogenic effect of *Achillea mellefolium* L. in mice, *Contraception* 58(5):309-313, 1998.

Tozyo T et al: Novel antitumor sesquiterpenoids in *Achillea millefolium*, *Chem Pharm Bull* 42(5):1096-1100, 1994.

Van der Weijden et al: The effect of herbal extracts in an experimental mouthrinse on established plaque and gingivitis, *J Clin Periodontol* 25(5):399-403, 1998.

Yellow Dock
(yeh-low dahk)

Scientific name: *Rumex crispus*

Other common names: Chin ch'iao mai, curled dock, curly dock, garden patience, hualtata, hummaidh, kivircik labada, narrow dock, niu she t'ou, oseille marron, sour dock, surale di bierdji   **Class 2d (Root)**

Origin: Yellow dock is a weed found in the United States, Europe, and Asia.

Uses

Reported Uses

Yellow dock is used primarily as a laxative or astringent. Topically, it may be used as an antidote to stinging nettle and to treat scabies and psoriasis. Traditionally it has been used internally as a blood cleanser and to treat sore throat and fever.

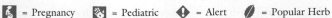

⚸ = Pregnancy   **🖐** = Pediatric   **◆** = Alert   **✇** = Popular Herb

Product Availability and Dosages
Available Forms
Capsules (ground root), extract, tea

Plant Parts Used: Root (dried and fresh), rhizome

Dosages and Routes
Adult
- PO: 2.5-5 mg qd

Precautionary Information
Contraindications
Because it can cause spontaneous abortion, yellow dock should not be used during pregnancy. Until more research is available, this herb should not be used during lactation and should not be given to children. Persons with renal disease, hepatic disease, electrolyte imbalances, or hypersensitivity to this herb should not use yellow dock, and persons with diabetes mellitus, poor nutritional status, or dehydration should use it with caution. Class 2d herb (root).

Side Effects/Adverse Reactions
Endocrine: SEVERE ELECTROLYTE IMBALANCES (HYPOCALCEMIA, METABOLIC ACIDOSIS)
Gastrointestinal: Nausea, vomiting, anorexia, cramps, diarrhea
Integumentary: Hypersensitivity reactions

Interactions with Yellow Dock

Drug
Yellow dock may cause increased hypocalcemia when used with calcitonin, diuretics, mithramycin, and phenytoin; do not use concurrently (theoretical).
Iron salts: Yellow dock tea may decrease the absorption of iron salts; separate by 2 hr.

Food	Herb	Lab Test
None known	None known	None known

🍀 Endangered Herb   Adverse effects: BOLD = life-threatening

Client Considerations

Assess

- Assess for hypersensitivity reactions. If present, discontinue use of yellow dock and administer antihistamine or other appropriate therapy.
- Determine whether the client is taking prescription drugs or other herbal products. Yellow dock should not be used with diuretics, phenytoin, mithramycin, or calcitonin (see Interactions).

Administer

- Instruct the client to store yellow dock products away from moisture and light.

Teach Client/Family

- Because it can cause spontaneous abortion, caution the client not to use yellow dock during pregnancy. Until more research is available, caution the client not to use this herb during lactation and not to give it to children.

Pharmacology

Pharmacokinetics

Pharmacokinetics and pharmacodynamics are unknown.

Primary Chemical Components of Yellow Dock and Their Possible Actions		
Chemical Class	**Individual Component**	**Possible Action**
Chrysophanic acid		
Rumicin		
Calcium oxalate		
Tannin		Astringent
Flavonoid	Quercetin	Antiinflammatory
Anthracene	Emodin	Laxative
	Chrysophanol; Aloe-emodin; Rhein	
Naphthalene	Lapodin; Neopodin	

Actions

The available research on yellow dock focuses on its toxicology. One study investigated acute oxalate poisoning in sheep that

 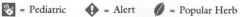

had ingested *Rumex crispus.* Symptoms of toxic reactions included tremors, ataxia, and increased salivation (Panciera, 1990). Another study focused on the fatal poisoning of a 53-year-old man who died 72 hours after simply ingesting *Rumex crispus* (Reig, 1990).

References

Panciera RJ et al: Acute oxalate poisoning attributable to ingestion of curly dock *(Rumex crispus)* in sheep, *J Am Vet Med Assoc* 196(12): 1981-1984, 1990.

Reig R et al: Fatal poisoning by *Rumex crispus* (curled dock): pathological findings and application of scanning electron microscopy, *Vet Hum Toxicol* 32(5):468-470, 1990.

Yellow Lady's Slipper
(yeh'low lay'deez sli-puhr)

Scientific names: *Cypripedium pubescens, Cypripedium calceolus*

Other common names: American valerian, moccasin flower, nerveroot, Noah's ark, whippoorwill's shoe, yellow Indian shoe

Origin: Yellow lady's slipper is an orchid found in the forests of Europe and the United States. It is considered an endangered species.

Uses

Reported Uses

Yellow lady's slipper traditionally has been used as a treatment for anxiety and insomnia and as a sedative. It has also been used to prevent seizures and as an antispasmodic and antidepressant.

Product Availability and Dosages

Available Forms

Extract, powdered root, rhizome, tea, tincture; component of various combination products

Plant Parts Used: Rhizome, roots

 Endangered Herb   Adverse effects: BOLD = life-threatening

Dosages and Routes

No consensus on dosage exists. Because it is on the endangered species list, yellow lady's slipper is not recommended for use.

Precautionary Information

Contraindications

Until more research is available, yellow lady's slipper should not be used during pregnancy and lactation and should not be given to children. Persons with psychosis, severe anxiety reactions, severe depression, migraines, cluster headaches, or hypersensitivity to this herb should not use it.

Side Effects/Adverse Reactions

Central Nervous System: Headache, insomnia, restlessness, stimulation
Gastrointestinal: Nausea, vomiting, anorexia
Integumentary: Hypersensitivity reactions, contact dermatitis

Interactions with Yellow Lady's Slipper

Drug	Food	Herb	Lab Test
None known	None known	None known	None known

Client Considerations

Assess

- Assess for hypersensitivity reactions and contact dermatitis. If these are present, discontinue use of yellow lady's slipper and administer antihistamine or other appropriate therapy.

Administer

- Instruct the client to store yellow lady's slipper products in a cool, dry place, away from heat and moisture.
- Inform the client that this herb is on the endangered species list and is illegal to collect.

Teach Client/Family

- Until more research is available, caution the client not to use this herb during pregnancy and lactation and not to give it to children.

 = Pregnancy   = Pediatric   = Alert 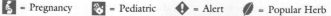 = Popular Herb

Pharmacology

Pharmacokinetics

Pharmacokinetics and pharmacodynamics are unknown.

Primary Chemical Components of Yellow Lady's Slipper and Their Possible Actions		
Chemical Class	**Individual Component**	**Possible Action**
Resinoid	Cypripedin	
Glycoside		
Quinone	Cypripedi	
Acid	Tannic acid; Gallic acid	

Actions

No research studies support any actions of or uses for yellow lady's slipper. Therefore this herb is not recommended for any use.

Yerba Maté

(yehr'buh mah-tay')

Scientific name: *Ilex paraguariensis*

Other common names: Armino, Bartholomew's tea, boca juniors, campeche, el agricultor, elacy, flor de lis, gaucho, jaguar, Jesuit's tea, la hoja, la mulata, la tranquera, lonjazo, madrugada, maté, nobleza gaucha, oro verde, Paraguay tea, payadito, rosamonte, safira, union, yi-yi, zerboni

Class 2d (Leaf)

Origin: Yerba maté is an evergreen found in South America.

Uses

Reported Uses

Yerba maté is used as a diuretic and to treat depression, lethargy, fatigue, constipation, arthritis, diabetes, gastrointestinal disorders, urinary tract infections, cardiac insufficiency, arrhyth-

🌿 Endangered Herb   Adverse effects: BOLD = life-threatening

mias, kidney or bladder stones. In China it is used parenterally as an antihypertensive.

Product Availability and Dosages

Available Forms
Fluid extract, leaves, tea

Plant Parts Used: Dried leaves

Dosages and Routes
Adult
- PO fluid extract: 2-4 ml tid (1:1 dilution in 25% alcohol)
- PO tea: 2-4 g tid

Precautionary Information

Contraindications
Until more research is available, yerba maté should not be used during pregnancy and lactation and should not be given to children. Persons with anxiety disorders, hypertension, or hypersensitivity to this herb should not use it. Class 2d herb (leaf).

Side Effects/Adverse Reactions
Central Nervous System: Anxiety, nervousness, insomnia, restlessness, irritability, headache
Gastrointestinal: Nausea, vomiting, anorexia, HEPATOTOXICITY
Integumentary: Hypersensitivity reactions
Systemic: CARCINOGENIC (long-term use)

Interactions with Yerba Maté

Drug
Central nervous system depressants (alcohol, sedatives/hypnotics, opiates, barbiturates, benzodiazepines): Use of central nervous system depressants with yerba maté may produce an antagonistic effect; avoid concurrent use.
Central nervous system stimulants: Yerba maté may increase the effects of central nervous system stimulants; use together cautiously.
Diuretics: Yerba maté may increase the effects of diuretics; avoid concurrent use.

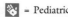 = Pregnancy   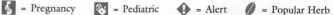 = Pediatric    = Alert   ✦ = Popular Herb

Interactions with Yerba Maté—cont'd	
Food	
Caffeine-containing products: Caffeinated foods and drinks may increase the effects of yerba maté; avoid concurrent use.	
Herb	Lab Test
None known	None known

Client Considerations

Assess

- Assess for hypersensitivity reactions. If these are present, discontinue use of yerba maté and administer antihistamine or other appropriate therapy.
- Assess for use of central nervous system stimulants, central nervous system depressants, diuretics, and products that contain caffeine (see Interactions).
- Assess for right upper-quadrant pain. Assess liver function studies (AST, ALT, bilirubin). If results are elevated, discontinue use of yerba maté.

Administer

- Instruct the client to store yerba maté products in a cool, dry place, away from heat and moisture.

Teach Client/Family

- Until more research is available, caution the client not to use yerba maté during pregnancy and lactation and not to give it to children.
- Advise the client not to use yerba maté if he or she is allergic to other plants in the Aquifoliaceae family (e.g., holly).
- Inform the client that using large amounts of yerba maté for a long period can lead to cancers of the gastrointestinal and urinary tracts.

Pharmacology

Pharmacokinetics

Yerba maté stimulates the central nervous system; possesses diuretic, analeptic, positive inotropic, and chronotropic effects; and is lipolytic and glycogenolytic.

Primary Chemical Components of Yerba Maté and Their Possible Actions

Chemical Class	Individual Component	Possible Action
Methylxanthine	Caffeine; Theobromine; Theophylline	Central nervous system stimulant
Sterol		
Fat		
Ursolic acid		Antitumor
Mineral	Iron; Calcium; Manganese; Magnesium; Sodium; Potassium; Zinc; Copper	
Flavonoid	Rutin; Isoquercitrin; Kaempferol glycosides	

Actions

Primary research has focused on several actions of yerba maté, including vasodilation, antioxidant, and antiobesity actions.

Vasodilation Action

One study has evaluated the vasodilatory effects of *Ilex paraguariensis* leaves in rats. Investigators documented a vasorelaxing effect (Muccillo Baisch, 1998).

Antioxidant Action

Two studies have reported the antioxidant effects of yerba maté. One study (Schinella, 2000) showed the antioxidant effect against free radicals. The second study identified the antioxidant effect as comparable to that of ascorbic acid (vitamin C).

Antiobesity Action

One study investigated the usefulness of yerba maté in the reduction of obesity. However, results indicated no effect (Martinet, 1999).

References

Martinet A et al: Thermogenic effects of commercially available plant preparations aimed at treating human obesity, *Phytomedicine* 6(4):231-238, 1999.

 = Pregnancy   = Pediatric   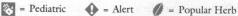 = Alert   = Popular Herb

Muccillo Baisch AL et al: Endothelium-dependent vasorelaxing activity of aqueous extracts of *Ilex paraguariensis* on mesenteric arterial bed of rats, *J Ethnopharmacol* 60(2):133-139, 1998.

Schinella GR et al: Antioxidant effects of an aqueous extract of *Ilex paraguariensis, Biochem Biophys Res Commun* 269(2):357-360, 2000.

Yerba Santa
(yehr′buh sahn′tuh)

Scientific name: *Eriodictyon californicum*

Other common names: Bear's weed, consumptive's weed, eriodictyon, gum bush, gum plant, holly herb, holy weed, mountain balm, sacred herb, tarweed

Class 1 (Whole Herb)

Origin: Yerba santa is an evergreen found in the southwestern region of the United States.

Uses

Reported Uses

Yerba santa traditionally has been used by Native Americans to decrease bruise and muscle inflammation. It has also been used to treat colds, asthma, congestion, allergies, arthritis, and rheumatism. The leaves are smoked or chewed to treat asthma.

Product Availability and Dosages

Available Forms

Dried leaves, fluid extract, liniment, powder, syrup, tea

Plant Parts Used: Dried leaves, roots

Dosages and Routes

Adult

- PO expectorant: dried powdered leaves
- PO tea: place dried leaves in water, boil, strain, drink prn
- Topical liniment: apply liniment of leaves to affected area prn
- Topical poultice: mix fresh leaves with water and apply to affected area prn

Y

Precautionary Information

Contraindications

Until more research is available, yerba santa should not be used during pregnancy and lactation. Persons with hypersensitivity to yerba santa should not use it. Class 1 herb (whole herb).

Side Effects/Adverse Reactions

Integumentary: Hypersensitivity reactions

Interactions with Yerba Santa			
Drug	Food	Herb	Lab Test
None known	None known	None known	None known

Client Considerations

Assess

- Assess for hypersensitivity reactions. If these are present, discontinue use of yerba santa and administer antihistamine or other appropriate therapy.

Administer

- Instruct the client to store yerba santa products in a cool, dry place, away from heat and moisture.

Teach Client/Family

- Until more research is available, caution the client not to use yerba santa during pregnancy and lactation.

Pharmacology

Pharmacokinetics

Pharmacokinetics and pharmacodynamics are unknown.

Primary Chemical Components of Yerba Santa and Their Possible Actions

Chemical Class	Individual Component	Possible Action
Flavonoid	Eriodictyol; Homoeriodictyol; Dimethoxyflavanone; Naringenin; Chrysoeriodictyol; Xanthoeriodictyol; Eriodict	
Flavone	Cirsimaritin; Chrysoeriol	Chemoprotective
	Hispidulin; Chrysin	
Tannin		
Volatile oil		
Acid	Formic acid; Butyric acid; Cerotinic acid	
Resin	Pentacontane; Priodonal; Xanthoeriodictytol	
Phenol		

Actions

Very little primary research is available for yerba santa. The only study found identified 12 new flavonoids that inhibited the metabolism of a carcinogen in hamster embryos. The chemical components cirsimaritan and chrysoeriol are thought to be chemoprotective (Liu, 1992).

References

Liu YL et al: Isolation of potential cancer chemopreventive agents from *Eriodictyon californicum, J Nat Prod* 55(3):357-363, 1992.

Y

Yew
(yew)

Scientific names: *Taxus brevifolia, Taxus baccata*

Other common names: American yew, California yew, chinwood, globeberry, ground hemlock, Oregon yew, western yew

Origin: Yew is found in Canada and the Pacific Northwest region of the United States.

Uses
Reported Uses

Yew is well known today as the plant used to manufacture the drug paclitaxel (Taxol), which is used to treat metastatic ovarian cancer. Native Americans have used yew to treat arthritis and other joint disorders, as well as fever. As a folk medicine, the cooked yew leaves were used as an abortifacient; to promote menstruation; and to treat diphtheria, epilepsy, tapeworms, and tonsillitis.

Product Availability and Dosages
Available Forms

Capsules, extract, salve

Plant Parts Used: Bark, branch tips

Dosages and Routes
Adult
- PO extract: 10-60 drops bid-qid
- PO tea: 8 oz qd
- Topical salve: apply to affected area prn

Precautionary Information
Contraindications

Until more research is available, yew should not be used during pregnancy and lactation and should not be given to children. Yew should not be used by persons who have hepatic disease or who are immunocompromised. Persons with hypersensitivity to yew should not use it. Yew is highly toxic and should be used only under the supervision of a skilled herbalist.

 = Pregnancy   = Pediatric   = Alert   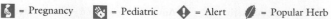 = Popular Herb

Precautionary Information—cont'd

Side Effects/Adverse Reactions

Cardiovascular: Hypotension, arrhythmias, elevated triglycerides and cholesterol

Gastrointestinal: Nausea, vomiting, anorexia, HEPATOTOXICITY

Hematologic: THROMBOCYTOPENIA, LEUKOPENIA, ANEMIA, NEUTROPENIA

Integumentary: Hypersensitivity reactions, alopecia

Musculoskeletal: Joint and muscle pain

Interactions with Yew

Drug

Antineoplastics: Use of yew with antineoplastics may cause increased myelosuppression; avoid concurrent use.

Food	Herb	Lab Test
None known	None known	None known

Client Considerations

Assess

- Assess for hypersensitivity reactions. If these are present, discontinue use of yew and administer antihistamine or other appropriate therapy.
- Monitor liver function studies (AST, ALT, bilirubin). If results are elevated, the client may need to discontinue using yew.
- Assess for the use of antineoplastics (see Interactions).

Administer

- Instruct the client to store yew products away from heat, light, and moisture.

Teach Client/Family

- Until more research is available, caution the client not to use yew during pregnancy and lactation and not to give it to children.
- Warn the client to use yew only under the supervision of a qualified herbalist. This herb is highly toxic.

Y

Pharmacology

Pharmacokinetics

Pharmacokinetics and pharmacodynamics are unknown.

Primary Chemical Components of Yew and Their Possible Actions		
Chemical Class	**Individual Component**	**Possible Action**
Alkaloid	Taxol	Antineoplastic
	Taxine A, B; Taxicatin; Milossine; Ephedrine	
Tannin		
Resin		
Lignan		
Flavonoid	Flavone; Sequoia; Ginkgetin; Sciadopytisin	

Actions

Antineoplastic Action

Yew is known for its antineoplastic properties. The main chemical component responsible for these effects is taxol, from which the drug paclitaxel (Taxol) is derived. This drug currently is used to inhibit metastatic breast cancer. It does so by inhibiting reorganization of the microtubule network needed for interphase in the cell division cycle and for mitotic cellular functions; it also causes abnormalities in bundles of microtubules during the cell cycle and multiple esters of microtubules during mitosis. Recent research has documented the efficacy of using Taxol in combination with radiation to treat head and neck cancers, cervical carcinomas, and breast adenocarcinomas (Pradier, 1999). Another study has evaluated the needles of different yew species for the presence of paclitaxel and related taxoids (Van Rozendaal, 2000). There appears to be a wide variation in taxane content in the different species found in different countries.

References

Pradier O et al: Effects of paclitaxel in combination with radiation on human head and neck cancer cells (ZMK-1), cervical squamous cell carcinoma (CaSki), and breast adenocarcinoma cells (MCF-7), *J Cancer Res Clin Oncol* 125(1):20-27, 1999.

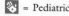 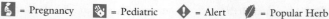

= Pregnancy   = Pediatric   = Alert   = Popular Herb

Van Rozendaal EL et al: Screening of the needles of different yew species and cultivars for paclitaxel and related taxoids, *Phytochemistry* 53(3): 383-389, 2000.

Yohimbe
(yoh-heem'buh)

Scientific name: *Pausinystalia yohimbe*

Other common names: Aphrodien, corynine, johimbe, quebrachine, yohimbehe, yohimbene, yohimbime, yohimbine

Class 2d (Bark)

Origin: Yohimbe is found in West Africa.

Uses

Reported Uses

Yohimbe traditionally has been used in Africa as an aphrodisiac. It is also used as a hallucinogenic.

Investigational Uses

Yohimbe is being studied for its use as a treatment for male erectile dysfunction, diabetes, orthostatic hypotension, and clonidine overdose.

Product Availability and Dosages

Available Forms

Tablets

Plant Parts Used: Bark

Dosages and Routes

Adult

Male Erectile Dysfunction
- PO tablets: 5.4 mg tid; dose may be adjusted to user's response

Orthostatic Hypotension
- PO tablets: 12.5 mg qd

Y

Precautionary Information
Contraindications

Until more research is available, yohimbe should not be used during pregnancy and lactation and should not be given to children. Persons with renal or hepatic disease, hypertension, angina pectoris, gastric or duodenal ulcers, bipolar disorder, anxiety disorder, schizophrenia, suicidal tendencies, prostatitis, or hypersensitivity to yohimbe should not use it. Prolonged use of this herb is contraindicated. Class 2d herb (bark).

Side Effects/Adverse Reactions

Cardiovascular: Hypertension, tachycardia, flushing
Central Nervous System: Headache, anxiety, restlessness, dizziness, tremors; manic reactions in psychiatric clients
Gastrointestinal: Nausea, vomiting, anorexia, diarrhea
Genitourinary: Dysuria, NEPHROTOXICITY
Integumentary: Hypersensitivity reactions

Interactions with Yohimbe

Drug

ACE inhibitors antihypertensives, beta-blockers, calcium channel blockers: Yohimbe may decrease or block the action of these drugs; avoid concurrent use (Musso, 1995).
Alpha-adrenergic blockers (phentolamine, phenoxybenzamine): Use of yohimbe with alpha-adrenergic blockers may result in increased toxicity; avoid concurrent use.
Central nervous system stimulants: Use of yohimbe with central nervous system stimulants may result in increased central nervous system stimulation; avoid concurrent use.
MAOIs (tranylcypromine, phenelzine): Yohimbe may increase the effects of MAOIs; avoid concurrent use (theoretical).
Phenothiazines (chlorpromazine, promazine, thioxanthene): Use of yohimbe with phenothiazines may result in increased toxicity; avoid concurrent use.
SSRIs: Use of yohimbe with SSRIs may cause increased central nervous system stimulation; do not use together.

Interactions with Yohimbe—cont'd

Drug—cont'd

Sympathomimetics (ephedrine, amphetamines, epinephrine):
Sympathomimetics increase yohimbe toxicity; avoid concurrent use (theoretical).

Tricyclic antidepressants (clomipramine, imipramine, amitriptyline): Use of yohimbe with tricyclic antidepressants may result in increased hypertension; dose may need to be lowered (Fugh-Berman, 2000).

Food

Caffeine-containing products: Use of yohimbe with products that contain caffeine may result in increased central nervous system stimulation; avoid concurrent use.

High-tyramine foods: Use of yohimbe with foods with a high tyramine content (e.g., wine, beer, aged cheese, liver) may cause increased blood pressure; avoid concurrent use.

Herb	Lab Test
None known	None known

Client Considerations

Assess

- Assess for hypersensitivity reactions. If these are present, discontinue use of yohimbe and administer antihistamine or other appropriate therapy.
- Assess for medication use. Yohimbe interacts with many types of medications (see Interactions).
- Assess for use of caffeine-containing products and high-tyramine foods (see Interactions).
- Monitor blood pressure and pulse if the client is using yohimbe for an extended period.

Administer

- Instruct the client to store yohimbe products in a cool, dry place, away from heat and moisture.
- Dosage may be increased to treat male erectile dysfunction; however, higher doses can lead to hypertension and tachycardia.

Y

Teach Client/Family

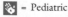

- Until more research is available, caution the client not to use yohimbe during pregnancy and lactation and not to give it to children. Yohimbe is usually used by males.

Pharmacology

Pharmacokinetics

Pharmacokinetics and pharmacodynamics are unknown.

Primary Chemical Components of Yohimbe and Their Possible Actions		
Chemical Class	**Individual Component**	**Possible Action**
Alkaloid	Yohimbine	Alpha-2 antagonist; increase blood pressure
	Alpha-yohimbine; Allo-yohimbine	

Actions

Chemically, yohimbe is similar in structure to reserpine and lysergic acid. One study found that commercial yohimbe products contain primarily the chemical component yohimbine and are devoid of other alkaloids. The high content of this component may increase the potential for toxicity (Betz, 1995).

Erectile Dysfunction

One study has evaluated the well-known use of yohimbe for the treatment of erectile disorders (Riley, 1994). It has shown a slight benefit in erectile disorder as compared with controls. However, yohimbe interacts with several drugs, which may lead to problems when taking this herb (see Interactions). One of the main actions of yohimbe is alpha-2 antagonism.

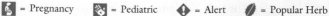

References

Betz JM et al: Gas chromatographic determination of yohimbine in commercial yohimbe products, *J AOAC Int* 78(5):1189-1194, 1995.

Fugh-Berman A: Herb-drug interactions, *Lancet* 355(9198):134-138, 2000.

Musso NR et al: Yohimbine effects on blood pressure and plasma catecholamines in human hypertension, *Am J Hypertens* 8:565-571, 1995.

Riley AJ: Yohimbine in the treatment of erectile disorder, *Br J Clin Pract* 48(3):133-136, 1994.

APPENDIX A
Herbal Resources

The following is a sampling of online resources that provide current, reliable information about herbal products, their uses, and their health effects. Some are consumer oriented, and others are intended for health professionals. The names of the sponsoring organizations' home pages are arranged alphabetically. URLs are provided for each individual site, or for the Internet portal through which the site may be accessed.

AGRICOLA (AGRICultural OnLine Access):
http://www.nal.usda.gov/ag98/

Alternative Herbal Index: Provides alphabetized monographs for more than 100 commonly used herbs, including information on usage, chemistry, interactions, and dosage, as well as a symptom-to-herb checker.
http://onhealth.webmd.com/alternative/resource/herbs/index.asp

Alternative Medicine Home Page, from the University of Pittsburgh: A compendium of resources to herbal and other alternative medicine information, broken into several categories. Each category includes a brief description of the linked material. Categories include:
- Databases
- Internet resources (divided into subject areas)
- Mailing lists & newsgroups
- AIDS and HIV
- Practitioner's directories
- Related resources
- Government resources
- Pennsylvania resources
http://www.pitt.edu/~cbw/altm.html

American Botanical Council:
http://www.herbalgram.org/

American Herbal Pharmacopoeia:
http://www.herbal-ahp.org/

American Herbalists Guild:
http://www.americanherbalistsguild.com/

American Society of Pharmacognosy:
http://www.phcog.org/

British Herbal Medicine Association:
   http://www.ex.ac.uk/phytonet/bhma.html

Dr. Duke's Phytochemical and Ethnobotanical Databases, from the Agricultural Research Service: A database of medicinal plants that allows the user to search by either common or scientific name. Provides information about the individual phytochemical components in each species, their biological actions, and relevant references.
   http://www.ars-grin.gov/duke/plants.html

European Scientific Cooperative on Phytotherapy (ESCOP):
   http://www.escop.com/

Herb Research Foundation (HRF): Contains an herbal question-and-answer column, an interface that allows the user to submit questions to the HRF foundation staff, herb news, herb references, and information about setting up media outreach and public education programs about safe and appropriate herb use. The HRF is a nonprofit research and education organization whose stated mission is to improve world health through the informed use of herbs. Some services are available free of charge, while others, such as custom botanical literature research and document delivery, involve a fee.
   http://www.herbs.org

Herbal Abstract Page: A compendium of links to Medline and other abstracts of articles about Western herbal and traditional Chinese medical therapies and their documented effects on human health.
   http://www.seanet.com/?vettf/Medline4.htm

Herbal Medicine, from MedlinePlus:
   http://www.nlm.nih.gov/medlineplus/herbalmedicine.html

Herbs for Health, from About.com: Offers a variety of consumer information about American Indian herbs, Ayurvedic medicinal products, Chinese herbs, ethnobotany, and Western herbs, along with daily updates on herbs and other alternative medicine issues in the news. Provides numerous links to other sites for information about herbs and alternative medicine.
   http://herbsforhealth.about.com/

Rocky Mountain Herbal Institute: Provides searchable general information about Chinese herbalism; describes continuing education courses available in Chinese herbal sciences and environmental health to medical and health professionals.

Provides a free, searchable database of 220 Chinese herbs and related sample course materials.
http://www.rmhiherbal.org/

RxList Alternatives, from allnurses.com: Provides searchable user monographs and frequently-asked-questions lists for commonly used Western herbs, Chinese herbal remedies, and homeopathic remedies.
http://www.rxlist.com/alternative.htm

Southwest School of Botanical Medicine: A comprehensive list of files containing botanical illustrations, including digitized photographs, color prints, lithographs, engravings, line drawings, and wood prints. Includes both .jpeg and .gif file formats.
http://www.swsbm.com/HOMEPAGE/HomePage.html

United States Pharmacopoeia (USP): Under "Dietary Supplements", includes detailed information on the status of USP-NF Botanical Monograph Development Project.
http://www.usp.org/

World Health Organization Herbal Monographs: Under "Development", see the entry for *Alternative Medicine Home Page, from the University of Pittsburgh.*
http://www.who.int/medicines/library/trm/medicinalplants/monographs.shtml

Centers for CAM Research

ADDICTIONS

Center for Addiction and Alternative Medicine Research (CAAMR)
Minneapolis Medical Research Foundation
914 South Eighth Street, Suite D917
Minneapolis, MN 55404

AGING AND WOMEN'S HEALTH

Botanical Center for Age-Related Diseases
Purdue University West Lafayette
Division of Sponsored Programs
West Lafayette, IN 47907-1021

Center for CAM Research in Aging and Women's Health
Columbia University
College of Physicians and Surgeons
630 West 168th Street
New York, NY 10032
URL: cpmcnet.columbia.edu/dept/rosenthal/

ARTHRITIS

Center for Alternative Medicine Research on Arthritis
University of Maryland School of Medicine
Division of Complementary Medicine
2200 Kernan Drive
Baltimore, MD 21207-6693

CANCER

Johns Hopkins Center for Cancer Complementary Medicine
Johns Hopkins University
720 Rutland Avenue
Baltimore, MD 21205
URL: www.hopkins-cam.org

Specialized Center of Research in Hyperbaric Oxygen Therapy
University of Pennsylvania
133 South 36th Street (6463801)
Research Services, Mezzanine
Philadelphia, PA 19104-3246

CARDIOVASCULAR DISEASE
Center for Complementary and Alternative Medicine Research in CVD
Adult Cardiac Surgery/Thoracic Transplantation
The University of Michigan Taubman Health Care Center
2120, Box 0344
Ann Arbor, MI 48109
URL: www.med.umich.edu/camrc/index.html

Center for Natural Medicine and Prevention
Maharishi University of Management
504 North 4th Street, Suite 207
Fairfield, IA 52557
URL: www.mum.edu/CNMP

CHIROPRACTIC
Consortial Center for Chiropractic Research
Palmer Center for Chiropractic Research
741 Brady Street
Davenport, IA 52803
URL: www.palmer.edu

CRANIOFACIAL DISORDERS
Center for Health Research
Kaiser Foundation Hospitals
3800 N. Interstate Avenue
Portland, OR 97227-1110

DIETARY SUPPLEMENTS
Botanical Dietary Supplements for Women's Health
University of Illinois at Chicago
809 S. Marshfield Avenue
Chicago, IL 60612-7205

UCLA Center for Dietary Supplements Research:
 Botanicals
University of California at Los Angeles
10945 Le Conte Avenue, Suite 1401
Box 951406
Los Angeles, CA 90095-1406

NEUROLOGIC DISORDERS
Oregon Center for Complementary and Alternative
 Medicine in Neurological Disorders
Oregon Health Sciences University
3181 SW Sam Jackson Park Road
Portland, OR 97201

NEURODEGENERATIVE DISORDERS
Center for CAM in Neurodegenerative Diseases
Department of Neurology
Emory University School of Medicine
1639 Pierce Drive
Atlanta, GA 30322
URL: www.emory.edu/WHSC/MED/NEUROLOGY/
 CAM/index.html

PEDIATRICS
University of Arizona Health Sciences Center
Department of Pediatrics
1501 N. Campbell Avenue
P.O. Box 245073
Tucson, AZ 85724-5073

PHYTOTHERAPY
Arizona Center for Phytomedicine Research
University of Arizona College of Pharmacy
1703 E. Mabel
P.O. Box 210207
Tucson, AZ 85721-0207

Selected CAM Training Programs

Academy of Oriental Medicine
In the Village Center
2700 West Anderson Lane, Suite 204
Austin, TX 78757
phone: (512) 454-1188
phone: (800) 824-9987
fax: (512) 454-7001
URL: www.aoma.edu/

Alchemy Botanicals
253 E. Main Street
Ashland, OR 97520
phone: (541) 488-4418
fax: (541) 488-4419

Alternative and Integrative Medical Society
University of British Columbia
400-2194 Health Sciences Mall
Vancouver, British Columbia
V6T 1Z3
CANADA
phone: (604) 822-7604
fax: (604) 822-2495
URL: www.aims.ubc.ca/

Alternative Medicine College of Canada
1120 East, Belanger Street
Montreal, Quebec
H2S 1H3
CANADA
phone: (800) 663-8380
fax: (514) 278-2637
URL: www.alternativemedicinecollege.com/

Alternative Medicines Research Institute
4995 James Walk, Suite 2
Vancouver, British Columbia
V5W2K3
CANADA
phone: (604) 325-7948
URL: www.altmedresearch.org/pages/armi.htm

American Institute of Vedic Studies
PO Box 8357
Santa Fe NM 87504-8357
phone: (505) 983-9385
fax: (505) 982-5807
URL: www.vedanet.com/

American Nutraceutical Association
5120 Selkirk Drive, Suite 100
Birmingham, AL 35242
phone: (205) 980-5710
fax: (205) 991-9302
URL: www.americanutra.com/

Association of Natural Medicine Pharmacists
P.O. Box 150727
San Rafael, CA 94915-0727
phone: (415) 868-1909
fax: (415) 868-1996
URL: www.anmp.org/

Ayurvedic Institute
P.O. Box 23445
Albuquerque, NM 87192-1445
phone: (505) 291-9698
URL: www.ayurveda.com/

Australasian College of Herbal Studies
5940 SW Hood Avenue
Portland, OR 97239
phone: (800) 487-8839
fax: (503) 244-0726

Bastyr University
14500 Juanita Drive NE
Kenmore, WA 98133
phone: (425) 602-3330
fax: (425) 602-3090
URL: www.bastyr.edu

Blue Crescent School of Botanical Medicine
P.O Box 983
Belfast, ME 04915
phone: (207) 338-1752
URL: www.bluecrescentschool.com

Blue Heron Academy
2040 Raybrook, SE, Suite 104
Grand Rapids, MI 49546
phone: (616) 285-9999
fax: (616) 956-7777
URL: www.blueheronacademy.com

Boston School of Herbal Energetics
12 Pelham Terrace
Arlington, MA 02174-6403
phone: (781) 646-6319
fax: (781) 641-4070
URL: www.herbalenergetics.com

British Institute of Homoeopathy
P.O. Box 23059
Ottawa, Ontario
K2A 4E2
CANADA
phone: (866) 866-3987
URL: http://www.bihcanada.ca/index.html

California College of Ayurveda
1117A East Main Street
Grass Valley, California 95945
phone: (530) 274-9100
URL: www.ayurvedacollege.com/services/index.htm

California School of Herbal Studies
PO Box 39 Physical: 9309 Hwy 116
Forestville, CA 95436
phone: (707) 887-7457
fax: (707) 887-1539
URL: www.cshs.com/

California Institute of the Healing Arts and Sciences
3550 Watt Avenue, Suite 140
Sacramento, California 95821, USA
phone: (916) 484-1700
fax: (916) 852-1310
URL: www.californiainstitute.net/

California School of Traditional Hispanic Herbalism
2801 Lincoln Avenue
Richmond, CA 94804
phone: (510) 233-5837
URL: www.hispanicherbs.com/

Canadian College of Naturopathic Medicine
1255 Sheppard Avenue East
Toronto, Ontario
M2K 1E2
CANADA
phone: (866) 241-2266
URL: www.ccnm.edu/

Centre for Natural Healing
300 N. Pioneer Street
Ashland, OR 97520
phone: (541) 201-1971
fax: (541) 488-6949
URL: www.centrehealing.com

Chicago College of Healings Arts
1622 West Devon Avenue
Chicago, IL 60660
phone: (773) 596-5012
URL: www.chicagocollegeofhealingarts.com/

Clayton College of Natural Health
2140 11th Ave. S. Suite 305
Birmingham, AL 35205
phone: (877) 782-8236
fax: (205) 323-8231
URL: www.ccnh.edu

**Complementary and Alternative Medicine Program
at Stanford**
Stanford Center for Research and Disease Prevention
Stanford University School of Medicine
phone: (650) 723-8628
URL: http://camps.stanford.edu/

Dominion Herbal College
7527 Kingsway
Burnaby, British Columbia
V3N 3C1
CANADA
phone: (604) 521-5822
fax: (604) 526-1561
URL: www.dominionherbal.com/

Duke Center for Integrative Medicine
phone: (919) 660-6801
phone: (866) 313-0959
URL: http://dukehealth.org/health_services/
    integrative_medicine.asp

EarthSong Herbals
10 Central Street
Marblehead, MA 01945
phone: (781) 631-4312
URL: www.earthsongherbals.com

East West School of Herbology
P.O. Box 275
Ben Lomond, CA 95005
phone: (800) 717-5010
fax: (831) 336-4548
URL: www.planetherbs.com

Foundations in Herbal Medicine
PO Box 4544
Albuquerque, NM 87196
phone: (888) 857-1976
fax: (505) 266-2160
URL: www.fihm.com

Greenfingers Foundation for Studies in Herbal Medicine
5515 North Seventh Street #119
Phoenix, AZ 85014
phone: (602) 277-8363
fax: (602) 997-2170

Heart of Herbs
48 Commonwealth Avenue
Springfield, VT 05156
phone: (866) 303-HERB
URL: www.heartofherbs.com

Herb Pharm HerbaCulture Work/Study Program
PO Box 116
Williams, OR 97544
phone: (541) 846-9121
fax: (541) 846-9259
URL: www.herb-pharm.com/Education/workstudy_fs.html

Homeopathy Vancouver
Vancouver Homeopathic Academy
PO Box 34095
Station D
Vancouver, British Columbia
V6J 4M1
CANADA
URL: www.homeopathyvancouver.com/index.html

Mind Body Medical Institute
824 Boylston Street
Chestnut Hill, MA 02467
phone: (617) 991-0102
phone: (866) 509-0732
fax: (617) 991-0112
URL: www.mbmi.org/default.asp

National Ayurvedic Medical Association
620 Cabrillo Avenue
Santa Cruz, CA. 95065
URL: www.ayurveda-nama.org/

National College of Naturopathic Medicine
049 Southwest Porter Street
Portland, Oregon 97201
phone: (503) 499-4343
URL: www.ncnm.edu/intro.html

Nature's Way Herbal Health Institute
2486 Hwy #6
Lumby, British Columbia
V0E 2G1
CANADA
phone: (250) 547-2281
fax: (250) 547-8911
URL: herbalistprograms.com

North American College of Botanical Medicine
1116 Park Avenue SW
Albuquerque, NM 87102
phone: (505) 873-8107
fax: (505) 873-4530
URL: www.swcp.com/botanicalmedicine

Northeast School of Botanical Medicine
PO Box 6626
Ithaca, NY 14851
phone: (607) 564-1023
URL: www.ph.utexas.edu/~wolfe/NSBM/NSBMcur.html

Oshio College of Acupuncture and Herbology
Suites 110/114-1595 McKenzie Avenue
Victoria, British Columbia
CANADA
V8N1A4
phone: (250) 472-6601
fax: (250) 472-6611

**Richard and Hinda Rosenthal Center for Complementary
& Alternative Medicine**
Columbia University, College of Physicians & Surgeons
630 W. 168th Street, Box 75
New York, NY 10032
phone: (212) 342-0101
fax: (212) 342-0100
URL: www.rosenthal.hs.columbia.edu/

Rocky Mountain Center for Botanical Studies
2639 Spruce Street
Boulder, CO 80302
phone: (303) 442-6861
fax: (303) 442-6294
URL: www.herbschool.com

School of Natural Healing
P.O. Box 412
Springville, UT 84663
phone: (800) 372-8255
fax: (801) 489-8341
URL: www.schoolofnaturalhealing.com/snh_cc.htm

Sierra Institute of Herbal Studies
P.O. Box 426
Big Oak Flat, CA 95305
phone: (209) 962-7425
fax: (209) 962-7717
URL: www.lodelink.com/sierrain

Southern California University of Health Sciences
College of Acupuncture and Oriental Medicine
16200 East Amber Valley Drive
Whittier, CA 90609
phone: (800) 221-5222
URL: www.lacc.edu/

Southwest College of Naturopathic Medicine
2140 E. Broadway Road
Tempe, AZ 85282
phone: (480) 858-9100
fax: (480) 858-9116
URL: www.scnm.edu/

Tai Sophia Institute for the Healing Arts
7750 Montpelier Road
Laurel, MD 20723
phone: (410) 888-9048
fax: (410) 888-9004
URL: www.tai.edu

Toronto School of Homeopathic Medicine
1246 Yonge Street, Suite 301
Toronto, Ontario
M4T 1W5
CANADA
phone: (416) 966-2350
phone: (800) 572-6001
URL: www.homeopathycanada.com/

Tree of Light
P.O. Box 911239
St. George, Utah 84791
phone: (888) 707-4372
fax: (435) 627-2367
URL: www.treelite.com

UCLA Collaborative Centers for Integrative Medicine
11301 Wilshire Boulevard
Building 115, Room 223
Los Angeles, California 90073
phone: (310) 825-5300
fax: (310) 794-2864
URL: www.mbcrc.med.ucla.edu/

University of Arizona Program in Integrative Medicine
URL: http://integrativemedicine.arizona.edu/

University of Bridgeport Naturopathic College Program
126 Park Avenue
Bridgeport, CT 06601
phone: (800) 392-3582)
URL: www.bridgeport.edu/default.cgi

University of Texas
MD Anderson Cancer Center
1515 Holcombe Boulevard
Houston, TX 77030
phone: (800) 392-1611
URL: www.mdanderson.org/departments/cimer/

Western Canadian Institute of TCM Practitioners
Student Services Branch
2nd Floor 1106 Cook Street
Victoria, British Columbia
V8V 3Z9
CANADA
phone: (250)387-6100
fax: (250)356-9455
URL: www.gov.bc.ca/aett

White Pine Healing Arts
86 Henry Street
Amherst, MA 01002
phone: (413) 549-4021
fax: (413) 549-2892
URL: www.whitepinehealingarts.com/

APPENDIX C
American Association
of Poison Control Centers

**U.S. Poison Control Center Members
(certified centers are in *italics*)**

ALABAMA

Alabama Poison Center
Emergency phone:
  (800) 222-1222

*Regional Poison Control
  Center*
Emergency phone:
  (800) 222-1222

ALASKA

Oregon Poison Center
Emergency phone:
  (800) 222-1222

ARIZONA

*Arizona Poison & Drug Info
  Center*
Emergency phone:
  (800) 222-1222

Banner Poison Control Center
Emergency phone:
  (800) 222-1222

ARKANSAS

Arkansas Poison & Drug
  Information Center
Emergency phone:
  (800) 222-1222
TDD/TTY:
  (800) 641-3805

CALIFORNIA

*California Poison Control
  System—Fresno/Madera
  Division*
Emergency phone:
  (800) 222-1222
TDD/TTY:
  (800) 972-3323

*California Poison Control
  System—Sacramento Division*
Emergency phone:
  (800) 222-1222
TDD/TTY:
  (800) 972-3323

*California Poison Control
  System—San Francisco
  Division*
Emergency phone:
  (800) 222-1222
TDD/TTY:
  (800) 972-3323

*California Poison Control
  System—San Diego Division*
Emergency phone:
  (800) 222-1222
TDD/TTY:
  (800) 972-3323

COLORADO

*Rocky Mountain Poison
& Drug Center*
Emergency phone:
(800) 222-1222
TDD/TTY:
(303) 739-1127

CONNECTICUT

*Connecticut Poison Control
Center*
Emergency phone:
(800) 222-1222

DELAWARE

The Poison Control Center
Emergency phone:
(800) 222-1222
TDD/TTY:
(215) 590-8789

DISTRICT OF COLUMBIA

*National Capital Poison
Center*
Emergency phone:
(800) 222-1222
TDD/TTY:
(800) 222-1222

FLORIDA

*Florida Poison Information
Center–Jacksonville*
Emergency phone:
(800) 222-1222
TDD/TTY:
(800) 222-1222
TDD/TTY:
(800) 282-3171
(Florida only)

*Florida Poison Information
Center–Miami*
Emergency phone:
(800) 222-1222

*Florida Poison Information
Center–Tampa*
Emergency phone:
(800) 222-1222

GEORGIA

Georgia Poison Center
Emergency phone:
(800) 222-1222
TDD/TTY:
(404) 616-9287

HAWAII

Hawaii Poison Center
Emergency phone:
(800) 222-1222

*Rocky Mountain Poison
& Drug Center*
Emergency phone:
(800) 222-1222
TDD/TTY:
(303) 739-1127

IDAHO

*Rocky Mountain Poison
& Drug Center*
Emergency phone:
(800) 222-1222
TDD/TTY:
(303) 739-1127

ILLINOIS

Illinois Poison Center
Emergency phone:
(800) 222-1222
TDD/TTY:
(312) 906-6185

INDIANA

Indiana Poison Center
Emergency phone:
    (800) 222-1222
TDD/TTY:
    (317) 962-2336

IOWA

Iowa Statewide Poison Control Center
Emergency phone:
    (800) 222-1222

KANSAS

Mid-America Poison Control Center
Emergency phone:
    (800) 222-1222
TDD/TTY:
    (913) 588-6639

KENTUCKY

Kentucky Regional Poison Center
Emergency phone:
    (800) 222-1222

LOUISIANA

Louisiana Drug and Poison Information Center
Emergency phone:
    (800) 222-1222

MAINE

Northern New England Poison Center
Emergency phone:
    (800) 222-1222
TDD/TTY:
    (877) 299-4447
TDD/TTY:
    (207) 871-2879
    (Maine only)

MARYLAND

Maryland Poison Center
Emergency phone:
    (800) 222-1222
TDD/TTY:
    (410) 706-1858 (TDD)

National Capital Poison Center
Emergency phone:
    (800) 222-1222
TDD/TTY:
    (800) 222-1222

MASSACHUSETTS

Regional Center for Poison Control and Prevention Serving Massachusetts and Rhode Island
Emergency phone:
    (800) 222-1222
TDD/TTY:
    (888) 244-5313

MICHIGAN

Children's Hospital of Michigan Regional Poison Control Center
Emergency phone:
    (800) 222-1222
TDD/TTY:
    (800) 356-3232

DeVos Children's Hospital Regional Poison Center
Emergency phone:
    (800) 222-1222
TDD/TTY:
    (800) 222-1222

MINNESOTA

Hennepin Regional Poison Center
Emergency phone:
(800) 222-1222
TDD/TTY:
(800) 222-1222
(612) 904-4691 (TTY)

MISSISSIPPI

Mississippi Regional Poison Control Center
Emergency phone:
(800) 222-1222

MISSOURI

Missouri Regional Poison Center
Emergency phone:
(800) 222-1222
TDD/TTY:
(314) 612-5705

MONTANA

Rocky Mountain Poison & Drug Center
Emergency phone:
(800) 222-1222
TDD/TTY:
(303) 739-1127

NEBRASKA

The Poison Center
Emergency phone:
(800) 222-1222

NEVADA

Oregon Poison Center
Emergency phone:
(800) 222-1222

Rocky Mountain Poison & Drug Center
Emergency phone:
(800) 222-1222
TDD/TTY:
(303) 739-1127

NEW HAMPSHIRE

New Hampshire Poison Information Center
Emergency phone:
(800) 222-1222

NEW JERSEY

New Jersey Poison Information and Education System
Emergency phone:
(800) 222-1222
TDD/TTY:
(973) 926-8008

NEW MEXICO

New Mexico Poison & Drug Info Center
Emergency phone:
(800) 222-1222

NEW YORK

Central New York Poison Center
Emergency phone:
(800) 222-1222

Finger Lakes Regional Poison & Drug Information Center
Emergency phone:
(800) 222-1222
TDD/TTY:
(585) 273-3854 (TTY)

Long Island Regional Poison and Drug Information Center
Emergency phone:
(800) 222-1222
TDD/TTY:
(516) 924-8811 (Suffolk)
TDD/TTY:
(516) 747-3323 (Nassau)

New York City Poison Control Center
Emergency phone:
(800) 222-1222
TDD/TTY:
(212) 689-9014

Western New York Poison Center
Emergency phone:
(800) 222-1222

NORTH CAROLINA

Carolinas Poison Center
Emergency phone:
(800) 222-1222

NORTH DAKOTA

Hennepin Regional Poison Center
Emergency phone:
(800) 222-1222
TDD/TTY:
(800) 222-1222
TDD/TTY:
(612) 904-4691

OHIO

Central Ohio Poison Center
Emergency phone:
(800) 222-1222
TDD/TTY:
(614) 228-2272

Cincinnati Drug & Poison Information Center
Emergency phone:
(800) 222-1222
TDD/TTY:
(800) 253-7955

Greater Cleveland Poison Control Center
Emergency phone:
(800) 222-1222

OKLAHOMA

Oklahoma Poison Control Center
Emergency phone:
(800) 222-1222
TDD/TTY:
(405) 271-1122

OREGON

Oregon Poison Center
Emergency phone:
(800) 222-1222

PENNSYLVANIA

Penn State Poison Center
Emergency phone:
(800) 222-1222
TDD/TTY:
(717) 531-8335

Pittsburgh Poison Center
Emergency phone:
(800) 222-1222

The Poison Control Center
Emergency phone:
(800) 222-1222
TDD/TTY:
(215) 590-8789

PUERTO RICO

San Jorge Children's Hospital
  Poison Center
Emergency phone:
  (800) 222-1222

RHODE ISLAND

Regional Center for Poison
  Control and Prevention
  Serving Massachusetts
  and Rhode Island
Emergency phone:
  (800) 222-1222
TDD/TTY:
  (888) 244-5313

SOUTH CAROLINA

Palmetto Poison Center
Emergency phone:
  (800) 222-1222

SOUTH DAKOTA

Hennepin Regional Poison
  Center
Emergency phone:
  (800) 222-1222
TDD/TTY:
  (800) 222-1222
TDD/TTY:
  (612) 904-4691

TENNESSEE

Middle Tennessee Poison
  Center
Emergency phone:
  (800) 222-1222
TDD/TTY:
  (615) 936-2047

Southern Poison Center
Emergency phone:
  (800) 222-1222

TEXAS

Central Texas Poison Center
Emergency phone:
  (800) 222-1222

North Texas Poison Center
Emergency phone:
  (800) 222-1222

Southeast Texas Poison Center
Emergency phone:
  (800) 222-1222

South Texas Poison Center
Emergency phone:
  (800) 222-1222

Texas Panhandle Poison
  Center
Emergency phone:
  (800) 222-1222

West Texas Regional Poison
  Center
Emergency phone:
  (800) 222-1222

UTAH

Utah Poison Control Center
Emergency phone:
  (800) 222-1222

VERMONT

Northern New England
  Poison Center
Emergency phone:
  (800) 222-1222
TDD/TTY:
  (877) 299-4447
TDD/TTY:
  (207) 871-2879
  (Maine only)

VIRGINIA

Blue Ridge Poison Center
Emergency phone:
(800) 222-1222

National Capital Poison Center
Emergency phone:
(800) 222-1222
TDD/TTY:
(800) 222-1222

Virginia Poison Center
Emergency phone:
(800) 222-1222

WASHINGTON

Washington Poison Center
Emergency phone:
(800) 222-1222
TDD/TTY:
(206) 517-2394
TDD/TTY:
(800) 572-0638
(Washington only)

WEST VIRGINIA

West Virginia Poison Center
Emergency phone:
(800) 222-1222
TDD/TTY:
(304) 388-9698

WISCONSIN

Children's Hospital of
Wisconsin Poison Center
Emergency phone:
(800) 222-1222
TDD/TTY:
(414) 266-2542

WYOMING

The Poison Center
Emergency phone:
(800) 222-1222

ANIMAL POISON CONTROL CENTER

American Society for the
Prevention of Cruelty to
Animals
Emergency phone:
(888) 426-4435

APPENDIX D
Drug/Herb Interactions

The table that follows lists known drug/herb interactions for herbs included in this handbook. The pharmaceuticals and drug classes that are known to interact with herbal products are listed in the first column in alphabetical order, beside the names of the herbs with which they interact.

The reader should not assume that an herbal product not included here may be taken safely with a given drug or class of drugs. Research into herbal products is changing constantly, and new interactions are becoming known every day. Caution is always necessary when using herbal products, particularly when the client is taking them concurrently with pharmaceuticals.

Drug/Drug Classes	Herb	Interaction
ACE inhibitors	Pill-bearing spurge	May ↑ hypotension, do not use concurrently
ACE inhibitors	Pineapple	May antagonize ACE inhibitor actions, do not use concurrently
ACE inhibitors	Yohimbe	May ↓ or block actions of these drugs, do not use concurrently
ACE inhibitors	St. John's wort	May lead to severe photosensitivity, do not use concurrently
Acetazolamide	Quinine	When used with acetazolamide may lead to toxicity, do not use concurrently
Adenosine	Guarana	May ↓ the adenosine response
Alcohol	Betel palm	↑ effects of alcohol
Alcohol	Catnip	May enhance the effects of alcohol
Alcohol	Chamomile	May ↑ the effects of alcohol
Alcohol	Clary	↑ the action of alcohol
Alcohol	Corkwood	May ↑ anticholinergic effect
Alcohol	Goldenseal	May ↑ the effects of alcohol
Alcohol	Hops	↑ CNS effects

Continued

Drug/Drug Classes	Herb	Interaction
Alcohol	Jamaican dogwood	↑ effects of alcohol, do not use concurrently
Alcohol	St. John's wort	May ↑ MAO inhibition, do not use concurrently
Alcohol	Lavender	↑ sedation when used with lavender, do not use concurrently
All medications	Fenugreek	May cause reduced absorption of all medications used concurrently
All medications	Glucomanan	May ↓ the absorption of all medications if taken concurrently; separate dosages by at least 2 hours
All medications	Kaolin	↓ absorption of all drugs
All medications	Karaya gum	↓ absorption of all drugs
All medications	Pectin	↓ absorption of all drugs, vitamins, and minerals if taken concurrently
All oral medications	Flax	Absorption may ↓ if taken concurrently
All oral medications	Ginger	May ↑ absorption of all medications taken orally
All oral medications	Guar gum	May ↓ the absorption of all oral medications
All oral medications	Marshmallow	May ↓ absorption of oral medications, do not use concurrently
All oral medications	Mullein	May ↓ absorption of oral medications
Alpha-adrenergic blockers	Yohimbe	May result in ↑ toxicity, do not use concurrently
Alpha-adrenergic blockers	Butcher's broom	May ↓ action of alpha-adrenergic blockers
Alpha-adrenergic blockers	Capsicum peppers	May ↓ the action of alpha-adrenergic blockers
Aluminium salts	Quinine	May cause ↓ absorption of quinine
Amantadine	Jimsonweed	↑ antocholinergic effects
Amphetamines	Eucalyptus	May ↓ the effectiveness of amphetamines
Amphetamines	Rauwolfia	May cause ↓ pressor effects, do not use concurrently

Drug/Drug Classes	Herb	Interaction
Amphetamines	St. John's wort	May cause serotonin syndrome
Amphetamines	Khat	↑ action
Analgesics	Cola tree	May ↑ the effect of analgesics
Anesthetics	Ephedra	Causes ↑ arrhythmias when used with halothane anesthetics
Antacids	Jimsonweed	↓ action of jimsonweed
Antacids	Buckthorn	May ↓ the action of buckthorn if taken within 1 hour of the herb
Antacids	Cascara sagrada	May ↓ the action of cascara if taken within 1 hour of the herb
Antacids	Castor	To prevent decreased absorption of castor, do not take within 1 hour of antacids
Antacids	Chinese rhubarb	May ↓ the effectiveness of Chinese rhubarb if taken within 1 hour of the herb
Antacids	Green tea	May ↓ the therapeutic effects of green tea
Antianginals	Blue cohosh	May ↓ the action of antianginals, causing chest pain
Antianxiety agents	Cowslip	May ↑ the effect of antianxiety agents
Antiarrhythmics	Buckthorn	Chronic buckthorn use can cause hypokalemia and enhance the effects of antiarrhythmics
Antiarrhythmics	Khat	↑ action
Antiarrhythmics	Broom	May ↑ the effect of antiarrhythmics
Antiarrhythmics	Cascara sagrada	Chronic cascara use can cause hypokalemia and enhance the effects of antiarrhythmics
Antiarrhythmics	Chinese rhubarb	Chronic use of Chinese rhubarb can cause hypokalemia and enhance the effects of antiarrhythmics
Antiarrhythmics	Figwort	May ↑ the effects of antiarrhythmics

Continued

Drug/Drug Classes	Herb	Interaction
Antiarrhythmics	Fumitory	May ↑ the effects of antiarrhythmics
Antiarrhythmics	Goldenseal	May ↑ the effects of antiarrhythmics
Antiarrhythmics	Horehound	↑ serotonin effect, do not use concurrently
Antiarrhythmics	Licorice	↑ cardiac effects of antiarrhythmics, do not use concurrently
Antiarrhythmics	Aconite	↑ toxicity
Antibiotics	Acidophilus	Do not use concurrently
Anticholinergics	Jaborandi tree	When taken internally may ↓ effects of anticholinergics
Anticholinergics	Butterbur	May enhance the effects of anticholinergics
Anticholinergics	Jimsonweed	↑ effects of anticholinergics
Anticholinergics	Pill-bearing spurge	May ↓ effects of anticholinergic, do not use concurrently
Anticoagulants	Agrimony	May ↓ clotting times
Anticoagulants	Alfalfa	May prolong bleeding
Anticoagulants	Angelica	May prolong bleeding
Anticoagulants	Bilberry	May ↑ action of anticoagulants
Anticoagulants	Black haw	↑ the action of anticoagulants
Anticoagulants	Bogbean	May ↑ risk of bleeding
Anticoagulants	Buchu	Can ↑ the action of anticoagulants, causing bleeding
Anticoagulants	Chamomile	May interfere with the actions of anticoagulants
Anticoagulants	Chondroitin	Can cause ↑ bleeding
Anticoagulants	Coenzyme q10	May ↓ the action of anticoagulants
Anticoagulants	Fenugreek	Risk of ↑ bleeding when used concurrently
Anticoagulants	Feverfew	May ↑ anticoagulant effects
Anticoagulants	Garlic	May ↑ bleeding when used concurrently
Anticoagulants	Ginger	May ↑ risk of bleeding when taken concurrently
Anticoagulants	Ginkgo	↑ risk of bleeding
Anticoagulants	Ginseng	May ↓ the action of anticoagulants

Drug/Drug Classes	Herb	Interaction
Anticoagulants	Goldenseal	May ↓ the effects of anticoagulants
Anticoagulants	Horse chestnut	↑ risk of severe bleeding, do not use concurrently
Anticoagulants	Irish moss	↑ effects of anticoagulants, do not use concurrently
Anticoagulants	Kelp	May pose ↑ risk of bleeding, do not use concurrently
Anticoagulants	Kelpware	May pose ↑ risk of bleeding, do not use concurrently
Anticoagulants	Khella	↑ risk of bleeding when used with anticoagulants, do not use concurrently
Anticoagulants	Lovage	May ↑ effects of anti-coagulants, do not use concurrently
Anticoagulants	Lungwort	May ↑ effects of anti-coagulants, do not use concurrently
Anticoagulants	Lysine	Use of large amounts of lysine causes ↑ aminoglyco-side toxicity, do not use concurrently
Anticoagulants	Meadowsweet	May ↑ risk of bleeding, do not use concurrently
Anticoagulants	Motherwort	May cause ↑ risk of bleeding, do not use concurrently
Anticoagulants	Mugwort	May cause ↑ risk of bleeding, do not use concurrently
Anticoagulants	Nettle	May ↓ effect of anti-coagulants, do not use concurrently
Anticoagulants	Parsley	Large amounts may interfere with anticoagulation therapy
Anticoagulants	Pau d'arco	May result in ↑ risk of bleeding, do not use concurrently
Anticoagulants	Pill-bearing spurge	May ↑ effects of anti-coagulants, do not use concurrently

Continued

Drug/Drug Classes	Herb	Interaction
Anticoagulants	Pineapple	May ↑ bleeding time when used with anticoagulants, do not use concurrently
Anticoagulants	Poplar	May ↑ bleeding time when used with anticoagulants, do not use concurrently
Anticoagulants	Prickly ash	May ↑ bleeding time when used with anticoagulants, do not use concurrently
Anticoagulants	Quinine	May ↑ action of anticoagulants, do not use concurrently
Anticoagulants	Safflower	May potentiate anticoagulant action, do not use concurrently
Anticoagulants	Saw palmetto	May potentiate anticoagulant effect of salicylants, do not use concurrently
Anticoagulants	Senega	May ↑ bleeding time, do not use concurrently
Anticoagulants	Tonka bean	May result in ↑ risk of bleeding, do not use concurrently
Anticoagulants	Turmeric	May result in ↑ risk of bleeding, do not use concurrently
Anticoagulants	Wintergreen	May cause ↑ risk of bleeding, do not use concurrently
Anticoagulants	Yarrow	May result in ↑ risk of bleeding, do not use concurrently
Anticoagulants, oral	Dong quai	May ↑ the effects of oral anticoagulants
Anticonvulsants	Ginkgo	May ↓ the anticonvulsant effect
Anticonvulsants	Ginseng	May provide an additive anticonvulsant action when taken concurrently
Anticonvulsants	Sage	May ↓ action of anticonvulsants, do not use concurrently
Antidepressants	Hops	↑ CNS effects

Drug/Drug Classes	Herb	Interaction
Antidepressants	Sam-e	Combining with antidepressants may lead to serotonin syndrome, do not use concurrently
Antidepressants	St. John's wort	Combined with these drugs may lead to severe photosensitivity, do not use concurrently
Antidiabetics	Alfalfa	May potentiate hypoglycemic action
Antidiabetics	Aloe	When taken internally may ↑ effects of antidiabetics
Antidiabetics	Blue cohosh	May ↓ the action of antidiabetics
Antidiabetics	Burdock	↑ hypoglycemic effect can occur
Antidiabetics	Elecampane	May ↓ blood glucose
Antidiabetics	Ephedra	May ↑ blood glucose
Antidiabetics	Eyebright	May ↑ the effects of antidiabetics when taken internally
Antidiabetics	Glucosamine	May ↑ the hypoglycemic effects of oral antidiabetics
Antidiabetics	Goat's rue	May ↑ the hypoglycemic effects of oral antidiabetics
Antidiabetics	Gotu kola	May ↓ the effectiveness of antidiabetics
Antidiabetics	Horehound	Enhance hypoglycemia, do not use concurrently
Antidiabetics	Horse chestnut	↑ hypoglycemic effects
Antidiabetics	Jambul	↑ effects of antidiabetics, do not use concurrently
Antidiabetics	Myrrh	May cause ↑ hypoglycemic effects, do not use concurrently
Antidiabetics	Myrtle	May cause ↑ hypoglycemic effects, do not use concurrently
Antidiabetics	Senega	May ↓ effects of antidiabetics, do not use concurrently
Antidiabetics	Raspberry	May ↑ hypoglycemia, monitor blood glucose levels
Antidiabetics	Siberian ginseng	May ↑ levels of antidiabetics, do not use concurrently
Antidiabetics, oral	Bay	May ↑ hypoglycemic effects

Continued

Drug/Drug Classes	Herb	Interaction
Antidiabetics, oral	Bee pollen	↓ effectiveness of antidiabetics, ↑ hyperglycemia
Antidiabetics, oral	Bilberry	May ↑ hypoglycemia
Antidiabetics, oral	Coenzyme q10	Oral antidiabetics may ↓ the action of coenzyme Q10 and deplete endogenous stores
Antidiabetics, oral	Coriander	May ↑ the effects of oral antidiabetics
Antidiabetics, oral	Dandelion	May ↑ the effects of oral antidiabetics
Antidiabetics, oral	Eucalyptus	May alter the effectiveness of antidiabetics
Antidiabetics, oral	Fenugreek	Hypoglycemial is possible when used concurrently
Antidiabetics, oral	Garlic	Because of hypoglycemic effects of garlic, oral antidiabetic dosages may need to be adjusted
Antidiabetics, oral	Ginseng	May ↑ the hypoglycemic effects of oral antidiabetics
Antidiabetics, oral	Glucomanan	May ↑ the hypoglycemic effects of oral antidiabetics
Antidiabetics, oral	Gymnema	May ↑ the action of oral antidiabetics
Antidiarrheals	Nutmeg	May be potentiated, monitor for constipation
Antidysrhythmics	Aloe	When taken internally may ↑ effects of antidysrhythmics
Antidysrhythmics	Coltsfoot	May antagonize antidysrhythmics
Antidysrhythmics	Devil's claw	Use cautiously because of possible inotropic and chronotropic effects
Antifungals	Gossypol	Concurrent use may cause nephrotoxicity
Antifungals, azole	Goldenseal	May slow the metabolism of azole antifungals
Antifungals, azole	Licorice	May ↑ levels of azole antifungals, do not use concurrently
Antiglaucoma agents	Betel palm	↓ effects of antiglaucoma agents

Drug/Drug Classes	Herb	Interaction
Antihistamines	Lavender	↑ sedation when used with lavender, do not use concurrently
Antihistamines	Khat	↑ action
Antihistamines	Corkwood	May ↑ anticholinergic effect
Antihistamines	Hops	↑ CNS effects
Antihistamines	Jamaican dogwood	May produce ↑ effect, do not use concurrently
Antihypertensives	Khat	↑ action
Antihypertensives	Aconite	↑ toxicity
Antihypertensives	Astragalus	May ↑ or ↓ action of antihypertensives
Antihypertensives	Barberry	May ↑ antihypertensive action
Antihypertensives	Betony	May ↑ action of antihypertensives
Antihypertensives	Black cohosh	↑ action of antihypertensives
Antihypertensives	Blood root	May ↑ hypotensive effects
Antihypertensives	Blue cohosh	↓ the action of antihypertensives and ↑ blood pressure
Antihypertensives	Broom	May ↑ the effect of antihypertensives
Antihypertensives	Burdock	May ↑ hypotensive effects
Antihypertensives	Cat's claw	May ↑ the hypotensive effects of antihypertensives
Antihypertensives	Coltsfoot	May antagonize antihypertensives
Antihypertensives	Dandelion	May ↑ the effects of antihypertensives
Antihypertensives	Goldenseal	May ↑ the effects of antihypertensives
Antihypertensives	Guarana	May ↓ the effects of antihypertensives
Antihypertensives	Hawthorn	May ↑ hypotension when used concurrently
Antihypertensives	Irish moss	↑ effects of antihypertensives, do not use concurrently
Antihypertensives	Jamaican dogwood	↑ effects of antihypertensive, do not use concurrently
Antihypertensives	Kelp	↑ hypotensive effects, do not use concurrently
Antihypertensives	Khella	↑ hypotension when used with antihypertensives, do not use concurrently

Continued

Drug/Drug Classes	Herb	Interaction
Antihypertensives	Licorice	May cause ↑ hypokalemia, do not use concurrently
Antihypertensives	Mistletoe	May cause ↑ hypotensive effect of antihypertensives, do not use concurrently
Antihypertensives	Queen Anne's lace	↑ hypotension when used with antihypertensives, use together cautiously
Antihypertensives	Rue	May cause ↑ vasodilation, do not use concurrently
Antihypertensives	Yarrow	May result in ↑ hypotension, do not use concurrently
Antilipidemics	Glucomanan	May ↑ the action of antilipidemics
Antilipidemics	Gotu kola	May ↓ the effectiveness of antilipidemics
Antimigraine agents	Butterbur	May enhance the effects of antimigraine agents
Antineoplastics	Yew	May cause ↑ myelosuppression, do not use concurrently
Antiparkinson agents	Kava	↑ symptoms of parkinsonism, do not use concurrently
Antiplatelet agents	Bilberry	May cause antiaggregation of platelets
Antiplatelet agents	Bogbean	May ↑ risk of bleeding
Antiplatelet agents	Dong quai	May ↑ the effects of antiplatelet agents
Antiplatelet agents	Feverfew	May ↑ the action of antiplatelet agents
Antiplatelet agents	Ginger	May ↑ risk of bleeding when taken concurrently
Antiplatelet agents	Saw palmetto	May lead to ↑ bleeding, do not use concurrently
Antiplatelet agents	Ginkgo	↑ risk of bleeding
Antipsychotics	Hops	↑ CNS effects
Antipsychotics	Kava	May result in neuroleptic disorder
Antiretrovirals	St. John's wort	When taken PO in combination with indinavir may ↓ the antiretroviral action.
Ascorbic acid	Chromium	Both chromium and ascorbic acid absorption ↑ when taken concurrently

Drug/Drug Classes	Herb	Interaction
Aspirin	Bilberry	May ↑ the anticoagulation action of aspirin
Aspirin	Bogbean	May ↑ risk of bleeding
Aspirin	Horse chestnut	↑ risk of severe bleeding, do not use concurrently
Atropine	Black root	Forms an insoluble complex with atropine; do not use concurrently
Barbiturates	Eucalyptus	May ↓ the effectiveness of barbiturates
Barbiturates	Jamaican dogwood	↑ effects of barbiturates, do not use concurrently
Barbiturates	Kava	↑ sedation
Barbiturates	Pill-bearing spurge	May ↑ effects of barbiturates, do not use concurrently
Barbiturates	Lemon balm	May potentiate the sedative effects of bariturates
Belladonna alkaloids	Mayapple	May ↓ laxative effects of mayapple, do not use concurrently
Benzodiazepines	Coffee	↓ the effect of benzodiazepines
Benzodiazepines	Cola tree	May ↓ the effect of cola tree products
Benzodiazepines	Goldenseal	May slow the metabolism of benzodiazepines
Benzodiazepines	Kava	↑ sedation and coma, do not use concurrently
Benzodiazepines	Melatonin	May ↑ anxiolytic effects of benzodiazepines, use cautiously
Beta-blockers	Betel palm	↑ action of beta-blockers
Beta-blockers	Butterbur	May enhance the effects of beta-blockers
Beta-blockers	Coenzyme q10	Beta-blockers may ↓ the action of coenzyme Q10 and deplete endogenous stores
Beta-blockers	Coffee	Caffeine in coffee ↑ blood pressure in those taking beta-blockers
Beta-blockers	Cola tree	May ↑ blood pressure when used with beta-blockers

Continued

Drug/Drug Classes	Herb	Interaction
Beta-blockers	Ephedra	Causes ↑ hypertension when used with beta-blockers
Beta-blockers	Figwort	May ↑ the effects of beta-blockers
Beta-blockers	Fumitory	May ↑ the effects of beta-blockers
Beta-blockers	Goldenseal	May ↑ the effects of beta-blockers
Beta-blockers	Guarana	May ↑ the effects of beta-blockers
Beta-blockers	Jaborandi tree	When used internally may ↑ adverse cardiovascular reactions, do not use concurrently
Beta-blockers	Khat	↑ action
Beta-blockers	Lily of the valley	May ↑ effects, do not use concurrently
Beta-blockers	Motherwort	May cause ↓ heart rate, do not use concurrently
Bethanechol	Jaborandi tree	When used internally, cholinergic effects ↑
Bronchodilators	Coffee	Large amounts of coffee may ↑ the action of some bronchodilators
Bronchodilators	Green tea	Large amounts of green tea ↑ the action of some bronchodilators
Bronchodilators	Guarana	May ↑ the action of bronchodilators
Caffeine	Creatine	May ↓ the effects of creatine
Calcitonin	Yellow dock	May cause ↑ hypocalcemia, do not use concurrently
Calcium supplements	Shark cartilage	May lead to ↑ calcium levels
Calcium-channel blockers	Khat	↑ action
Calcium-channel blockers	Lily of the valley	May ↑ effects, do not use concurrently
Calcium-channel blockers	Burdock	May ↑ hypotensive effects
Calcium-channel blockers	Goldenseal	May slow the metabolism of calcium-channel blockers

Drug/Drug Classes	Herb	Interaction
Calcium-channel blockers	Khella	↑ hypotension when used with calcium-channel blockers, do not use concurrently
Calcium-channel blockers	Barberry	May ↑ effect of calcium-channel blockers
Calcium-channel blockers	Betel palm	↑ action of calcium-channel blockers
Carbamazepine	Plantain	May ↓ effects of carbamazepine, do not use concurrently
Carbidopa	Octacosanol	May cause dyskinesia when used with carbidopa/levodopa, do not use concurrently
Cardiac agents	Squill	May ↑ effect of cardiac agents, causing life-threatening toxicity, do not use concurrently
Cardiac agents	Plantain	May ↑ effect of cardiac agents, do not use concurrently
Cardiac agents	Rauwolfia	May result in ↑ hypotension, do not use concurrently
Cardiac glycosides	Khat	↑ action
Cardiac glycosides	Lily of the valley	May ↑ effects, do not use concurrently
Cardiac glycosides	Aconite	↑ toxicity
Cardiac glycosides	Aloe	When taken internally may ↑ effects of cardiac glycosides
Cardiac glycosides	Betel palm	↑ action of cardiac glycosides
Cardiac glycosides	Beth root	May ↓ effects of cardiac glycosides
Cardiac glycosides	Black root	Forms an insoluble complex with cardiac glycosides; do not use concurrently
Cardiac glycosides	Broom	May ↑ the effect of cardiac glycosides
Cardiac glycosides	Buckthorn	Chronic buckthorn use can cause hypokalemia and enhance the effects of cardiac glycosides

Continued

Drug/Drug Classes	Herb	Interaction
Cardiac glycosides	Cascara sagrada	Chronic cascara use can cause hypokalemia and enhance the effects of cardiac glycosides
Cardiac glycosides	Chinese rhubarb	Chronic use of Chinese rhubarb can cause hypokalemia and enhance the effects of cardiac glycosides
Cardiac glycosides	Condurango	Absorption of digitoxin and digoxin may be ↓ when taken concurrently
Cardiac glycosides	Figwort	May ↑ the action of figwort
Cardiac glycosides	Fumitory	May ↑ the effects of cardiac glycosides
Cardiac glycosides	Goldenseal	May ↓ the effects of cardiac glycosides
Cardiac glycosides	Hawthorn	May ↑ the effects of cardiac glycosides
Cardiac glycosides	Horsetail	↑ toxicity and ↑ hypokalemia
Cardiac glycosides	Licorice	May cause ↑ toxicity and ↑ hypokalemia, do not use concurrently.
Cardiac glycosides	Mistletoe	May cause ↓ cardiac function, do not use concurrently
Cardiac glycosides	Motherwort	May cause ↓ heart rate, do not use concurrently
Cardiac glycosides	Night-blooming cereus	May ↑ actions of cardiac glycosides, do not use concurrently
Cardiac glycosides	Oleander	May cause fatal digitalis toxicity, do not use concurrently
Cardiac glycosides	Queen anne's lace	May ↑ cardiac depression, do not use concurrently
Cardiac glycosides	Quinine	May ↑ action of cardiac glycosides, do not use concurrently
Cardiac glycosides	Rauwolfia	Will cause severe bradycardia, do not use together
Cardiac glycosides	Rue	May cause ↑ inotropic effects, do not use concurrently
Cardiac glycosides	Senna	Chronic use may potentiate cardiac glycosides

Drug/Drug Classes	Herb	Interaction
Cardiac glycosides	Siberian ginseng	May ↑ levels of cardiac glycosides, do not use concurrently
Cardiac medications	Kudzu	Enhance effects of cardiac medications, do not use concurrently
Central nervous system depressants	Yarrow	May cause ↑ sedation, do not use concurrently
Central nervous system depressants	Goldenseal	May ↑ the effects of central nervous system depressants
Central nervous system depressants	Hawthorn	May ↑ the sedative effects of central nervous system depressants
Central nervous system depressants	Kava	↑ sedation, do not use concurrently
Central nervous system depressants	Mistletoe	May cause ↑ sedation, do not use concurrently
Central nervous system depressants	Passion flower	May cause ↑ sedation, do not use concurrently
Central nervous system depressants	Peyote	May ↑ effect of other CNS drugs, do not use concurrently
Central nervous system depressants	Hops	↑ CNS effects
Central nervous system depressants	Lemon balm	May potentiate the sedative effects of CNS depressants
Central nervous system depressants	Rauwolfia	May cause ↑ CNS depression, do not use concurrently
Central nervous system depressants	Skullcap	May potentiate sedation of CNS depressants, do not use concurrently
Central nervous system depressants	Senega	May cause ↑ CNS effects, do not use concurrently
Central nervous system depressants	Valerian	May ↑ effects of CNS depressants, do not use concurrently
Central nervous system depressants	Poppy	↑ CNS depression when use with CNS depressants, do not use concurrently
Central nervous system depressants	Nettle	May lead to ↑ CNS depression

Continued

Drug/Drug Classes	Herb	Interaction
Central nervous system depressants	Pokeweed	May ↑ action of CNS depressants, do not use concurrently
Central nervous system depressants	Yerba mate	May produce antagonistic effect, do not use concurrently
Central nervous system depressants	Queen Anne's lace	↑ action of CNS depressants, use together cautiously
Central nervous system stimulants	Squill	May ↑ effects of CNS stimulants, do not use concurrently
Central nervous system stimulants	Yerba mate	May ↑ effects CNS stimulants, use together cautiously
Central nervous system stimulants	Yohimbe	May result in ↑ CNS stimulation, do not use concurrently
Cerebral stimulants	Horsetail	↑ CNS effects, do not use concurrently
Cerebral stimulants	Melatonin	May have a synergistic effect and exacerbate insomnia, do not use concurrently
Cholinergics, ophthalmic	Jaborandi tree	When used internally cholinergic effects ↑
Cholinesterase inhibitors	Pill-bearing spurge	May ↑ effects of cholinesterase inhibitors
Ciprofloxacin	Fennel	Affects the absorption, distribution, and elimination of ciprofloxacin; dosages should be separated by at least 2 hours
Clonidine	Capsicum peppers	May ↓ the antihypertensive effects of clonidine
Contraceptives, oral	Alfalfa	May alter action
Contraceptives, oral	Black cohosh	May ↑ effects
Contraceptives, oral	Chaste tree	May interfere with the action of oral contraceptives
Contraceptives, oral	St. John's wort	When combined with oral contraceptives, may lead to severe photosensitivity, do not use concurrently
Corticosteroids	Buckthorn	Hypokalemia can result from use of buckthorn with corticosteroids

Drug/Drug Classes	Herb	Interaction
Corticosteroids	Cascara sagrada	Hypokalemia may result from concurrent use
Corticosteroids	Chinese rhubarb	Chronic use of Chinese rhubarb can cause hypokalemia and enhance the effects of corticosteroids
Corticosteroids	Licorice	May ↑ effects of corticosteroids, do not use concurrently
Corticosteroids	Perilla	May augment the effects of corticosteroids, do not use concurrently
CYP2A6, drugs metabolized by	Condurango	Use condurango with caution
CYP3A4, drugs metabolized by	Wild cherry	May slow metabolism, do not use concurrently
CYP450, drugs metabolized by	Myrtle	Do not use concurrently
CYP450, drugs metabolized by	Pennyroyal	Do not use concurrently with drugs metabolized by CYP450
CYP450, drugs metabolized by	Hops	↓ CYP450 levels
CYP450, drugs metabolized by	Milk thistle	Should not be used together
CYP450, drugs metabolized by	Black pepper	Avoid concurrent use
CYP450, drugs metabolized by	Condurango	Use condurango with caution, especially in clients with hepatic disorders
Decongestants	Khat	↑ action
Dhea	Melatonin	May ↓ cytokine production, do not use concurrently
Disulfiram	Pill-bearing spurge	Do not use concurrently
Disulfiram	Senna	Do not use with disulfiram
Diuretics	Yellow dock	May cause ↑ hypocalcemia, do not use concurrently
Diuretics	Bearberry	Concurrent use may lead to electrolyte loss, primarily hypokalemia
Diuretics	Cucumber	May ↑ the diuretic effect of other diuretics

Continued

Drug/Drug Classes	Herb	Interaction
Diuretics	Dandelion	May ↑ diuresis, leading to fluid loss and electrolyte imbalances
Diuretics	Gossypol	Concurrent use may cause severe hypokalemia
Diuretics	Horsetail	↑ effects of diuretics, do not use concurrently
Diuretics	Khella	↑ hypotension when used with diuretics, do not use concurrently
Diuretics	Licorice	May cause ↑ hypokalemia, do not use concurrently
Diuretics	Nettle	May ↑ effects of diuretics, resulting in dehydration and hypokalemia, do not use concurrently
Diuretics	Queen Anne's lace	↑ hypotension, use together cautiously
Diuretics	Yerba mate	May ↑ effects of diuretics, do not use concurrently
Diuretics, loop	St. John's wort	May lead to severe photosensitivity, do not use concurrently
Diuretics, loop	Aloe	When taken internally may ↑ effects of loop diuretics
Diuretics, thiazide	St. John's wort	May lead to severe photosensitivity, do not use concurrently
Diuretics, thiazide	Aloe	When taken internally may ↑ effects of thiazide diuretics
Diuretics, thiazide	Buckthorn	Hypokalemia can result from use of buckthorn with thiazide diuretics
Diuretics, thiazide	Cascara sagrada	Hypokalemia may result from concurrent use
Diuretics, thiazide	Chinese rhubarb	Chronic use of Chinese rhubarb can cause hypokalemia and enhance the effects of thiazide diuretics
Econazole vaginal cream	Echinacea	May ↓ the action of this cream
Electrolyte solutions	Agar	↑ dehydration

Drug/Drug Classes	Herb	Interaction
Emetics	Horehound	Granisetron and ondansetron ↑ serotonin effect, do not use concurrently
Ephedrine	Rauwolfia	May cause ↓ pressor effects, do not use concurrently
Epinephrine	Rauwolfia	May cause ↓ pressor effects, do not use concurrently
Ergots	Horehound	↑ serotonin effect, do not use concurrently
Estrogens	Alfalfa	May alter action
Estrogens	Hops	↑ hormonal levels
Furoquinolones	Cola tree	May ↑ the effect of cola tree products
Glucocorticoids	Squill	May ↑ effects of glucocorticoids, do not use concurrently
Glucose	Creatine	May ↑ the storage of creatine in muscle tissue
Guanethidine	Ephedra	May ↓ the effect of guanethidine
Hepatotoxic agents	Black root	Avoid concurrent use
HMG-coa reductase inhibitors	Coenzyme Q10	HMG-coa reductase inhibitors may ↓ the action of coenzyme Q10 and deplete endogenous stores
Hormone replacement therapy	Black cohosh	May alter the effects of other hormone replacement therapies
Hormone replacement therapy	Dhea	DHEA may interfere with estrogen and androgen therapy
Hormones	Saw palmetto	May antagonize hormone therapy, do not use concurrently
Hormones (animal)	Cat's claw	May interact with hormones made from animal products
Hypnotics	Clary	↑ the action of hypnotics
Hypoglycemics, oral	Bitter melon	May ↑ effects of oral hypoglycemics
Immune serum	Safflower	May cause ↑ immunosuppression, do not use concurrently

Continued

Drug/Drug Classes	Herb	Interaction
Immunomodulators	Echinacea	May ↓ the effects of immunosuppressants; should not be used immediately before, during, or after transplant surgery
Immunostimulants	Cat's claw	Do not use concurrently
Immunosuppressants	Ginseng	May diminish the effect of immunosuppressants; do not use before, during, or after transplant surgery
Immunosuppressants	Schisandra	May ↓ effectiveness of immunosuppressants, avoid use before, during, or after transplant surgery
Immunosuppressants	Safflower	May cause ↑ immunosuppression, do not use concurrently
Immunosuppressants	Mistletoe	May stimulate immunity, do not use concurrently
Immunosuppressants	St. John's wort	Rejection of transplanted hearts has occurred when taken PO with cyclosporine. Other immunosuppressants may have same interaction in this and other transplants
Immunosuppressants	Saw palmetto	May ↑ or ↓ immunostimulant effects, do not use concurrently
Immunosuppressants	Skullcap	May ↓ effects of immunosuppressants, do not use concurrently
Immunosuppressants	Turmeric	May ↓ effectiveness of immunosuppressants, do not use concurrently
Immunosuppressants	Maitake	May ↓ effects of immunosuppressants, do not use immediately before, during, or after transplant surgery.
Insulin	Basil	May ↑ hypoglycemic effects
Insulin	Bay	May ↑ hypoglycemic effects
Insulin	Bee pollen	↓ effectiveness of insulin, ↑ hyperglycemia

Drug/Drug Classes	Herb	Interaction
Insulin	Bilberry	May significantly ↓ blood sugar levels—monitor carefully
Insulin	Cat's claw	May interact with insulin
Insulin	Dandelion	May ↑ the effects of insulin
Insulin	Eucalyptus	May alter the effectiveness of insulin
Insulin	Garlic	Because of hypoglycemic effects of garlic, insulin dosages may need to be adjusted
Insulin	Ginseng	May ↑ the hypoglycemic effects of insulin
Insulin	Glucomanan	May ↑ the hypoglycemic effects of insulin
Insulin	Guar gum	May delay glucose absorption when used concurrently; insulin dose may need to be decreased
Insulin	Gymnema	May ↑ the action of insulin
Interferon	Astragalus	May prevent or shorten upper respiratory infections
Interleukin-2	Astragalus	May ↑ or ↓ effect of drugs such as interleukin-2
Ipecac	Mayapple	May ↓ laxative effects of mayapple, do not use concurrently
Iron salts	Bilberry	Interferes with iron absorption
Iron salts	Chromium	↓ chromium absorption when taken concurrently
Iron salts	Condurango	Iron absorption may be ↓
Iron salts	Ground ivy	May ↓ the absorption of iron salts
Iron salts	Hawthorn	May ↓ the absorption of iron salts; separate dosages by at least 2 hours
Iron salts	Hops	↓ absorption of iron salts
Iron salts	Horehound	↓ absorption of iron salts
Iron salts	Horse chestnut	↓ absorption of iron salts
Iron salts	Lady's mantle	↓ absorption of iron salts
Iron salts	Lavender	↓ absorption of iron salts
Iron salts	Lemon balm	↓ absorption of iron salts

Continued

Drug/Drug Classes	Herb	Interaction
Iron salts	Marshmallow	May ↓ absorption of iron salts
Iron salts	Meadowsweet	May ↓ absorption of iron salts
Iron salts	Mistletoe	May ↓ absorption of iron salts
Iron salts	Motherwort	May ↓ absorption of iron salts
Iron salts	Nettle	May interfere with absorption of iron salts
Iron salts	Oak	May ↓ absorption of iron salts
Iron salts	Plantain	May ↓ absorption of iron salts
Iron salts	Poplar	May ↓ absorption of iron salts
Iron salts	Prickly ash	May ↓ absorption of iron salts
Iron salts	Raspberry	May ↓ absorption of iron salts
Iron salts	Sage	May ↓ absorption of iron salts
Iron salts	Slippery elm	May ↓ absorption of iron salts
Iron salts	Squill	May ↓ absorption of iron salts
Iron salts	Valerian	May interfere with absorption of iron salts
Iron salts	Witch hazel	May ↓ absorption of iron salts
Iron salts	Yellow dock	May ↓ absorption of iron salts
Isoproterenol	Rauwolfia	May cause ↓ pressor effects, do not use concurrently
Kanamycin	Siberian ginseng	May ↑ action of kanamycin
Laxatives	Flax	May ↑ the action of laxatives
Laxatives	Senna	Additive effect can occur, do not use concurrently
Laxatives	Squill	May ↑ effects of laxatives, do not use concurrently

Drug/Drug Classes	Herb	Interaction
Levodopa	Octacosanol	May cause dyskinesia when used with carbidopa/levodopa, do not use concurrently
Levodopa	Rauwolfia	↓ effect of levodopa, with ↑ extrapyramidal motor symptoms
Lithium	Coffee	↓ levels of lithium
Lithium	Cola tree	May ↓ the effect of cola tree products
Lithium	Dandelion	Toxicity may occur if used concurrently
Lithium	Goldenrod	May result in dehydration and lithium toxicity
Lithium	Horsetail	Dehydration and lithium toxicity
Lithium	Juniper	Dehydration and lithium toxicity
Lithium	Nettle	May result in dehydration, lithium toxicity
Lithium	Parsley	May lead to dehydration, lithium toxicity
Lithium	Plantain	May ↓ effects of lithium, do not use concurrently
Magnesium	Melatonin	↑ inhibition of N-methyl-D-aspartate receptors, do not use concurrently
Magnesium	Quinine	May cause ↓ absorption of quinine
MAOIs	Khat	↑ action
MAOIs	Betel palm	May ↑ chance of hypertensive crisis
MAOIs	Butcher's broom	May ↑ action of MAOIs and precipitate a hypertensive crisis
MAOIs	Cacao tree	May ↑ the vasopressor effect of MAOIs
MAOIs	Capsicum peppers	May precipitate hypertensive crisis
MAOIs	Coffee	Large amounts of coffee should be avoided; hypertensive actions may occur

Continued

Drug/Drug Classes	Herb	Interaction
MAOIs	Cola tree	May ↑ blood pressure when used with phenelzine and tranylcypromine
MAOIs	Ephedra	Hypertensive crisis can occur when used concurrently
MAOIs	Galanthamine	Hypertensive crisis may occur
MAOIs	Ginkgo	May ↑ action of MAOIs
MAOIs	Ginseng	Concurrent use may result in manic-like syndrome
MAOIs	Green tea	Large amounts of green tea taken concurrently with MAOIs can cause hypertensive crisis
MAOIs	Guarana	Large amounts of guarana taken with MAOIs can result in hypertensive crisis
MAOIs	Jimsonweed	↑ anticholinergic effects
MAOIs	Night-blooming cereus	May ↑ cardiac effects, do not use concurrently
MAOIs	Nutmeg	May be potentiated, do not use concurrently
MAOIs	Parsley	When used with tricyclics or SSRIs may lead to serotonin syndrome, do not use concurrently
MAOIs	Passion flower	May cause ↑ MAOI activity, do not use concurrently
MAOIs	Rauwolfia	May cause excitation and/or hypertension, do not use concurrently
MAOIs	St. John's wort	May ↑ MAO inhibition, do not use concurrently
MAOIs	Valerian	May negate therapeutic effects of MAOIs, do not use concurrently
MAOIs	Yohimbe	May ↑ effects of MAOIs, do not use concurrently
Methyldopa	Capsicum peppers	May ↓ the antihypertensive effects of methyldopa
Minerals	Allspice	May interfere with absorption of minerals
Minerals	Pipsissewa	Should be taken 2 hrs before or after pipsissewa

Drug/Drug Classes	Herb	Interaction
Mithramycin	Yellow dock	May cause ↑ hypocalcemia, do not use concurrently
Morphine	Oats	May ↓ effect of morphine, do not use concurrently
Neuromuscular blockers	Quinine	May ↑ action of neuromuscular blockers, do not use concurrently
Nicotine	Lobelia	↑ effects of nicotine-containing products, do not use concurrently
Nicotine	Oats	May ↓ hypertensive effects of nicotine
Norepinephrine	Rauwolfia	May cause ↓ pressor effects, do not use concurrently
NSAIDs	Bearberry	May ↑ effect of NSAIDs
NSAIDs	Bilberry	May ↑ action of NSAIDs
NSAIDs	Bogbean	May ↑ risk of bleeding
NSAIDs	Chondroitin	Can ↑ bleeding
NSAIDs	Gossypol	Concurrent use may result in gastrointestinal distress and gastrointestinal tissue damage
NSAIDs	St. John's wort	When combined may lead to severe photosensitivity, do not use concurrently
NSAIDs	Turmeric	May result in ↑ risk of bleeding, do not use concurrently
NSAIDs	Saw palmetto	May lead to ↑ bleeding time, do not use concurrently
NSAIDs, topical	Jaborandi tree	Jaborandi tree action ↓ when used with topical NSAIDs, do not use concurrently
Opioids	Lavender	↑ sedation when used with lavender, do not use concurrently
Opioids	Parsley	May cause serotonin syndrome, do not use concurrently
Opioids	Corkwood	May ↑ anticholinergic effect
Opioids	Jamaican dogwood	↑ effects of opioids, do not use concurrently
Oxytocics	Ephedra	Causes severe hypertension when used with oxytocics

Continued

Drug/Drug Classes	Herb	Interaction
Paroxetine	St. John's wort	↑ sedation
Phenothiazines	Coenzyme q10	Some phenothiazines may ↓ the action of coenzyme Q10 and deplete endogenous stores
Phenothiazines	Corkwood	May ↑ anticholinergic effect
Phenothiazines	Ephedra	Tachycardia may result if used concurrently
Phenothiazines	Evening primrose oil	May cause seizures
Phenothiazines	Jimsonweed	↓ action of phenothiazines
Phenothiazines	Yohimbe	May result in ↑ toxicity, do not use concurrently
Phenytoin	Yellow dock	May cause ↑ hypocalcemia, do not use concurrently
Phenytoin	Valerian	May negate therapeutic effects of meds containing phenytoin, do not use concurrently
Plasma, fresh	Cat's claw	May interact with fresh plasma
Potassium-wasting drugs	Aloe	When taken internally may ↑ effects of potassium-wasting drugs
Psychoanaleptic agents	Cola tree	May ↑ the effects of psychoanaleptic agents
Psychotropic agents	Nutmeg	May be potentiated, do not use concurrently
Radioactive isotopes	Bugleweed	Can interfere with the action of radioactive isotopes
Salicylates	Horse chestnut	↑ risk of severe bleeding, do not use concurrently
Salicylates	Chondroitin	Can cause ↑ bleeding
Salicylates	Cola tree	May ↑ the effect of cola tree products
Salicylates	Gossypol	Concurrent use may result in tissue damage
Salicylates	Irish moss	↑ risk of bleeding, do not use concurrently
Salicylates	Pansy	May ↑ actions of salicylates
Scopolamine	Black root	Forms an insoluble complex with scopolamine; do not use concurrently

Drug/Drug Classes	Herb	Interaction
Sedative/hypnotics	Lavender	↑ sedation when used with lavender, do not use concurrently
Sedative/hypnotics	Cowslip	May ↑ the effect of sedative/hypnotics
Sedative/hypnotics	Catnip	May enhance the effects of sedatives
Sedative/hypnotics	Chamomile	May ↑ the effects of sedatives
Sedatives/hypnotics	Black cohosh	May ↑ hypotensive effects
Sodium bicarbonate	Quinine	May lead to toxicity, do not use concurrently
SSRIs	St. John's wort	Serotonin syndrome and an additive effect may occur. Concurrent use may lead to coma, do not use concurrently
SSRIs	Yohimbe	May cause ↑ CNS stimulation, do not use together
Statins	Goldenseal	May slow the metabolism of statins
Stimulants	Ginseng	Overstimulation may occur with concurrent use
Stimulants	Siberian ginseng	Concurrent use is not recommended, overstimulation may occur
Succinylcholine	Melatonin	↑ blocking properties of succinylcholine, do not use concurrently
Sumatriptan	Horehound	↑ serotonin effect, do not use concurrently
Sympathomimetics	Ephedra	↑ the effect of sympathomimetics and causes hypertension
Sympathomimetics	Rauwolfia	Will ↑ blood pressure, do not use concurrently
Sympathomimetics	Yohimbe	↑ yohimbe toxicity, do not use concurrently
Systemic steroids	Aloe	When taken internally may ↑ effects of systemic steroids
Tannic acids	Agar	↑ dehydration
Thyroid hormones	Soy	May interfere with thyroid hormone absorption, do not use concurrently

Continued

Drug/Drug Classes	Herb	Interaction
Thyroid hormones	Kelpware	May ↓ effects of thyroid hormones, do not use concurrently
Thyroid hormones	Spirulina	High iodine content of spirulina may ↓ action of thyroid hormones, do not use concurrently
Thyroid preparations	Bugleweed	Can interfere with the action of thyroid preparations
Thyroid preparations	Agar	Avoid concurrent use because of high iodine content in agar
Tolbutamide	Angelica	May delay elimination of tolbutamide
Toxoids	Safflower	May cause ↑ immunosuppression, do not use concurrently
Trazodone	St. John's wort	May cause serotonin syndrome
Tricyclic antidepressants	Coenzyme q10	Tricyclic antidepressants ay ↓ the action of coenzyme Q10 and deplete endogenous stores
Tricyclic antidepressants	Jimsonweed	↑ anticholinergic effects when jimsonweed used with tricyclics
Tricyclic antidepressants	Yohimbe	May result in ↑ hypertension, doses may need to be ↓
Tricyclic antidepressants	Corkwood	May ↑ anticholinergic effect
Tricyclic antidepressants	Ephedra	Hypertensive crisis can occur when used concurrently
Urinary alkalizers	Ephedra	↑ the effect of urinary alkalizers
Urine acidifiers	Bearberry	May inactivate bearberry
Vaccines	Safflower	May cause ↑ immunosuppression, do not use concurrently
Vaccines (passive)	Cat's claw	May interact with passive vaccines composed of animal sera
Vitamin B	Goldenseal	May ↓ absorption of vitamin B
Warfarin	Acidophilus	↓ warfarin action

Drug/Drug Classes	Herb	Interaction
Warfarin	Anise	May ↑ action of warfarin
Warfarin	Valerian	May negate therapeutic effects of warfarin, do not use concurrently
Xanthines	Cacao tree	May ↓ the metabolism of xanthines such as theophylline
Xanthines	Coffee	Large amounts of coffee ↑ the action of xanthines such as theophylline
Xanthines	Cola tree	May ↑ the action of xanthines
Xanthines	Ephedra	Causes ↑ central nervous system stimulation
Xanthines	Green tea	Large amounts of green tea ↑ the action of xanthines
Xanthines	Guarana	May ↑ pulse rate, blood pressure, and arrhythmias when taken concurrently
Zinc	Chromium	↓ chromium absorption when taken concurrently
Zinc	Melatonin	↑ inhibition of NMDA receptors, do not use concurrently

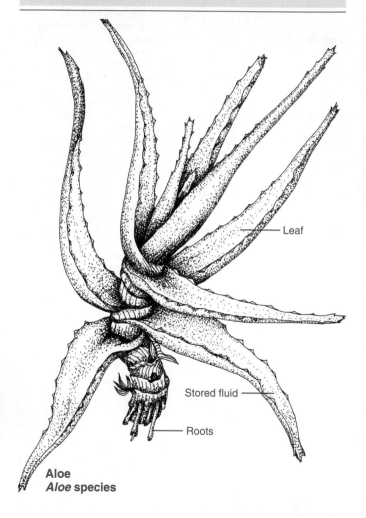

Leaf

Stored fluid

Roots

Aloe
Aloe species

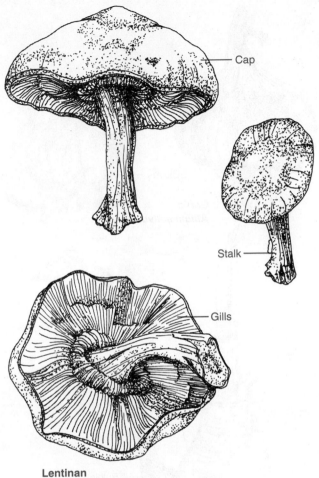

Lentinan
Lentinula edodes

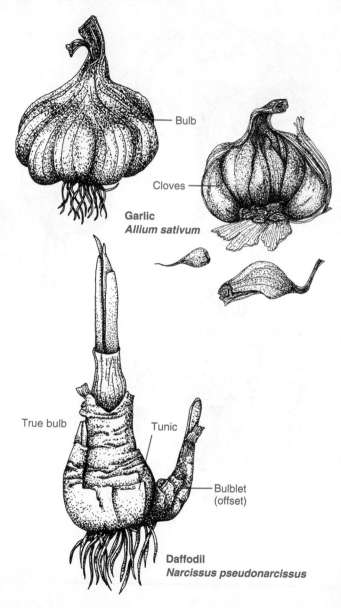

Bulb

Cloves

Garlic
Allium sativum

True bulb

Tunic

Bulblet
(offset)

Daffodil
Narcissus pseudonarcissus

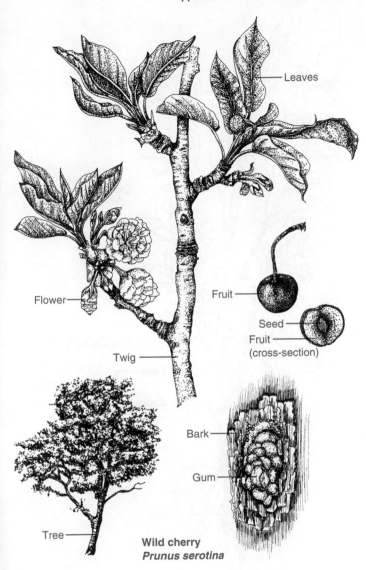

Leaves

Flower

Fruit

Seed

Fruit
(cross-section)

Twig

Bark

Gum

Tree

Wild cherry
Prunus serotina

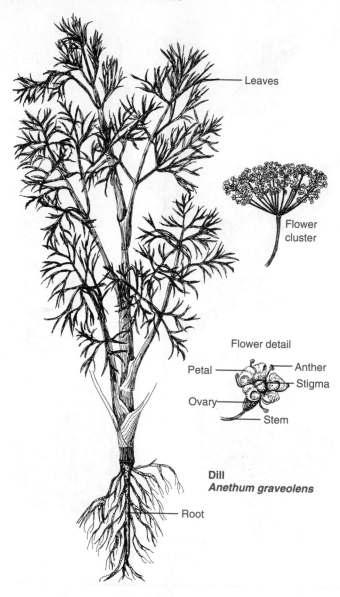

Leaves

Flower cluster

Flower detail

Petal — — Anther

— Stigma

Ovary —

— Stem

Dill
Anethum graveolens

Root

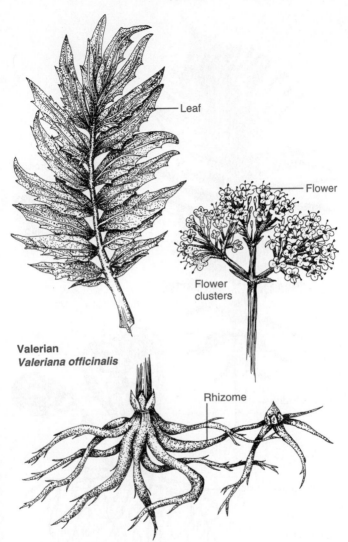

Leaf

Flower

Flower clusters

Valerian
Valeriana officinalis

Rhizome

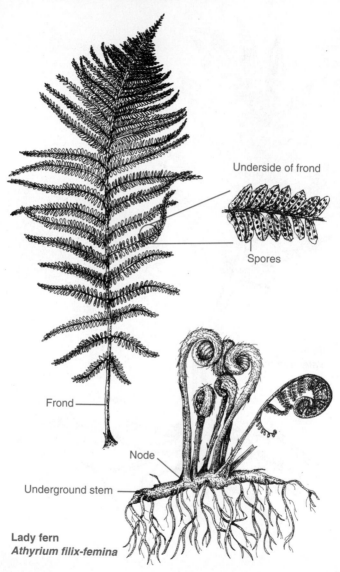

Underside of frond

Spores

Frond

Node

Underground stem

Lady fern
Athyrium filix-femina

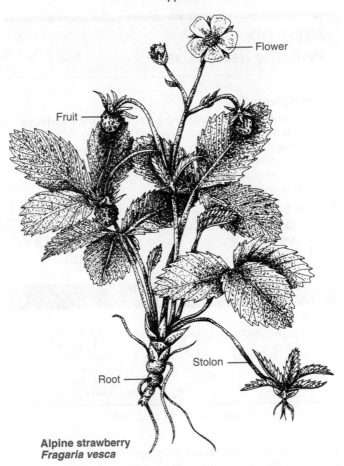

Alpine strawberry
Fragaria vesca

APPENDIX F
Pediatric Herbal Use

General Precautions
1. Because childproof packaging is not required for herbs, be sure to store them out of children's reach.
2. Although herbs have commonly been combined for use, the synergistic effects of multiple herbs—potentially positive as well as negative—are only beginning to be studied (Williamson, 2001).

Dosage Guidelines
Start with the lowest dose in the range and work up. Frequency and consistency: 1 large dose per day is not as effective as 3-4 small doses.

Tea Dosage Guidelines*

Age of Child	Dosage
<1 yr	1 tsp qd, working up to 1 tsp tid
1-2 yrs	1 oz-¼ cup qd, working up to ¼ cup tid
3-6 yrs	¼-½ cup qd, working up to tid
7-11 yrs	Up to 6 oz qd, working up to tid-qid
12 yrs-adult	1 cup qd, working up to tid-qid

*(Kemper, 1996; Scott, 2003; White, 1998; Zand, 1994)

How to Make Herbal Teas (Infusions)
(Kemper, 1996; Scott, 2003; White, 1998)
- 1 cup boiling water
- 1 tsp *dried* or 3 tsp *fresh* leaves, stems, or flowers

Steep together 3-5 min in a covered pot; strain; serve the liquid tea when temperature is appropriate.

Tincture Dosage Guidelines*	
Age of Child	**Dosage**
≤2 yrs	Not recommended for use
3-6 yrs	2-10 drops in ¼ cup water qd, working up to tid
7-11 yrs	10-20 drops in 6 oz water qd, working up to tid-qid
12 yrs-adult	20-50 drops up to tid-qid

*(Scott, 2003; White, 1998; Zand 1994)

How to Make Herbal Decoctions
(Kemper, 1996; Scott, 2003; White, 1998)
• 2 tsp *dried* herb **or** up to 6 tsp *fresh* herb
• 2 cups water

Combine and simmer gently 5-15 min; strain; cool before serving the liquid.

Decoction dose guidelines are listed with each herb.

Acidophilus

Uses
Prevention of diarrhea and stunted growth (Saran, 2002) after antibiotics or antimicrobial herbs, treatment of oral thrush through competitive inhibition, colic (Gladstar, 2001), treatment of diarrhea (Elmer, 2001)

Precautions
Be sure no lactose intolerance or allergy exists before prescribing yogurt. Do not give in the presence of high fever.

Dosage/Administration
• Acidophilus supplements: follow directions on product label (Zand, 1994)
• Yogurt with live active cultures: use topically after each feeding in infants
• ¼ tsp, 4-5 times/day for colic (Gladstar, 2001)
• Diarrhea prevention: 50 ml curd containing *L. acidophilus* daily (Saran 2002)

Aloe

Uses
Topical treatment of minor burns, sunburn, cuts, abrasions, insect bites, acne, poison ivy, frostbite, itching of chicken pox (Vessey, 2001). Not recommended for internal use in children.

Decreased bowel transit time reduces absorption of other medications (Gardiner, 2000).

Research/Future Possibilities

A clinical observation in 31 pediatric patients ages 6-14 yrs showed the use of a bioadhesive patch of aloe vera hydrogel to improve the condition of aphthous stomatitis in 80% of patients (Andriani, 2000). Another study showed decreased incidence of alveolar osteitis after treatment with a patch containing the clear inner gel from aloe vera, compared with a clindamycin-soaked gel foam. (Poor, 2002)

Precautions

For external use only in children <12 yrs

Dosage/Administration

- Topical: break off leaf, split lengthwise, apply gel to affected skin (White, 1998)

Anise

Uses

Cough, expectorant, colic

Precautions

Do not give the essential oil to children

Dosage/Administration

- Decoct 1 tsp seed in 1 cup water; strain and serve several times/day. (White, 1998)
- Tea: see tea dosage guidelines (Gladstar, 2001; Romm, 2000; Scott, 2003)

Arnica

Uses

Muscle strains, bruises, minor bumps, sports injuries, sprains. May be used before an athletic event to reduce pain and stiffness (Balch, 2002)

Precautions

Salve and infused oils for external use only; not for open wounds

Dosage/Administration

- Topical analgesic and antiinflammatory; rub directly on un-open skin. (Romm, 2000; White, 1998)
- Homeopathic remedy for internal use: 3-5 pellets of 30X as needed. (Romm, 2000)

Astragalus

Uses

Immune system support

Precautions

Do not use during fevers; use only *Astragalus membranaceus* sp.; do not use wild species of American astragalus.

Dosage/Administration

- Capsules/extract: follow package directions
- Cooked: drop 1 stick of herb into cooking pot when making soup or cooked grains
- Tea: use 1 stick herb decocted in 1 cup water (White, 1998); see tea dosage guidelines

Barberry

Uses

Nausea, diarrhea, mucous conditions such as coughs

Precautions

At first, barberry increases the amount of mucus being expelled, so start with small doses; do not take for more than 10 days at a time because extended consumption may decrease B-vitamin absorption and utilization; do not give barberry if the child has high blood pressure

Dosage/Administration

- Extract (strength of 1:1): use ⅛ tsp in 4 oz water, sipped slowly over an hour (Kemper, 1996)
- Tincture (strength of 1:5): use 2-3 drops in 4 oz water, sipped slowly over an hour (Kemper, 1996)

Benzoin

Uses

Topically as an antiseptic; as an inhalant and expectorant for bronchial disorders

Precautions

Allergy to benzoin can develop and cross-react with Mastisol; discontinue use if any hypersensitivity reactions occur (James, 1984)

Dosage/Administration

- Inhalant: 5 ml benzoin gum/1 pt water; breathe vapors
- Topical: apply to affected area every 2-4 hrs; test a small area before applying to larger one

Black Haw

Uses

Relieves muscle cramps or spasms, including irritable bladder muscles; menstrual pain

Precautions

Do not use if history of kidney stones or kidney disease

Dosage/Administration

- Capsule/decoction: for a 50-lb child (age approx 7 yrs) use ½ capsule or ½ cup decoction up to qid (White, 1998)
- Cream: apply topically to relieve muscle cramps (Ody, 1993)
- Tea: see tea dosage guidelines (White, 1998)

Boneset

Uses

Colds and flu, to promote sweating, expectorant, antispasmodic

Precautions

High doses can cause vomiting; not for children <1 yr; do not administer for longer than 7 days; can cause contact dermatitis in those hypersensitive to Asteraceae (Brinker, 1998)

Dosage/Administration

- Tea: ¾ cup for 40-lb child, tid up to 3 days; adjust quantity by weight of child; better too little than too much (White, 1998); see tea dosage guidelines

Burdock

Uses

Skin irritations, eczema, psoriasis

Precautions

Insulin dose may need to be adjusted because of hypoglycemic effect of burdock (Brinker, 1998); commercial sample may be adulterated with belladonna; do not give for longer than 2 wks; take a 1-wk break after a 2-wk regimen

Dosage/Administration

- Capsule/tea: 1 capsule/day or 1 cup tea /day for a 50-lb child (White, 1998); see tea dosage guidelines

Catnip

Uses

Colic, relaxes spasms and cramps, clears flatulence, sleeplessness, minor fevers

Precautions

None known when using a reasonable amount (Vessey, 2001);
There is a potential additive effect with drugs that sedate,
such as anticonvulsants, antianxiety medications, and tricyclic
antidepressants. (Harkness, 2001)

Dosage/Administration

- Tea (internal): nursing mothers can take adult dose to ease baby's colic; a few oz qd for infants—can give in dropper along-
  side nipple; 1 cup qd for toddlers; see tea dosage guidelines
  for older children (White, 1998)

Chamomile

Uses

Anxiety, teething, stomach upsets, muscle and digestive spasms,
nausea, colic

Precautions

Avoid if allergic to daisy family (Asteraceae), including ragweed;
anaphylaxis to chamomile is well known (Subiza, 1989;
Reider, 2000); to avoid contamination, use only commercial
preparations

NOTE: Filling up infant on tea leaves less room for milk. *Do
not substitute tea for milk or formula!*

**Dosage/Administration (Balch, 2002; Kemper, 1996;
Scott, 2003; White, 1998)**

- Capsule: ½ capsule tid for 50-lb child
- Glycerites/tinctures: follow package directions or ¼-1 tsp, up
  to qid (Romm, 2000)
- Tea: infant: 1-3 tsp/day; toddler: ½ cup/day; 50-lb child:
  1 cup tea or 1 dropperful extract/day
- Tea: colic: start slowly at 1 oz/day; watch for side effects
  before increasing to 3-4 oz/day

Topically as a wash or salve

Dandelion

Uses

Internal: diuretic (bladder irritations), mild laxative, increases
bile secretion (liver disorders)
External: warts (White, 1998), acne

Precautions

Do not use in children with acute gall bladder problems.

Dosage/Administration

Fresh greens as a vegetable in season, can be steamed, or steamed and marinated

- Root infusion: ¼-1 cup daily or as a skin wash for acne (Romm, 2000)
- Root tincture: ¼-1 tsp bid
- Dandelion juice for warts: squeeze white juice from stems directly on wart several times/day for several weeks (White, 1998)

Echinacea

Uses

Immune system support, childhood fevers, colds, flu, sore throats and coughs; externally for wounds, eczema, chicken pox/herpes

Precautions

Not for use during immune disorders such as lupus, tuberculosis, multiple sclerosis or HIV infection (Brinker, 1998; Vessey, 2001); rarely, patients with asthma, eczema or hay fever have shown allergic reactions; not for children with allergy to daisy family (Asteraceae); limit use to 10 days at a time, then take a 5-day break; for eczema (external use), take only a 2-day break. Do not give to children younger than 2 years of age.

Research/Future Possibilities

The University of Arizona has initiated a study of the use of Echinacea in the prevention of recurrent otitis media (Mark, 2001)

Dosage/Administration

- Capsule/glycerite/tincture: 50-lb child: 1 dropperful glycerite or tincture; 1 capsule (White, 1998)
- Tincture: ½ tsp bid to prevent colds and infections; for acute infections ½-1 tsp as often as every 2 hours (Romm, 2000)
- For skin infections, make a topical tincture of 1 tablespoon root per ¼ cup water to use as a rinse (Romm, 2000)
- Tea: See tea dosage guidelines

Elderberry

Uses

Fevers, stimulate the immune system, antiviral, flu, infections, asthma

Precautions

Use only blue-black elderberries; the red ones are toxic. Do NOT ingest the stem because of its cyanide content; do not use the leaves, roots, or bark internally. Only use cooked berries. Uncooked berries can cause nausea and vomiting. Large doses of elderberry juice can cause diarrhea.

Dosage/Administration

- Tea: ½-1 cup up to qid, taken hot.
- Prepared Syrup: 2 tablespoons/day or 1-2 tsp up to tid.

To make syrup, use 1 cup fresh *or* ½ cup dried elderberries, 3 cups water and 1 cup honey. Boil the berries in water, reduce heat and simmer 30-45 minutes. Smash the berries, strain them and add the honey to the strained liquid. Bottle and store in the refrigerator up to 2-3 months (Gladstar, 2001).

- Tincture: ½-1 tsp up to qid.

Eucalyptus

Uses

Decongestant for coughs and chest infections

Precautions

Essential oil is *not* for internal use (Burkhard PR, 1999); child must be 2 yrs of age to use eucalyptus; do *not* apply to face of small children; not for patients with liver, gallbladder, or digestive diseases

Dosage/Administration

- Chest rub: dilute 0.5-2 ml eucalyptus oil in 25 ml almond oil; apply to chest (Ody, 1993)

Evening Primrose Oil

Uses

Eczema and atopic dermatitis (Yoon, 2002), PMS, mastalgia, ADHD (Vessey, 2001), ADHD with borderline zinc deficiency (Arnold, 2000)

Precautions

May trigger temporal lobe epilepsy, especially in schizophrenics receiving phenothiazines; side effects include nausea, stomach pain, and headache. Do not give to children who have a seizure disorder.

Dosage/Administration

- Eczema: 1-2 g/day from capsules (Ody, 1993)

- Mastalgia: 3-4 g/day (1 g tid-qid) from capsules (Integrative Medicine, 2000)
- PMS: 3 g/day (1 g tid) from capsules (Integrative Medicine, 2000)

Fennel

Uses

Stomach upsets, gas, colic, cramps from diarrhea, to promote milk flow in nursing mothers

Precautions

Large doses may cause nausea, vomiting, and skin irritation; essential oil is *not* for infants or small children (Burkhard PR, 1999; Brinker, 1998). Food allergy has been reported, although it is rare (Moneret-Vautrin, 2002)

NOTE: Filling up infant on tea leaves less room for milk. *Do not substitute tea for milk or formula!*

Dosage/Administration

- Infant colic: 3-4 oz tea/day (Kemper, 1996)
- Other conditions: See tea dosage guidelines

Garlic

Uses

Respiratory infections, ear infections

Research/Future Possibilities

Concentrations of garlic extract supplement were able to inhibit formation of dense red cells of sickle cell anemia that trigger vaso-occlusion (Ohnishi, 2000)

Precautions

Large quantities can irritate mouth or stomach (Brinker, 1998); use sparingly for children younger than 2 years of age. May interact with drugs used to alter platelet function and coagulation (Tomassoni, 2001; Harkness, 2000)

Caution: Topical application can result in garlic skin burns (Parish, 1987; Rafaat, 2000)

Dosage/Administration

- Cooked: children can eat rice or other foods flavored with garlic or can eat ½-3 cloves daily
- Garlic oil: a 50-lb child can take ½ capsule garlic oil several times a day with food (White, 1998)
- Tea: see tea dosage guidelines; up to 4 cups daily can be used during colds

- Syrup: 1-2 tsp/day (Romm, 2000)
- Supplements: per package dosages

NOTE: Nurslings spent more time at the breast when mothers who didn't usually consume garlic did so (Menella, 1993)

Ginger

Uses

Nausea, motion sickness, vomiting (Langner, 1998), digestive cramping, stomach upsets, muscle aches, menstrual cramps, headaches

Precautions

Do not use during childhood fevers or in children with gallstones; in large doses over long periods, ginger can cause inflammation and weakness. Although a theoretical additive effect to warfarin has not been investigated in humans, it may be best to avoid this combination.

Dosage/Administration

- Fresh herb/extract/capsule: grate fresh ginger into teas or follow package directions for extract or capsule (White, 1998)
- Ginger root: <3 yrs: 25 mg qid; 3-6 yrs: 50-75 mg qid; 7-11 yrs: 125 mg qid; ≥12 yrs: 250 mg qid (Kemper, 1996)
- Tea: 2 slices ginger in 1 cup water (Kemper, 1996); see tea dosage guidelines
- Tincture: 5-25 drops in water as needed (Romm, 2000)

Hops

Uses

Restlessness, hyperactivity, insomnia, headaches, pain

Precautions

Not for those with estrogen-dependent disorders; not appropriate in children with bedwetting, lethargy, or depression; not for long-term use; may cause skin irritation. There is a potential additive effect with drugs that sedate, such as anticonvulsants, antianxiety medications, and tricyclic antidepressants (Harkness, 2001)

Dosage/Administration

- Bath: add a few drops of oil or dried herbs in a stocking to bath water (Kemper, 1996)
- Tea: See tea dosage guidelines

Hyssop

Uses

Coughing, colds and flu, chronic phlegm

Precautions

Do not give to children <2 yrs of age; use essential oil in very small quantities only for children.

Research/Future Possibilities

Muscle-relaxing activity of the essential oil has been shown on guinea pig and rabbit intestine (Lu, 2002)

Dosage/Administration

- Tea: can be combined with lemongrass and elderberry as tea to treat childhood fevers (White, 1998); see tea dosage guidelines

Juniper

Uses

Diuretic, stomach upsets, menstrual pain, urinary tract infection

Precautions

Do not give to children <2 yrs; contraindicated for those with kidney infection and inflammation (Brinker, 1998); do not use longer than 4 wks because of potential kidney damage

Dosage/Administration

- Menstrual pain: use a weak tea of 15 g berries in 500 ml water (Ody, 1993)
- Urinary tract infection: PO berry juice: dilute in water
- Other conditions: see tea dosage guidelines

Lemon Balm

Uses

Nervousness, anxiety, hyperactivity, sleep disorders, irritability, tension, antiviral

Precautions

There is a potential additive effect with drugs that sedate, such as anticonvulsants, antianxiety medications, and tricyclic anti-depressants. (Harkness, 2001)

Dosage/Administration

- Tea
  - Infants ¼ cup tid
  - Young children up to 50 lbs: up to 5 oz tid
  - Older children: 1-3 cups/day

- Tincture: ¼-1 tsp up to tid
- Cream: topically as needed
- Massage oil: dilute 2-3 drops per tablespoon of carrier oil

Lemongrass
Uses
Childhood fevers

Precautions
None identified

Dosage/Administration
- Tea: use in tea with hyssop and elderberry (White, 1998); see tea dosage guidelines

Lobelia
Uses
Expectorant, coughs, asthma

Precautions
Do not administer during shock or nervous prostration, low blood pressure or paralysis, or with dyspnea from heart disease (Brinker, 1998); small quantities may cause slight nausea or a tight sensation in throat; give to children ≥5 yrs only; expect expectoration! Do not use large doses.

Dosage/Administration
- Tea: infuse no more than ¼ tsp dried herb/1 cup hot water; a 50-lb child can drink up to 1 cup tid (White, 1998); see tea dosage guidelines

Nettle
Uses
Allergies, hay fever, colds, coughs

Precautions
Do not give to children <2 yrs; do not give to those with severe allergies, especially during anaphylactic shock; excessive use may interfere with these drugs: hypoglycemics, hyperglycemics, antidiabetics, and central nervous system depressants

Dosage/Administration
- Capsule/tea: a 50-lb child can have ½ capsule/day or ½ cup tea/day to begin, increasing to tid during allergy season (White, 1998); see tea dosage guidelines
- Cooked: can serve as steamed fresh greens, but be careful of the nettles; use gloves when gathering and preparing

Plantain

Uses

Externally for bee stings, poison oak or ivy rash, chicken pox, scrapes; internally for urinary tract inflammation or respiratory inflammation (Wegener, 1999)

Precautions

Internal use may cause nausea, vomiting, anorexia, flatus, diarrhea, bloating or obstruction

Dosage/Administration

- Tea (internal): for urinary or lung disorders, make a tea of ½ tsp dried herb; administer as often as q2h (Scott, 2003)
- Topical: apply fresh poultice of leaves, or apply leaves directly

Tea Tree Oil

Uses

Acne, athlete's foot

Precautions

Oil may burn if it gets into eyes, nose, mouth, or tender areas. Do not give internally. Do not give to individuals allergic to celery or thyme because they share a potential allergen.

Dosage/Administration

- Dilute for use in small children: 1-2 drops per teaspoon of carrier oil, such as almond or olive (White, 1998)
- 5% oil gel was used effectively on acne (Fugh-Berman, 2002)

Thyme

Uses

Antiinflammatory, coughs, bronchitis, upper respiratory mucus, sore throats, colic

Research/Future Possibilities

Genital vulvar lichen sclerosis has been treated successfully with a cream containing thyme extract in prepubertal girls (Hagedorn, 1989). Essential oils have potent mosquito repellent activity for hairless mice (Choi, 2002)

Precautions

Never use essential oil internally or near eyes or sensitive mucous membranes (Romm, 2000). In large doses can cause diarrhea. One case of allergy has been reported (Benito, 1996); cross reaction occurred within the Lamiaceae family, which includes Hyssop.

Dosage/Administration
- Bath: for infants, add strained tea to bath water (Scott, 2003)
- Chest rub: add 10 drops thyme oil diluted in 20 ml almond or sunflower oil (Ody, 1993); or 5-10 drops diluted with 2 tablespoons almond oil for topical application (Romm, 2000)
- Tea: see tea dosage guidelines or use ¼-1 cup up to tid
- Tincture: 10 drops to ½ tsp up to tid

Valerian

Uses

Insomnia, anxiety, hyperactivity (Berdonces, 2001), ADHD (Vessey, 2001), muscle or digestive cramps, flatulence, sleep difficulties in children with intellectual deficits (Francis, 2002)

Precautions

For some children, valerian can have a slight simulating effect—discontinue if this occurs (Gladstar, 2002). Withdrawal syndrome can occur after chronic use (Tomassoni, 2001); can be mentally habit forming; in large doses (>100 g daily) can cause muscle pain and heart palpitations; may be toxic to liver when used for an extended period. There is a potential additive effect with drugs that sedate, such as anticonvulsants, antianxiety medications, and tricyclic antidepressants. (Harkness, 2001)

Dosage/Administration
- Capsules: Follow package directions
- Tea/tincture: See dosage guidelines

Yarrow

Uses

Externally for inflammatory skin conditions such as chicken pox, poison ivy and oak rashes; internally for fever, colds, and flu

Precautions

Contraindicated for children allergic to daisy family (Asteraceae) (Brinker, 1998)

Dosage/Administration
- Tea: See tea dosage guidelines

References

Andriani E, et al: The effectiveness and acceptance of a medical device for the treatment of aphthous stomatitis: clinical observation in pediatric age, *Minerva Pediatr* 52(1-2):15-20, 2000.

Arnold LE, Pinkham SM, Votolato N: Does zinc moderate essential fatty acid and amphetamine treatment of attention deficit hyperactivity disorder? J Child Adolesc Psychopharmacol 2000 summer; 100(2) 111-7.

Balch PA: Prescription for Herbal Healing, 2000, Avery, New York.

Benito M, Jorro G, Morales C, Pelaez A, Fernandez A: Labiatae allergy: systemic reactions due to ingestion of oregano and thyme. Ann Allergy Asthma Immunol 1996 May; 76(5): 416-8.

Berdonces JL: Attention deficit and infantile hyperactivity, *Rev Enferm* 24(1):11-14, 2001.

Brinker F: *Herb contraindications and drug interactions,* Sandy, Ore, 1998, Eclectic Medical.

Burkhard PR, Burkhardt K, Haenggeli CA, Landis T: Plant-induced seizures: reappearance of an old problem, *J Neurol* 246(8):667-670, 1999.

Choi WS, Park BS, Ku SK, Lee SE: Repellent activities of essential oils and monoterpenes against Culex pipiens pallens. J Am Mosq Control Assoc 2002 Dec; 18(4): 348-51.

Elmer GW, McFarland LV: Biotherapeutic Agents in the Treatment of Infectious Diarrhea. Gastroenterology Clinics of North America, vol. 30 (3), 837-854, September, 2001.

Francis AJ, Dempster RJ: Effect of valerian, Valeriana edulis, on sleep difficulties in children with intellectual deficits: randomised trial. Phytomedicine 2002 May;9(4): 273-9.

Fugh-Berman A: Herbal Supplements: Indications, clinical concerns, and safety. Nutrition Today 2002;37:122-4.

Gardiner P and Kemper KJ: Herbs in Pediatric and Adolescent Medicine. Pediatrics in Review. 2000, Feb:21(2): 44-57.

Gladstar R: Family Herbal: A Guide to Living Life with Energy, Health and Vitality. Storey, 2001.

Hagedorn M: Genital vulvar lichen sclerosis in 2 siblings, *Z Hautkr* 64(9):810, 813-814, 1989.

Harkness R, Bratman S: Drug-Herb-Vitamin Interactions Bible. 2000, Prima.

Integrative Medicine: *Quick access professional guide to conditions, herbs* & supplements, Newton, Mass, 2000, Integrative Medicine Communications.

James WD, White SW, Yanklowitz B: Allergic contact dermatitis to compound tincture of benzoin, *J Am Acad Dermatol* 11(5 Pt 1):847-850, 1984.

Kemper KJ: *The holistic pediatrician,* New York, 1996, Harper Collins.

Langner E, Greifenberg S, Gruenwald J: Ginger: history and use, *Adv Ther* 15(1):25-44, 1998.

Lu M, Battinelli L, Daniele C, Melchioni C, Salvatore G, Mazzanti G: Muscle relaxing activity of Hyssopus officinalis essential oil on isolated intestinal preparations. Planta Med 2002 Mar;68(3)213-6.

Mark JD, Grant KL, Barton LL: The use of dietary supplements in pediatrics; a study of echinacea. Clin Pediatr (Phila) 2001 May; 40(5): 265-9.

Menella JA, Beauchamp GK: The effects of repeated exposure to garlic-flavored milk on the nursling's behavior, *Pediatr Res* 34(6):805-808, 1993.

Moneret-Vautrin DA et al: Food allergy and IgE sensitization caused by spices: CICBAA data. Allerg Immunol (Paris) 2002 Apr; 34(4):135-40.

Ody P: *The complete medicinal herbal,* London, 1993, DK.

Ohnishi ST, Ohnishi T, Ogunmola GB: Sickle cell anemia: a potential nutritional approach for a molecular disease, *Nutrition* 16(5):330-338, 2000.

Parish RA, McIntire S, Heimbach DM: Garlic burns: a naturopathic remedy gone awry, *Pediatr Emerg Care* 3(4):258-260, 1987.

Poor MR, Hall JE, Poor AS: Reduction in the Incidence of Alveolar Osteitis in Patients Treated with the SaliCept Patch, Containing Acemannan Hydrogel. J Oral Maxillofac Surg 60:374-9, 2002.

Rafaat M, Leung AK: Garlic burns, *Pediatr Dermatol* 17(6):475-476, 2000.

Reider N, Sepp N, Fritsch P, Weinlich G, Jensen-Jarolim E: Anaphylaxis to camomile: clinical features and allergen cross-reactivity, *Clin Exp Allergy* 30(10):1436-1443, 2000.

Romm A: 2000 Guide to Children's Supplements. Better Nutrition (suppl), October 2000, pp 38-43.

Saran S, Gopalan S and Krishna TP: Use of Fermented Foods to Combat Stunting and Failure to Thrive. Nutrition 2002: 18: 393-6.

Scott J, Barlow T, Chilingar GV: Herbs in the Treatment of Children: Leading a Child to Health, [copy editor: please insert city] 2003, Churchill-Livingstone.

Subiza J, et al: Anaphylactic reaction after the ingestion of chamomile tea: a study of cross-reactivity with other composite pollens, *J Allergy Clin Immunol* 84(3):353-358, 1989.

Tomassoni AJ, Simone K: Herbal medicines for children: an illusion of safety? Current Opinion in Pediatrics 2001, 13:162-9.

Vessey JA, Rechkemmer A: Natural Approaches to Children's Health: Herbals and Complementary and Alternative Medicine. Pediatric Nursing 2001 Jan-Feb: 27(1): 61-7.

Wegener T, Kraft K: Plantain (Plantago lanceolata L.): anti-inflammatory action in upper respiratory tract infections. Wien Med Wochenschr 1999;149(8-10):211-6.

White S, Mavor S: *Kids, herbs & health,* Loveland, Colorado, 1998, Interweave Press.

Williamson EM: Synergy and other interactions in phytomedicines. Phytomedicine 2001 Sep; 8(5): 401-9.

Yoon S, Lee J, Lee S: The therapeutic effect of evening primrose oil in atopic dermatitis patients with dry scaly skin lesions is associated with the normalization of serum gamma-interferon levels. Skin Pharmacol Appl Skin Physiol 2002 Jan-Feb; 15(1):20-5.

Zand J, Walton R, Rountree B: *Smart medicine for a healthier child,* Garden City Park, NY, 1994, Avery.

APPENDIX G
Herbal Safety

Toward a Consensus on Safety

The American Herbal Products Association (AHPA) is taking an active role in the area of herb regulation and product safety. The AHPA is the national trade association that represents the herb industry. It was founded in 1983 by a group of botanical companies, and its stated mission is to "promote responsible commerce of herbal products" (AHPA, 2000). The ongoing activities of the AHPA include coordinating educational events on herbal products, working with state and federal legislative and regulatory agencies, and disseminating information to the public. In 1992 the organization published *Herbs of Commerce* to help alleviate the confusion surrounding the numerous common names of herbs. The FDA then incorporated this standard naming system into federal label regulation in 1997.

The AHPA supports standardization of the labeling of commercial herbal products as a means of achieving product safety, and it has created a unique rating system that classifies herbal products into four categories according to their relative safety and potential toxicity. In 1997 the AHPA published the *Botanical Safety Handbook,* which is based on case reports; toxicologic, pharmacologic, and clinical studies; and information drawn from a number of books considered to be authoritative references on botanicals. This publication provides data on hundreds of herbs and plant-based products sold in the United States. Each product included in the *Botanical Safety Handbook* has been assigned an AHPA safety rating.

The AHPA Herb Safety Rating System*

The AHPA assigns a safety rating to all herbal products included in the *Botanical Safety Handbook* based on the following four categories. The classification of an herb in any given category is dependent upon the reasonable use of the herb.

---

*Used with permission from the American Herbal Products Association: *Botanical Safety Handbook,* Boca Raton, Fla, 1997, CRC Press.

Class 1   Herbs that can be safely consumed when used appropriately.

Class 2   Herbs for which the following use restrictions apply, unless otherwise directed by an expert qualified in the use of the described substance:
2a For external use only.
2b Not to be used during pregnancy.
2c Not to be used while nursing.
2d Other specific use restrictions as noted.

Class 3   Herbs for which significant data exist to recommend the following labeling: "To be used only under the supervision of an expert qualified in the appropriate use of this substance." Labeling must include proper use information as follows: dosage, contraindications, potential adverse effects and drug interactions, and any other relevant information related to the safe use of the substance.

Class 4   Herbs for which insufficient data are available for classification.

The AHPA safety classifications assume the following: (1) that the product is composed of dehydrated plant matter, unless otherwise noted; (2) that the herb is used alone and not in combination with other herbs; and (3) that amounts taken do not exceed those recommended to achieve a therapeutic effect. The AHPA specifically excludes the following conditions from consideration:

- Excessive consumption
- Safety or toxicity concerns based on isolated constituents
- Toxicity data based solely on intravenous or intraperitoneal administration
- Traditional Chinese and Ayurvedic contraindications
- Gastrointestinal disturbances
- Potential drug interactions
- Idiosyncratic reactions
- Allergic reactions
- Contact dermatitis
- Well-known toxic plants which are not found in trade
- Homeopathic herbal preparations
- Essential oils
- Herbal products to which chemically defined active sub-

stances, including chemically defined isolated constituents
of an herb, have been added
- Environmental factors, additives, or contaminants

U.S. Food and Drug Administration Center for Food Safety and Applied Nutrition

The Food and Drug Administration (FDA) provides and
updates a Poisonous Plant Database. This list includes vascular
plants that the authors of individual studies in the database have
concluded are associated with toxic effects. The FDA advises
that this list is best used only as a preliminary screening of potentially poisonous plants, not as a definitive conclusion of
safety or toxicity for the following reasons:

- In compiling the Poisonous Plant Database, the FDA did
  not attempt to evaluate the validity, reliability, or scientific merits of the individual reports cited in the database.
- Because the FDA has included in the list only those plants
  that are noted in papers that are referenced in the Poisonous Plant Database, the list is neither comprehensive nor
  complete.
- Conditions of use by consumers of the composition of
  marketed products can significantly affect the safety or toxicity of an ingredient. The database does not adequately
  address these issues.
- Any definitive determination of the safety or toxicity of a
  vascular plant used as an ingredient in a marketed product
  should be based on a comprehensive and critical review
  of the scientific literature and on test conditions that can
  be generalized appropriately to conditions of use.*

Poisonous Plant Database (Plant List)

The following plants appear in *Mosby's Handbook of Herbs and
Natural Supplements, second edition* and also appear in the
FDA's Poisonous Plant Database.

Aconite	Angelica
Agrimony	Arnica
Alfalfa	Ash
Aloe	Balsam of Peru
American hellebore	Barberry

---

*U.S. Food & Drug Administration Center for Food Safety & Applied
Nutrition Poisonous Plant Database, http://vm.cfsan.fda.gov/~djw (accessed 12/8/2000).

Barley
Bayberry
Bearberry
Betel palm
Beth root
Birch
Bistort
Bitter melon
Bitter orange
Black catechu
Black cohosh
Black haw
Black hellebore
Black pepper
Black root
Blue cohosh
Blue flag
Bogbean
Borage
Broom
Buckthorn
Burdock
Butcher's broom
Butterbur
Cacao tree
Capsicum peppers
Carline thistle
Cascara sagrada
Castor
Catnip
Celandine
Celery
Chamomile
Chaparral
Chaulmoogra oil
Chicory
Chinese cucumber
Clematis
Coffee
Coltsfoot
Comfrey
Condurango
Corkwood

Couchgrass
Cowslip
Daffodil
Elderberry
Ephedra
Eucalyptus
Fenugreek
Feverfew
Figwort
Flax
Fo-ti
Fumitory
Galanthamine
Garcinia
Garlic
Ginger
Ginkgo
Ginseng
Goat's rue
Goldenrod
Goldenseal
Gossypol
Gotu kola
Ground ivy
Guarana
Gum arabic
Gymnema
Hawthorn
Hops
Horse chestnut
Horseradish
Horsetail
Hyssop
Indigo
Jaborandi tree
Jamaican dogwood
Jimsonweed
Juniper
Karaya gum
Kava
Khat
Khella
Licorice

Lily of the valley
Lobelia
Male fern
Mallow
Marjoram
Mayapple
Meadowsweet
Milk thistle
Mistletoe
Morinda
Motherwort
Mugwort
Mullein
Mustard
Myrtle
Neem
Nettle
Nutmeg
Oak
Oats
Oleander
Oregano
Pansy
Papaya
Passion flower
Peach
Pennyroyal
Perilla
Peyote
Pill-bearing spurge
Pineapple
Pipsissewa
Pokeweed

Pomegranate
Poplar
Poppy
Prickly ash
Pulsatilla
Pumpkin
Pygeum
Queen Anne's lace
Quince
Rauwolfia
Rose hips
Rue
Saffron
Sage
St. John's wort
Sassafras
Senega
Senna
Skullcap
Sorrel
Soy
Squill
Tonka bean
Valerian
White cohosh
Wild cherry
Wild yam
Wintergreen
Yarrow
Yellow dock
Yellow lady's slipper
Yew

INDEX

common name, *Scientific name*, DISORDER

common name, *Scientific name*, DISORDER

common name, *Scientific name*, DISORDER

common name, *Scientific name*, DISORDER

common name, *Scientific name,* DISORDER

common name, *Scientific name,* DISORDER

common name, *Scientific name*, DISORDER

common name, *Scientific name,* DISORDER

common name, *Scientific name*, DISORDER

common name, *Scientific name,* DISORDER

common name, *Scientific name,* DISORDER

common name, *Scientific name,* DISORDER

common name, *Scientific name,* DISORDER

common name, *Scientific name,* DISORDER

common name, *Scientific name,* DISORDER

common name, *Scientific name*, DISORDER

common name, *Scientific name,* DISORDER

common name, *Scientific name*, DISORDER

common name, *Scientific name,* DISORDER

common name, *Scientific name*, DISORDER

common name, *Scientific name*, DISORDER

common name, *Scientific name*, DISORDER

common name, *Scientific name*, DISORDER

common name, *Scientific name,* DISORDER

common name, *Scientific name,* DISORDER

common name, *Scientific name,* DISORDER

common name, *Scientific name*, DISORDER

common name, *Scientific name*, DISORDER

common name, *Scientific name*, DISORDER

common name, *Scientific name*, DISORDER